THE TREATMENT OF EATING DISORDERS

The Treatment of Eating Disorders

A CLINICAL HANDBOOK

Edited by

Carlos M. Grilo
James E. Mitchell

THE GUILFORD PRESS
New York   London

© 2010 The Guilford Press
A Division of Guilford Publications, Inc.
72 Spring Street, New York, NY 10012
www.guilford.com

Printed in the United States of America

This book is printed on acid-free paper.

Last digit is print number: 9   8   7   6   5   4   3   2   1

The authors have checked with sources believed to be reliable in their efforts to provide
information that is complete and generally in accord with the standards of practice that
are accepted at the time of publication. However, in view of the possibility of human
error or changes in medical sciences, neither the authors, nor the editors and publisher,
nor any other party who has been involved in the preparation or publication of this work
warrants that the information contained herein is in every respect accurate or complete,
and they are not responsible for any errors or omissions or the results obtained from the
use of such information. Readers are encouraged to confirm the information contained
in this book with other sources.

Library of Congress Cataloging-in-Publication Data

The treatment of eating disorders : a clinical handbook / edited by Carlos M. Grilo,
James E. Mitchell.
    p. ; cm.
  Includes bibliographical references and index.
  ISBN 978-1-60623-446-4 (hardcover : alk. paper)
  1. Eating disorders—Treatment.   I. Grilo, Carlos (Carlos M.)   II. Mitchell, James E.
(James Edward), 1947–
  [DNLM: 1. Eating Disorders—therapy.   WM 175 T7849 2010]
  RC552.E18T744 2010
  616.85′26—dc22
                                     2009016122

My deepest gratitude goes to three generations of Grilo women:
To my mother, Eduarda, who immigrated to the United States for opportunity.
Not only did she provide me with education and opportunity, she did it with love.
To my wife and best friend, Diana, for who she is and her 25 years
of constant love, support, and encouragement. To my wonderful daughters,
Christina and Stephanie, both college students, who see a world without limits
and imagine endless possibilities.

—CARLOS M. GRILO

I would like to also express my great gratitude to the women in my life:
To my mother, Elisabeth, who has been a source of encouragement
my entire life. To my wife, Karen, whose love, friendship, and deep moral character
have sustained me and our family for 40 years. To my daughter, Katherine,
who has always been such an absolute joy and now, as an adult,
such a source of wisdom. And to my three granddaughters,
ranging in age from 5 years to 6 weeks as of this writing—
may their lives be filled with purpose, with dreams realized,
and with much happiness.

—JAMES E. MITCHELL

About the Editors

Carlos M. Grilo, PhD, is Professor of Psychiatry and Director of the Program for Obesity, Weight, and Eating Research at Yale University School of Medicine. He is also Professor of Psychology at Yale University. Dr. Grilo completed his undergraduate education at Brown University and received his doctorate in clinical psychology from the University of Pittsburgh. Following an internship and a fellowship at Harvard Medical School and McLean Hospital and postdoctoral training at Yale University, he joined Yale's faculty and served as Director of Psychology at the Yale Psychiatric Institute until 2000. Dr. Grilo's primary research focus is on eating disorders and obesity, and his secondary interests include personality disorders and psychopathology. He has received numerous research grants and has served as Principal Investigator on eight grants from the National Institutes of Health. Dr. Grilo serves on the editorial boards of the *Journal of Consulting and Clinical Psychology, Behaviour Research and Therapy, Obesity, Obesity Surgery, International Journal of Eating Disorders, Journal of Psychiatric Practice,* and *International Journal of Clinical and Health Psychology*. He has written over 260 peer-reviewed journal articles and one book, *Eating and Weight Disorders*.

James E. Mitchell, MD, is the NRI/Lee A. Christofferson, MD, Professor and Chair of the Department of Clinical Neuroscience at the University of North Dakota School of Medicine and Health Sciences. He is also the Chester Fritz Distinguished University Professor and President and Scientific Director of the Neuropsychiatric Research Institute. Dr. Mitchell completed his undergraduate education at Indiana University and medical school at Northwestern University. Following an internship in internal medicine, he completed his residency in psychiatry and a fellowship in consultation/liaison psychiatry at the University of Minnesota. Dr. Mitchell's research activities focus on the areas of eating disorders, obesity, and bariatric surgery. He is past president of the Academy for Eating Disorders and the Eating Disorders Research Society; has received the Award for Research in the Field of Eating Disorders from the Academy for Eating Disorders, the Visionary Award from the Eating Disorders Research Society, the National Eating Disorders Association Price Foundation Award for Research Excellence, and the National Eating Disorders Coalition Award for Research Leadership. He has served as Principal Investigator on 11 grants from the National Institutes of Health. Dr. Mitchell is on the editorial boards of the *International Journal of Eating Disorders, Eating Disorders Review,* and *Obesity Reviews*. He has written over 350 scientific articles and is coauthor or editor of 14 books.

Contributors

W. Stewart Agras, MD, Department of Psychiatry and Behavioral Sciences, Stanford University, Stanford, California

Kelly C. Allison, PhD, Department of Psychiatry, University of Pennsylvania, Philadelphia, Pennsylvania

Laura A. Berner, AB, Eating Disorders Research Unit, New York State Psychiatric Institute, New York, New York

C. Laird Birmingham, MD, Department of Psychiatry, University of British Columbia, Vancouver, British Columbia, Canada

Lindsay P. Bodell, BA, Eating Disorders Research Unit, New York State Psychiatric Institute, New York, New York

Beth Brandenburg, MD, Department of Psychiatry, University of Minnesota Twin Cities, Minneapolis, Minnesota

Allegra Broft, MD, Department of Psychiatry, Columbia University, New York, New York

Rachel Bryant-Waugh, DPhil, Department of Child and Adolescent Mental Health, Great Ormond Street Hospital, London, United Kingdom

Cynthia M. Bulik, PhD, Department of Psychiatry, University of North Carolina at Chapel Hill, Chapel Hill, North Carolina

Terry Carney, PhD, Sydney Law School, University of Sydney, Sydney, Australia

Jacqueline C. Carter, PhD, Department of Psychiatry, University of Toronto, Toronto, Ontario, Canada

Eunice Y. Chen, PhD, Department of Psychiatry and Behavioral Neuroscience, University of Chicago, Chicago, Illinois

Zafra Cooper, DPhil, DipClinPsych, Department of Psychiatry, Oxford University, Oxford, United Kingdom

Anita P. Courcoulas, MD, Department of Surgery, University of Pittsburgh Medical Center, Pittsburgh, Pennsylvania

Ross D. Crosby, PhD, Department of Clinical Neuroscience, University of North Dakota School of Medicine and Health Sciences, Fargo, North Dakota

Scott J. Crow, MD, Department of Psychiatry, University of Minnesota Twin Cities, Minneapolis, Minnesota

Michael J. Devlin, MD, Department of Psychiatry, Columbia University, New York, New York

Martina de Zwaan, MD, Department of Psychosomatic Medicine and Psychotherapy, University of Erlangen-Nuremberg, Erlangen, Germany

Gina Dimitropoulos, PhD, Department of Psychiatry, University of Toronto, Toronto, Ontario, Canada

Ivan Eisler, PhD, Section of Family Therapy, Institute of Psychiatry, King's College London, London, United Kingdom

Scott G. Engel, PhD, Neuropsychiatric Research Institute and Department of Clinical Neuroscience, University of North Dakota School of Medicine and Health Sciences, Fargo, North Dakota

Christopher G. Fairburn, DM, FMedSci, FRCPsych, Department of Psychiatry, Oxford University, Oxford, United Kingdom

Elizabeth Goddard, MSc, Division of Psychological Medicine and Psychiatry, Institute of Psychiatry, King's College London, London, United Kingdom

Carlos M. Grilo, PhD, Departments of Psychiatry and Psychology, Yale University, New Haven, Connecticut

David Hambrook, MSc, Department of Psychological Medicine and Psychiatry, Institute of Psychiatry, King's College London, London, United Kingdom

Andrew Howlett, MD, Department of Psychiatry, University of Toronto, Toronto, Ontario, Canada

Mimi Israel, MD, Department of Psychiatry, McGill University, Montreal, Quebec, Canada

Joel P. Jahraus, MD, Eating Disorders Institute, Park Nicollet Health Services, Minneapolis, Minnesota

Jennifer Jordan, PhD, Department of Psychological Medicine, University of Otago, Dunedin, New Zealand

Melissa A. Kalarchian, PhD, Departments of Psychiatry and Psychology, Western Psychiatric Institute and Clinic, University of Pittsburgh Medical Center, Pittsburgh, Pennsylvania

Allan S. Kaplan, MD, FRCP(c), Department of Psychiatry, University of Toronto, Toronto, Ontario, Canada

Pamela K. Keel, PhD, Department of Psychology, Florida State University, Tallahassee, Florida

Marj Klein, PhD, Department of Psychiatry, University of Wisconsin–Madison, Madison, Wisconsin

Bryan Lask, FRCPsych, FRCPCH, Great Ormond Street Hospital for Children and Ellern Mede Centre, London, United Kingdom; Oslo University Hospital, Oslo, Norway

Daniel le Grange, PhD, Department of Psychiatry and Behavioral Neuroscience, University of Chicago, Chicago, Illinois

James Lock, MD, PhD, Department of Psychiatry and Behavioral Sciences, Stanford University, Stanford, California

Pam Macdonald, MSc, Division of Psychological Medicine and Psychiatry, Institute of Psychiatry, King's College London, London, United Kingdom

Marsha D. Marcus, PhD, Department of Psychiatry, Western Psychiatric Institute and Clinic, University of Pittsburgh Medical Center, and Department of Psychology, University of Pittsburgh, Pittsburgh, Pennsylvania

Laurie McCormick, MD, Department of Psychiatry, University of Iowa Hospitals and Clinics, Iowa City, Iowa

Traci L. McFarlane, PhD, Department of Psychiatry, University of Toronto, Toronto, Ontario, Canada

Virginia V. W. McIntosh, PhD, Department of Psychological Medicine, University of Otago, Dunedin, New Zealand

Siân A. McLean, BSc, Department of Psychological Science, La Trobe University, Victoria, Australia

Philip S. Mehler, MD, ACUTE Eating Disorders Program, Denver Health, Denver, Colorado

James E. Mitchell, MD, Neuropsychiatric Research Institute and Department of Clinical Neuroscience, University of North Dakota School of Medicine and Health Sciences, Fargo, North Dakota

Marion P. Olmsted, PhD, Department of Psychiatry, University of Toronto, Toronto, Ontario, Canada

Susan J. Paxton, PhD, Department of Psychological Science, La Trobe University, Victoria, Australia

Carol B. Peterson, PhD, Department of Psychiatry, University of Minnesota Twin Cities, Minneapolis, Minnesota

Kathleen M. Pike, PhD, Department of Psychology, Temple University, Japan Campus, Tokyo, Japan

Athena Hagler Robinson, PhD, Department of Psychiatry and Behavioral Sciences, Stanford University, Stanford, California

Cheryl L. Rock, PhD, RD, Department of Family and Preventive Medicine, University of California San Diego, La Jolla, California

Debra L. Safer, MD, Department of Psychiatry and Behavioral Sciences, Stanford University, Stanford, California

Varinia C. Sánchez-Ortiz, PhD, Department of Psychological Medicine and Psychiatry, Institute of Psychiatry, King's College London, London, United Kingdom

Ulrike Schmidt, MD, Department of Psychological Medicine and Psychiatry, Institute of Psychiatry, King's College London, London, United Kingdom

Tracey L. Smith, PhD, Department of Psychiatry, University of Wisconsin, and William S. Middleton Memorial Veterans Hospital, Madison, Wisconsin

Howard Steiger, PhD, Department of Psychiatry, McGill University, Montreal, Quebec, Canada

Michael Strober, PhD, Department of Psychiatry, University of California, Los Angeles, Los Angeles, California

Albert J. Stunkard, MD, Department of Psychiatry, University of Pennsylvania, Philadelphia, Pennsylvania

Marian Tanofsky-Kraff, PhD, Department of Medical and Clinical Psychology, Uniformed Services University of the Health Sciences, Bethesda, Maryland

Kate Tchanturia, PhD, Department of Psychological Medicine and Psychiatry, Institute of Psychiatry, King's College London, London, United Kingdom

Stephen W. Touyz, PhD, School of Psychology, University of Sydney, Sydney, Australia

Janet Treasure, MD, Eating Disorders Research Unit, Department of Academic Psychiatry, Institute of Psychiatry, King's College London, London, United Kingdom

Kathryn Trottier, PhD, Department of Psychiatry, University of Toronto, Toronto, Ontario, Canada

B. Timothy Walsh, MD, Department of Psychiatry, Columbia University, New York, New York

Jennifer E. Wildes, PhD, Department of Psychiatry, University of Pittsburgh School of Medicine and Western Psychiatric Institute and Clinic, Pittsburgh, Pennsylvania

Denise E. Wilfley, PhD, Departments of Psychiatry and Psychology, Washington University in St. Louis, St. Louis, Missouri

G. Terence Wilson, PhD, Graduate School of Applied and Professional Psychology, Rutgers, The State University of New Jersey, Piscataway, New Jersey

Stephen A. Wonderlich, PhD, Neuropsychiatric Research Institute and Department of Clinical Neuroscience, University of North Dakota School of Medicine and Health Sciences, Fargo, North Dakota

D. Blake Woodside, MD, Department of Psychiatry, University of Toronto, Toronto, Ontario, Canada

Kathryn J. Zerbe, MD, Department of Psychiatry, Oregon Health and Science University, Portland, Oregon

Overview and Introduction

Our goal was to create an authoritative clinical handbook that comprehensively addresses what is known about the treatment of eating disorders. We hoped to work with our colleagues to produce a volume that was useful to clinicians, researchers, and teachers. We approached colleagues who are leading experts on each topic, in most cases including the developers of the specific treatment approaches, and asked for state-of-the-art chapters. Our objective was to bring together authoritative coverage combined with practical clinical guidance for clinicians. We were most fortunate. Our colleagues responded positively and contributed 35 chapters that comprehensively cover what we know about treating eating disorders, how to deliver such therapies, and what we need to learn to improve our therapies.

One feature of this book is the inclusion of "mini-manuals" describing specific treatment approaches. A total of 11 mini-manuals are included. These mini-manuals provide the reader with information and guidance about how the treatments are administered and give examples about the use of specific techniques. Clinical examples are provided to elucidate further the interventions. We hope that clinicians and educators will find these presentations helpful. We also hope that the contributors' critical and cogent overviews will stimulate continued research on the treatment of eating disorders.

We thank our esteemed colleagues and contributors to this clinical handbook. We thank our patients and research participants for sharing their struggles in the hopes that we may learn from them to help others.

CARLOS M. GRILO
JAMES E. MITCHELL

Contents

PART I

Overview of Eating Disorders

CHAPTER 1

Diagnosis, Assessment, and Treatment Planning for Anorexia Nervosa

Pamela K. Keel and Laurie McCormick

Overview of Anorexia Nervosa

Description and Diagnostic Criteria

The term "anorexia nervosa" (AN) was first introduced into the medical literature by Sir William Gull in 1874 (Gull, 1874). However, an illness strikingly similar to AN appears in various historical accounts of fasting girls and Catholic saints dating back to the 14th century (Keel & Klump, 2003). Across accounts, common features have included deliberate self-starvation resulting in low weight, denial of the seriousness of weight loss, excessive activity, amenorrhea, and, in modern Western cultures, a morbid fear of weight gain or being fat. The DSM-IV-TR (American Psychiatric Association [APA], 2000, p. 589) criteria for AN include:

A. Refusal to maintain body weight at or above a minimally normal weight for age and height (e.g., weight loss leading to maintenance of body weight less than 85% of that expected; or failure to make expected weight gain during period of growth, leading to body weight less than 85% of that expected).
B. Intense fear of gaining weight or becoming fat, even though underweight.
C. Disturbance in the way in which one's body weight or shape is experienced, undue influence of body weight or shape on self-evaluation, or denial of the seriousness of current low body weight.
D. In postmenarcheal females, amenorrhea, i.e., the absence of at least three consecutive menstrual cycles. (A woman is considered to have amenorrhea if her periods occur only following hormone, e.g., estrogen, administration.)

DSM-IV-TR also includes subtype specifications for individuals who do not regularly engage in binge-eating or purging behaviors (the restricting subtype) as well as those who do regularly engage in binge-eating or purging behaviors (the binge–purge subtype).

3

In addition to patients who meet full DSM-IV-TR criteria for AN are many patients who meet partial criteria and would be diagnosed with an eating disorder not otherwise specified (EDNOS) (Dalle Grave & Calugi, 2007). Examples include females who meet all criteria for AN with the exception that they do not experience amenorrhea as well as individuals whose weight loss, though significant, is not considered to be below a "minimally normal" threshold for their age and height. Importantly, the DSM-IV-TR does not provide a strict threshold for low weight. Instead, 85% below expected weight is provided as a guideline, and no standard approach for determining expected weight has been provided. Thus, a patient diagnosed with DSM-IV-TR AN in one setting might receive a diagnosis of EDNOS in another, depending on how "low weight" is defined (Thomas, Roberto, & Brownell, 2009).

Differential Diagnosis

Medical conditions leading to significant weight loss should be excluded when making a diagnosis of AN, because low weight in these conditions is not deliberate. Such general medical conditions may include, but are not restricted to, gastrointestinal diseases, brain tumors, and acquired immunodeficiency syndrome (AIDS) (APA, 2000). Gastrointestinal disorders may be more common among individuals with AN due to the consequences of starvation and purging on gastrointestinal function. Thus, a second feature that may distinguish patients with a diagnosis of AN is the presence of body image disturbance in the forms of fear of weight gain or denial of the seriousness of low weight. Significant body image disturbance and reluctance to gain weight should be absent in individuals whose weight loss is attributable to a gastrointestinal disease.

Mental disorders that lead to significant weight loss also should be considered when making a diagnosis of AN. Major depressive disorder can be associated with significant weight loss and is a common comorbid disorder for individuals with AN. The primary distinction is whether or not weight loss is intentional. In major depressive disorder weight loss is unintentional and attributable to a loss in appetite. Importantly, individuals with AN often report a loss of appetite that may be secondary to prolonged starvation or problems in interoceptive awareness. However, these individuals may demonstrate resistance to the idea that they need to gain weight in order to be healthy, which would distinguish them from those with a sole diagnosis of major depressive disorder. Individuals with schizophrenia who have delusions regarding food and eating also may lose substantial weight. For example, an individual with a paranoid delusion that her husband is trying to poison her may refuse to eat food in the household, resulting in substantial weight loss. However, the motivation behind food refusal would differ between this individual and one with AN. A patient with AN may express near-delusional beliefs regarding the effects of eating on her weight or shape; however, the theme of beliefs will center around weight and shape concerns.

Brief Overview of Research

Epidemiology

AN affects approximately 1 in 200 girls and women over their lifetime and 1 in 2,000 boys and men (APA, 2000). Two recent population-based epidemiological studies have reported higher lifetime prevalence estimates for AN in women, including a lifetime prevalence of 0.9% in the United States (Hudson, Hiripi, Pope, & Kessler, 2007) and 2.2% in Finland (Keski-Rahkonen et al., 2007). In addition, one recent study reported a less dramatic, though still statistically significant, gender difference in prevalence between women and men in the United States (Hudson et al., 2007). Results from these studies may reflect detection of cases that are missed when ascertainment is based on clinical referral (Keski-Rahkonen et al., 2007). Alternatively, results may reflect an increasing prevalence of the syndrome. A meta-analysis of incidence studies indicated that the number of new cases per 100,000 population per year increased over the 20th century (Keel & Klump, 2003), suggesting that the disorder has become increasingly common. However, the size of this increase, though statistically significant, was modest, reflecting the extent to which AN remains a relatively rare illness rather than an epidemic, as sometimes suggested in the popular media.

Associated Features and Comorbidity

Individuals with AN often display disturbances in affect, including depressed mood and anxiety. Both mood and anxiety disorders are more common among individuals with AN compared to age-matched comparison samples (Hudson et al., 2006). Some characteristics of these comorbid disorders may be explained or exacerbated by the effects of starvation in AN. Specifically, depressed mood, anhedonia, and insomnia may result from malnutrition (Keys, Brozek, Henschel, Mickelson, & Taylor, 1950). Similarly, preoccupations with food and rituals around food and eating may emerge as a consequence of starvation (Keys et al., 1950). Thus, a diagnosis of a mood or anxiety disorder should be made when the symptoms do not appear to be explained by starvation and do not appear to be related to the primary diagnosis of AN. For example, compulsions related to the need to repeatedly calculate caloric intake and expenditure may be better conceptualized as a feature of AN, whereas compulsions related to the need to keep belongings in a certain order may be better conceptualized as a feature of obsessive–compulsive disorder or obsessive–compulsive personality disorder.

The diagnosis of social phobia may be particularly challenging in AN because some patients may report discomfort when eating in public for fear that they will be judged for eating too little. In such instances, the fear of judgment may not be irrational or excessive, given that friends and family sometimes adopt the role of "food police" when they are with a loved one who suffers from AN. Patients may also report a fear of being judged for eating too much when eating in public. If this fear centers on others observing their binge-eating episodes, it may not represent an irrational fear— given that binge-eating episodes, by definition, involve an amount of food that is definitely more than others would eat. Notably, patients with AN may fear judgment for eating too much even when they are eating a normal or small amount of food. In these instances, the fear may be judged excessive; however, the content of the fear may be better explained by a diagnosis of AN, given that individuals with the disorder may have disrupted perceptions of what constitutes a normal amount of food and would judge themselves as eating excessively even if no one else were observing them. Importantly, many patients with AN endorse premorbid fears of eating in public related to concerns of being critically evaluated or judged by others in ways that are not thematically related to others judging what or how much they eat. Instead, they are concerned that others will experience disgust in simply watching them engage in the act of eating. In such cases, the relationship between anxiety disorders and AN may reflect shared risk factors for these syndromes (Keel, Klump, Miller, McGue, & Iacono, 2005).

Cultural Influences

A recent review of eating disorders in a cross-cultural context (Keel & Klump, 2003) indicated that AN was not a culturally bound syndrome, although certain features of the illness appear to be culturally bound. Specifically, the endorsement of fear of gaining weight or becoming fat as a motivation for starvation appeared to be restricted to individuals exposed to ideals from a modern Western context. Of note, this feature was not included in the description of AN when it was first introduced into the medical literature in the late 19th century. However, research suggests that individuals who meet all criteria for AN with the exception of criterion B may have a less severe presentation and a better prognosis compared to those who meet full criteria (Strober, Freeman, & Morrell, 1999). Thus, debate continues on the centrality of this feature to the definition of the syndrome.

Significant differences have been observed between ethnic groups in prevalence estimates and incidence rates for AN. Research within the United States has indicated that the lifetime prevalence of AN is significantly lower in African American women than in European American women (Striegel-Moore et al., 2003). Similarly, research in Curacao has supported significant differences in the incidence of AN in the white/mixed population versus the black population (Hoek et al., 2005), with an incidence of 9.08 per 100,000 population per year versus 0 per 100,000 population per year, respectively. Overall, the incidence of AN in the mixed/white population of Curacao was similar to that observed in the United States and the Netherlands (Hoek et al., 2005).

Gender Influences

As noted in the section on epidemiology, AN is approximately 10 times more common in women compared to men. Some of this prevalence difference can be understood in terms of gender differences in body image ideals. In modern Western cultures, thinness represents an aesthetic ideal for women whereas muscularity represents an aesthetic ideal for men. Of interest, a preponderance of cases in women appears to be present in cross-historical and cross-cultural descriptions of the syndrome (Keel & Klump, 2003), suggesting that factors other than culturally bound ideals of beauty may contribute to the observed gender difference.

An emerging line of research is beginning to examine the role of gonadal steroid hormones in contributing to possible sex differences in risk for developing eating disorders (EDs). This work has demonstrated that genetic effects on the development of EDs are activated at puberty (Klump, Burt, McGue, & Iacono, 2007) and that prenatal exposure to testosterone may serve an organizational role in protecting individuals from the development of disordered eating (Culbert, Breedlove, Burt, & Klump, 2008). Of note, these studies have examined a broadly defined phenotype of disordered eating rather than AN.

Course and Outcome

AN has a variable course. A minority of patients achieves remission early in the course of illness (i.e., within 1 year) and sustains recovery throughout life. This course appears to be most likely to occur in individuals diagnosed at a younger age, who experience a shorter delay between onset of illness and initiation of treatment (Steinhausen, 2002). Indeed, the only evidence-based treatment identified for AN, a specific form ("Maudsley model") of family-based therapy (Russell, Szmukler, Dare, & Eisler, 1987), has demonstrated efficacy in the treatment of children and adolescents (Keel & Haedt, 2008). In contrast, no evidence-based treatment has been consistently supported for the treatment of AN in adults (Bulik, Berkman, Brownley, Sedway, & Lohr, 2007; Wilson, Grilo, & Vitousek, 2007). Although a better prognosis is associated with an earlier age of onset, most cases first develop in mid- to late adolescence (APA, 2000).

With longer durations of follow-up, such as 10–20 years following diagnosis, just under half of patients achieve full recovery, another third remain symptomatic but demonstrate some improvement, and 20% remain chronically ill (Steinhausen, 2002). Complicating the attempt to interpret findings across studies is the variability in how recovery is defined, with some studies defining full recovery by 8 consecutive weeks of no or minimal symptom levels (Herzog et al., 1999). In addition, there is variability in how changing clinical presentation is defined. Longitudinal studies suggest that a majority of patients who do not recover from the restricting subtype of AN go on to develop binge-eating or purging behaviors (Eddy et al., 2002). Among these, some experience weight gain resulting in a shift in diagnosis (i.e., "diagnostic crossover") from AN to bulimia nervosa (BN). Although these individuals may be considered "improved" because they no longer meet full criteria for the binge–purge subtype of AN, it is difficult to consider them recovered. Similar issues emerge for those whose illness changes over time to meet partial criteria for AN. Such individuals may be viewed as partially recovered (Herzog et al., 1999), or they may be viewed as having an EDNOS.

Mortality has been observed in approximately 1 in 20 patients (Steinhausen, 2002; Sullivan, 1995) across studies, reflecting a standardized mortality ratio of approximately 10.0—or a 10-fold increase in risk of premature death (Keel et al., 2003; Löwe et al., 2001). Primary causes of death include the physical consequences of starvation and suicide (Nielsen et al., 1998). Predictors of fatal outcome include poor psychosocial functioning, longer duration of follow-up, and severity of alcohol use disorders (Keel et al., 2003).

Psychobiology

Symptoms and associated features of AN can have a profound impact on neuroanatomical structures and function. Several studies have demonstrated brain matter reductions in patients with AN, compared to controls, that appear to result from starvation (Keel, 2005). Recent work has focused on reductions in the right dorsal anterior cingulate cortex (ACC) that are related to both weight loss and weight recovery and prospectively predict eating disorder outcome, independently of body mass index (BMI) (McCormick et al., 2008). This region is of particular interest because it is a phylogenetically recent structure, containing a category of spindle-shaped neurons distinct to humans and great apes. This structure integrates cognitive and emotional information—

particularly with regard to reward-based learning. In a study comparing women ill with AN, recovered from AN, and healthy control women, Uher and colleagues (2003) found increased activation of the dorsal ACC specifically in response to food stimuli in recovered women, compared to both controls and ill patients, and increased dorsal ACC activation in women with a lifetime history of AN (ill and recovered), compared to controls. Consistent with structural changes related to weight recovery reported by McCormick and colleagues (2008), Uher and colleagues (2003) found that dorsal ACC activity was positively correlated with current body weight—explaining activation differences between recovered and ill patients. However, this finding does not explain differences found between recovered and control participants who did not differ in BMI, nor does it explain why differences were specific to food stimuli versus aversive emotional stimuli. Overall, results suggest some potential involvement of the dorsal ACC in the processing of information, which may leave individuals vulnerable to develop AN. This hypothesis is supported by the prospective association found between right dorsal ACC volume following weight recovery and risk for relapse in patients treated for AN (McCormick et al., 2008).

Considerable work has focused on neurotransmitters and neuropeptides that regulate eating and weight. Studies generally find reduced levels of neurochemicals that inhibit food intake (e.g., serotonin, leptin, melanocortin-stimulating hormone, and brain-derived neurotrophic factor) and increased levels of neurochemicals that promote food intake (e.g., ghrelin and neuropeptide-Y) in patients with AN, compared to controls (Favaro, Monteleone, Santonastaso, & Maj, 2008; Keel, 2005). Thus, when differences have been found, they have suggested that the bodies of patients with AN may respond to starvation by reducing signals that might inhibit food intake and increasing signals that would stimulate food intake. This interpretation is supported by normalization of most of these alterations with weight restoration (Favaro et al., 2008).

The serotonin system has received considerable attention in the search to understand the psychobiology of AN and has produced findings that deviate somewhat from that described for other neurochemicals. Specifically, serotonin levels do appear to be reduced during illness with AN. However, some evidence suggests elevated activity of this neurotransmitter system following weight recovery (Favaro et al., 2008). One interpretation of this pattern of findings is that individuals vulnerable to developing AN may have increased serotonin receptor activity, particularly the serotonin 1A receptor, which contributes to premorbidly higher levels of anxiety and harm avoidance. When individuals with these features initiate a weight loss diet, they may find that reducing their food intake helps to regulate their anxiety (Kaye, Frank, Bailer, & Henry, 2005). Of note, a key challenge to this model is that patients who are actively ill with AN report high levels of anxiety and harm avoidance (Klump et al., 2004), suggesting that starvation does not ameliorate these features.

Behavior and Molecular Genetic Findings

Family studies support the hypothesis that AN runs in families affected by eating disorders (Becker, Keel, Anderson-Fye, & Thomas, 2004). There is also evidence of shared familial transmission of obsessive–compulsive personality disorder (Lilenfeld et al., 1998) and anxiety disorders (Keel, Klump, et al., 2005). Twin studies further support the role of genes in explaining why AN runs in families. Specifically, twin concordance for broadly defined AN is greater in monozygotic compared to dizygotic twins (Becker et al., 2004). Molecular genetic studies have pointed to a number of possible genetic variations that may be linked to risk for development of AN. However, most findings have not been replicated. An exception to this pattern are findings related to the serotonin 2A receptor gene (Becker et al., 2004; Klump & Culbert, 2007), for which multiple independent association studies have supported increased A allele frequency in probands with AN. The functional significance of this finding has yet to be determined.

Risk and Maintenance Factors

Some risk factors for the development of AN have been covered in previous sections, specifically those concerning epidemiology, psychobiology, and genetic findings. For example, being an adolescent or young adult female represents a risk factor for the development of AN. Genes confer risk for developing the disorder as well, though it is unclear exactly which genes are key in the diathesis or what these genes influence. A vulnerability to perturbations in the function of the right dorsal ACC also may increase risk for developing the disorder. In support of AN as a neurodevelopmental disease, several studies have demonstrated a link between obstetric complications during the perinatal period and later development of AN, with a recent study demonstrating that the number of obstetric complications was inversely associated with age of AN onset (Favaro, Tenconi, & Santonastaso, 2006).

Beyond these considerations, there has also been a search to understand psychosocial risk factors for the development of AN. Perfectionism has been associated specifically with the development of AN and related syndromes in retrospective (Fairburn, Cooper, Doll, & Welch, 1999) and prospective longitudinal studies (Tyrka, Waldron, Graber, & Brooks-Gunn, 2002). Most other studies have examined prospective risk factors for the development of disordered eating, which is heavily weighted toward syndromes characterized by binge eating at normal or elevated weight, or have been cross-sectional studies that examined correlates of AN (Jacobi, Hayward, de Zwaan, Kraemer, & Agras, 2004). This latter set of studies cannot provide information regarding the temporal association between a posited risk factor and the development of AN. Thus, correlates may reflect consequences of the illness. Among a host of correlates that may contribute to risk for developing AN are a parenting style marked by high concern, difficulties with sleeping or eating during infancy and early childhood, childhood anxiety disorders, negative self-evaluation, and adverse life events (Jacobi et al., 2004).

Assessment

Interview at Intake Assessment

Clinical interviews are a central part of any intake assessment because they identify the problem for which patients are seeking treatment, and they form the basis of a treatment plan. This interview also is crucial for determining whether a given treatment setting can offer the services needed for the patient or whether a referral to another treatment facility would be needed. Different approaches may be employed for the intake interview, ranging from an unstructured case-history interview to a structured diagnostic interview. In practice, clinicians may adopt a combination of these approaches to obtain information about patient background (age, education, employment, relationship status, family history, medical history, legal history) and life events (e.g., transitions that may have preceded the onset of the eating disorder, traumatic events) as well as more detailed information about specific mental disorders that might be the focus of treatment.

In addition to structured interviews designed to obtain diagnoses across of range of mental disorders, such as the *Structured Clinical Interview for DSM-IV Axis I Disorders* (SCID; First, Spitzer, Gibbon, & Williams, 1996), there are also structured clinical interviews designed specifically for the assessment of eating disorders, such as the *Eating Disorders Examination* (Fairburn & Cooper, 1993). Structured clinical interviews require intensive training in order to be administered reliably. Because of this requirement, full structured clinical interviews are most often obtained within research settings. Outside of a research setting, clinicians may prefer to supplement unstructured clinical interviews with psychometrically validated self-report assessments (discussed below).

Key features to assess during an interview to determine presence of AN include:

1. Current body weight and height, objectively measured
2. Attitudes about gaining weight, if underweight
3. Perception of current weight/amount of body fat, influence of weight and shape on self worth, concern over medical consequences of low weight if weight is extremely low
4. If female and after the age of menarche, pattern of current menstrual cycles and use of hormonal contraception

In addition to assessing for these features to evaluate the presence of AN, it is important to assess related eating disorder features, including:

1. Presence and frequency of binge-eating episodes—that is, episodes in which the person feels a loss of control over eating and consumes more food than most people would under similar circumstances (excluding fasting behavior as a circumstance surrounding binge eating)
2. Presence of purging behavior, including use and frequency of self-induced vomiting, ipecac, laxatives for weight control, diuretics for weight control, enemas, or omission of insulin if diabetic
3. Presence of nonpurging weight control behaviors such as frequency, period, and intensity of fasting and exercise
4. Misuse of prescription or over-the-counter medications to promote weight loss, including diet pills, herbal agents, stimulants, or medications that stimulate the thyroid

Although weight and height can be objectively measured and signs of purging may be detected through physical examination, detection of other features relies on accurate self-report. Patients with AN are not always able or willing to provide accurate information about their illness for a variety of reasons including, resistance to treatment that might result in weight gain, fear of being stigmatized, and genuine belief that their thoughts and behaviors are healthy. Clinicians should be aware of the impact of secrecy or denial on accuracy of assessments that rely on patients as the sole source of information. Repeating assessments throughout treatment is a good way to recheck information because patients may become more willing to reveal symptoms as they improve and develop greater trust in their therapists. Repeating assessments also is crucial for determining whether patients are making progress in treatment.

Following thorough assessment of eating disorder features, including onset and course of disordered eating symptoms leading up to the intake assessment, it is important to assess for presence of comorbid syndromes that may require clinical attention. As noted above, AN is associated with elevated risk of mortality due to suicide (Keel et al., 2003). Thus, it is important to evaluate for the presence of passive thoughts of death, active suicidal thoughts, plans, availability of means, and intentions—whether or not the patient endorses depressed mood or meets criteria for a major depressive episode. Given that comorbid substance use disorders significantly increase the risk of fatal outcome (Keel et al., 2003), a careful assessment of drug and alcohol use should be completed as well. Information regarding evaluation of medical stability is provided in the following section.

Recent work has supported the utility of motivational interviewing during intake assessment as a predictor of changes during treatment and maintenance of changes after treatment (Geller, Drab-Hudson, Whisenhunt, & Srikameswaran, 2004). Proponents of this approach note that motivational interviewing is useful both for assessment and for enhancing outcomes by addressing the need for patients to be in the action phase of making a change before therapists implement interventions designed to effect changes.

Medical Evaluation

A medical evaluation is advisable for any patient diagnosed with AN, given the risk of medical complications associated with the illness. This type of evaluation is particularly important for patients with low weight (BMI < 16.0) or frequent purging (purging on a daily basis) who may require inpatient treatment to achieve medical stabilization. In addition to objective assessment of height and weight, medical evaluations should include:

1. Vital signs (pulse, blood pressure, temperature, respiration)
2. Electrolytes, glucose, calcium, magnesium, phosporus
3. Amylase
4. Complete blood count with differential
5. Thyroid function tests (T3, T4, and TSH)
6. Albumin, transferrin
7. BUN/creatinine
8. Urinalysis, stool guaiac
9. Liver function tests (SGOT, SGPT, bilirubin)
10. Bone densitometry
11. Electrocardiogram

In cases of unstable vital signs and EKG abnormalities or very low potassium levels (hypokalemia) or other signs of medical instability (kidney or liver dysfunction), inpatient treatment is warranted to achieve medical stability. Inpatient treatment is also warranted when weight is extremely low and cannot be safely normalized on an outpatient basis. Thresholds for determining treatment setting are discussed in more detail in the treatment planning section.

Psychological Assessment

Several widely used self-report measures can be administered to determine psychological functioning related to eating disorders and other disorders. Table 1.1 provides a list of measures and what they are designed to assess based on information provided in Carter, McFarlane, and Olmsted (2004). This list is not exhaustive but does provide an indication of some of the most widely used measures and their length. As noted above, it is important to repeat assessments to determine whether improvements are occurring with treatment, and this is more feasible with shorter assessments. Measures included in Table 1.1 have reasonably straightforward scoring systems and interpretation. However, it is worth noting that several measures use reverse-scored items to avoid response pattern bias. In addition, one of the more widely used eating disorder assessments, the Eating Disorders Inventory (EDI), measures features specific to eating disorders (in three subscales) as well as associated personality and psychopathology features (in five subscales). For all self-report measures, it is important to determine that a patient has an adequate reading level (usually eighth grade) to complete these measures.

Nutritional Assessment

A referral to a dietician is an important component of assessment and is crucial for developing a treatment plan (see Treatment Team Members below). A nutritional assessment can establish the patient's current pattern of eating and rules around what he/she eats, when he/she eats, and how much he/she eats. This assessment can also focus on what physical sensations the patient experiences before, during, and after eating and how he/she interprets these signals. For example, does the patient interpret feelings of hunger as being "good" or as a sign that he/she is losing weight rather than as a signal that it is time to eat? Do feelings of hunger trigger a fear of losing control over eating? These experiences suggest a perturbation in the association between biological drives to eat and interpretation of these drives, which may contribute to disordered-eating behaviors. How quickly does a patient feel full once he/she commences eating? Premature feelings of extreme fullness may reflect delays in gastric emptying that are a consequence of long periods of fasting. These feelings may contribute to reduced food intake or self-induced vomiting. Does the patient believe certain myths regarding the effects of food on body weight or composition? What are the patient's feelings and thoughts (e.g., rules) about different food groups (carbohydrates, fats, dairy)? Does the patient follow a special diet for medical, religious, or cultural reasons?

There is likely to be considerable overlap in content of assessment for planning nutritional rehabilitation and psychological intervention. However, it is important to note that a psychologist may help a patient notice and challenge patterns of thinking about his/her eating, weight, and self-worth (e.g., dichotomous thinking—"I am only a person of worth if my weight remains below 100"), whereas a dietician's role is to provide healthy eating guidelines and to serve as the expert on what patterns of food intake result in healthy weight and nutritional status.

TABLE 1.1. Self-Report Measures Used in the Psychological Assessment of AN

Measure (authors)	Construct assessed	Age	Scoring and interpretation
Eating Attitudes Test (EAT) (Garner & Garfinkel, 1979); EAT-26 (Garner, Olmsted, Borh & Garfinkel, 1982)	Anorexia nervosa symptoms Dieting (EAT-26) Bulimia (EAT-26) Oral Control (EAT-26)	≥ 16 years	Items (40 or 26) with responses ranging from "never" to "always" on 6-point Likert scale; least pathological responses receive 0 points and remaining items scored 1, 2, and 3 to denote increasing severity; on EAT-26, cutoff > 20 indicative of an eating disorder
Eating Disorders Inventory (EDI) (Garner, Olmsted & Polivy, 1983); EDI-2 (Garner, 1991)	Drive for Thinness Bulimia Body Dissatisfaction Ineffectiveness Perfectionism Interpersonal Distrust Interoceptive Awareness Maturity Fears Asceticism (EDI-2) Impulse Regulation (EDI-2) Social Insecurity (EDI-2)	≥ 12 years	Scored similarly to EAT and EAT-26; a cutoff of 14 for Drive for Thinness recommended for screening purposes
Eating Disorders Examination Questionnaire (EDE-Q) (Fairburn & Beglin, 1994)	Global eating disorder severity Restraint Eating Concern Shape Concern Weight Concern	Older adolescents and adults	36 items with responses ranging from 0 "never" to 6 "every day" over previous 28 days; item scores averaged, and scores between 4 and 6 are considered to be clinically significant
Mizes Anorectic Cognitions Scale (MACS-R) (Mizes, Christiano, Madison et al., 2000)	Self-control self-esteem Weight and approval Rigid weight regulation/ fear of weight gain	Adults	Items rated from "strongly disagree" to "strongly agree" on 5-point Likert scale
Shape- and Weight-Based Self-Esteem Inventory (Geller, Johnson, Madson, 1997)	Influence of weight and shape on self-evaluation	≥ 13 years	Patient completes pie chart indicating size of self-esteem pie influenced by different domains, including weight shape; score is determined by angle of pie shape that reflects influence of shape and weight on self-esteem
Beck Depression Inventory–2 (BDI-2) (Beck, Steer & Brown, 1996)	Depression severity	≥ 13 years	21 items endorsed for degree of depressive symptoms in previous 2 weeks; total score determined by sum of highest response to each item; cutoff of 29 and higher indicates severe depression; 20–28 moderate depression; 14–19 moderate depression

(cont.)

TABLE 1.1. *(cont.)*

Measure (authors)	Construct assessed	Age	Scoring and interpretation
Beck Anxiety Inventory (BAI) (Beck, Epstein, Brown & Steer, 1988)	Anxiety severity	Older adolescents and adults	21 items endorsed for degree of anxiety symptoms in previous week; total score determined by sum of highest response to each item
Rosenberg Self-Esteem Scale (RSE) (Rosenberg, 1965)	Self-esteem	Older adolescents and adults	10 items endorsed for feelings of self-worth; higher scores indicate higher self-esteem

Family Assessment

In the preceding sections we have emphasized assessing the patient, assuming in some cases that the patient is an adult. Indeed, many of the psychological assessments included in Table 1.1 are validated specifically in adult populations. For younger patients still living with parents or guardians, family assessment can provide information about the family environment and about the patient.

First, family assessment gives information about the patient's immediate living environment, which may not be available through traditional, patient-focused assessments. For example, the Family Assessment Measure–III (FAM-III; Skinner, Steinhauer, & Santa-Barbara, 1995) is a self-report questionnaire that is completed by each family member, including children and siblings 10 years of age or older. The FAM-III produces three subscale scores: the General Scale taps the family system; the Dyadic Relationships Scale assesses relationship quality between pairs within a family (e.g., Mother–Daughter Dyad); and the Self-Rating Scale measures how the individual completing the scale perceives his/her function within a family (Carter et al., 2004).

Second, family assessment can provide additional information about the patient. Indeed, regardless of a patient's age, any assessment can be significantly enhanced by talking with a family member, spouse, or friend of the patient. This family inclusion is particularly important for younger patients because minors are more likely to have been brought into treatment by their family rather than being self-referred. Thus, younger patients may not believe that they have a problem that requires intervention and may be less forthcoming with their thoughts, feelings, and behaviors. Conducting assessments with the family can reveal behavioral patterns that provide crucial information for understanding the patient's motivations and fears.

As noted above, a specific family-based intervention (Russell et al., 1987) has demonstrated efficacy in treating AN in younger patients. This intervention requires a careful assessment of family processes to identify how the child's illness has impacted family functioning and ways in which these alterations serve to maintain the illness. Initially, assessment focuses on factors that would directly impact the patient's ability to eat and gain weight. One part of this assessment occurs during a family meal in which the therapist observes what foods are prepared, how they are presented, and interactions among family members around eating (or the lack thereof). Of note, this is not a purely observational assessment. The therapist uses this event to coach parents *in vivo* in ways to improve their child's food intake. Later sessions of family-based therapy focus on how the eating disorder impacts not only the patient's medical and psychological well-being but also family interactions and developmental processes that should occur during adolescence. Again, this assessment occurs within the context of intervention to improve patient outcome.

Treatment Planning

Treatment Setting Options

Services available for treating EDs range from intensive inpatient programs (in which general medical care is readily available), to residential and partial hospitalization programs, to varying levels of outpatient care (in which the patient receives general medical treatment, nutritional counseling, and/or individual, group, and family psychotherapy). Specialized ED programs are unavailable in many geographic areas, and the financial burden associated with specialized multidisciplinary treatment is significant. Thus, many patients and health professionals face the dilemma of identifying the best treatment available, given treatment needs and resources available.

Recent work by Gowers and colleagues (2007) found no outcome differences when comparing adolescent patients with AN who had been initially randomized to inpatient treatment, specialized outpatient treatment, or general outpatient treatment. Instead, greater differences were found for those who transitioned from their assigned treatment condition. Specifically, those randomized to inpatient treatment who gained weight and "bargained their way out" of inpatient treatment had better outcomes compared to those who remained in that treatment arm. Conversely, those randomized to either outpatient arm but subsequently transferred to inpatient treatment had worse outcomes compared to those who remained in outpatient treatment. Generally, Gowers and colleagues' findings paint a bleak picture for the effectiveness of inpatient treatment for adolescent patients with AN. However, their findings should be interpreted in light of the impact of patient factors (specifically, severity of illness) on treatment utilization (Keel et al., 2002).

Inpatient Treatment

Factors suggesting that hospitalization may be appropriate include rapid or persistent decline in oral intake, a decline in weight despite maximally intensive outpatient or partial hospitalization interventions, the presence of additional stressors that may interfere with the patient's ability to eat, reaching a weight at which instability previously occurred in the patient, co-occurring psychiatric problems that merit hospitalization (e.g., suicidality), and the degree of the patient's denial and resistance to participate in his/her own care in less intensively supervised settings. Legal interventions, including involuntary hospitalization and legal guardianship, may be necessary to address the safety of treatment-reluctant adult patients who have developed, or are at imminent risk for developing, life-threatening medical sequelae from starvation. Many adult patients with AN have considerable difficulty gaining weight outside of a highly structured program, such as that provided by an inpatient program. Within an inpatient program, patients are initially prescribed 1,200–1,500 calories per day, depending on their weight at admission, and then intake is increased by 500 calories every 4–5 days until patients are consuming between 3,500–4,500 calories per day (Bowers, Andersen,

& Evans, 2004). This schedule is designed to achieve weight gain of 3 pounds per week in females and 4 pounds per week in males without risk of medical complications of refeeding.

Partial Hospitalization

Although studies suggest that weight restoration is more efficient during inpatient hospitalization, growing pressure from insurance companies to transition patients to an outpatient setting once they are medically stabilized has placed more emphasis on partial hospitalization to provide intensive treatment over extended periods (Howard, Evans, Quintero-Howard, Bowers, & Andersen, 1999; Treat, McCabe, Gaskill, & Marcus, 2008). This pressure has caused a shift in focus from long-term inpatient programs with outpatient follow-up to day treatment care with hospital backup. A partial hospitalization program is appropriate for individuals discharged from inpatient care who have achieved at least 85% of their expected body weight but who still require intensive treatment to regain 95–100% of their body weight (Bowers et al., 2004). Partial hospitalization is also useful for addressing the cognitive features of AN that persist after weight restoration and increase risk of relapse (Keel, Dorer, Franko, Jackson, & Herzog, 2005). A partial hospital program offers a structured environment for most of the day—typically from 8:00 A.M. to 6:00 P.M.—and thus offers patients the opportunity to consume two to three meals and snacks to achieve continued weight gain. For example, within a partial hospital program, patients may consume 3,500 calories per day in order to gain approximately 2 pounds per week (Bowers et al., 2004). However, steady gains of even 0.5 pounds per week have been associated with better outcome at 6-month follow-up (Treat et al., 2008). Partial hospital treatment may be appropriate for patients who have not responded to outpatient treatment but who remain medically stable.

Outpatient Treatment

Although weight restoration may be faster in inpatient settings (Howard et al., 1999; Treat et al., 2008), findings from Gowers and colleagues (2007) suggest that inpatient and outpatient treatment achieve similar levels of weight gain and recovery. In addition, outpatient treatment provides more socialization, interactions in a real-world setting, and greater opportunities for patients to improve feelings of self-efficacy. However, in order to achieve weight restoration, it is important for outpatient treatment to provide repeated assessments of weight. Specifically, monitoring of weight should be done at least weekly (and often two to three times a week). Weight should be objectively measured in the same setting (same scale) after the patient voids and while the patient is wearing the same class of garment (e.g., hospital gown or standard clothing with pockets emptied and without shoes or heavy outer wear). In patients who purge, it is important to routinely monitor serum electrolytes. Urine-specific gravity, orthostatic vital signs, and oral temperatures may need to be measured on a regular basis as well.

Treatment Setting Transitions

Relapse occurs in 30% of patients with AN (Keel, Dorer, et al., 2005), and, as a result, patients may transition between inpatient, partial hospitalization, and outpatient treatment and back again throughout the course of their recovery. Shorter duration of illness and higher BMI at the time of transition from inpatient to partial hospitalization predict better outcome (Howard et al., 1999; Treat et al., 2008), reinforcing the importance of patient variables in predicting treatment response. If the patient is going from one treatment setting to another, transition planning requires that the care team in the new setting be identified and that specific patient appointments be made. Similar guidelines apply to changes in locale that occur when patients require more intensive specialized treatment than is available to them locally. Changes in locale are particularly likely to occur in college-age patients who may initiate treatment where they attend school, return home for more intensive care, and then return to school when they are judged to be medically stable and able to benefit from a less intensive treatment approach. It is preferable that a specific clinician on the team be designated as the primary coordinator of care to ensure continuity and attention to important aspects of treatment.

Treatment Choices

Medications

At this time there is no empirical support for attempting to treat AN with medication alone. The decision about whether to use psychotropic medications and, if so, which medications to choose is based on the patient's clinical presentation. The limited empirical data on malnourished patients indicate that selective serotonin reuptake inhibitors (SSRIs) do not appear to confer advantage over placebo regarding maintenance of healthy weight (Walsh et al., 2006) or any advantage over psychotherapy for preventing relapse (Treasure & Schmidt, 2005). However, antidepressant medications are often used to treat comorbid depressive, anxiety, or obsessive–compulsive symptoms and for bulimic symptoms in weight-restored patients. Psychiatrists should evaluate the possible role of starvation in producing symptoms of depression and anxiety prior to initiating treatment with an antidepressant. Adverse reactions to tricyclic antidepressants and monoamine oxidase inhibitors are more pronounced in malnourished individuals, and these medications should generally be avoided in this patient population.

Recent randomized controlled trials of olanzapine (an antipsychotic) in AN have shown that weight restoration is faster when this medication is utilized (Attia, Kaplan, Haynos, Yilmaz, & Musante, 2008; Bissada, Tasca, Barber, & Bradwejn, 2008). There are mixed results for cyproheptadine's (an antihistamine) improvement of appetite, and other strategies that have not been investigated yet include the use of megastrol acetate (a steroid) or mirtazapine (an antidepressant), which have appetite-stimulating effects. Antianxiety agents used selectively before meals may be useful to reduce patients' anticipatory anxiety before eating. However, within the anxiety disorders literature, anxiolytics have been shown to reduce the efficacy of interventions that employ exposure and response prevention. Thus, the short-term benefits of using antianxiety medications may be offset by their potential to undermine long-term benefits of psychotherapeutic interventions. Promotility agents such as metoclopramide may be useful for bloating and abdominal pains that occur during refeeding in some patients. However, the risk of side effects such as sedation and motor abnormalities should be considered and discussed with patients before initiating medication use.

Although no specific hormone treatments or vitamin supplements have been shown to be helpful, supplemental calcium, vitamins, and hormones are often used. Calcium has been used in the hope that it will reduce problems with osteoporosis, but data have not substantiated this effect. Vitamin supplements have been used to balance nutritional deficiencies associated with prior food restriction. Finally, hormonal contraceptives have been used to trigger menstrual bleeding. However, given the lack of evidence that any of these improve patient outcomes, they are not a recommended part of treatment. Instead, emphasis should be placed on increasing food intake and achieving weight restoration.

Psychotherapy

During the acute phase of treatment, the efficacy of specific psychotherapeutic interventions for facilitating weight gain remains uncertain. Table 1.2 includes randomized control treatment trials conducted in younger-adolescent as well as late-adolescent and adult samples with AN. Several observations can be made of the studies listed in this table. First, for younger patients, a specific family-based therapy has demonstrated superiority to alternative treatments in independent studies (Robin et al., 1999; Russell et al., 1987), making it a well-established evidence-based treatment for adolescents with AN (Keel & Haedt, 2008). However, this does not generalize to older patients with AN. Second, based on findings from two studies in Table 1.2 (Pike, Walsh, Vitousek, Wilson, & Bauer, 2003; Serfaty, Turkington, Heap, Ledsham, & Jolley, 1999), nutritional counseling alone is not beneficial for patients with AN compared to alternative interventions.

Third, few randomized controlled studies of psychosocial interventions have been conducted on AN in late-adolescent/adult samples, despite the fact that AN has been recognized as a form of mental illness for more than a century (Gull, 1874). Fourth, with few exceptions (Crisp et al., 1991), studies have compared two or more alternative treatments rather than using wait-list control or assessment-only conditions, due to ethnical constraints of withholding treatment from severely ill patients. As a consequence, studies have been unable to establish possible efficacy of a treatment in comparison to a no-treatment control (Chambless & Ollendick, 2001). Instead, treatments have been held to the highest standard of having to demonstrate superiority to alternative interventions. Fifth, sample sizes assigned to each treatment condition have been small and then further reduced by noncompletion, such that an average of 13 patients completed each treatment condition included in Table 1.2. These patterns contribute to a final, almost inevitable observation: The majority of comparisons from controlled treatment studies fail to identify any psychotherapy as being superior to another for the treatment of adult patients with AN.

In practice, modes of therapy (e.g., individual psychotherapies, family therapies, nutritional counseling, and group therapies) are often combined during hospital treatment and in comprehensive follow-up care. In addition, clinicians frequently attempt to blend features of different intervention models (cognitive-behavioral techniques, 12-step abstinence approaches, interpersonal, dialectical, and psychodynamic frameworks) resulting in an eclectic treatment approach (e.g., Johnson & Taylor, 1996). Although clinicians often view combined approaches as superior to a single-therapy approach and would endorse their effectiveness, no systematic data have been published regarding outcomes of using these combined integrated approaches to allow

TABLE 1.2. Randomized Controlled Treatment Studies of AN in Young Adolescent Samples (Mean Age < 17 Years) and Late Adolescent/Adult Patients (Mean Age > 17 Years)

Study	N	Sex (%F)	Age (M or range)	Inclusion criteria	Therapy conditions: N (% complete)	Results summary
Young adolescent (M age < 17 years)						
Eisler, Dare, Hodes, et al. (2000)	40	97.5	15.5	DSM-IV; ICD-10 AN	Conjoint family therapy (CFT): 19 (89.5%) Separated family therapy (SFT): 21 (90.5%)	*CFT > SFT* on EDI *CFT = SFT* on BMI, bulimic symptoms EAT, M-R scales, and outcome *CFT > SFT* on Depression, Obsessionality SMFQ *CFT = SFT* MOCI, RSE, Tension
Geist, Heinmaa, Stephens, et al. (2000)	25	100	14.6	Female Ages 12–17.4 yr Weight < 90% IBW Self-imposed food restriction	Family therapy (FT): 12 (100%) Family group psychoeducation (FPE): 13 (100%)	FT = FPE
Le Grange, Eisler, Dare, & Russell (1992)	18	88.9	15.3	DSM-III-R AN Age < 18 yr Duration of illness shorter than 3 yr	CFT: 9 (100%) SFT: 9 (100%)	CFT = SFT
Lock, Agras, Bryson, & Kraemer (2005)	86	89.5	15.2	DSM-IV AN Some partially weight restored Loss of one menstrual cycle	Short-term FT (STFT): 44 (96%) Long-term FT (LTFT): 42 (84%)	STFT = LTFT
Robin et al. (1999)	41	100	14.2	DSM-III-R AN Females Ages 11–20 yr Residing at home with one or both parents	Behavioral family systems therapy (BFST): 19 Ego-oriented individual therapy (EOIT): 18 90.2% completion across conditions	*BFST > EOIT* on BMI *BFST = EOIT* on EAT, EDI *BFST = EOIT* on BDI, CBCL
Russell, Szmukler, Dare, & Eisler (1987)[a]	21	91.3	16.6	DSM-III AN Extreme loss of weight, no purging following overeating Amenorrhea or loss of sex interest/potency	FT: 10 (100%) Nonspecific individual treatment (NST): 11 (100%)	*FT > NST* on % ABW MR scales MR outcome

(cont.)

TABLE 1.2. (cont.)

Study	N	Sex (%F)	Age (M or range)	Inclusion criteria	Therapy conditions: N (% complete)	Results summary
Late adolescent/adult (M age > 17 years)						
Bachar, Latzer, Kreitler, & Berry (1999)	13	100	18.1	DSM-IV AN	Self-psychological treatment (SPT): 7 (85.7%) Cognitive orientation treatment (COT): 6 (33.3%)	N too small for inferential statistics
Channon, de Silva, Hemsley, & Perkins (1989)	24	100	23.8	Russell's AN (17) Female	Cognitive-behavioral therapy (CBT): 8 (100%) Behavioral therapy (BT): 8 (87.5%) Routine outpatient: 8 (75%)	CBT = BT on All measures Routine > CBT, BT on Maturity fears
Crisp et al. (1991)	90	100	22	DSM-III-R AN Female Duration of illness < 10 yr Living near the service	Inpatient (IP): 30 (60%) Outpatient individual/family (OI): 20 (90%) Outpatient group (OG): 20 (85%) No further treatment (NT): 20 (100%)	IP, OI, OG > NT on Weight IP = OI = OG = NT on MR scales
Dare, Eisler, Russell, Treasure, & Dodge (2001)	84	98	26.3	DSM-IV AN Age > 18 yr	FT: 22 (72.7%) Focal psychoanalytic therapy (FP): 21 (57.1%) Cognitive-analytic therapy (CAT): 22 (59.1%) Routine treatment (RT): 19 (68.4%)	FT, FP > RT on BMI FT = FP = CAT = RT MR Scales

20

Study	N	%	Age	Diagnostic criteria	Treatment conditions	Results
McIntosh et al. (2005)	56	100	17–40	Female, Ages 17–40 yr, DSM-IV AN or lenient AN (BMI 17.5–19)—without amenorrhea criterion	CBT: 19 (63%), Interpersonal psychotherapy (IPT): 21 (57%), NST: 16 (69%)	$NST > IPT$ on EDE restraint, Global outcome, GAF; $CBT > IPT$ on EDE restraint; $CBT = IPT$ on Global outcome, GAF; $CBT = IPT = NST$ on BMI, EDE (exc. restraint), EDI, HAM-D
Pike, Walsh, Vitousek, Wilson, & Bauer (2003)	33	100	25.2	DSM-IV AN–posthospitalization, Lived within commuting distance	CBT: 18 (100%), Nutritional counseling (NC): 15 (80%)	$CBT > NC$
Russell et al. (1987)[a]	36	91	24.2	DSM-III AN, Extreme weight loss, amenorrhea/ loss of sex interest, posthospitalization	FT: 19 (84.2%), NST: 17 (94.1%)	$NST > FT$ for Weight gain; $NST = FT$ for MR outcome
Serfaty, Turkington, Heap, Lesham, & Jolley (1999)	35	94	20.9	Ages > 16 yr, DSM-III-R AN	CBT: 25 (92%), Dietician control (DC): 10 (0%)	$CBT > DC$ on % remitted; $CBT = DC$ on BMI
Treasure et al. (1995)	30	97	25.0	Ages > 18 yr, ICD-10 AN	CAT: 14 (71.4%), Educational behavior therapy (EBT): 16 (62.5%)	$CAT > EBT$ on Subjective rating; $CAT = EBT$ on BMI, MR Scales

Note: ABW, average body weight; BDI, Beck Depression Inventory; BMI, body mass index; CBCL, Child Behavior Checklist; EDE, Eating Disorder Examination; EDI, Eating Disorder Inventory; GAF, Global Assessment of Functioning; HAM-D, Hamilton Depression Rating Scale; IBW, ideal body weight; ICD, International Classification of Diseases; MOCI, Maudsley Obsessional Compulsive Index; MR Outcome, Morgan and Russell outcome; MR Scales, Morgan and Russell scales; RSE, Rosenberg Self-Esteem Scale; SMFQ, Short Mood and Feelings Questionnaire.

[a]Russell et al. (1987) included a group of young-adolescent patients with AN and adult patients with AN and is included in the table twice.

evaluation of their efficacy (i.e., their superiority in a randomized control trial) or their effectiveness (i.e., their success when employed in clinical settings).

Involvement of Family and Caregivers

A specific form of family therapy has demonstrated success in reducing symptoms in adolescent patients (Russell et al., 1987). Adolescent patients have been shown to improve most with conjoint family therapy (see Table 1.2), except in cases of highly critical parents, for which separate family groups may be more effective (Eisler et al., 2000). Patients with higher levels of obsessive–compulsive symptoms or those who come from a nonintact family have demonstrated improved outcomes when assigned to a 12-month, compared to a 6-month, family-based treatment (Lock, Agras, Bryson, & Kraemer, 2005).

Despite evidence supporting the importance of involving family and caregivers in the treatment of adolescents with AN, limited data support this approach in adult patients. In the original trial supporting the use of family-based treatment for younger patients with a shorter duration of illness (Russell et al., 1987), individual psychotherapy was associated with superior outcomes compared to family-based therapy in adult patients with AN (Russell et al., 1987). Of note, involving family and caregivers in the treatment of adult patients is complicated by ethical considerations to protect the confidentiality of information shared during treatment. However, given the potential for treatment resistance, family and caregivers often look to clinicians to provide them with tools they may use to support patients' efforts to make progress in treatment. Family and caregivers also may benefit from affiliation with support groups designed to acknowledge the stress of caring for an ill child, regardless of the age of that child. Goddard, MacDonald, and Treasure (Chapter 29, this volume) examine recent work addressing the needs of AN caregivers (see also Sepulveda, Lopez, Todd, Whitaker, & Treasure, 2008; Whitney et al., 2006).

Treatment Team Members

Among various forms of mental disorders, AN presents one of the greatest challenges because the illness impacts multiple domains of function. As such, a multidisciplinary team is required to address the various aspects of the illness. This treatment team should consist of at least a medical professional, a mental health professional, and a dietician.

The role of the medical professional is to monitor physical health and safety and ensure involvement of medical specialists as indicated. AN can trigger medical sequelae that require attention from specialists in endocrinology, cardiology, nephrology, gastroenterology, and orthopedics. The role of the mental health professional is to address disturbances in thoughts, feelings, and behaviors that form the core of the illness. A range of professions may fulfill this role, including psychiatrists, licensed clinical psychologists, clinical social workers, marriage and family therapists, and psychiatric nurses. While individuals in each of these professions are trained to provide psychotherapeutic interventions, a psychiatrist also may manage psychopharmacological treatments. The role of the dietician is to assess nutritional needs for healthy weight gain and maintenance, create an appropriate dietary plan, and assist in implementation of the plan.

Aside from these three team members, additional professions may be involved in the treatment of inpatients—who are often more severely impacted by illness than those who are seen on an outpatient basis. Occupational therapists are involved with inpatient and partial hospitalization programs to assist patients in learning how to prepare healthy meals, go grocery shopping, attend restaurant outings with peers, and engage in family meals. Recreational therapists have been utilized in inpatient and partial hospital settings to help patients learn to incorporate healthy exercise, as well as creative relaxation strategies to improve more balanced living. The components of the treatment team should be guided by the patient's needs. However, it is important for health professionals to fully appreciate the limits of their own professional training with respect to treating a patient with AN.

References

American Psychiatric Association. (2000). *Diagnostic and statistical manual of mental disorders* (4th ed., text rev.). Washington, DC: Author.

Attia E, Kaplan AS, Haynos A, Yilmaz Z, & Musante D. (2008, September). *Olanzapine vs. placebo for outpatients with anorexia nervosa: A pilot study.* Paper presented at the 14th Annual Eating Disorders Research Society Meeting, Montreal, QB.

Bachar E, Latzer Y, Kreitler S, & Berry EM. (1999). Empirical comparison of two psychological therapies: Self psychology and cognitive orientation in the treatment of anorexia and bulimia. *Journal of Psychotherapy Practice and Research*, 8:115–128.

Beck AT, Epstein N, Brown G, & Steer RA. (1988). An inventory for measuring clinical anxiety: Psychometric properties. *Journal of Consulting and Clinical Psychology*, 56:893–897.

Beck AT, Steer RA, & Brown GK. (1996). *The Beck Depression Inventory Manual* (2nd ed.). San Antonio, TX: Psychological Corporation Harcourt & Brace.

Becker AE, Keel PK, Anderson-Fye EP, & Thomas JJ. (2004). Genes (and/or) jeans?: Genetic and socio-cultural contributions to risk for eating disorders. *Journal of Addictive Diseases*, 23:81–103.

Bissada H, Tasca GA, Barber AM, & Bradwejn J. (2008). Olanzapine in the treatment of low body weight and obsessive thinking in women with anorexia nervosa: A randomized, double-blind, placebo controlled trial. *American Journal of Psychiatry*, 165:1281–1288.

Bowers WA, Andersen AE, & Evans K. (2004). Management for eating disorders: Inpatient and partial hospital programs. In TD Brewerton (Ed.), *Clinical handbook of eating disorders: An integrated approach* (pp. 349–376). New York: Marcel Dekker.

Bulik CM, Berkman ND, Brownley KA, Sedway JA, & Lohr KN. (2007). Anorexia nervosa treatment: A systematic review of randomized controlled trials. *International Journal of Eating Disorders*, 40:310–320.

Carter JC, McFarlane TL, & Olmsted MP. (2004). Psychometric assessment of eating disorders. In TD Brewerton (Ed.), *Clinical handbook of eating disorders: An integrated approach* (pp. 21–46). New York: Marcel Dekker.

Chambless DL, & Ollendick TH. (2001). Empirically supported psychological interventions: Controversies and evidence. *Annual Review of Psychology*, 52:685–716.

Channon S, de Silva P, Hemsley D, & Perkins R. (1989). A controlled trial of cognitive-behavioural and behavioural treatment of anorexia nervosa. *Behaviour Research and Therapy*, 27:529–535.

Crisp AH, Norton K, Gowers S, Halek C, Bowyer C, Yeldham D, et al. (1991). A controlled study of the effect of therapies aimed at adolescent and family psychopathology in anorexia nervosa. *British Journal of Psychiatry*, 159:325–333.

Culbert KM, Breedlove SM, Burt SA, & Klump KL. (2008). Prenatal hormone exposure and risk for eating disorders: A comparison of opposite-sex and same-sex twins. *Archives of General Psychiatry*, 65:329–336.

Dalle Grave R, & Calugi S. (2007). Eating disorder not otherwise specified in an inpatient unit: The impact of altering the DSM-IV criteria for anorexia and bulimia nervosa. *European Eating Disorders Review*, 15:340–349.

Dare C, Eisler I, Russell G, Treasure J, & Dodge L. (2001). Psychological therapies for adults with anorexia nervosa: Randomized controlled trial of out-patient treatments. *British Journal of Psychiatry*, 178:216–221.

Eddy KT, Keel PK, Dorer DJ, Delinsky SS, Franko DL, & Herzog DB. (2002). A longitudinal comparison of anorexia nervosa subtypes. *International Journal of Eating Disorders*, 31:191–201.

Eisler I, Dare C, Hodes M, Russell G, Dodge E, & Le Grange D. (2000). Family therapy for adolescent anorexia nervosa: The results of a controlled comparison of two family interventions. *Journal of Child Psychology and Psychiatry*, 41:727–736.

Fairburn CG, & Beglin SJ. (1994). Assessment of eating disorders: Interview or self-report questionnaire. *International Journal of Eating Disorders*, 16:363–370.

Fairburn CG, & Cooper Z. (1993). The Eating Disorder Examination (12th ed.). In C Fairburn & GT Wilson (Eds.), *Binge eating: Nature, assessment, and treatment* (pp. 317–331). New York: Guilford Press.

Fairburn CG, Cooper Z, Doll HA, & Welch SL. (1999). Risk factors for anorexia nervosa: Three integrated case-control comparisons. *Archives of General Psychiatry*, 56:468–476.

Favaro A, Monteleone P, Santonastaso P, & Maj M. (2008). Psychobiology of eating disorders. *Annual Review of Eating Disorders* (Part 2). Oxford, UK: Radcliffe.

Favaro A, Tenconi E, & Santonastaso P. (2006). Perinatal factors and the risk of developing anorexia nervosa and bulimia nervosa. *Archives of General Psychiatry*, 63:82–88.

First MB, Spitzer RL, Gibbon M, & Williams JB. (1996). *Structured Clinical Interview for Axis I DSM-IV Disorders*. New York: Biometrics Research Department, New York State Psychiatric Institute.

Garner DM. (1991). *Eating Disorder Inventory–2: Professional manual*. Odessa, FL: Psychological Assessment Resources.

Garner DM, & Garfinkel PE. (1979). The Eating Attitudes Test: An index of the symptoms of anorexia nervosa. *Psychological Medicine*, 9:273–279.

Garner DM, Olmsted MP, Bohr Y, & Garfinkel PE. (1982). The Eating Attitudes Test: Psychometric features and clinical correlates. *Psychological Medicine*, 12:871–878.

Garner DM, Olmsted MP, & Polivy J. (1983). Development and validation of a multidimensional Eating Disorder Inventory for anorexia nervosa and bulimia. *International Journal of Eating Disorders*, 2:15–34.

Geist R, Heinmaa M, Stephens D, Davis R, & Katzman DK. (2000). Comparison of family therapy and family group psychoeducation in adolescents with anorexia nervosa. *Canadian Journal of Psychiatry*, 45:173–178.

Geller J, Drab-Hudson DL, Whisenhunt BL, & Srikameswaran S. (2004). Readiness to change dietary restriction predicts outcomes in eating disorders. *Eating Disorders*, 12:209–224.

Geller J, Srikameswaran S, Cockell S, & Zaitsoff Z. (2000). Assessment of shape- and weight-based self-esteem in adolescents. *International Journal of Eating Disorders*, 28:339–345.

Gowers SG, Clark A, Roberts C, Griffiths A, Edwards V, Bryan C, et al. (2007). Clinical effectiveness of treatments for anorexia nervosa in adolescents: Randomised controlled trial. *British Journal of Psychiatry*, 191:427–435.

Gull WW. (1874). Anorexia nervosa (apepsia hysterica, anorexia hysterica). *Transactions of the Clinical Society of London*, 7:22–28.

Herzog DB, Dorer DJ, Keel PK, Selwyn SE, Ekeblad ER, Flores AT, et al. (1999). Recovery and relapse in anorexia nervosa and bulimia nervosa: A 7.5 year follow-up study. *Journal of the American Academy of Child and Adolescent Psychiatry*, 38:829–837.

Hoek HW, van Harten PN, Hermans KM, Katzman MA, Matroos GE, & Susser ES. (2005). The incidence of anorexia nervosa in Curacao. *American Journal of Psychiatry*, 162:748–752.

Howard WT, Evans KK, Quintero-Howard C, Bowers WA, & Andersen AE. (1999). Predictors of success or failure of transition to day hospital treatment for inpatients with anorexia nervosa. *American Journal of Psychiatry*, 156:1697–1702.

Hudson JI, Hiripi E, Pope HG, & Kessler RC. (2007). The prevalence and correlates of eating disorders in the National Comorbidity Survey Replication. *Biological Psychiatry*, 61:348–358.

Jacobi C, Hayward C, de Zwaan M, Kraemer HC, & Agras WS. (2004). Coming to terms with risk factors for eating disorders: Application of risk terminology and suggestions for general taxonomy. *Psychological Bulletin*, 130:19–65.

Johnson CL, & Taylor C. (1996). Working with difficult-to-treat eating disorders using an integration of twelve-step and traditional psychotherapies. *Psychiatric Clinics of North America*, 19:829–841.

Kaye SH, Frank GK, Bailer UF, & Henry SE. (2005). Neurobiology of anorexia nervosa: Clinical implications of alterations of the function of serotonin and other neuronal systems. *International Journal of Eating Disorders*, 37:S15–S19.

Keel PK. (2005). *Eating disorders.* Upper Saddle River, NJ: Pearson Prentice-Hall.

Keel PK, Dorer DJ, Eddy KT, Delinsky SS, Franko DL, Blais MA, et al. (2002). Predictors of treatment utilization among women with anorexia and bulimia nervosa. *American Journal of Psychiatry*, 159:140–142.

Keel PK, Dorer DJ, Eddy KT, Franko DL, Charatan D, & Herzog DB. (2003). Predictors of mortality in eating disorders. *Archives of General Psychiatry*, 60:179–183.

Keel PK, Dorer DJ, Franko DL, Jackson SC, & Herzog DB. (2005). Post-remission predictors of relapse in eating disorders. *American Journal of Psychiatry*, 162:2263–2268.

Keel PK, & Haedt A. (2008). Evidence-based psychosocial treatments for eating problems and eating disorders. *Journal of Clinical Child and Adolescent Psychology*, 37:39–61.

Keel PK, & Klump KL. (2003). Are eating disorders culture-bound syndromes?: Implications for conceptualizing their etiology. *Psychological Bulletin*, 129:747–769.

Keel PK, Klump KL, Miller KB, McGue M, & Iacono WG. (2005). Shared transmission of eating disorders and anxiety disorders. *International Journal of Eating Disorders*, 38:99–105.

Keski-Rahkonen A, Hoek HW, Susser ES, Linna MS, Sihvola E, Raevuori A, et al. (2007). Epidemiology and course of anorexia nervosa in the community. *American Journal of Psychiatry*, 164:1259–1265.

Keys A, Brozek J, Henschel A, Mickelson O, & Taylor HL. (1950). *The biology of human starvation.* Minneapolis: University of Minnesota Press.

Klump KL, Burt SA, McGue M, & Iacono WG. (2007). Changes in genetic and environmental influences on disordered eating across adolescence: A longitudinal twin study. *Archives of General Psychiatry*, 64:1409–1415.

Klump KL, & Culbert KM. (2007). Molecular genetic studies of eating disorders. *Current Directions in Psychological Science*, 16:37–41.

Klump KL, Strober M, Bulik CM, Thornton L, Johnson C, Devlin B, et al. (2004). Personality characteristics of women before and after recovery from an eating disorder. *Psychological Medicine*, 34:1407–1418.

Le Grange D, Eisler I, Dare C, & Russell GFM. (1992). Evaluation of family treatments in adolescent anorexia nervosa: A pilot study. *International Journal of Eating Disorders*, 12:347–357.

Lilenfeld LR, Kaye WH, Greeno CG, Merikangas KR, Plotnicov K, Pollice C, et al. (1998). A controlled family study of anorexia nervosa and bulimia nervosa: Psychiatric disorders in first-degree relatives and effects of proband comorbidity. *Archives of General Psychiatry*, 55:603–610.

Lock J, Agras WS, Bryson S, & Kraemer HC. (2005). A comparison of short- and long-term family therapy for adolescent anorexia nervosa. *Journal of the American Academy of Child and Adolescent Psychiatry*, 44:632–639.

Lock J, & Le Grange D. (2005). Family-based treatment of eating disorders. *International Journal of Eating Disorders*, 37:26–30.

Löwe B, Zipfel S, Buchholz C, Dupont Y, Reas DL, & Herzog W. (2001). Long-term outcome of anorexia nervosa in a prospective 21-year follow-up study. *Psychological Medicine*, 31:881–890.

McCormick LM, Keel PK, Brumm MC, Bowers W, Swayze V, Andersen A, et al. (2008). Implications of starvation-induced change in right dorsal anterior cingulate volume in anorexia nervosa. *International Journal of Eating Disorders*, 41:602–610.

McIntosh VW, Jordan J, Carter FA, Luty SE, McKenzie JM, Bulik CM, et al. (2005). Three psychotherapies for anorexia nervosa: A randomized, controlled trial. *American Journal of Psychiatry*, 162:741–747.

Mizes JS, Christiano B, Madison J, Post G, Seime R, & Varnado P. (2000). Development of the Mizes Anorectic Cognitions Questionnaire—Revised: Psychometric properties and factor structure in a large sample of eating disorder patients. *International Journal of Eating Disorders*, 28:415–421.

Nielsen S, Moller-Madsen S, Isager T, Jorgensen J, Pagsberg K, & Theander S. (1998). Standardized mortality in eating disorders: A quantitative summary of previously published and new evidence. *Journal of Psychosomatic Research*, 44:413–434.

Pike KM, Walsh BT, Vitousek K, Wilson GT, & Bauer J. (2003). Cognitive behavior therapy in the posthospitalization treatment of anorexia nervosa. *American Journal of Psychiatry*, 160:2046–2049.

Robin AL, Siegel PT, Moye AW, Gilroy M, Dennis AB, & Sikand A. (1999). A controlled comparison of family versus individual therapy for adolescents with anorexia nervosa. *Journal of the American Academy of Child and Adolescent Psychiatry*, 38:1482–1489.

Rosenberg M. (1979). *Conceiving of the self*. New York: Basic Books.

Russell GFM, Szmukler GI, Dare C, & Eisler I. (1987). An evaluation of family therapy in anorexia nervosa and bulimia nervosa. *Archives of General Psychiatry*, 44:1047–1056.

Sepulveda AR, Lopez C, Todd G, Whitaker W, & Treasure J. (2008). An examination of the impact of "the Maudsley eating disorder collaborative care skills workshops" on the well being of carers: A pilot study. *Social Psychiatry and Psychiatric Epidemiology*, 43:584–591.

Serfaty MA, Turkington D, Heap M, Ledsham L, & Jolley E. (1999). Cognitive therapy versus dietary counseling in the outpatient treatment of anorexia nervosa: Effects of the treatment phase. *European Eating Disorders Review*, 7:334–350.

Skinner HA, Steinhauer PD, & Santa-Barbara J. (1995). *Family Assessment Measure–III*. Toronto: Multi-Health Systems.

Steinhausen HC. (2002). The outcome of anorexia nervosa in the 20th century. *American Journal of Psychiatry*, 159:1284–1293.

Striegel-Moore RH, Dohm FA, Kraemer HC, Taylor CB, Daniels S, Crawford PB, et al. (2003). Eating disorders in white and black women. *American Journal of Psychiatry*, 160:1326–1331.

Strober M, Freeman R, & Morrell W. (1999). Atypical anorexia nervosa: Separation from typical cases in course and outcome in a long-term prospective study. *International Journal of Eating Disorders*, 25:135–142.

Sullivan PF. (1995). Mortality in anorexia nervosa. *American Journal of Psychiatry*, 152:1073–1074.

Thomas JJ, Roberto CA, & Brownell KD. (2009). Eighty-five per cent of what? Discrepancies in the weight cut-off for anorexia nervosa substantially affect the prevalence of underweight. *Psychological Medicine*, 39:833–843.

Treasure J, & Schmidt U. (2005). Anorexia nervosa. *Clinical Evidence*, 14:1140–1148.

Treasure J, Todd G, Brolly M, Tiller J, Nehmed A, & Denman F. (1995). A pilot study of a randomised trial of cognitive analytical therapy vs educational behavioural therapy for adult anorexia nervosa. *Behaviour Research and Therapy*, 33:363–367.

Treat TA, McCabe EB, Gaskill JA, & Marcus MD. (2008). Treatment of anorexia nervosa in a specialty care continuum. *International Journal of Eating Disorders*, 41:564–572.

Tyrka AR, Waldron I, Graber JA, & Brooks-Gunn J. (2002). Prospective predictors of the onset of anorexic and bulimic syndromes. *International Journal of Eating Disorders*, 32:282–290.

Uher R, Brammer MJ, Murphy T, Campbell IC, Ng VW, Williams SCR, et al. (2003). Recovery and chronicity in anorexia nervosa: Brain activity associated with differential outcomes. *Biological Psychiatry*, 54:934–942.

Walsh BT, Kaplan AS, Attia E, Olmsted M, Parides M, Carter JC, et al. (2006). Fluoxetine after weight restoration in anorexia nervosa: A randomized controlled trial. *Journal of the American Medical Association*, 295:2605–2612.

Whitney J, Murray J, Gavan K, Todd G, Whitaker W, & Treasure J. (2004). Experience of caring for someone with anorexia nervosa: Qualitative study. *British Journal of Psychiatry*, 187:444–449.

Wilson GT, Grilo CM, & Vitousek KM. (2007). Psychological treatment of eating disorders. *American Psychologist*, 62:199–216.

CHAPTER 2

Diagnosis, Assessment, and Treatment Planning for Bulimia Nervosa

Scott J. Crow and Beth Brandenburg

Bulimia nervosa (BN) was initially described as distinct from anorexia nervosa (AN) by Russell in 1979. Since that time, BN has emerged as an important diagnostic entity with well-recognized medical, psychological, and social comorbidities and complications. Much is now known about its associated features, complications, and course. Risk factors and appropriate treatments are also increasingly well understood. This chapter provides a broad overview of BN, discusses appropriate assessment approaches, and describes a basic approach to treatment planning.

Diagnostic Criteria for and Differential Diagnosis of BN

Two sets of diagnostic criteria for BN currently exist. The diagnostic criteria included in the text revision of the fourth edition of the *Diagnostic and Statistical Manual of Mental Disorders* (DSM-IV-TR; American Psychiatric Association [APA], 2000) are as follows:

A. Recurrent episodes of binge eating. An episode of binge eating is characterized by both of the following:
   1. Eating, in a discrete period of time (e.g., within any 2-hour period), an amount of food that is definitely larger than most people would eat during a similar period of time and under similar circumstances.
   2. A sense of lack of control over eating during the episode (e.g., a feeling that one cannot stop eating or control what or how much one is eating).
B. Recurrent inappropriate compensatory behavior in order to prevent weight gain, such as self-induced vomiting; misuse of laxatives, diuretics, enemas, or other medications; fasting or excessive exercise.
C. The binge eating and inappropriate compensatory behaviors both occur, on average, at least twice a week for 3 months.
D. Self-evaluation is unduly influenced by body shape and weight.

E. The disturbance does not occur exclusively during episodes of AN.
    Specify type:
    1. **Purging Type:** During the current episode of BN, the person has regularly engaged
        in self-induced vomiting or the misuse of laxatives, diuretics, or enemas.
    2. **Nonpurging Type:** During the current episode of BN, the person has used other
        inappropriate compensatory behaviors, such as fasting or excessive exercise, but
        has not engaged in self-induced vomiting or the misuse of laxatives, diuretics, or
        enemas. (p. 550)

The ICD-10 classification of mental and behavioral disorders (World Health Organization, 1992) lays out similar diagnostic guidelines, though the focus of the cognitive
criterion is "morbid fear of fatness," not self-evaluation as per DSM-IV-TR. In addition,
purging and nonpurging types are not recognized in ICD-10.

These two sets of diagnostic criteria, if rigorously applied, will lead to some diagnostic discrepancy for certain individuals, but each criterion set captures the broad concept of disordered eating characterized by binge eating, compensatory behaviors, and a
disturbance in attitudes about weight, shape, and eating. A substantial number of individuals with disordered eating have symptoms reminiscent of BN but do not meet either
DSM-IV-TR or ICD-10 criteria for BN, often because they lack the required frequency
of binge eating, compensatory behaviors, or both. Under current diagnostic guidelines,
such individuals would likely receive a diagnosis of eating disorder not otherwise specified (EDNOS). At this writing the DSM criteria for eating disorder (ED) diagnoses are
being critically examined in anticipation of a new DSM to be published in 2012. In light
of these efforts, these diagnostic criteria for BN (and the corresponding differential
diagnosis for those not meeting full criteria for BN) may be subject to change. Another
differential diagnostic consideration is AN: Individuals with AN can present with binge-
eating and purging behavior and typically have similar disturbances regarding body
shape, weight, and eating. The DSM-IV-TR stipulates that if someone has such symptoms
but is at sufficiently low weight to meet diagnostic criteria for AN, then that diagnosis
would supersede BN, with the AN binge–purge subtype specification.

On rare occasion, other medical entities should be considered in the differential
diagnosis. For example, some types of upper gastrointestinal pathology can be associated with recurrent vomiting. Similarly, other gastrointestinal pathology (e.g., celiac
sprue) can be associated with weight loss and persistent diarrhea, thus mimicking purging by laxative abuse.

Brief Overview of BN

Epidemiology

Estimates of the prevalence of BN have varied widely since it was introduced as a diagnostic category in 1980. This variation has been attributed to changing definitions of
the illness, differences in the populations studied, and possible changes in illness prevalence over time. DSM-III did not include a frequency requirement for binge-eating
episodes. Prevalence estimates based on DSM-III were therefore quite high, as the
diagnostic criteria did not distinguish occasional binge episodes from a more serious
disorder. DSM-III-R established a minimum number of weekly eating binges, resulting

in lower prevalence estimates. Currently, the general consensus is that approximately 2–3% of young women meet criteria for BN as defined in DSM-IV-TR. However, most of the epidemiological studies of BN have been conducted on school- or college-age populations. Based on surveys of a large, nationally representative sample of randomly chosen U.S. adults, the National Comorbidity Survey Replication study reported a lifetime prevalence of BN as 1.5% among females and 0.5% among males (Hudson, Hiripi, Pope, & Kessler, 2007). The median age of onset reported was 18, which is consistent with previous studies.

It is unclear whether the prevalence of BN has changed over time; evidence exists for decreased, increased, and stable prevalence. Keel, Heatherton, Dorer, Joiner, and Zalta (2006) found that the point prevalence of BN (based on DSM-III criteria) among college females decreased significantly from 4.2% in 1982 to 1.3% in 1992, then stabilized to 1.7% in 2002. A survey of adolescent girls conducted at a suburban high school in 1981 and again in 1986 showed a significant decrease in point prevalence of BN from 4.1 to 2.0% (Johnson, Tobin, & Lipkin, 1989). Heatherton, Nichols, Mahamedi, and Keel (1995) conducted a survey of college students in 1982 and again in 1992. They found that the point prevalence of BN (based on DSM-III criteria) had decreased from 7.2 to 5.1% in women and from 1.1 to 0.4% in men. Several more recent studies found no significant change in the prevalence of BN (Crowther, Armey, Luce, Dalton, & Leahey, 2008; van Son, van Hoeken, Bartelds, van Furth, & Hoek, 2006; Zachrisson, Vedul-Kjelsas, Gotestam, & Mykletun, 2008). Still other studies have argued for increased risk with successive birth cohorts (e.g., Hudson et al., 2007; Kendler et al., 1991). Interpretation of these various studies is limited by changes in diagnostic criteria over time and between studies. Possible explanations for any changes observed might include true changes in prevalence, growing awareness of the disease after it was described, changes in media portrayal of eating disorders since that time, or recall bias.

Associated Features/Comorbidity

A striking feature associated with BN is the high rate of co-occurring psychopathology. Most prominent is depression, which occurs in the majority of patients with BN at some point during the illness (Herzog, Keller, Sacks, Yeh, & Lavori, 1992; Hudson et al., 2007); studies suggest rates of 50–70% or more. At one time, BN was hypothesized to be a variant of depression (Hudson, Pope, Jonas, & Yurgelun-Todd, 1983; Hudson, Pope, Yurgelun-Todd, Jonas, & Frankenburg, 1987; Kassett et al., 1989), although this hypothesis seems no longer tenable. Whether this comorbidity with mood disorders is confined to unipolar mood disorder is somewhat unclear. Historically, the focus has been mostly on major depression, but recent reports suggest that rates of bipolar illness may be elevated as well (Baldassano et al., 2005; Hudson et al., 2007; Ramacciotti et al., 2005). Mood disorders have their own, independent clinical significance, of course. The presence of comorbid mood problems portends a less favorable outcome in some studies (Keel, Mitchell, Miller, Davis, & Crow, 1999) but not others (e.g., Fichter, Quadflieg, & Hedlund, 2008).

A wide variety of anxiety disorders is also quite common (Kaye, Bulik, Thornton, Barbarich, & Masters, 2004). Obsessive–compulsive disorder (OCD) is sometimes viewed as being more strongly related to AN (Swinbourne & Touyz, 2007), although in some samples rates in AN and BN are similar (e.g., Kaye et al., 2004). OCD symptoms may persist long after recovery from BN (von Ranson, Kaye, Weltzin, Rao, & Matsunaga, 1999). Substance use disorders are also quite common. Alcohol and other types of substance dependence appear to impact a substantial minority of patients with BN (Bulik et al., 2004; Holderness, Brooks-Gunn, & Warren, 1994), and tobacco dependence is also quite common (Anzengruber et al., 2006; Welch & Fairburn, 1998). The relationship between BN and personality disorders also has been widely explored. A number of reports have cited elevated rates of personality disorders, including particularly those in Cluster B (for a review, see Grilo, 2002).

Cultural Factors

Cultural factors are thought to play an important role in BN, as in other EDs (Keel & Klump, 2003). Prevailing cultural attitudes regarding thinness, the importance of shape, and the high positive value placed on low weight are widely prevalent in Western societies at this time. Many observers have commented on the fact that the seeming appearance of BN as an important diagnostic entity in the latter half of the 20th century coincides with a growing cultural emphasis on thinness. This seems evident from a casual examination of the evolution of popular culture over several decades, whether reflected in popular media, in advertising and fashion, or in the depiction of ideal body types in art. Some investigators have also provided objective evidence for this change (e.g., in the form of changes in the body mass index (BMI) of beauty contest winners; Rubinstein & Caballero, 2000). One might interpret the birth cohort effects on BN prevalence (found in some BN prevalence studies, reviewed above) as supporting the role of culture in BN.

There is also growing evidence supporting the impact of cultural change on the prevalence of both disordered-eating attitudes and EDs. One example comes from studies conducted by Becker and colleagues in Fiji, both prior to, and shortly following, the introduction of Western TV broadcasting (Becker, Burwell, Navara, & Gilman, 2003). This work has documented very low rates of disordered eating prior to the introduction of Westernized TV and the rapid development of attitudes toward weight and shape similar to those found in Western culture within just a few years of the introduction of Western media. This natural experiment vividly highlights the potent role of culture in the development of BN and other EDs.

Gender

BN primarily affects women. This fact has been known from the earliest descriptive samples (Fairburn, Cooper, Doll, Norman, & O'Connor, 2000), and historically, gender ratios of 10:1 or greater have been cited (e.g., see DSM-IV). On the other hand, more recent samples (e.g., from the National Comorbidity Survey; Hudson et al., 2007) have found that although in community samples BN is still more prevalent in women than men, the ratio may be closer to 3:1. One possibility is that this finding reflects a radical shift in prevalence, but it seems more likely that it results from a higher prevalence of treatment seeking among women with BN than among men.

This gender disparity raises the interesting question as to the reason for such a divergence. The answer remains somewhat unclear, and a number of hypotheses have been advanced. Certainly, cultural messages about weight and shape are focused mostly (though not entirely) on females, which might account for part of the discrepancy. Biological factors might also help to explain this difference. There is evidence to suggest that changes in gonadal hormone status with puberty may impact eating behavior (Klump, Keel, Culbert, & Edler, 2008). Furthermore, there is now evidence to suggest that the impact of familial, presumably genetic, variables on eating behavior may be highly dependent on changes in gonadal hormone status associated with the onset of puberty (Klump, Burt, McGue, & Iacono, 2007). Intrauterine hormonal exposure (assessed using co-twin gender in twin studies) influences disordered eating in adulthood (Culbert, Breedlove, Burt, & Klump, 2008). These results raise the possibility that biological factors may play a far greater role in the gender disparity and prevalence of BN than was previously thought.

Course

The course of BN is increasingly well understood. A wide variety of studies has now described this course, though many have been of relatively short duration (Keel & Mitchell, 1997). One study examined outcome in a cohort 10–15 years after participants initially presented for treatment (Keel et al., 1999). In this study of 222 women (80.5%) agreed to participate. At a mean follow-up of 11.5 years, only 11% still had full BN and about 70% were in full remission. Other studies using somewhat smaller samples have also described outcomes using repeated assessments (rather than a single time point). Examples include studies of 4 years' duration (Agras, in press), 5 years' duration (Grilo et al., 2007), 7.5 years' duration (Herzog et al., 1999), and 12 years' duration (Fichter et al., 2008). All these studies found partial remission or full recovery at follow-up in the majority of participants. At the same time the pattern observed en route to recovery involves remission and relapse for many people, and frequent diagnostic crossover (most often to EDNOS or binge-eating disorder, but rarely to AN). Thus, it appears that the overall course of BN is more favorable than that seen in AN, and this appears to be true both in clinical (Keel et al., 1999) and community (Fairburn et al., 2000) samples.

One important aspect is mortality, and here the data are somewhat surprising. For example, in the Keel et al. study, mortality was 0.5%. In this and other studies, mortality rates have been low and standardized mortality ratios (i.e., the mortality reported in the population divided by the expected mortality rate, based on age, gender, and ethnicity) have generally not been elevated. This finding is surprising for two reasons: (1) the medical complications known to be associated with BN, and (2) the strong association of BN with other psychiatric illnesses known to confer increased risk for suicide. Whether this finding accurately represents mortality in BN or is due to a variety of confounding factors (e.g., the secretive nature of the illness, the inadequacy of mortality reporting, methods used to ascertain vital status) is unknown.

Psychobiology

Efforts to understand the psychobiology of BN have evolved along several lines. First, a variety of studies has attempted to examine neurotransmitters and neuromodulators known to be involved in the control of feeding, mood, or anxiety. A main focus of this work has been serotonin (Kaye, 2008). In brief, there is evidence for diminished serotonergic neurotransmission, reflected by diminished serotonin metabolite levels in acutely ill women with BN (Jimerson, Lesem, Kaye, & Brewerton, 1992), which appears, conversely, high in recovered women (Kaye et al., 1998). Platelet paroxetine binding, another measure of serotonin function, is also altered in BN (Steiger et al., 2005), and response to serotonergic probes is blunted (Brewerton, Lydiard, Laraia, Shook, & Ballenger, 1992; Jimerson et al., 1997). These findings intersect with positron emission tomography (PET) studies that have shown altered serotonin receptor 1A and 2A activity after recovery from BN (Kaye, 2008; Kaye et al., 2001) and diminished serotonin transporter levels in ill individuals (Tauscher et al., 2001).

Functional magnetic resonance imaging (fMRI) studies have also been conducted, examining patterns of brain activation and response to salient stimuli. The stimuli have included drawings of varying body shapes (Schienle, Schafer, Hermann, & Vaitl, 2008; Uher et al., 2005), visual images of food (Schienle et al., 2008; Uher, 2004), and ingestion of glucose (Frank et al., 2006). Increased activation of structures such as the anterior cingulate cortex (ACC) and insula, in conjunction with diminished activity in other cortical regions, has been frequently observed in acutely ill participants, with persistent diminished ACC activities in recovered participants. PET studies have also pointed to alterations in regional cerebral blood flow (rCBF) (Andreason et al., 1992) which may normalize with recovery (Frank, Kaye, Greer, Meltzer, & Price, 2000).

Taken together, this work suggests state-dependent alterations in brain function at neurochemical and circuitry levels. Whether these represent an underlying predisposition to BN, the acute effects of BN symptoms, or aftereffects of the illness (in recovered individuals) is unclear, and the implications for treatment or prevention are not known. Of potential importance, it is not known whether alterations observed in recovered women are associated with risk for relapse.

Genetics/Familial Issues

A wide variety of studies has now examined the familial and genetic bases for BN. This work has evolved as follows. First, there is clear evidence that BN is a familial entity, as are other EDs. For example, the risk of having BN, if one has a female relative with an ED, has been reported to be 4.4 times the risk in the general population (Strober, Freeman, Lampert, Diamond, & Kaye, 2000). The results of twin registry studies comparing monozygotic and dizygotic twins have also shown that disordered eating appears to be not merely familial but in fact genetic; that is, symptoms occur more commonly in the sibling of an affected identical cotwin than in the sibling of an affected fraternal cotwin. Different analyses have yielded different heritability estimates, often in the range of 50–80% (Kendler et al., 1991). Examination of behaviors seen in BN separately has shown both binge eating and vomiting to be heritable (Sullivan, Bulik, & Kendler, 1998). More recently, Wade et al. have reported both common and distinct risk factors for these two BN symptoms (Wade, Treloar, & Martin, 2008). At this point, active work is underway to understand the specific genetic bases for this heritable risk (Kaye, Devlin, et al., 2004). Linkage analyses and candidate gene studies are now beginning to identify potential target regions for consideration for a variety of quantitative traits observed in EDs (Bacanu et al., 2005).

Etiology

The forgoing provides a complex but potentially somewhat contradictory series of factors to be considered when thinking about the etiology of BN. Evidence of a genetic basis for BN is strong, consistent, and, at this point, widely accepted. On the other hand, studies suggest an important role for cultural factors. Furthermore, it is difficult to reconcile a simple genetic basis for BN with the apparent emergence of this diagnostic entity over the last half century (during which time the genome could not have changed sufficiently to account for the rise of a new, purely genetic illness). The most likely explanation of the etiology of BN, which addresses all of these conflicting factors, is one in which gene–environment interactions are posited. Specifically, genes of importance in BN may code for behavioral traits important in, but probably not specific to, BN. These likely include anxiety, perfectionism, impulsivity, and food obsessions. In the absence of the critically necessary environment, these genes may have a different behavioral presentation or may have very little observable behavioral impact. When provided with a critically important environment—in this case, an environment that places extreme salience on weight, shape, and appearance—many of those carrying these genes develop BN. This appealingly parsimonious explanation is consistent with a number of observations, including the relatively recent appearance of BN; the important contributions of both genetic and environmental factors; the development of disordered-eating attitudes in substantial numbers of individuals after relatively brief exposure to Westernized culture; and the fact that, although disordered attitudes toward eating, weight, and shape are relatively common in a society that exposes everyone to messages about weight and shape, full-blown eating disorders do not occur in most individuals. This conceptualization also fits well with existing literature that has examined factors that provide risk for the onset of disordered eating (including BN). These include a variety of prospective studies (Bearman, Martinez, & Stice, 2006; Fairburn, Cooper, Doll, & Davies, 2005; McKnight Investigators, 2003; Neumark-Sztainer et al., 2007; Wade, Bulik, Prescott, & Kendler, 2004). From this literature, a number of important factors, particularly risk factors for onset, has emerged, including constructs such as thin ideal internalization, higher BMI, neuroticism, weight teasing, social pressure, and negative life events. Most would be consistent with the forgoing model of etiology

Maintenance Factors

BN symptoms typically persist for years, raising the question: What factors maintain these symptoms? Generally, work in this area has focused on psychological mechanisms. A limited amount of work has hypothesized potential biological maintenance mechanisms, such as vagal nerve dysfunction (Faris et al., 2008); other psychobiological changes (discussed elsewhere in this chapter) might also play an important maintaining role. None of these potential biological changes has yet been incorporated into a well-developed maintenance model that has been formally tested, however.

The best developed model for the maintenance of BN symptoms has been described by Fairburn and has received some empirical support (Fairburn et al., 2003). In this model a critical factor is extreme concern about weight and shape, which results in severely restrictive eating behavior, in turn leading to binge eating followed by compensatory purging behavior. Binge eating and purging tend to lead to one another in a cyclical fashion. In addition, both are thought to increase concern about weight and shape, leading to further restrictive eating, further binge eating and purging, and so on.

Fairburn and colleagues (2003) examined this potential model in a 5-year longitudinal study. Predictors of persistent BN symptoms were overvaluation of shape and weight, a history of childhood obesity, poor social adjustment, and duration of eating disturbance. Also in keeping with the model, persistent binge eating and persistent purging predicted one another.

Thus, it appears that cognitive symptoms of the eating disorder lead to behavioral symptoms, which in turn reinforce the cognitive symptoms. There is every possibility that biological maintenance factors also tend to perpetuate this cycle, although this hypothesis remains untested.

Assessment

Initial Interview and Data Gathering

Aspects of effective interview techniques are directly applicable to the assessment of individuals with BN. This disorder is frequently a secretive illness in which most individuals have symptoms for a number of years prior to acknowledging the problem and first seeking assessment and treatment. Some individuals present in an open fashion, eager to receive treatment, but others are more guarded and reluctant to divulge BN symptoms unless specifically asked. Traditional, open-ended initial questioning often yields little information regarding BN symptoms, about which many patients feel much shame. More directed, focused questions are then useful. Conveying an open, accepting, nonjudgmental, and knowledgeable attitude is particularly useful. It is often necessary to ask about BN symptoms at repeat visits because patients may only gradually become willing to reveal some symptoms.

A number of ED-specific factors should be addressed as they help to inform treatment, predict course, and assess for possible complications. For example, understanding the time course of symptoms leading up to presentation is quite useful. A specific evaluation of the severity of symptoms (including the size of eating binges and their frequency, the nature and frequency of compensatory behaviors, eating patterns, dietary restraint, and body image/body dissatisfaction) is also needed. A careful assessment of laxative and ipecac use is important, as the presence of these factors influence risk of medical complications and helps inform management. The use of diuretics, diet pills, and over-the-counter weight loss medications is not uncommon, but their use is not often volunteered. It is important to inquire about a history of AN in the past, as this information will help to clarify the risk for osteoporosis. Finally, a critical part of initial data gathering involves the measurement of weight. Careful information about the frequency of self-weighing by subjects should also be collected.

Psychological Assessment

Because other psychiatric problems frequently co-occur with BN, a thorough assessment for comorbid psychopathology is also indicated. Most prominent among the comorbid problems are mood disorders, particularly unipolar depression. Clinical assessment for unipolar depression can be aided by the use of an instrument that quantifies severity of depressive symptoms, such as the Beck Depression Inventory (BDI; Beck, Ward, Mendelson, Mock, & Erbaugh, 1961). Repeated use of such measures will allow the clinician to track the severity of depression throughout treatment. Moreover, there is increased interest in subtyping those with BN based on the presence of even subdiagnostic levels of depression symptoms (Stice & Fairburn, 2003), and the BDI allows for this. Of note, ED treatment is often associated with improvement in mood symptoms, independent of using medications or psychotherapies that directly target depressed mood. Thus, monitoring mood is helpful for identifying those instances in which adding definitive treatment for mood disorder is necessary.

Anxiety disorders are similarly very common in people with BN; these too should be evaluated in everyone presenting for BN treatment. As with depression, treatments for BN can improve anxiety, and some BN treatments are treatments for anxiety in their own right, such as selective serotonin reuptake inhibitors (SSRIs). Conversely, improvements in eating behavior are sometimes associated with the short-term exacerbation of anxiety symptoms. Finally, comorbid substance abuse and dependence should be assessed at intake.

Medical Evaluation

Because medical complications are common in BN, a physical examination is often indicated. BN occurs most frequently at an age when contacts with the medical system are relatively uncommon, so such contact typically must be specifically recommended. Early in the course of treatment when symptom levels are high, medical monitoring is appropriate and useful. In many treatment settings individuals are referred to their regular medical provider when they first present for BN treatment.

One of the most common complications is electrolyte disturbance, particularly hypokalemia, which is a fairly specific but not particularly sensitive method for detecting the presence of purging (Crow, Salisbury, Crosby, & Mitchell, 1997). Electrolytes should be measured at intake and then intermittently when they are abnormal at intake, or when purging symptoms persist during treatment. Dental evaluation is often overlooked but can be quite helpful, because dental complications are common in BN. Also, clear identification of any existing dental complications can form an important part of the rationale for change for some patients. Finally, osteoporosis evaluation should be considered in those with a prior history of AN. There is evidence to suggest that a history of depression may also increase osteoporosis risk (Konstantynowicz et al., 2005).

Nutritional Assessment

The major measure used to inform nutritional assessment in most patients with BN is that of weight. This measure is vital for ascertaining a patient's overall level of physical and nutritional health, and it serves as critically important information for providing feedback that addresses eating disorder–related cognitions, in particular, as they may worsen with the resumption of standard patterned eating. Usually, an assessment of meal patterning is obtained through self-monitoring. For some individuals, this occurs as an independent aspect of treatment; for others, this may be an integral part of psychotherapy. In particular, empirically supported therapies for the treatment of BN, such as cognitive-behavioral therapy (CBT) (Fairburn, Marcus, & Wilson, 1993), target self-monitoring of both weight and meal pattern. For patients at relatively "normal" body weights, further nutritional assessment beyond that described above is typically not indicated.

Treatment Planning

Treatment should provide the patient with sufficient structure and support to resume normal meal patterning and cease binge eating and purging. Most often, these goals can be effectively accomplished in outpatient treatment. There is evidence to suggest that an early treatment focus on symptom interruption may provide a greater chance of eventual abstinence (Mitchell, et al., 1993). In turn, symptom interruption may be facilitated by a higher frequency of sessions early in treatment; in fact, many specialized outpatient treatments for BN now include a greater frequency of treatment visits (often twice per week) in the first several weeks.

For patients who require more intensive treatment, partial hospitalization or day programming may be a useful alternative. Most often such programs involve living at home and attending treatment several hours a day, several days per week. Many patients struggle most with urges to binge-eat and purge later in the day, so these programs often meet later in the day and provide structured meal interventions. Hospitalization is generally reserved as an option when less intensive treatments fail or when severe co-occurring psychopathology (particularly suicidality) is present.

One other possible indication for a more intensive treatment setting is the presence of co-occurring substance or alcohol use dependence (SAUD). When EDs and SAUD co-occur, it would seem ideal to provide an integrated treatment program that actively addresses both of these issues. Unfortunately, the question of how best to treat such co-occurring problems has received little research attention, and combined programs are rare. One recent controlled trial found that for alcohol-dependent women with concurrent ED, participation in treatment for alcoholism (behavioral coping skills therapy) was associated with reductions in both alcohol and ED problems, although the addition of the opiate antagonist naltrexone did not further substantially enhance outcomes (O'Malley et al., 2007). In the absence of such an integrated program, arguments can be made favoring the initial treatment of either the BN or the SAUD; practically speaking, sequencing of treatment is usually decided partly by the availability of each of these treatment resources, and also by the relative severity of the BN and the substance or alcohol use (and their attendant medical complications).

Treatment Choices

A substantial literature provides empirical support for several approaches to treating BN (National Institute for Health and Clinical Excellence [NICE], 2004; Wilson, Grilo, & Vitousek, 2007), including CBT, interpersonal therapy (IPT), and antidepressant pharmacotherapy. Among the best studied of these treatments is CBT, which received an "A" evidence grade in the NICE guidelines (2004). Currently, CBT is viewed as the treatment of choice for BN; it can be delivered using individual, group, and guided self-help approaches (Hay et al., 2008). However, delivery of CBT via group therapy methods is mostly confined to specialty ED settings, as most practitioners who do not specialize in ED treatment will not have a critical mass of patients at any given time to allow for group treatment. In studies with BN, CBT generally achieves abstinence in one-third to one-half of patients. There is also empirical support for IPT, another focal psychological treatment, which received a "B" grade in the NICE guidelines (2004). In two studies IPT resulted in lower abstinence rates than CBT at end of treatment, but did not differ from CBT at later follow-up (Agras, Walsh, Fairburn, Wilson, & Kraemer, 2000; Fairburn, Jones, Peveler, Hope, & O'Connor, 1993).

An extensive body of literature also has examined pharmacotherapy for BN, with antidepressants by far the most studied agents. Most antidepressants have been studied, and most trials have reported positive results relative to placebo. Overall, response rates to antidepressant medications are generally lower than those seen in psychotherapy trials (typically, end-of-treatment abstinence rates of 20–35%). The SSRI fluoxetine in high doses (i.e., 60 mg/day) is often described as the "gold standard" pharmacotherapy treatment, given significant findings reported in the largest trial to date (Fluoxetine Bulimia Nervosa Collaborative Study Group, 1992; Goldstein, Wilson, Thompson, Potvin, & Rampey, 1995), and it has received a Food and Drug Administration (FDA) indication for BN treatment in the United States. Less is known about the relative or combined effects of CBT and pharmacotherapy. Studies have found that CBT alone is superior to pharmacotherapy alone (Agras et al., 1992; Walsh et al, 1997). Combined treatments seem to be better than pharmacotherapy alone but not substantially better than CBT alone, although the combined approach may have an added benefit for associated problems such as depressed affect (Agras et al., 1992; Walsh et al., 1997).

A major practical challenge in the treatment of BN is the fact that most therapists have not received specific training in these therapies (Mussell et al., 2000), and it appears that these treatments are rarely used (Crow, Mussell, Peterson, Knopke, & Mitchell, 1999). This reality raises questions about the potential utility of more generalizable treatments such as medications, self-help approaches, and stepped-care approaches. Guided self-help CBT appears to be an option with some literature support (see Wilson, Grilo, & Vitousek, 2007, for a review), although effective implementation of self-help treatments in real-world controlled trials has been challenging (Walsh, Fairburn, Mickley, Sysko, & Parides, 2004). Alternatively, a treatment plan employing an increasingly intensive series of interventions could be considered. There is some evidence that simple sequential treatment approaches for nonresponders to a first full course of treatment may be associated with limited further response and low retention rates (Mitchell et al., 2002). This finding has spurred interest in stepped-care treatment approaches, which make more rapid transitions between treatments involving increasing intensity, specialization, and cost. For example, a stepped-care approach of guided self-help, followed by fluoxetine, followed by CBT may be more cost-effective and more therapeutically effective than starting with the most cost- and time-intensive treatments, such as CBT (Crow et al., 2008; Mitchell et al., 2008).

Treatment Team

Many treatment configurations are used in ED treatment. These span the spectrum from an individual physician prescribing antidepressant treatment as the sole treatment approach to a specialty center treatment team consisting of a psychotherapist, a psychiatrist for medication management, a dietician for nutritional assessment and recommendations, an occupational therapist for group cooking activities, and a primary care physician for medical monitoring. In practice, decisions as to the makeup of the treatment team are driven by several practical factors, including the local availability of clinicians. Due to the scarcity of specialized eating disorder services, many (perhaps most) patients live in areas where this full spectrum treatment team is unavailable. If somewhat less than that full spectrum is available, then the secondary question should be: What functions are most critically necessary? First, obtain initial medical assessment and ongoing monitoring of medical stability as needed. Second, obtain initial psychiatric/psychological assessment. Third, identify someone to provide initial specific treatment for BN (medication treatment or psychotherapy).

References

Agras WS, Crow S, Mitchell JE, Halmi KA, & Bryson S. (in press). A 4-year prospective study of Eating Disorder NOS compared with full eating disorder syndromes. *International Journal of Eating Disorders.*

Agras WS, Rossiter EM, Arnow B, Schneider JA, Telch CF, Raeburn SD, et al. (1992). Pharmacologic and cognitive-behavioral treatment for bulimia nervosa: A controlled comparison. *American Journal of Psychiatry,* 149:82–87.

Agras WS, Walsh T, Fairburn CG, Wilson GT, & Kraemer HC. (2000). A multicenter comparison of cognitive-behavioral therapy and interpersonal psychotherapy for bulimia nervosa. *Archives of General Psychiatry,* 57:459–466.

American Psychiatric Association. (2000). *Diagnostic and statistical manual of mental disorders* (4th ed., text rev.). Washington, DC: Author.

Andreason PJ, Altemus M, Zametkin AJ, King AC, Lucinio J, & Cohen RM. (1992). Regional cerebral glucose metabolism in bulimia nervosa. *American Journal of Psychiatry,* 149:1506–1513.

Anzengruber D, Klump KL, Thornton L, Brandt H, Crawford S, Fichter MM, et al. (2006). Smoking in eating disorders. *Eating Behaviors,* 7:291–299.

Bacanu SA, Bulik CM, Klump KL, Fichter MM, Halmi KA, Keel P, et al. (2005). Linkage analysis of anorexia and bulimia nervosa cohorts using selected behavioral phenotypes as quantitative traits or covariates. *American Journal of Medical Genetics, Part B, Neuropsychiatric Genetics,* 139:61–68.

Baldassano CF, Marangell LB, Gyulai L, Nassir Ghaemi S, Joffe H, Kim DR, et al. (2005). Gender differences in bipolar disorder: Retrospective data from the first 500 STEP-BD participants. *Bipolar Disorders,* 7:465–470.

Bearman SK, Martinez E, & Stice E. (2006). The skinny on body dissatisfaction: A longitudinal study of adolescent girls and boys. *Journal of Youth Adolescents,* 35:217–229.

Beck AT, Ward CH, Mendelson M, Mock J, & Erbaugh J. (1961). An inventory for measuring depression. *Archives of General Psychiatry,* 4:561–571.

Becker AE, Burwell RA, Navara K, & Gilman SE. (2003). Binge eating and binge eating disorder in a small-scale, indigenous society: The view from Fiji. *International Journal of Eating Disorders,* 34:423–431.

Brewerton TD, Lydiard RB, Laraia MT, Shook JE, & Ballenger JC. (1992). CSF beta-endorphin and dynorphin in bulimia nervosa. *American Journal of Psychiatry,* 149:1086–1090.

Bulik CM, Klump KL, Thornton L, Kaplan AS, Devlin B, Fichter MM, et al. (2004). Alcohol use disorder comorbidity in eating disorders: A multicenter study. *Journal of Clinical Psychiatry,* 65:1000–1006.

Crow SJ, Agras WS, Halmi KA, Fairburn, CG, Mitchell JE, & Nyman JA. (2008). *A cost effectiveness analysis of stepped care treatment for bulimia nervosa.* Manuscript submitted for publication.

Crow SJ, Mussell MP, Peterson C, Knopke A, & Mitchell J. (1999). Prior treatment received by patients with bulimia nervosa. *International Journal of Eating Disorders*, 25:39–44.

Crow SJ, Salisbury JJ, Crosby RD, & Mitchell JE. (1997). Serum electrolytes as markers of vomiting in bulimia nervosa. *International Journal of Eating Disorders*, 21:95–98.

Crowther JH, Armey M, Luce KH, Dalton GR, & Leahey T. (2008). The point prevalence of bulimic disorders from 1990 to 2004. *International Journal of Eating Disorders*, 41:491–497.

Culbert KM, Breedlove SM, Burt SA, & Klump KL. (2008). Prenatal hormone exposure and risk for eating disorders: A comparison of opposite-sex and same-sex twins. *Archives of General Psychiatry*, 65:329–336.

Fairburn CG, Cooper Z, Doll HA, & Davies BA. (2005). Identifying dieters who will develop an eating disorder: A prospective, population-based study. *American Journal of Psychiatry*, 162:2249–2255.

Fairburn CG, Cooper Z, Doll HA, Norman P, & O'Connor M. (2000). The natural course of bulimia nervosa and binge eating disorder in young women. *Archives of General Psychiatry*, 57:659–665.

Fairburn CG, Jones R, Peveler RC, Hope RA, & O'Connor M. (1993). Psychotherapy and bulimia nervosa: Longer-term effects of interpersonal psychotherapy, behavior therapy, and cognitive behavior therapy. *Archives of General Psychiatry*, 50:419–428.

Fairburn CG, Marcus MD, & Wilson GT. (1993). *Cognitive-behavioral therapy for binge eating and bulimia nervosa: A comprehensive treatment manual*. New York: Guilford Press.

Fairburn CG, Stice E, Cooper Z, Doll HA, Norman PA, & O'Connor ME. (2003). Understanding persistence in bulimia nervosa: A 5-year naturalistic study. *Journal of Consulting and Clinical Psychology*, 71:103–109.

Faris PL, Hofbauer RD, Daughters R, Vandenlangenberg E, Iversen L, Goodale RL, et al. (2008). De-stabilization of the positive vago–vagal reflex in bulimia nervosa. *Physiology and Behavior*, 94:136–153.

Fichter, M. M., Quadflieg, N., & Hedlund, S. (2008). Long-term course of binge eating disorder and bulimia nervosa: Relevance for nosology and diagnostic criteria. *International Journal of Eating Disorders, 41*, 577–586.

Fluoxetine Bulimia Nervosa Collaborative Study Group. (1992). Fluoxetine in the treatment of bulimia nervosa: A multicenter double-blind trial. *Archives of General Psychiatry*, 49:139–147.

Frank GK, Kaye WH, Greer P, Meltzer CC, & Price JC. (2000). Regional cerebral blood flow after recovery from bulimia nervosa. *Psychiatry Research*, 100:31–39.

Frank GK, Wagner A, Achenbach S, McConaha C, Skovira K, Aizenstein H, et al. (2006). Altered brain activity in women recovered from bulimic-type eating disorders after a glucose challenge: A pilot study. *International Journal of Eating Disorders*, 39:76–79.

Goldstein DJ, Wilson MG, Thompson VL, Potvin JH, & Rampey AH, Jr. (1995). Long-term fluoxetine treatment of bulimia nervosa: Fluoxetine Bulimia Nervosa Research Group. *British Journal of Psychiatry*, 166:660–666.

Grilo CM. (2002). Recent research of relationships among eating disorders and personality disorders. *Current Psychiatry Reports*, 4:18–24.

Grilo CM, Pagano ME, Skodol AE, Sanislow CA, McGlashan TH, Gunderson JG, et al. (2007). Natural course of bulimia nervosa and of eating disorder not otherwise specified: 5-year prospective study of remissions, relapses, and the effects of personality disorder psychopathology. *American Journal of Clinical Psychiatry*, 68:738–746.

Hay PPJ, Bacaltchuk J, Byrnes RT, Claudino AM, Ekmejian AA, & Yong PY. (2008). Individual psychotherapy in the outpatient treatment of adults with anorexia nervosa. *Cochrane Database Systematic Review*, Issue 1 (Article No. CD003909), DOI: 10.1002/14651858.CD003909.

Heatherton TF, Nichols P, Mahamedi F, & Keel P. (1995). Body weight, dieting, and eating disorder symptoms among college students, 1982 to 1992. *American Journal of Psychiatry*, 152:1623–1629.

Herzog DB, Dorer DJ, Keel PK, Selwyn SE, Ekeblad ER, Flores AT, et al. (1999). Recovery and relapse in anorexia and bulimia nervosa: A 7.5-year follow-up study. *Journal of the American Academy of Child and Adolescent Psychiatry*, 38:829–837.

Herzog DB, Keller MB, Sacks NR, Yeh CJ, & Lavori PW. (1992). Psychiatric comorbidity in treatment-seeking anorexics and bulimics. *Journal of the American Academy of Child and Adolescent Psychiatry*, 31:810–818.

Holderness CC, Brooks-Gunn J, & Warren MP. (1994). Co-morbidity of eating disorders and substance abuse review of the literature. *International Journal of Eating Disorders*, 16:1–34.

Hudson JI, Hiripi E, Pope HG, Jr, & Kessler RC. (2007). The prevalence and correlates of eating disorders in the National Comorbidity Survey Replication. *Biological Psychiatry*, 61:348–358.

Hudson JI, Pope HG, Jr, Jonas JM, & Yurgelun-Todd D. (1983). Phenomenologic relationship of eating disorders to major affective disorder. *Psychiatry Research*, 9:345–354.

Hudson JI, Pope HG, Jr, Yurgelun-Todd D, Jonas JM, & Frankenburg FR. (1987). A controlled study of lifetime prevalence of affective and other psychiatric disorders in bulimic outpatients. *American Journal of Psychiatry*, 144:1283–1287.

Jimerson DC, Lesem MD, Kaye WH, & Brewerton TD. (1992). Low serotonin and dopamine metabolite concentrations in cerebrospinal fluid from bulimic patients with frequent binge episodes. *Archives of General Psychiatry*, 49:132–138.

Jimerson DC, Wolfe BE, Metzger ED, Finkelstein DM, Cooper TB, & Levine JM. (1997). Decreased serotonin function in bulimia nervosa. *Archives of General Psychiatry*, 54:529–534.

Johnson C, Tobin DL, & Lipkin J. (1989). Epidemiologic changes in bulimic behavior among female adolescents over a five-year period. *International Journal of Eating Disorders*, 8:647–655.

Kassett JA, Gershon ES, Maxwell ME, Guroff JJ, Kazuba DM, Smith AL, et al. (1989). Psychiatric disorders in the first-degree relatives of probands with bulimia nervosa. *American Journal of Psychiatry*, 146:1468–1471.

Kaye WH. (2008). Neurobiology of anorexia and bulimia nervosa. *Physiology and Behavior*, 94:121–135.

Kaye WH, Bulik CM, Thornton L, Barbarich N, & Masters K. (2004). Comorbidity of anxiety disorders with anorexia and bulimia nervosa. *American Journal of Psychiatry*, 161:2215–2221.

Kaye WH, Devlin B, Barbarich N, Bulik CM, Thornton L, Bacanu SA, et al. (2004). Genetic analysis of bulimia nervosa: Methods and sample description. *International Journal of Eating Disorders*, 35:556–570.

Kaye WH, Frank GK, Meltzer CC, Price JC, McConaha CW, Crossan PJ, et al. (2001). Altered serotonin 2A receptor activity in women who have recovered from bulimia nervosa. *American Journal of Psychiatry*, 158:1152–1155.

Kaye WH, Greeno CG, Moss H, Fernstrom J, Fernstrom M, Lilenfeld LR, et al. (1998). Alterations in serotonin activity and psychiatric symptoms after recovery from bulimia nervosa. *Archives of General Psychiatry*, 55:927–935.

Keel PK, Heatherton TF, Dorer DJ, Joiner TE, & Zalta AK. (2006). Point prevalence of bulimia nervosa in 1982, 1992, and 2002. *Psychological Medicine*, 36:19–127.

Keel PK, & Klump KL. (2003). Are eating disorders culture-bound syndromes? Implications for conceptualizing their etiology. *Psychological Bulletin*, 129:747–769.

Keel PK, & Mitchell JE. (1997). Outcome in bulimia nervosa. *American Journal of Psychiatry*, 154:313–321.

Keel PK, Mitchell JE, Miller KB, Davis TL, & Crow SJ. (1999). Long-term outcome of bulimia nervosa. *Archives of General Psychiatry*, 56:63–69.

Kendler KS, MacLean C, Neale M, Kessler R, Heath A, & Eaves L. (1991). The genetic epidemiology of bulimia nervosa. *American Journal of Psychiatry*, 148:1627–1637.

Klump KL, Burt SA, McGue M, & Iacono WG. (2007). Changes in genetic and environmental influences on disordered eating across adolescence: A longitudinal twin study. *Archives of General Psychiatry*, 64:1409–1415.

Klump KL, Keel PK, Culbert KM, & Edler C. (2008). Ovarian hormones and binge eating: Exploring associations in community samples. *Psychological Medicine*, 38:1749–1757.

Konstantynowicz J, Kadziela-Olech H, Kaczmarski M, Zebaze RM, Iuliano-Burns S, Piotrowska-Jastrzebska J, et al. (2005). Depression in anorexia nervosa: A risk factor for osteoporosis. *Journal of Clinical Endocrinology and Metabolism*, 90:5382–5385.

McKnight Investigators. (2003). Risk factors for the onset of eating disorders in adolescent girls: Results of the McKnight longitudinal risk factor study. *American Journal of Psychiatry*, 160:248–254.

Mitchell JE, Agras S, Crow S, Halmi K, Fairburn CG, Bryson S, et al. (2008). *A multi-center randomized trial comparing the efficacy of cognitive behavioral therapy for bulimia nervosa to a stepped-care approach.* Manuscript submitted for publication.

Mitchell JE, Halmi K, Wilson GT, Agras WS, Kraemer H, & Crow S. (2002). A randomized secondary treatment study of women with bulimia nervosa who fail to respond to CBT. *International Journal of Eating Disorders*, 32:271–281.

Mitchell JE, Pyle RL, Pomeroy C, Zollman M, Crosby R, Seim H, et al. (1993). Cognitive-behavioral group psychotherapy of bulimia nervosa: Importance of logistical variables. *International Journal of Eating Disorders*, 14:277–287.

Mussell MP, Crosby RD, Crow SJ, Knopke AJ, Peterson CB, Wonderlich SA, et al. (2000). Utilization of empirically supported psychotherapy treatments for individuals with eating disorders: A survey of psychologists. *International Journal of Eating Disorders*, 27:230–237.

National Institute for Health and Clinical Excellence. (2004). *Eating disorders: Core interventions in the treatment and management of anorexia nervosa, bulimia nervosa and related eating disorders.* London: Author.

Neumark-Sztainer DR, Wall MM, Haines JI, Story MT, Sherwood NE, & van den Berg PA. (2007). Shared risk and protective factors for overweight and disordered eating in adolescents. *American Journal of Preventive Medicine*, 33:359–369.

O'Malley SS, Sinha R, Grilo CM, Capone C, Farren CK, McKee SA, et al. (2007). Naltrexone and cognitive behavioral coping skills therapy for the treatment of alcohol drinking and eating disorder features in alcohol-dependent women: A randomized controlled trial. *Alcoholism: Clinical Experimental Research*, 31:625–634.

Ramacciotti CE, Paoli RA, Marcacci G, Piccinni A, Burgalassi A, Dell'Osso L, et al. (2005). Relationship between bipolar illness and binge-eating disorders. *Psychiatry Research*, 135:165–170.

Rubinstein S, & Caballero B. (2000). Is Miss America an undernourished role model? *Journal of the American Medical Association*, 283:1569.

Russell G. (1979). Bulimia nervosa: An ominous variant of anorexia nervosa. *Psychological Medicine*, 9:429–448.

Schienle A, Schafer A, Hermann A, & Vaitl D. (2008). Binge-eating disorder: Reward sensitivity and brain activation to images of food. *Biological Psychiatry*, 65(8):654–661.

Steiger H, Richardson J, Israel M, Ng Ying Kin NM, Bruce K, Mansour S, et al. (2005). Reduced density of platelet-binding sites for [3H]paroxetine in remitted bulimic women. *Neuropsychopharmacology*, 30:1028–1032.

Stice E, & Fairburn CG. (2003). Dietary and dietary-depressive subtypes of bulimia nervosa show differential symptom presentation, social impairment, comorbidity, and course of illness. *Journal of Consulting and Clinical Psychology*, 71:1090–1094.

Strober M, Freeman R, Lampert C, Diamond J, & Kaye W. (2000). Controlled family study of anorexia nervosa and bulimia nervosa: Evidence of shared liability and transmission of partial syndromes. *American Journal of Psychiatry*, 157:393–401.

Sullivan PF, Bulik CM, & Kendler KS. (1998). Genetic epidemiology of bingeing and vomiting. *British Journal of Psychiatry*, 173:75–79.

Swinbourne JM, & Touyz SW. (2007). The co-morbidity of eating disorders and anxiety disorders: A review. *European Eating Disorders Review*, 15:253–274.

Tauscher J, Pirker W, Willeit M, de Zwaan M, Bailer U, Neumeister A, et al. (2001). [123I] Beta-CIT and single photon emission computed tomography reveal reduced brain serotonin transporter availability in bulimia nervosa. *Biological Psychiatry*, 49:326–332.

Uher R, Murphy T, Brammer MJ, Dalgleish T, Phillips ML, Ng VW, et al. (2004). Medial prefrontal cortex activity associated with symptom provocation in eating disorders. *American Journal of Psychiatry*, 161:1238–1246.

Uher R, Murphy T, Friederich HC, Dalgleish T, Brammer MJ, Giampietro V, et al. (2005). Functional neuroanatomy of body shape perception in healthy and eating-disordered women. *Biological Psychiatry*, 58:990–997.

van Son GE, van Hoeken D, Bartelds AI, van Furth EF, & Hoek HW. (2006). Time trends in the incidence of eating disorders: A primary care study in the Netherlands. *International Journal of Eating Disorders*, 39:565–569.

von Ranson KM, Kaye WH, Weltzin TE, Rao R, & Matsunaga H. (1999). Obsessive–compulsive disorder symptoms before and after recovery from bulimia nervosa. *American Journal of Psychiatry*, 156:1703–1708.

Wade TD, Bulik CM, Prescott CA, & Kendler KS. (2004). Sex influences on shared risk factors for bulimia nervosa and other psychiatric disorders. *Archives of General Psychiatry*, 61:251–256.

Wade TD, Treloar S, & Martin NG. (2008). Shared and unique risk factors between lifetime purging and objective binge eating: A twin study. *Psychological Medicine*, 38:1455–1464.

Walsh BT, Fairburn CG, Mickley D, Sysko R, & Parides MK. (2004). Treatment of bulimia nervosa in a primary care setting. *American Journal of Psychiatry*, 161:556–561.

Walsh BT, Wilson GT, Loeb KL, Devlin MJ, Pike KM, Roose SP, et al. (1997). Medication and psychotherapy in the treatment of bulimia nervosa. *American Journal of Psychiatry*, 154:523–531.

Welch SL, & Fairburn CG. (1998). Smoking and bulimia nervosa. *International Journal of Eating Disorders*, 23:433–437.

Wilson GT, Grilo CM, & Vitousek KM. (2007). Psychological treatment of eating disorders. *American Psychologist*, 62:199–216.

World Health Organization. (1992). *The ICD-10 classification of mental and behavioural disorders.* Geneva: Author.

Zachrisson HD, Vedul-Kjelsas E, Gotestam KG, & Mykletun A. (2008). Time trends in obesity and eating disorders. *International Journal of Eating Disorders*, 41:673–680.

CHAPTER 3

Diagnosis, Assessment, and Treatment Planning for Binge-Eating Disorder and Eating Disorder Not Otherwise Specified

Jennifer E. Wildes and Marsha D. Marcus

According to the fourth edition of the *Diagnostic and Statistical Manual of Mental Disorders* (DSM-IV; American Psychiatric Association, 1994), individuals presenting with "disorders of eating that do not meet the criteria for any specific eating disorder" (p. 550), that is, individuals with clinically significant eating disorder psychopathology that does not meet DSM-IV criteria for anorexia nervosa (AN) or bulimia nervosa (BN), are classified as having an eating disorder not otherwise specified (EDNOS). Because EDNOS is, by definition, a residual diagnostic category, there are numerous presentations, and little is known about specific variants, with a few notable exceptions. Chief among these is binge-eating disorder (BED), for which research criteria are included in an appendix to the DSM-IV. Investigators also have proposed diagnostic criteria for two additional forms of EDNOS: purging disorder (PD) (Keel, 2007) and night-eating syndrome (Stunkard, Allison, & Lundgren, 2008). Although the limitations of categorical approaches to conceptualizing psychiatric diagnosis have been discussed widely (see, e.g., Widiger & Samuel, 2005), one advantage of defining specific EDNOS syndromes has been to promote research that may inform approaches to the evaluation and treatment of these conditions. Thus, in this chapter, we focus primarily on issues pertaining to the diagnosis, assessment, and treatment of BED, as this is by far the best-studied EDNOS variant. Second, we address forms of EDNOS that are more closely related to AN and BN, including PD. Because night-eating syndrome is covered in another chapter in this volume (see Allison & Stunkard, Chapter 27, this volume), we do not discuss it further here.

Binge-Eating Disorder

Diagnostic Considerations

Diagnostic Criteria

Binge-eating disorder (BED) is characterized by recurrent episodes of binge eating (i.e., the ingestion of a large amount of food accompanied by a sense of loss of control over when, what, or the amount that one is eating) that occur in the absence of the regular compensatory behaviors (e.g., purging, fasting, excessive exercise) seen in BN and the binge-eating/purging subtype of AN. DSM-IV criteria for BED require that binge-eating episodes be associated with "marked distress" and three or more of the following features: (1) eating much more rapidly than normal; (2) eating until uncomfortably full; (3) eating in the absence of hunger; (4) eating alone because of embarrassment over the amount eaten; and (5) feelings of disgust, depression, or guilt after overeating. Finally, the DSM-IV stipulates that for individuals with BED, binge eating occurs at least 2 days per week, on average, for a 6-month period. However, research findings are mixed with respect to the clinical validity of the 2-day-per-week frequency criterion (Latner & Clyne, 2008), and there is no empirical basis for the 6-month duration requirement.

Epidemiology

Recent studies indicate that BED is at least as common as AN and BN in the general population (Hudson, Hiripi, Pope, & Kessler, 2007; Striegel-Moore et al., 2003; Wade, Bergin, Tiggemann, Bulik, & Fairburn, 2006). For example, using data from the National Comorbidity Survey Replication, Hudson and colleagues (2007) reported lifetime prevalence estimates for BED of 3.5% in women and 2.0% in men; these rates were nearly twice as high as those reported for AN and BN combined. Prevalence estimates for BED are even higher among obese individuals, ranging from 4 to 8% in community samples, and up to 30% among patients seeking bariatric surgery or other weight loss interventions (Kalarchian et al., 2007; Marcus & Levine, 2004).

Demographic Correlates

Although eating disorders (EDs) often are thought of as "culture-bound syndromes" that affect young, white females primarily (Keel & Klump, 2003), epidemiological data suggest that BED may occur more widely in the general population. For example, studies using structured diagnostic interviews to evaluate rates of binge eating in black women have documented lifetime prevalence estimates for BED that are similar to those of white women (Taylor, Caldwell, Baser, Faison, & Jackson, 2007), although one report indicates that rates of BED still are higher in whites compared to blacks (Striegel-Moore et al., 2003). Sex differences in rates of BED also are less pronounced than those for AN and BN. Indeed, epidemiological data indicate that although full-syndrome BED is approximately 1.75 times more common in women than in men, the prevalence of recurrent binge eating is at least as high among males as compared to females (Hudson et al., 2007). This discrepancy may be due, in part, to the fact that men are less likely than women to endorse distress related to binge-eating episodes (Hudson et al., 2007), and thus fail to meet the threshold for BED diagnosis. Finally, it appears that threshold and subthreshold forms of BED may be more common in adults as compared to children and adolescents (Favaro, Ferrara, & Santonastaso, 2003). However, this discrepancy may be due, in part, to the current definition of binge eating, which requires the intake of an objectively large amount of food. Indeed, research has indicated that loss of control is more salient to disordered eating in children than is the amount of food eaten (Tanofsky-Kraff et al., 2007). Similarly, among adolescents, loss of control over eating is associated with heightened ED psychopathology and depression independent of overeating (Goldschmidt et al., 2008).

Other Associated Features and Comorbidity

The clinical correlates of BED are well documented and include high rates of medical and psychiatric comorbidity, elevated distress related to weight, shape, and eating, and diminished quality of life relative to comparison groups. Individuals with BED are significantly more likely than controls to be obese (Hudson et al., 2007) and to have chronic medical problems such as irritable bowel syndrome, fibromyalgia, and insomnia (Javaras, Pope, et al., 2008). Patients with BED also have higher rates of most major psychiatric disorders, including major depressive disorder, bipolar disorder, anxiety disorders, BN, substance use, and personality disorders, compared to individuals without clinically significant binge eating (Cassin & von Ranson, 2005; Hudson et al., 2007; Javaras, Pope, et al., 2008). Studies focusing on the cognitive correlates of disordered eating have documented that concerns about weight, shape, and eating are elevated in individuals with BED relative to obese and nonobese controls, including other disordered-eating groups (Allison, Grilo, Masheb, & Stunkard, 2005; Pike, Dohm, Striegel-Moore, Wilfley, & Fairburn, 2001). Furthermore, overvaluation of shape and weight, a diagnostic requirement for BN but not a diagnostic criterion for BED, is a commonly occurring cognitive feature in BED that has been found to be associated with greater levels of ED psychopathology, higher depression, and lower self-esteem (Grilo et al., 2008; Hrabosky, Masheb, White, & Grilo, 2007). Finally, there is evidence that obese individuals with BED have significantly greater impairment in psychosocial aspects of quality of life (e.g., work, sexual life, self-esteem) relative to obese individuals without binge-eating problems (Hudson et al., 2007; Rieger, Wilfley, Stein, Marino, & Crow, 2005).

Etiology

Although the exact causes remain unknown, BED almost certainly arises from a complex cascade of genetic, biological, and environmental factors. Studies using twin data and advanced statistical techniques have indicated that the heritability of BED lies somewhere between 30 and 80%, most likely in the middle of this range (Javaras, Laird, et al., 2008). Moreover, family interview data have shown that BED aggregates in families independently of obesity (Hudson et al., 2006).

With respect to biological mechanisms, there is evidence that individuals with binge-eating problems have functional alterations in several central and peripheral systems that are associated with the regulation of appetite and eating behavior (for a review, see Steiger & Bruce, 2007). However, the role of these biological correlates in the pathogenesis of BED has not been well established. For example, although decreased serotonin availability has been implicated in animal models of binge eating (Blundell, 1986), as well as in studies focusing on the pathophysiology of BN (Steiger & Bruce, 2007), one report examining prolactin response to *d*-fenfluramine in individuals with BED found no evidence that the hypothalamic serotonin system is altered in this group (Monteleone, Brambilla, Bortolotti, & Maj, 2000). Similarly, research has failed to document an association between level of brain-derived neurotrophic factor (BDNF) and BED, although BDNF has been shown to modulate eating behavior both in animals and in humans, and decreased levels of BDNF have been found in other disordered-eating groups (e.g., underweight individuals with AN, individuals with BN) (Monteleone et al., 2005). Finally, studies examining the role of appetite-regulating hormones (e.g., cholecystokinin [CCK], leptin, ghrelin) in BED have produced mixed results. Although alterations in CCK and leptin generally have not been observed in individuals with BED (for review, see Steiger & Bruce, 2007), there is some evidence that levels of fasting ghrelin may be diminished in this group (Geliebter, Gluck, & Hashim, 2005; Geliebter, Yahav, Gluck, & Hashim, 2004). However, studies examining ghrelin gene polymorphisms in relation to BN and BED have produced equivocal findings (Monteleone, Tortorella, Castaldo, Di Filippo, & Maj, 2006, 2007), leading some investigators to conclude that ghrelin alterations in patients with BED are a consequence rather than a cause of binge eating (Steiger & Bruce, 2007).

Finally, studies using case-control methodology have identified several potential genetic and environmental risk factors for BED. Examples include childhood obesity, family overeating, low parental contact and high parental demands, and negative comments about weight, shape, and eating (Fairburn et al., 1998; Striegel-Moore et al., 2005). One study using signal detection analysis to identify potential risk factors for BED and BN reported that an elevated level of perceived stress prior to age 14 preceded the onset of binge eating in a significant minority of individuals (Striegel-Moore et al., 2007). Finally, some research has indicated that rates of childhood physical and sexual abuse and bullying by peers are higher in women with BED compared to healthy control women; however, with the exception of sexual abuse in black women, these factors generally do not distinguish women with BED from psychiatric comparison women, suggesting that they are associated with an increased risk for psychiatric disorders, in general, rather than binge eating more specifically (Striegel-Moore, Dohm, Pike, Wilfley, & Fairburn, 2002).

Course of Illness

With notable exceptions (i.e., Cachelin et al., 1999; Fairburn, Cooper, Doll, Norman, & O'Connor, 2000), research evidence indicates that BED is a chronic condition associated with morbidity, mortality, and duration of illness comparable to BN. For example, using data from the National Comorbidity Survey Replication, Hudson and colleagues (2007) reported a mean lifetime duration of illness for BED that was roughly equivalent to BN (i.e., 8.1 vs. 8.3 years) and significantly longer than AN (1.7 years). Similarly, Pope and colleagues (2006) found that individuals with BED reported a significantly longer mean duration of illness (i.e., 14.4 years) than did individuals with AN (5.7 years) or BN (5.8 years) in a community sample of 888 relatives of overweight and obese probands.

Finally, Fichter, Quadflieg, and Hedlund (2008) followed a clinical sample for 12 years after discharge from an inpatient ED program and found no differences between individuals initially diagnosed with BED and individuals initially diagnosed with BN on rates of current ED diagnoses (36% of patients with BED and 28% of patients with BN met criteria for an ED at follow-up), rates of current and lifetime mood and anxiety disorder diagnoses, and number of inpatient treatment days during the follow-up period. The standardized mortality ratios for BED and BN were low (i.e., 2.29 and 2.36, respectively) and did not differ significantly (Fichter et al., 2008). Taken together, these findings highlight the clinical significance of BED as a chronic syndrome, requiring a similar degree of long-term care and follow-up to other EDs.

Assessment

Psychological Evaluation and Data Gathering

BED is a complicated syndrome with behavioral (i.e., binge eating) and psychological (e.g., depression, guilt) components, and a comprehensive assessment may require multimodal methods (Grilo, Masheb, & Wilson, 2001). An interview format generally is the preferred method of diagnostic evaluation. Although self-report questionnaires can be used to screen for BED symptoms, these instruments are not appropriate for assigning diagnoses due to limited specificity—that is, high rates of false-positive diagnoses in persons who do not actually meet criteria for BED (Celio, Wilfley, Crow, Mitchell, & Walsh, 2004). Similarly, although self-report measures can be used to screen for associated psychological problems that may influence treatment formulation and planning, such as mood, anxiety, and substance use disorder comorbidities, interviews are required to arrive at firmer diagnostic impressions. Finally, it is important to keep in mind that although self-report measures can provide useful information about ED psychopathology, their results sometimes differ from those generated by interview-based assessments (Grilo et al., 2001).

In research settings BED often is assessed using standardized interview schedules such as the Structured Diagnostic Interview for DSM-IV Axis I Disorders (SCID-I) (First, Spitzer, Gibbon, & Williams, 1995) or the Eating Disorder Examination (EDE) (Fairburn & Cooper, 1993). However, these instruments require extensive training and considerable time to administer and thus are impractical in many clinical settings. Nevertheless, a careful psychiatric evaluation is important for all individuals seeking treatment for BED. Because binge eating is the cardinal feature of BED, particular attention should be given to the assessment of this behavior. It may be helpful to ask patients to recall details of specific overeating and loss-of-control eating episodes, or to request a description of a "typical binge." Self-monitoring methods, in which patients record information about overeating or loss-of-control eating prospectively for a specified of period time (e.g., the week prior to the interview), also can provide detailed assessment information without introducing the bias of retrospective self-report; however, self-monitoring has been shown to affect eating behavior and frequently is employed in clinical treatment.

It is important to recognize that unlike BN, the BED diagnosis is based on the number of binge-eating "days" rather than "episodes." However, recent data suggest that individuals with BED are able to delineate binges into discrete episodes (e.g., Grilo &

Masheb, 2005; Hilbert et al., 2007), and assessment of binge eating–episode frequency may provide useful clinical information. Finally, many observers have concluded that loss of control over eating, rather than the amount of food ingested, is the hallmark of binge eating (e.g., Latner, Hildebrandt, Rosewall, Chisholm, & Hayashi, 2007); thus, the patient's subjective experience of loss of control is of particular salience.

Medical Evaluation

There is no standard indication for the medical evaluation of individuals with BED independent of the assessment of obesity-related comorbidities. However, because many patients with BED are overweight or obese, medical evaluation may be necessary to ensure that comorbid conditions are managed appropriately. Obesity is associated with numerous medical problems including cardiovascular disease, diabetes, hypertension, kidney disease, obstructive sleep apnea, and several forms of cancer (i.e., colon, breast, esophageal, uterine, ovarian, kidney, and pancreatic) (Eckel, 2008). Thus, it is important that clinicians involved in the evaluation and treatment of obese patients with BED attend to the possibility that these individuals may require referral for assessment and management of coexisting medical problems.

Nutrition Assessment

Nutrition rehabilitation generally is not a major focus of BED treatment. Individuals with BED typically do not engage in severe dietary restriction, and thus the prescription of a healthy diet is of less concern than it might be in other disordered-eating groups (e.g., underweight patients with AN). Nevertheless, because overeating and overweight are common in patients with BED (Allison et al., 2005; Hudson et al., 2007), a nutrition evaluation that focuses on the tailoring of a balanced eating plan that reflects individual preferences may have considerable utility for this group.

Treatment Planning

Treatment Setting

Treatment for BED typically occurs in an outpatient setting. Inpatient or partial hospitalization programs rarely are warranted unless there are significant psychiatric or medical comorbidities that require more intensive intervention. For patients with relatively uncomplicated presentations and no history of prior treatment, it may be appropriate to suggest a stepped-care approach in which a course of self-help is undertaken prior to initiating more intensive intervention. Several studies have documented the benefits of therapist-guided self-help programs relative to waiting-list controls in the treatment of BN and BED (for a review, see Sysko & Walsh, 2008). Moreover, results from a recent study indicate that self-help guided by brief (i.e., six 15- to 20-minute sessions conducted individually over a 12-week period) cognitive-behavioral therapy (CBT) is superior to self-help guided by behavioral weight control in the management of BED (Grilo & Masheb, 2005). Recent work also has documented the promise of computerized technologies (e.g., CD-ROM and Internet-based interventions) as a means of disseminating therapist-guided self-help for BED (Ljotsson et al., 2007; Shapiro, Reba-Harrelson, et al., 2007).

Treatment Options

Several forms of treatment, including individual and group psychotherapy, behavioral weight control, and pharmacotherapy, have demonstrated efficacy in the management of BED. Because empirical support for these interventions has been derived primarily from clinical trials conducted in specialized research centers, their effectiveness in "real-world" settings remains unknown (Wilson, Grilo, & Vitousek, 2007). Nevertheless, evidence-based treatments represent the best first-line approaches to managing BED.

With respect to psychotherapeutic interventions, CBT, conducted individually or in a group format, has the strongest empirical support in the treatment of BED. Indeed, guidelines published by the National Institute for Health and Clinical Excellence (NICE; 2004) in the United Kingdom state that CBT is the treatment of choice for this disorder. Controlled trials have shown that CBT is effective in reducing the frequency of binge days and episodes and also leads to improvements in associated behavioral and cognitive features of disordered eating (e.g., hunger, restraint, disinhibition; for a review, see Brownley, Berkman, Sedway, Lohr, & Bulik, 2007). Moreover, research has documented that these improvements are well maintained over 12-month follow-up (Wilson et al., 2007). Nevertheless, one limitation of CBT as a treatment for BED is that it generally does not produce significant weight loss, despite high rates of abstinence from binge eating at treatment completion. In addition, the superiority of CBT for BED relative to other active interventions remains uncertain. As detailed below, although some research has shown that CBT is more effective than fluoxetine in the treatment of individuals with BED (Grilo, Masheb, & Wilson, 2005; Ricca et al., 2001), there is no evidence that CBT performs better than interpersonal psychotherapy (IPT) in the management of these patients.

Other specialized psychotherapies that have shown promise in the treatment of BED include IPT and dialectical behavior therapy (DBT). As noted above, IPT produces improvements in binge eating, the cognitive correlates of disordered eating, self-esteem, depressive symptoms, and interpersonal functioning that are comparable to CBT (Wilfley et al., 1993, 2002). Likewise, a study comparing group DBT skills training to a wait-list control found that DBT was associated with high rates of abstinence from binge eating at treatment completion that were well-maintained over a 6-month follow-up (Telch, Agras, & Linehan, 2001). However, despite its emphasis on emotion regulation, DBT did not demonstrate superiority relative to the wait-list control in reducing negative affect or enhancing adaptive affect regulation skills—which raises some question about the mechanisms by which this intervention effects change in BED symptoms.

Because most individuals seeking treatment for BED are overweight or obese, there has been considerable interest in the role of behavioral weight control in the management of this illness. Weight management interventions focusing both on moderate calorie restriction and very-low-calorie diets (i.e., approximately 800 kilocalories [kcal] per day) have been utilized in the treatment of obese patients with BED. These interventions differ from psychotherapeutic approaches in that the focus is on weight loss rather than amelioration of binge eating. Although caloric restriction and weight loss do not appear to exacerbate binge eating in patients with BED (for a review, see Marcus & Levine, 2004), support for the efficacy of behavioral weight control in this group has been equivocal.

Several studies have documented that participation in a behavioral weight control program is associated with improvements in binge eating and mood among obese patients with BED. For example, de Zwaan and colleagues (2005) randomized 71 obese women with BED to a very-low-calorie diet program with or without the addition of group CBT for binge eating. They found no differences between the two conditions with respect to weight loss or abstinence from binge eating. Participants in both groups lost a significant amount of weight (i.e., 35.2 pounds, on average), and 66% were free of binge eating at treatment completion (de Zwaan et al., 2005). These findings are consistent with work from our research group, which found no benefit for CBT over behavioral weight loss in ameliorating binge eating and associated ED psychopathology among obese patients with BED (Marcus & Levine, 2004). Moreover, results from our study indicated that behavioral weight control using a moderate-calorie diet (i.e., 1,200–1,500 kcal/day) was associated with significantly more weight loss at posttreatment compared to CBT in obese individuals with BED. Taken together, these findings suggest that behavioral weight control interventions may be the optimal approach for treating individuals with comorbid obesity and BED.

However, some investigators have raised questions about the utility of behavioral weight control for obese patients with BED. Of particular concern are high rates of weight regain posttreatment in most studies (for a review, see Wilson et al., 2007), as well as research indicating that behavioral weight loss interventions may not be as effective as CBT and IPT in reducing binge eating among patients with BED (Grilo & Masheb, 2005; Wilfley, Wilson, & Agras, 2008). For example, a recently completed multisite randomized controlled trial comparing IPT, behavioral weight loss, and guided self-help CBT for BED found that rates of remission from binge eating at 2 years posttreatment were significantly lower among patients who received the behavioral weight loss intervention compared to those who received IPT or guided self-help CBT (Wilfley, Wilson, et al., 2008). Moreover, results of this study suggested that behavioral weight control was particularly ineffective for patients with BED who had more severe ED and general psychopathology (Wilfley, Wilson, et al., 2008).

Finally, several classes of medication, including antidepressants, anticonvulsants, and antiobesity agents, have demonstrated efficacy relative to placebo in reducing the frequency of binge-eating episodes and promoting weight loss in patients with BED (for a review, see Brownley et al., 2007; Reas & Grilo, 2008). Because pharmacological interventions require considerably less investment of time by patient and clinician than do psychotherapeutic approaches or behavioral weight loss programs, medication may be an attractive first-line treatment for BED in many clinical settings. However, it is important to consider that most controlled trials of pharmacological treatments for BED have been of short duration (i.e., 6–14 weeks), and the long-term benefits of these approaches following medication discontinuation are unknown, as no controlled pharmacotherapy-only trials have reported follow-up data (Reas & Grilo, 2008). Although two recent studies have documented the efficacy of an anticonvulsant (i.e., topiramate) and an antiobesity agent (i.e., sibutramine) relative to placebo in ameliorating BED symptoms and reducing body weight over longer periods of active treatment (i.e., 21 and 24 weeks, respectively), neither report included posttreatment follow-up data (Claudino et al., 2007; Wilfley, Crow, et al., 2008).

One approach that often is suggested for the management of patients with BED is the combination of psychotherapeutic and pharmacological interventions. This strategy may be particularly useful for treating obese patients with BED, given that psychotherapies for BED generally have a limited impact on body weight (Wilson et al., 2007).

However, the few studies that have examined the effects of adding pharmacological treatments to psychotherapeutic and behavioral approaches have produced equivocal findings (Reas & Grilo, 2008). For example, although early reports indicated that adding antidepressant medication (i.e., fluoxetine, desipramine, imipramine) to CBT or behavioral weight control interventions was associated with a greater short-term reduction in the frequency of binge eating (imipramine only) and improved weight loss in overweight individuals with binge eating (Agras et al., 1994; Laederach-Hofmann et al., 1999; Marcus et al., 1990), two recent double-blind randomized controlled trials found no benefit of augmenting CBT (Grilo, Masheb, & Wilson, 2005) or behavioral weight control (Devlin et al., 2005) with fluoxetine for either weight loss or remission of binge eating in patients with BED. Findings for anticonvulsant and antiobesity agents are somewhat more promising. For example, one recent study found that augmenting group CBT for BED with the anticonvulsant medication topiramate produced significantly greater reductions in body weight and higher rates of remission from binge eating over a 21-week course of treatment, relative to CBT with placebo (Claudino et al., 2007). Similarly, another report showed that adding the antiobesity agent orlistat to guided self-help CBT led to increased weight loss and higher rates of remission from binge eating at the completion of a 12-week course of treatment; moreover, reductions in body weight were maintained at a 3-month posttreatment follow-up (Grilo, Masheb, & Salant, 2005). These results require replication with longer-term follow-up to determine whether reduction in binge eating and weight loss persist after drug withdrawal. Nevertheless, they provide tentative support for the notion that augmenting empirically supported psychosocial treatments with medications designed specifically to target overweight is an effective approach to managing obese patients with BED.

In summary, treatment options for patients with BED include individual and group psychotherapies, behavioral weight loss interventions, and medication. Although CBT has been recommended as the treatment of choice for BED by some evidence-based expert guidelines (i.e., NICE, 2004), no available intervention is effective for all patients. There is an emerging literature on factors that predict treatment response and outcome in patients with BED. For example, research has shown that comorbid personality disorders and increased interpersonal problems, higher levels of shape and weight concern (among patients with low interpersonal problems), and greater negative affect are associated with poor treatment outcome in BED (Hilbert et al., 2007; Masheb & Grilo, 2008). In contrast, it appears that rapid response to treatment, defined as 65% or greater reduction in binge eating by the fourth week of treatment, is associated with superior outcomes in patients with BED, although the prognostic significance of rapid response depends, to some degree, on the treatment studied (Grilo, Masheb, & Wilson, 2006; Masheb & Grilo, 2007). Moderators of treatment outcome (i.e., variables that predict for whom or under what conditions a specific treatment works; Kraemer, Wilson, Fairburn, & Agras, 2002) for BED have yet to be identified (Masheb & Grilo, 2008). Thus, the selection of a specific treatment approach for an individual with BED must be based on a careful assessment by the clinician or treatment team, as well as a discussion of the pros and cons of available options with each patient.

Involvement of Family and Caregivers

Only one study has examined the impact of involving family members or supportive others in the treatment of BED. The results indicate that spouse involvement does not improve the efficacy of group CBT for BED (Gorin, Le Grange, & Stone, 2003). Nonetheless, there is some evidence that including a support partner improves the efficacy of behavioral weight control programs for obese individuals without BED (Black, Gleser, & Kooyers, 1990; Wing & Jeffery, 1999). Furthermore, including support partners in behavioral weight loss treatment is one of the few strategies that has been shown to improve weight loss maintenance (Gorin et al., 2005). Thus, the involvement of family members or other supportive persons may offer some benefit in the management of obese patients with BED, particularly those enrolled in behavioral weight control programs.

Treatment Team

The treatment team for an individual with BED depends, in large part, on the choice of intervention. Specialized psychotherapies such as CBT, IPT, and DBT require involvement of clinicians with specific training and experience in these modalities, which may be difficult to obtain in some settings. Behavioral weight control programs are available in a variety of contexts (e.g., academic centers, commercial weight loss programs, self-help manuals) and from providers of numerous backgrounds (e.g., dietitians, nutritionists, health psychologists). However, the extent to which weight management provided in the community resembles interventions tested in clinical research may vary widely. Finally, pharmacological interventions require a physician or nurse practitioner to prescribe medication; however, because pharmacotherapy can be performed in a primary care setting by nonspecialists, these treatments may hold the greatest promise in terms of widespread dissemination (Wilson et al., 2007).

Summary

BED is a chronic disorder associated with significant medical and psychiatric morbidity. It also is a relatively common condition, especially among obese individuals. Thus, treatment for BED often focuses on promoting weight loss as well as ameliorating disordered-eating symptoms. Effective interventions include individual and group psychotherapy, behavioral weight control, and pharmacotherapy. However, each of these treatments has disadvantages (e.g., psychotherapy for BED generally does not lead to weight loss; long-term benefits of behavioral weight control and pharmacotherapy are unknown), and no intervention is effective for all patients. Thus, decisions about the treatment of BED must be based on a careful assessment of each patient's presenting symptomatology, including medical and psychiatric comorbidities, review of the benefits and disadvantages of different therapies, and consideration of the availability of trained professionals to provide care.

NOS Variants of AN and BN

In the second part of this chapter we review issues pertaining to the diagnosis, assessment, and treatment of individuals presenting with EDNOS variants that resemble, but do not meet the criteria for, AN and BN. As detailed below, such presentations often represent either a prodromal or residual phase of threshold-level illness, and as such, their management is identical to that of full-syndrome AN or BN. In cases in which

EDNOS symptomatology is atypical or does not resemble a DSM-defined ED, best clinical judgment and consultation are recommended.

Diagnostic Considerations

Diagnostic Criteria

Although the DSM-IV provides no specific criteria for NOS variants of AN and BN, clinicians and researchers working in the ED field are familiar with several common examples of these EDNOS subgroups. Frequently cited NOS presentations of AN include (1) all criteria for AN are met except amenorrhea; (2) all criteria for AN are met except the individual denies fear of fat or concerns about body weight and shape; and (3) all criteria for AN are met; however, despite significant weight loss, current weight is in the normal range. With respect to BN, NOS variants generally are diagnosed in cases in which an individual does not meet the two-episode-per-week frequency criterion for binge eating or compensatory behaviors, or in situations in which the size of the binge-eating episodes is not objectively large. Keel and colleagues (Keel, 2007; Keel, Haedt, & Edler, 2005) have termed this latter EDNOS variant "purging disorder"; others have called it EDNOS—purging type (EDNOS-p; Binford & Le Grange, 2005; Wade, 2007) and EDNOS-BN (Le Grange et al., 2006). In the remainder of this chapter, we use the term *purging disorder* (PD) to denote an EDNOS variant characterized by recurrent episodes of purging (i.e., self-induced vomiting, laxative misuse, diuretic misuse) in the absence of objectively large binge-eating episodes among individuals who are normal weight or overweight.

With the recent formation of the Eating Disorders Work Group for DSM-V, there has been considerable interest in the utility of amending the diagnostic criteria for AN and BN to encompass some of the above-mentioned EDNOS variants. One possibility for change is deletion of amenorrhea from the diagnostic criteria set for AN, as research has consistently failed to document that amenorrhea increases the specificity of this diagnosis (e.g., Andersen, Bowers, & Watson, 2001; Garfinkel et al., 1996). Other proposed changes include modifying "arbitrary" diagnostic criteria such as the suggested minimal body weight criterion for AN (i.e., maintenance of body weight that is < 85% of that expected) and the twice-weekly frequency criterion for BN (Wilfley, Bishop, Wilson, & Agras, 2007). Finally, PD has been proposed as a new diagnostic category for DSM-V (Keel, 2007); however, the ongoing debate over the validity of the large-amount-of-food criterion for binge eating coupled with high numbers of subjective binge-eating episodes in samples of patients with PD (e.g., Keel et al., 2005) raise questions about whether this group could be encompassed more appropriately within the BN spectrum.

Epidemiology

Individuals with EDNOS comprise the majority of patients seeking treatment for disordered eating (for a review, see Fairburn & Bohn, 2005). Moreover, with few exceptions (e.g., Fairburn et al., 2007), clinical data have indicated that most of these patients present with atypical or subthreshold forms of AN and BN. For example, Andersen and colleagues (2001) reported that of 119 individuals with EDNOS admitted to the ED unit of a large university hospital, 78% met all but one criterion for AN ($n = 89$) or

BN ($n = 4$). Similarly, Eddy, Doyle, Hoste, Herzog, and Le Grange (2008) reported that three-quarters of a sample of treatment-seeking adolescents with EDNOS ($N = 166$) had subthreshold AN ($n = 46$) or subthreshold BN, including PD ($n = 79$). High rates of EDNOS also have been reported in general psychiatric settings. For example, Zimmerman, Francione-Witt, Chelminski, Young, and Tortolani (2008) found that 51% ($N = 84/164$) of individuals with a current ED presenting to a nonspecialty psychiatric service had EDNOS. Moreover, 40% of these patients met criteria for subthreshold AN ($n = 17$) or BN ($n = 17$). Finally, studies examining rates of ED psychopathology in community samples have documented that 2–5% of individuals have a lifetime diagnosis of subsyndromal AN or BN (Favaro et al., 2003; Wade et al., 2006).

Demographic Correlates

Consistent with the demographic characteristics of threshold-level EDs, available data suggest that NOS variants of AN and BN occur more frequently in whites compared to nonwhites and in females compared to males (Eddy et al., 2008; Fairburn & Bohn, 2005). A notable exception may be extreme dietary restriction in the absence of fear of fat or weight concern, as this AN variant often is observed in non-Western groups (Keel & Klump, 2003).

Other Associated Features and Comorbidity

In general, NOS variants of AN and BN are similar in presentation to full-syndrome EDs. Affected individuals endorse significantly more ED symptomatology, Axis I and II psychiatric comorbidity—particularly mood and anxiety disorder comorbidity—and impairment in psychosocial functioning than do non-eating-disordered groups (Keel et al., 2005; Wade, 2007). Furthermore, studies comparing individuals with NOS variants of AN and BN to their threshold-level counterparts have found few differences on measures of comorbid psychopathology or psychosocial impairment (Binford & Le Grange, 2005; Fairburn et al., 2007; Garfinkel et al., 1996; Keel et al., 2005). There is some evidence that threshold-level BN is associated with greater ED symptomatology relative to PD and other NOS presentations of BN (Binford & Le Grange, 2005; Keel et al., 2005; Le Grange et al., 2006; Wade, 2007); however, differences relate primarily to lower levels of disinhibition and hunger in individuals with PD compared to those with BN, which is consistent with the absence of objective binge-eating episodes in the former group (Keel, 2007).

Etiology

Although there has been considerable interest in identifying factors that may influence the onset of threshold-level EDs, few studies have focused specifically on the etiology of NOS variants of AN and BN. The limitations of assuming etiological continuity across full- and partial-syndrome presentations notwithstanding (for a review, see Striegel-Moore & Bulik, 2007), longitudinal data indicate that NOS variants of AN and BN often represent stages in the long-term course of threshold-level EDs (Milos, Spindler, Schnyder, & Fairburn, 2005), and thus it is likely that they arise from many of the same factors as their DSM-defined counterparts. Indeed, risk-factor studies have identified several variables that are associated with the onset of both threshold and subthreshold ED psychopathology; examples include childhood feeding problems, sexual abuse and other early adverse experiences, dieting and weight concerns, negative self-evaluation, and general psychiatric morbidity (for a review, see Jacobi, Hayward, de Zwaan, Kraemer, & Agras, 2004). Furthermore, family history data have shown that rates of subthreshold EDs (defined as meeting all but one diagnostic criterion for AN, BN, or BED) are significantly higher in the first-degree relatives of women with threshold-level EDs, as compared to the first-degree relatives of non-eating-disordered probands (Stein et al., 1999), indicating that EDNOS aggregates in the families of individuals with DSM-defined eating disturbance.

Because, by definition, individuals with PD do not report objective binge-eating episodes, there has been some recent speculation that the physiological mechanisms underlying this EDNOS variant may differ from those associated with threshold-level BN. In particular, research has documented that women with PD do not exhibit the blunted postprandial CCK response that has been found in patients with BN (Keel, Wolfe, Liddle, De Young, & Jimerson, 2007). Moreover, when compared to women with BN and healthy controls, women with PD report greater subjective feelings of fullness, nausea, and stomachache following a test meal, which may suggest that other neuropeptide systems involved in the regulation of food intake or delayed gastric emptying are involved in the pathophysiology of this illness (Keel et al., 2007). However, future research is needed to determine whether physiological differences between PD and BN represent a distinction in the causes, consequences, or maintenance factors for these conditions. In addition, studies are needed to identify biological factors that may be associated with the presentation and course of other NOS variants of AN and BN.

Course of Illness

Available data suggest that NOS variants of AN and BN are characterized by a variable course of illness, with frequent diagnostic crossover to threshold-level ED psychopathology and high rates of remission from disordered-eating symptoms. For example, Milos and colleagues (2005) reported that of 29 patients initially diagnosed with EDNOS, only 8 (27.6%) retained this status at 12-month follow-up; 5 (17.2%) were diagnosed with AN, 7 (24.1%) with BN, and 9 (31.0%) no longer met criteria for an ED. Furthermore, at the 30-month follow-up assessment, more than half of the patients initially diagnosed with EDNOS no longer met criteria for an ED. Fichter and Quadfleig (2007) found similar results in a longitudinal study of inpatients with EDs. Specifically, they reported that more than two-thirds of patients with an EDNOS diagnosis (excluding BED) crossed over to "no eating disorder" at some point during their course of illness; the next highest remission rate was from BED (62.7%) followed by BN (53.0%) and AN (37.6%). Finally, Grilo and colleagues (2007) reported that 83% of a sample of 69 patients with EDNOS experienced remission from threshold-level ED symptoms during a 5-year follow-up, compared to 74% of individuals with BN ($n = 23$); however, relapse rates were high for both groups, with 42% of remitted EDNOS patients and 47% of remitted BN patients experiencing a return of threshold-level ED symptoms. These findings are consistent with the results of other longitudinal studies that have documented similarities between EDNOS and BN with respect to course of illness (Ben-Tovim et al., 2001).

Assessment

Psychological Evaluation and Data Gathering

As in other EDs, a clinical interview by a trained professional is the preferred method of assessment for NOS variants of AN and BN. Interviews should focus particular attention on the individual's history of ED symptoms and weight, as this may help to determine whether the NOS presentation represents a residual phase in the course of a threshold-level illness, a newer onset of disordered-eating symptoms, or a distinct pattern of symptomatology altogether (e.g., PD). Psychological evaluations of individuals presenting with NOS variants of AN and BN also should address psychiatric comorbidities frequently seen in patients with EDs (e.g., depression, anxiety, substance use), as well as history of past treatment for disordered eating and other mental illness.

Medical Evaluation

The medical evaluation of individuals with NOS variants of AN and BN generally is identical to that recommended for threshold-level EDs. Individuals presenting with NOS variants of AN should receive the standard protocol for DSM-defined AN; individuals with bulimic symptoms should be evaluated in the same manner as patients with BN.

Nutrition Assessment

Nutrition concerns for patients with NOS variants of AN and BN generally are similar to those for individuals with threshold-level EDs. Thus, nutrition assessment should follow guidelines recommended for the DSM-defined disorder that the patient's presenting symptomatology resembles most closely.

Treatment Planning

Although individuals with NOS variants of AN and BN have been included in some recent clinical trials (e.g., Fairburn & Grave, 2008), no studies have focused specifically on the treatment of these patients. Thus, there are limited empirical data to guide decisions about the management of NOS variants of AN and BN. As detailed below, in the absence of specific treatment guidelines, individuals presenting with NOS variants of AN and BN typically receive care that is identical to that of individuals with the DSM-defined ED that their symptoms resemble most closely (see Figure 3.1).

Treatment Setting

Decisions about the appropriate level of care for individuals with NOS variants of AN and BN are based largely on the nature and severity of the presenting psychopathology. For underweight patients, acute weight restoration treatment in an inpatient or day hospital setting often is warranted to normalize eating and decrease the frequency of unhealthy compensatory behaviors (e.g., purging, excessive exercise). Normal-weight individuals typically are treated in an outpatient setting; however, brief hospital stays may be required to address medical abnormalities consequent to disordered-eating

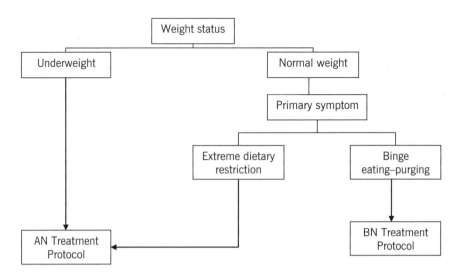

FIGURE 3.1. Treatment algorithm for patients presenting with NOS variants of AN and BN.

behaviors (e.g., electrolyte imbalances due to frequent purging) or severe psychiatric comorbidities (e.g., suicidal behaviors).

Treatment Options

The choice of treatment for individuals with NOS variants of AN and BN depends on the nature of the disordered-eating psychopathology. For underweight individuals, nutrition rehabilitation aimed at normalizing eating and restoring a healthy body weight is a critical component of treatment. However, there is consensus in the field that nutrition rehabilitation alone is insufficient to promote lasting recovery from disordered-eating symptoms (Agras et al., 2004), and thus there is a need for research to develop effective psychotherapeutic and pharmacological interventions for individuals with NOS variants of AN. As reviewed in detail elsewhere (Bulik, Berkman, Brownley, Sedway, & Lohr, 2007), very few controlled trials have focused on the treatment of patients with DSM-defined AN, and they have produced inconsistent findings. Consequently, there is limited evidence on which to base even tentative suggestions for the management of individuals with NOS variants of the disorder. Interventions that may hold promise for the treatment of patients with NOS variants of AN include family therapy for adolescents and individual psychotherapy, particularly for weight-restored patients. Few empirical data support the efficacy of pharmacological interventions for underweight individuals with anorexic psychopathology (Bulik et al., 2007).

Treatment options for patients presenting with NOS variants of BN include individual and group psychotherapies and medication. CBT appears to be particularly effective for individuals with bulimic psychopathology, although there also is evidence that IPT, DBT, and guided imagery are associated with significant and sustained reductions in the frequency of binge-eating and compensatory behaviors (for a review, see Shapiro, Berkman, et al., 2007). With respect to pharamacological interventions, there is strong support for the utility of fluoxetine in the management of patients with BN, and preliminary evidence suggests that several other medications (e.g., trazodone, topiramate, desipramine) are effective in reducing bulimic symptomatology (Shapiro, Berkman, et al., 2007). Finally, some investigators have suggested that differences in the psychobiology of BN and PD may indicate the need for novel pharmacological treatments for individuals who purge in the absence of objective binge-eating episodes (e.g., Keel et al., 2007); however, no empirical studies have addressed the treatment of individuals with PD.

Involvement of Family and Caregivers

For adolescents living at home, parental involvement is standard in the treatment of disordered eating. Empirical studies that have included adolescents with NOS variants of AN and BN have documented the efficacy of family-based interventions for this group (Le Grange, Crosby, Rathouz, & Leventhal, 2007; Lock, Agras, Bryson, & Kraemer, 2005). In contrast, research generally has not supported the utility of family-based treatment for adults with EDs (Bulik et al., 2007); however, clinical experience suggests that some adults with EDNOS may benefit from including family members or other supportive individuals in treatment.

Treatment Team

Professionals involved in the care of patients with NOS variants of AN and BN include psychiatrists, psychologists, social workers, and dietitians. The specific treatment team for an individual with EDNOS depends on the required level of care and the choice of intervention.

Summary

EDNOS is the most common diagnosis assigned to patients seeking treatment for disordered eating, and data suggest that many of these individuals have NOS variants of AN and BN. Although clinical research has found few differences between patients with EDNOS and patients with DSM-defined EDs on measures of clinical severity, including course of illness, little is known about the specific needs of this group. In the absence of empirical data on which to guide treatment planning decisions, the management of EDNOS generally is identical to the management of threshold-level EDs. Future research is needed to characterize EDNOS subgroups more clearly and to develop strategies for their evaluation and treatment.

References

Agras WS, Brandt HA, Bulik CM, Dolan-Sewell R, Fairburn CG, Halmi KA, et al. (2004). Report of the National Institutes of Health workshop on overcoming barriers to treatment research in anorexia nervosa. *International Journal of Eating Disorders*, 35:509–521.

Agras WS, Telch CF, Arnow B, Eldredge K, Wilfley DE, Raeburn SD, et al. (1994). Weight loss, cognitive-behavioral, and desipramine treatments in binge eating disorder: An additive design. *Behavior Therapy*, 25:225–238.

Allison KC, Grilo CM, Masheb RM, & Stunkard AJ. (2005). Binge eating disorder and night eating syndrome: A comparative study of disordered eating. *Journal of Consulting and Clinical Psychology*, 73:1107–1115.

American Psychiatric Association. (1994). *Diagnostic and statistical manual of mental disorders* (4th ed.). Washington, DC: Author.

Andersen AE, Bowers WA, & Watson T. (2001). A slimming program for eating disorders not otherwise specified: Reconceptualizing a confusing, residual diagnostic category. *Psychiatric Clinics of North America*, 24:271–280.

Ben-Tovim DI, Walker K, Gilchrist P, Freeman R, Kalucy R, & Esterman A. (2001). Outcome in patients with eating disorders: A 5-year study. *The Lancet*, 357:1254–1257.

Binford RB, & Le Grange D. (2005). Adolescents with bulimia nervosa and eating disorder not otherwise specified—purging only. *International Journal of Eating Disorders*, 38:157–161.

Black DR, Gleser LJ, & Kooyers KJ. (1990). A meta-analytic evaluation of couples weight-loss programs. *Health Psychology*, 9:330–347.

Blundell JE. (1986). Serotonin manipulations and the structure of feeding behavior. *Appetite*, 7:39–56.

Brownley KA, Berkman ND, Sedway JA, Lohr KN, & Bulik CM. (2007). Binge eating disorder treatment: A systematic review of randomized controlled trials. *International Journal of Eating Disorders*, 40:337–348.

Bulik CM, Berkman ND, Brownley KA, Sedway JA, & Lohr KN. (2007). Anorexia nervosa treatment: A systematic review of randomized controlled trials. *International Journal of Eating Disorders*, 40:310–320.

Cachelin FM, Striegel-Moore RH, Elder KA, Pike KM, Wilfley DE, & Fairburn CG. (1999). Natural course of a community sample of women with binge eating disorder. *International Journal of Eating Disorders*, 25:45–54.

Cassin SE, & von Ranson KM. (2005). Personality and eating disorders: A decade in review. *Clinical Psychology Review*, 25:895–916.

Celio AA, Wilfley DE, Crow SJ, Mitchell J, & Walsh BT. (2004). A comparison of the Binge Eating Scale, Questionnaire for Eating and Weight Patterns-Revised, and Eating Disorder Examination Questionnaire with Instructions with the Eating Disorder Examination in the assessment of binge eating disorder and its symptoms. *International Journal of Eating Disorders*, 36:434–444.

Claudino AM, de Oliveira IR, Appolinario JC, Cordás TA, Duchesne M, Sichieri R, et al. (2007). Double-blind, placebo-controlled trial of topiramate plus cognitive-behavior therapy in binge-eating disorder. *Journal of Clinical Psychiatry*, 68:1324–1332.

Devlin MJ, Goldfein JA, Petkova E, Jiang H, Raizman PS, Wolk S, et al. (2005). Cognitive behavioral therapy and fluoxetine as adjuncts to group behavioral therapy for binge eating disorder. *Obesity Research*, 13:1077–1088.

de Zwaan M, Mitchell JE, Crosby RD, Mussell MP, Raymond NC, Specker SM, et al. (2005). Short-term cognitive-behavioral treatment does not improve outcome of a comprehensive very-low-calorie diet program in obese women with binge eating disorder. *Behavior Therapy*, 36:89–99.

Eckel RH. (2008). Nonsurgical management of obesity in adults. *New England Journal of Medicine*, 358:1941–1950.

Eddy KT, Doyle AC, Hoste RR, Herzog DB, & Le Grange D. (2008). Eating disorder not otherwise specified in adolescents. *Journal of the American Academy of Child and Adolescent Psychiatry*, 47:156–164.

Fairburn CG, & Bohn K. (2005). Eating disorder NOS (EDNOS): An example of the troublesome "not otherwise specified" (NOS) category in DSM-IV. *Behaviour Research and Therapy*, 43:691–701.

Fairburn CG, & Cooper Z. (1993). The Eating Disorder Examination (12th ed.). In CG Fairburn & GT Wilson (Eds.), *Binge eating: Nature, treatment, and assessment* (pp. 317–360). New York: Guilford Press.

Fairburn CG, Cooper Z, Bohn K, O'Connor ME, Doll HA, & Palmer RL. (2007). The severity and status of eating disorder NOS: Implications for DSM-V. *Behaviour Research and Therapy*, 45:1705–1715.

Fairburn CG, Cooper Z, Doll HA, Norman P, & O'Connor M. (2000). The natural course of bulimia nervosa and binge eating disorder in young women. *Archives of General Psychiatry*, 57:659–665.

Fairburn CG, Doll HA, Welch SL, Hay PJ, Davies BA, & O'Connor ME. (1998). Risk factors for binge eating disorder. *Archives of General Psychiatry*, 55:425–432.

Fairburn CG, & Grave RD. (2008, September). "Enhanced" CBT for anorexia nervosa: Findings from Oxford, Leicester and Verona. In M Marcus (Chair), *Psychotherapy contexts, processes, and outcomes*. Symposium conducted at the 14th annual meeting of the Eating Disorders Research Society, Montreal, Quebec, Canada.

Favaro A, Ferrara S, & Santonastaso P. (2003). The spectrum of eating disorders in young women: A prevalence study in a general population sample. *Psychosomatic Medicine*, 65:701–708.

Fichter MM, & Quadflieg N. (2007). Long-term stability of eating disorder diagnoses. *International Journal of Eating Disorders*, 40:S61–S66.

Fichter MM, Quadflieg N, & Hedlund S. (2008). Long-term course of binge eating disorder and bulimia nervosa: Relevance for nosology and diagnostic criteria. *International Journal of Eating Disorders*, 41:577–586.

First MB, Spitzer R, Gibbon M, & Williams JBW. (1995). *Structured clinical interview for DSM-IV Axis I disorders—patient edition* (SCID-I/P). New York: Biometrics.

Garfinkel PE, Lin E, Goering P, Spegg C, Goldbloom DS, Kennedy S, et al. (1996). Should amenorrhea be necessary for the diagnosis of anorexia nervosa? *British Journal of Psychiatry*, 168:500–506.

Geliebter A, Gluck ME, & Hashim SA. (2005). Plasma ghrelin concentrations are lower in binge-eating disorder. *Journal of Nutrition*, 135:1326–1330.

Geliebter A, Yahav EK, Gluck ME, & Hashim SA. (2004). Gastric capacity, test meal intake, and appetitive hormones in binge eating disorder. *Physiology and Behavior*, 81:735–740.

Goldschmidt AB, Jones M, Manwaring JL, Luce KH, Osborne MI, Cunning D, et al. (2008). The clinical significance of loss of control over eating in overweight adolescents. *International Journal of Eating Disorders*, 41:153–158.

Gorin A, Phelan S, Tate D, Sherwood N, Jeffrey R, & Wing R. (2005). Involving support partners in obesity treatment. *Journal of Consulting and Clinical Psychology*, 73:341–343.

Gorin AA, Le Grange D, & Stone AA. (2003). Effectiveness of spouse involvement in cognitive behavioral therapy for binge eating disorder. *International Journal of Eating Disorders*, 33:421–433.

Grilo CM, Hrabosky JI, White MA, Allison KC, Stunkard AJ, & Masheb RM. (2008). Overvaluation of shape and weight in binge eating disorder and overweight controls: Refinement of a diagnostic construct. *Journal of Abnormal Psychology*, 117:414–419.

Grilo CM, & Masheb RM. (2005). A randomized controlled comparison of guided self-help cognitive behavioral therapy and behavioral weight loss for binge eating disorder. *Behaviour Research and Therapy*, 43:1509–1525.

Grilo CM, Masheb RM, & Salant SL. (2005). Cognitive behavioral therapy guided self-help and orlistat for the treatment of binge eating disorder: A randomized, double-blind, placebo-controlled trial. *Biological Psychiatry*, 57:1193–1201.

Grilo CM, Masheb RM, & Wilson GT. (2001). A comparison of different methods for assessing the features of eating disorders in patients with binge eating disorder. *Journal of Consulting and Clinical Psychology*, 69:317–322.

Grilo CM, Masheb RM, & Wilson GT. (2005). Efficacy of cognitive behavioral therapy and flu-oxetine for the treatment of binge eating disorder: A randomized double-blind placebo-controlled comparison. *Biological Psychiatry*, 57:301–309.

Grilo CM, Masheb RM, & Wilson GT. (2006). Rapid response to treatment for binge eating disorder. *Journal of Consulting and Clinical Psychology*, 74:602–613.

Grilo CM, Pagano ME, Skodol AE, Sanislow CA, McGlashan TH, Gunderson JG, et al. (2007). Natural course of bulimia nervosa and eating disorder not otherwise specified: 5-year pro-spective study of remissions, relapses, and the effects of personality disorder psychopathol-ogy. *Journal of Clinical Psychiatry*, 68:738–746.

Hilbert A, Saelens BE, Stein RI, Mockus DS, Welch RR, Matt GE, et al. (2007). Pretreatment and process predictors of outcome in interpersonal and cognitive behavioral psychotherapy for binge eating disorder. *Journal of Consulting and Clinical Psychology*, 75:645–651.

Hrabrosky JI, Masheb RM, White MA, & Grilo CM. (2007). Overvaluation of shape and weight in binge eating disorder. *Journal of Consulting and Clinical Psychology*, 75:175–180.

Hudson JI, Hiripi E, Pope HG, & Kessler RC. (2007). The prevalence and correlates of eating dis-orders in the National Comorbidity Survey Replication. *Biological Psychiatry*, 61:348–358.

Hudson JI, Lalonde JK, Berry JM, Pindyck LJ, Bulik CM, Crow SJ, et al. (2006). Binge-eating disorder as a distinct familial phenotype in obese individuals. *Archives of General Psychiatry*, 63:313–319.

Jacobi C, Hayward C, de Zwaan M, Kraemer HC, & Agras WS. (2004). Coming to terms with risk factors for eating disorders: Application of risk terminology and suggestions for a general taxonomy. *Psychological Bulletin*, 130:19–65.

Javaras KN, Laird NM, Reichborn-Kjennerud T, Bulik CM, Pope HG, & Hudson JI. (2008). Familiality and heritability of binge eating disorder: Results of a case-control family study and a twin study. *International Journal of Eating Disorders*, 41:174–179.

Javaras KN, Pope HG, Lalonde JK, Roberts JL, Nillni YI, Laird NM, et al. (2008). Co-occurrence of binge eating disorder with psychiatric and medical disorders. *Journal of Clinical Psychia-try*, 69:266–273.

Kalarchian MA, Marcus MD, Levine MD, Courcoulas AP, Pilkonis PA, Ringham RM, et al. (2007). Psychiatric disorders among bariatric surgery candidates: Relationship to obesity and functional health status. *American Journal of Psychiatry*, 164:328–334.

Keel PK. (2007). Purging disorder: Subthreshold variant or full-threshold eating disorder? *Inter-national Journal of Eating Disorders*, 40:S89–S94.

Keel PK, Haedt A, & Edler C. (2005). Purging disorder: An ominous variant of bulimia nervosa? *International Journal of Eating Disorders*, 38:191–199.

Keel PK, & Klump KL. (2003). Are eating disorders culture-bound syndromes? Implications for conceptualizing their etiology. *Psychological Bulletin*, 129:747–769.

Keel PK, Wolfe BE, Liddle RA, De Young KP, & Jimerson DC. (2007). Clinical features and physiological response to a test meal in purging disorder and bulimia nervosa. *Archives of General Psychiatry*, 64:1058–1066.

Kraemer HC, Wilson GT, Fairburn CG, & Agras WS. (2002). Mediators and moderators of treat-ment effects in randomized clinical trials. *Archives of General Psychiatry*, 59:877–883.

Laederach-Hofmann K, Graf C, Horber F, Lippuner K, Lederer S, Michel R, et al. (1999). Imi-pramine and diet counseling with psychological support in the treatment of obese binge eaters: A randomized, placebo-controlled double-blind study. *International Journal of Eating Disorders*, 26:231–244.

Latner JD, & Clyne C. (2008). The diagnostic validity of the criteria for binge eating disorder. *International Journal of Eating Disorders*, 41:1–14.

Latner JD, Hildebrandt T, Rosewall JK, Chisholm AM, & Hayashi K. (2007). Loss of control over eating reflects eating disturbances and general psychopathology. *Behaviour Research and Therapy*, 45:2203–2211.

Le Grange D, Binford RB, Peterson CB, Crow SJ, Crosby RD, Klein MH, et al. (2006). DSM-IV threshold versus subthreshold bulimia nervosa. *International Journal of Eating Disorders*, 39:462–467.

Le Grange D, Crosby RD, Rathouz PJ, & Leventhal BL. (2007). A randomized controlled comparison of family-based treatment and supportive psychotherapy for adolescent bulimia nervosa. *Archives of General Psychiatry*, 64:1049–1056.

Ljotsson B, Lundin C, Mitsell K, Carlbring P, Ramklint M, & Ghaderi A. (2007). Remote treatment of bulimia nervosa and binge eating disorder: A randomized trial of Internet-assisted cognitive behavioural therapy. *Behaviour Research and Therapy*, 45:649–661.

Lock J, Agras WS, Bryson S, & Kraemer HC. (2005). A comparison of short- and long-term family therapy for adolescent anorexia nervosa. *Journal of the American Academy of Child and Adolescent Psychiatry*, 44:632–639.

Marcus MD, Kalarchian MA, & Levine M. (2005). Eating disorders: Binge eating. In B Caballero, L Allen, & A Prentice (Eds.), *Encyclopedia of human nutrition* (2nd ed., pp. 80–85). Oxford, UK: Elsevier.

Marcus MD, & Levine MD. (2004). Obese patients with binge-eating disorder. In DJ Goldstein (Ed.), *The management of eating disorders and obesity* (2nd ed., pp. 143–160). Totowa, NJ: Humana Press.

Marcus MD, Wing RR, Ewing L, Kern E, McDermott M, & Gooding W. (1990). A double-blind, placebo-controlled trial of fluoxetine plus behavior modification in the treatment of obese binge-eaters and non-binge-eaters. *American Journal of Psychiatry*, 147:876–881.

Masheb RM, & Grilo CM. (2007). Rapid response predicts treatment outcomes in binge eating disorder: Implications for stepped care. *Journal of Consulting and Clinical Psychology*, 75:639–644.

Masheb RM, & Grilo CM. (2008). Examination of predictors and moderators for self-help treatments of binge-eating disorder. *Journal of Consulting and Clinical Psychology*, 76:900–904.

Milos G, Spindler A, Schnyder U, & Fairburn CG. (2005). Instability of eating disorder diagnoses: Prospective study. *British Journal of Psychiatry*, 187:573–578.

Monteleone P, Brambilla F, Bortolotti F, & Maj M. (2000). Serotonergic dysfunction across the eating disorders: Relationship to eating behaviour, purging behaviour, nutritional status, and general psychopathology. *Psychological Medicine*, 30:1099–1110.

Monteleone P, Fabrazzo M, Martiadis V, Serritella C, Pannuto M, & Maj M. (2005). Circulating brain-derived neurotrophic factor is decreased in women with anorexia and bulimia nervosa but not in women with binge-eating disorder: Relationships to co-morbid depression, psychopathology, and hormonal variables. *Psychological Medicine*, 35:897–905.

Monteleone P, Tortorella A, Castaldo, Di Filippo C, & Maj M. (2006). No association of the Arg-51Gln and Leu72Met polymorphisms of the ghrelin gene with anorexia nervosa or bulimia nervosa. *Neuroscience Letters*, 398:325–327.

Monteleone P, Tortorella A, Castaldo, Di Filippo C, & Maj M. (2007). The Leu72Met polymorphism of the ghrelin gene is significantly associated with binge eating disorder. *Psychiatric Genetics*, 17:13–16.

National Institute for Clinical Excellence. (2004). *Eating disorders: Core interventions in the treatment and management of anorexia nervosa, bulimia nervosa and related eating disorders* (Clinical Guideline No. 9). London: Author. (Available at *www.nice.org.uk/guidance/CG9*)

Pike KM, Dohm FA, Striegel-Moore RH, Wilfley DE, & Fairburn CG. (2001). A comparison of black and white women with binge eating disorder. *American Journal of Psychiatry*, 158:1455–1460.

Pope HG, Lalonde JK, Pindyck LJ, Walsh T, Bulik CM, Crow SJ, et al. (2006). Binge eating disorder: A stable syndrome. *American Journal of Psychiatry*, 163:2181–2183.

Reas DL, & Grilo CM. (2008). Review and meta-analysis of pharmacotherapy for binge-eating disorder. *Obesity*, 16:2024–2038.

Ricca V, Mannucci E, Mezzani B, Moretti S, Di Bernardo M, Bertelli M, et al. (2001). Fluoxetine and fluvoxamine combined with individual cognitive-behaviour therapy in binge eating disorder: A one-year follow-up study. *Psychotherapy and Psychosomatics*, 70:298–306.

Rieger E, Wilfley DE, Stein RI, Marino V, & Crow SJ. (2005). A comparison of quality of life in obese individuals with and without binge eating disorder. *International Journal of Eating Disorders*, 37:234–240.

Shapiro JR, Berkman ND, Brownley KA, Sedway JA, Lohr KN, & Bulik CM. (2007). Bulimia nervosa treatment: A systematic review of randomized controlled trials. *International Journal of Eating Disorders*, 40:321–336.

Shapiro JR, Reba-Harrelson L, Dymek-Valentine M, Woolson SL, Hamer RM, & Bulik CM. (2007). Feasibility and acceptability of CD-ROM-based cognitive behavioural treatment for binge-eating disorder. *European Eating Disorders Review*, 15:175–184.

Steiger H, & Bruce KR. (2007). Phenotypes, endophenotypes, and genotypes in bulimia spectrum eating disorders. *Canadian Journal of Psychiatry*, 52:220–227.

Stein D, Lilenfeld LR, Plotnicov K, Pollice C, Rao R, Strober M, et al. (1999). Familial aggregation of eating disorders: Results from a controlled family study of bulimia nervosa. *International Journal of Eating Disorders*, 26:211–215.

Striegel-Moore RH, & Bulik CM. (2007). Risk factors for eating disorders. *American Psychologist*, 62:181–198.

Striegel-Moore RH, Dohm FA, Kraemer HC, Schreiber GB, Taylor CB, & Daniels SR. (2007). Risk factors for binge-eating disorders: An exploratory study. *International Journal of Eating Disorders*, 40:481–487.

Striegel-Moore RH, Dohm FA, Kraemer HC, Taylor CB, Daniels S, Crawford PB, et al. (2003). Eating disorders in white and black women. *American Journal of Psychiatry*, 160:1326–1331.

Striegel-Moore RH, Dohm FA, Pike KM, Wilfley DE, & Fairburn CG. (2002). Abuse, bullying, and discrimination as risk factors for binge eating disorder. *American Journal of Psychiatry*, 159:1902–1907.

Striegel-Moore RH, Fairburn CG, Wilfley DE, Pike KM, Dohm FA, & Kraemer HC. (2005). Toward an understanding of risk factors for binge-eating in black and white women: A community-based case-control study. *Psychological Medicine*, 35:907–917.

Stunkard A, Allison K, & Lundgren J. (2008). Issues for DSM-V: Night eating syndrome. *American Journal of Psychiatry*, 165:4.

Sysko R, & Walsh BT. (2008). A critical evaluation of the efficacy of self-help interventions for the treatment of bulimia nervosa and binge-eating disorder. *International Journal of Eating Disorders*, 41:97–112.

Tanofsky-Kraff M, Goossens L, Eddy KT, Ringham R, Goldschmidt A, Yanovski SZ, et al. (2007). A multisite investigation of binge eating behaviors in children and adolescents. *Journal of Consulting and Clinical Psychology*, 75:901–913.

Taylor JY, Caldwell CH, Baser RE, Faison N, & Jackson JS. (2007). Prevalence of eating disorders among blacks in the National Survey of American Life. *International Journal of Eating Disorders*, 40:S10–S14.

Telch CF, Agras WS, & Linehan MM. (2001). Dialectical behavior therapy for binge eating disorder. *Journal of Consulting and Clinical Psychology*, 69:1061–1065.

Wade TD. (2007). A retrospective comparison of purging type disorders: Eating disorder not otherwise specified and bulimia nervosa. *International Journal of Eating Disorders*, 40:1–6.

Wade TD, Bergin JL, Tiggemann M, Bulik CM, & Fairburn CG. (2006). Prevalence and long-term course of lifetime eating disorders in an adult Australian twin cohort. *Australian and New Zealand Journal of Psychiatry*, 40:121–128.

Widiger TA, & Samuel DB. (2005). Diagnostic categories or dimensions?: A question for the *Diagnostic and Statistical Manual of Mental Disorders—Fifth Edition*. *Journal of Abnormal Psychology*, 114:494–504.

Wilfley DE, Agras WS, Telch CF, Rossiter EM, Schneider JA, Golomb-Cole AE, et al. (1993). Group cognitive-behavioral therapy and group interpersonal psychotherapy for the non-purging bulimic individual: A controlled comparison. *Journal of Consulting and Clinical Psychology*, 61:296–305.

Wilfley DE, Bishop ME, Wilson GT, & Agras WS. (2007). Classification of eating disorders: Toward DSM-V. *International Journal of Eating Disorders*, 40:S123–S129.

Wilfley DE, Crow SJ, Hudson JI, Mitchell JE, Berkowitz RI, Blakesley V, et al. (2008). Efficacy of sibutramine in the treatment of binge eating disorder: A randomized multicenter placebo-controlled double-blind study. *American Journal of Psychiatry*, 165:51–58.

Wilfley DE, Welch RR, Stein RI, Spurrell EB, Cohen LR, Saelens BE, et al. (2002). A randomized comparison of group cognitive-behavioral therapy and group interpersonal psychotherapy for the treatment of overweight individuals with binge-eating disorder. *Archives of General Psychiatry*, 59:713–721.

Wilfley DE, Wilson GT, & Agras WS. (2008, September). Psychological treatments for binge eating disorder: A multi-site randomized controlled trial. In M Marcus (Chair), *Psychotherapy contexts, processes, and outcomes*. Symposium conducted at the 14th annual meeting of the Eating Disorders Research Society, Montreal, Quebec, Canada.

Wilson GT, Grilo CM, & Vitousek KM. (2007). Psychological treatment of eating disorders. *American Psychologist*, 62:199–216.

Wing RR, & Jeffery RW. (1999). Benefits of recruiting participants with friends and increasing social support for weight loss and maintenance. *Journal of Consulting and Clinical Psychology*, 67:132–138.

Zimmerman M, Francione-Witt C, Chelminski I, Young D, & Tortolani C. (2008). Problems applying the DSM-IV eating disorders diagnostic criteria in a general psychiatric outpatient practice. *Journal of Clinical Psychiatry*, 69:381–384.

CHAPTER 4

Medical Complications of Eating Disorders

Philip S. Mehler, Laird C. Birmingham, Scott J. Crow,
and Joel P. Jahraus

Anorexia Nervosa and Bulimia Nervosa

Medical complications are common among patients with anorexia nervosa (AN), bulimia nervosa (BN), and binge-eating disorder (BED). In this chapter we review the medical complications of these three eating disorders (EDs) in detail, focusing on the signs and symptoms and the medical assessment and management of the specific complications that arise. We mainly discuss medical issues in patients with AN and BN. We cover BED more briefly toward the end of the chapter, focusing on medical issues unique to BED rather than those seen in obesity, in general, since a review of the medical issues associated with obesity is beyond the scope of this chapter.

Signs Associated with AN and BN

Most patients with AN and BN are females in their teens or 20s, and they often present for medical care with nonspecific complaints of feeling "bloated," experiencing constipation, infertility problems, swelling of the hands and feet, or nonspecific cardiopulmonary symptoms such as exertional fatigue, palpitations, or syncope (fainting). A summary of the most common signs associated with AN and BN are presented in Table 4.1 (Pomeroy, Mitchell, Roerig, & Crow, 2002).

In severe AN the emaciation of the patient usually alerts the clinician to the diagnosis. However, many patients with AN try to conceal their low weight. Common strategies include wearing large pants and sweaters to mask their thinness, carrying objects hidden in their clothes, and/or drinking water to artificially inflate their weight. Patients with BN also may hide their symptoms from medical professionals and can be quite difficult to diagnose because of the lack of overt changes in physical appearance.

Next we review medical issues by organ system, including further explanations for many of the physical signs noted in Table 4.1. We also briefly discuss the medical management of these complications.

TABLE 4.1. Physical Signs Present in Patients with Eating Disorders

Anorexia nervosa	Bulimia nervosa
Emaciation[a]	Hypotension (< 9 0 mm Hg systolic)[a]
Hypothermia[a]	Dry skin[a]
Bradycardia (Heart rate < 60 beats/minute)[a]	Parotid gland swelling[a]
Hypotension (< 90 mm Hg systolic)[a]	Erosion of dental enamel[a]
Hypoactive bowel sounds[a]	Tachycardia (heart rate >100 beats/minute)[a]
Dry skin[a]	Hair loss
Brittle hair and scalp hair loss[a]	"Russell's sign"
Hyperactivity	Edema
Brittle nails	
Pressure sores	
"Yellow" skin, especially palms	
Lanugo hair	
Cyanotic (blue) and cold hands and feet	
Edema (ankle, periorbital)	
Heart murmur (mitral valve prolapse)	

[a]Common.

Dermatological Problems

Patients with AN have thinning scalp hair and often develop lanugo hair growth (downy, fine hair), particularly on the face, neck, arms, back, and legs (Yager & Andersen, 2008). They can have a yellowish tinge to the skin (carotodermia) secondary to excess ingestion of carotenoids in vegetables. The hands and feet can become purplish-blue (acrocyanosis), and abnormalities of temperature regulation can occur (Yager & Andersen, 2008). Dermatological findings in BN, though usually less pronounced, can include "Russell's sign": a thickening or scarring over the back of the hand caused by pressing the fingers against the teeth while inducing vomiting. The lesion can become permanent. This sign is usually seen in the early stage of the illness. Chronic patients are more likely to induce vomiting by pressing on their abdomen or "willing" themselves to vomit.

Self-injurious behaviors (SIBs) are sometimes seen in patients with AN or BN. SIBs may be overt or covert, miniscule or extensive, acute or chronic, and involve any part of the body. SIBs may produce one or more types of trauma: burns (e.g., cigarette burns), needle marks, round or elliptical marks (cup marks), or cuts. Routine wound care is the immediate treatment (Pomeroy et al., 2002).

Gastrointestinal Problems

Erosion of dental enamel and sensitivity of the teeth to hot and cold temperatures in foods and drinks are common in BN and in AN (if patients vomit) (Milosevic, Brodie, & Slade, 1997). Gastric acid causes enamel to soften temporarily. Patients should be instructed to reduce the loss of enamel by washing out their mouth after vomiting, alkalinizing their mouth (gargling with baking soda in water) and waiting a minimum of 30 minutes before brushing. Hot and cold foods and fluids should be avoided if they cause pain. A dentist should be consulted, as dental restoration can have a positive psychological effect on the patient. Restoration should not be attempted, however, until purging is under control. Gum disease is also very common.

The parotid and submandibular glands are commonly symmetrically enlarged and can be slightly tender (Lo Russo et al., 2000). The face may appear swollen or "fat." Parotid and submandibular gland hypertrophy may be due to purging behavior, malnutrition, and autonomic dysfunction. The main way to prevent parotid hypertrophy is to abstain from self-induced vomiting. The parotids and submandibular glands will then gradually decrease in size over several months. Treatment involves applying hot packs to the swollen glands, sucking on hard candies, and if refractory, a trial of oral pilocarpine to stimulate salivary flow. In contrast, parotitis is an inflammation of the parotid gland, which becomes swollen, tender, and may be warm (usually caused by bacterial infection). An increase in pain, tenderness, and asymmetric swelling of the parotids should lead to inspection and culture of Stensen's duct (the parotid duct) above the second upper molar. The proper treatment is the use of antibiotics chosen for the bacterium cultured and its sensitivity pattern.

As a side note, erythema of the conjunctivae (white part of the eye), occasionally accompanied by subconjunctival hemorrhage, can be caused by vomiting (Weinstein & Halabis, 1986). This condition results from the marked elevation in venous pressure when vomiting; no treatment is needed.

Gastroparesis (slowing of gastric emptying) is common in AN. Once weight loss of approximately 10–20 pounds occurs, there is almost universal development of gastroparesis (Kamel et al., 1991). Bloating, particularly after eating, is the main symptom, and may be severe. The bloating can be worsened by a high-fiber diet, such as a vegetarian diet or the use of fiber-based laxatives. This bloating may hamper the food intake necessary for weight restoration.

Useful approaches to the problem of gastroparesis include (1) using liquid food supplements as one source of daily calories for the first week or two of refeeding; (2) taking in liquid components as opposed to solids earlier in the meal, which generally results in less bloating; and (3) dividing the daily caloric intake into two to three snacks and three smaller meals per day. Metachlorpramide is useful in low doses to treat gastroparesis, but can be associated with tardive dyskinesia. Gastroparesis induced by weight loss will generally improve with partial weight restoration.

Gallstone disease should also be considered in the differential diagnosis of patients with either AN or BN who complain of vomiting and/or right upper quadrant pain. This pain, due to gallstones, shows an increased incidence in patients who experience weight loss (Nogou & Suter, 2008). A painless, right upper quadrant abdominal ultrasound is a simple way to exclude the presence of gallstones.

Constipation invariably accompanies the weight loss in AN and is also common in BN (Pomeroy et al., 2002). Patients complain of bowel movements that are both infrequent and small and may respond to their perceived problem by starting treatment with high-dose bulking, fiber-containing laxatives, or dangerous stimulant laxatives. These may worsen their constipation. Because some patients take laxatives in the mistaken belief that they will cause weight loss, it is also useful to educate them that laxatives have their site of action in the colon, *after* caloric absorption has already occurred. Generally, with weight restoration and refeeding comes a resumption of normal bowel transit time within 3 weeks. Treatment options for constipation, in addition to education and progressive weight restoration, include (1) adequate water intake (six to eight glasses of water per day), (2) fiber in low doses (10 grams per day), (3) one to three tablespoons of polyethylene glycol powder (PEG) daily, and (4) lactulose, a nonabsorbable synthetic disaccharide, 30–60 ml one to two times per day (similar to PEG products in its efficacy and mode of action). It is useful to tell patients that, although this latter medication tastes extremely sweet, it is devoid of calories because it is not absorbed. It is best to avoid the use of any stimulant laxative that contains senna, cascara, or bisocodyl because of the potential for long-term abuse and dependence.

In patients with AN one other rare syndrome to be aware of is the superior mesenteric artery (SMA) syndrome (Merrett, Wilson, Cosman, & Biankin, 2008), which results from compression of the third portion of the duodenum between the aorta and the vertebral column posteriorly and the SMA anteriorly. Any factor that narrows the angle can cause entrapment of the duodenum as it passes between these vessels. The SMA is normally covered with fatty tissue; reduction in the fat pad narrows the angle. Weight loss can thus cause the syndrome. These patients typically present with intermittent vomiting and abdominal pain soon after eating. The diagnosis is made by an upper gastrointestinal X-ray series (i.e., upper GI series).

Forceful vomiting may tear the surface of the esophagus (Overby & Litt, 1988), usually at the junction of the esophagus and the stomach. Bright red blood may be vomited, initially with gastric contents. In Boerhaave's syndrome a complete rupture of the wall of the esophagus results from forceful vomiting. This condition is extremely rare but quite dangerous. The rupture usually occurs at the level of the lower chest, resulting in extreme pain due to immediate inflammation and bacterial contamination of the tissues of the mediastinum and lung. Treatment is immediate transfer for emergency care: intravenous fluids and consideration of endoscopy and surgery.

"Ruminative behavior" refers to the conscious regurgitation of gastric contents that are then chewed and swallowed again (Attri, Ravipati, Agrawal, Healy, & Feller, 2008). This symptom can result in rapid erosion of the teeth, aspiration, and Barrett's esophagus (a precancerous lesion of the lower esophagus). The diagnosis is often missed because clinicians frequently fail to ask about ruminative behavior, and patients rarely volunteer the history.

There is no evidence that pancreatitis is caused by AN or BN per se, but pancreatitis is more common in both groups who use alcohol to excess (Morris, Stephenson, Herring, & Marti, 2004). More importantly, the diagnosis of pancreatitis may be missed because its symptoms may be confused with the nonspecific abdominal symptoms seen in AN and BN. Although fractionated amylase may be slightly increased with purging, serum amylase is usually much higher in pancreatitis. Ultrasound can help confirm pancreatitis by demonstrating pancreatic inflammation (fluid within the pancreas). Routine treatment of pancreatitis is indicated including transfer to a medicine unit, rest, nasogastric suction, taking in nothing by mouth, intravenous saline, as well thiamine administration.

Cardiovascular Problems

Cardiac abnormalities can occur in patients with either AN or BN, and indeed do commonly occur in those with AN. Indeed, AN has the highest mortality rate of any psychiatric disorder (Roche et al., 2005). Initially, there were concerns that patients with AN were dying as a result of myocardial infarction due to elevated cholesterol levels and atherosclerosis. However, autopsy studies, published over 20 years ago, did not reveal evidence of obstructive coronary disease (Isner, Roberts, Heymsfield, & Yager, 1985).

Studies then focused on QT interval prolongation as an etiology, since this predisposes patients to *torsade de pointes*, a serious, life-threatening, ventricular arrhythmia that can degenerate into fatal ventricular tachycardia and fibrillation. Studies subsequently have documented QT interval prolongation in severe AN (Cooke et al., 1994)—not, however, consistently (Facchini et al., 2006). Current thinking is that the QT interval may not be inherently prolonged in AN, nor is it independently the cause of sudden death in these patients. Thus, if the QT interval is found to be prolonged in a patient with AN, it should prompt a search for potential independent contributing causes such as electrolyte disturbances involving potassium or magnesium or congenital long-QT syndrome.

Another marker of increased arrhythmic risk in patients with AN is QT dispersion. This condition is defined by interlead variation in the QT segment length on a routine 12-lead electrocardiogram (EKG). QT dispersion reflects heterogeneous ventricular depolarization and may indicate a heightened propensity for the development of serious ventricular arrhythmias (Krantz, Donahoo, Melanson, & Mehler, 2005). Increased QT dispersion has been found in young women with AN before refeeding (Mont et al., 2003). Patients with AN may have a twofold or greater increase in QT dispersion, which correlates with the severity of their weight loss and reduced metabolic rate. Measuring QT dispersion is a widely available and inexpensive procedure and may provide information on both metabolic status and arrhythmia potential. QT dispersion normalizes with refeeding.

With substantial weight loss there is a concomitant skeletal and cardiac muscle shrinkage, specifically, a reduction in cardiac chamber volumes and a decrease in cardiac mass and cardiac output. A state of reduced exercise capacity, an attenuated blood pressure response to exercise, and subjective fatigue result from the shrinkage and thinning of the cardiac muscle cells and the decreased cardiac output. These abnormalities improve with weight gain and generally normalize with clinical recovery. Most of these changes become significant only once the patient is below 20% of ideal body weight (Olivares et al., 2005).

Two of the most prominent and consistent findings seen in patients with AN are bradycardia (heart rates less then 60 beats per minute) and hypotension (defined as a systolic blood pressure less than 90 mm Hg and/or a diastolic blood pressure less than 50 mm Hg).

The progressive bradycardia seen with increasing severity of AN has been an area of scientific inquiry with regard to the influence of the parasympathetic and sympathetic nervous systems on cardiac function. Some studies have shown a marked reduction in both parasympathetic and sympathetic tone (e.g., Rechlin, Weis, Ott, Bleichner, & Joraschky, 1998), whereas others have found an increase in parasympathetic activity with unchanged sympathetic tone (Galetta et al., 2003). This increased parasympathetic tone is the accepted prevailing explanation for the bradycardia commonly seen with AN.

The bradycardia of AN generally increases into the normal range of 60–90 beats per minute with weight restoration to a level greater than 80% of ideal body weight, or once a stable pattern of nutritional replenishment and progressive weight gain ensues (Shamim, Golden, Arden, Filiberto, & Shenker, 2003). However, although clinicians might find comfort in a "normal" heart rate, it is worth noting that a "relative tachycardia" (pulse of 70–100) in a patient with moderate to severe AN may actually have more sinister implications (Derman & Szabo, 2006). Indeed because the bradycardia of AN is such a constant finding in nutritionally deplete patients with AN, these "normal" heart rates, even if not strictly in the elevated range (pulse > 100), are likely due to medication side effects, anxiety, or an impending medical complication and should be viewed as a warning sign in need of further evaluation, particularly for the refeeding syndrome discussed later (Krantz & Mehler, 2004).

An additional sequelae of the aforementioned state of abnormal autonomic nervous system function found in patients with AN is diminished heart rate variability. Emerging data demonstrate lower heart rate variability in AN (Melanson, Donahoo, Krantz, Poirier, & Mehler, 2004). This reduced heart rate variability is a known predictor of sudden death in patients who have the kind of heart failure seen in coronary artery disease.

An important clinical dilemma is what degree of bradycardia necessitates treatment on an intensive care unit or telemetry-based cardiac monitoring? There is general agreement that a heart rate of less than 30 beats per minute mandates hospital admission and, at minimum, telemetry monitoring. Some treatment facilities extend this practice to any patient with AN with a heart rate less than 40 beats per minute. Certainly the presence of any cardiac rhythm other than sinus bradycardia, or a heart rate between 30 and 40 beats per minute and hypotension or symptoms of lightheadedness, mandate formal cardiac monitoring. Marked orthostatic hypotension, with an increase in pulse of 20 beats per minute or a drop in blood pressure of 20 mm Hg upon standing, may also be indicative of the need for acute care hospitalization (Yager et al., 2006).

Cardiac complications are usually rare in those with BN. Palpitations are often due to a sinus tachycardia (normal increase in heart rate) in response to purging. Hypokalemia, hypomagnesaemia, and dehydration can also cause palpitations. Any associated cause (e.g., hypokalemia) should be treated. Cardiology consultation should be sought if palpitations continue despite correction of deficiencies and volume depletion, or if they are associated with chest pain, shortness of breath, dizziness, or loss of consciousness.

Other fluid and electrolyte abnormalities also occur in both AN and BN patients. Most commonly seen are hypochloremia, hypokalemia, and metabolic alkalosis (because of volume contraction). In terms of the management of fluid and electrolyte abnormalities, one should expand the intravascular fluid with saline. If the patient is an outpatient, use salt-containing liquids such as salt cubes in water or chicken broth. Begin with three cups a day and increase as needed. Assess response by an increase in urine output associated with lighter-colored urine and by increased jugular venous pressure and absence of postural change in heart rate and blood pressure on physical examination. If the patient is hospitalized, use intravenous normal saline, but caution must be exercised due to a propensity toward edema formation as a manifestation of pseudo-Bartter's syndrome and high aldosterone levels from the volume contraction.

On occasion the patient with AN will complain of chest pain. The organic cardiac cause for chest pain in these patients is due to the presence of mitral valve prolapse, which may be seen in 30–50% of patients with severe AN. This syndrome is defined by prolapse of the mitral valve due to the heart muscle decreasing in size with weight loss, while the structural supporting tissues that comprise the mitral valve do not decrease in size (Johnson, Humphries, Shirley, Mazzoleni, & Noonan, 1986). Often a systolic murmur and "click" are heard when a cardiac examination is performed on a patient with mitral valve prolapse, but there are no associated EKG findings.

Refeeding Syndrome

The refeeding syndrome is a multifactorial metabolic complication that can develop early in refeeding significantly malnourished patients during the early phase of nutritional replenishment. The risk of the refeeding syndrome is directly correlated with the degree of weight loss that has occurred as a result of the AN. Thus, it is self-evident why those patients who are more than 30% below their ideal body weight (IBW) should be initially refed during an inpatient hospitalization (Bermudez & Beightol, 2004; Solomon & Kirby, 1990).

The mechanism of the potential cardiovascular collapse that occurs with the refeeding syndrome is multifactorial. First, the reduced heart mass that accompanies weight loss makes it difficult for the heart to handle the increase in total circulatory blood volume seen with refeeding. Even though the heart mass does revert toward normal with weight gain, the first few weeks of refeeding require close attention to a patient's cardiovascular status until this normalization process has occurred.

Changes in serum levels of phosphorus as well as potassium and magnesium are important in the refeeding syndrome. Low phosphorus levels, hypophosphatemia, develop during refeeding due to the glucose content of the food substrate. The glucose load increases insulin release, which in turn produces shifts of phosphate and potassium into the intracellular space. There is also an incorporation of phosphate into newly synthesized tissues during refeeding. The resultant low phosphate levels are accompanied by depletion of the high-energy chemical adenosine triphosphate (ATP), which impairs the contractile properties of the heart and can evolve into congestive heart failure. Other sequealae of refeeding-induced hypophosphatemia include red and white blood cell dysfunction, skeletal muscle breakdown (rhabdomyolysis), and seizures. Rhabdomyolysis is diagnosed in response to an abnormally high level of the muscle enzyme creatinine phosphokinase (CPK). Low levels of serum potassium and magnesium can also cause cardiac irritability and arrhythmias along with skeletal muscle weakness.

From a clinical standpoint, rates of weight gain greater than 2–3 pounds per week are usually not nutritionally sound. Aside from this numeric guide to weight gain, there are clinical parameters that are worthy of being followed closely. Specifically, vital signs contribute useful daily information. Individuals with AN generally are bradycardic (heart rate < 60 beats/minute). Although there are other potential reasons for tachycardia (heart rate > 100 beats/minute), the presence of an elevated heart rate, even if just in the 80–90 range, during refeeding can be a harbinger of the refeeding syndrome as discussed previously. In addition, patients with AN should be examined for the presence of edema in the ankle and shin areas during early refeeding.

Endocrine Problems

All major endocrine functions are dysregulated in AN. Such changes, if seen, are usually more modest in those with BN. One endocrine system that is profoundly altered in AN and commonly altered as well in BN is the reproductive system. The neuroendocrine regulation of normal female reproductive functions depends on a rhythm of nerve impulses, generated within the medial basal hypothalamus, which governs the pulsatile release of gonadotropin-releasing hormone (GnRH) from nerve terminals. Pulsatile GnRH release is the central controller of pituitary luteinizing hormone (LH) and follicle-stimulating hormone (FSH) secretion, which determine the timely onset of normal menstrual function (Doufas & Mastorakos, 2000). At puberty, there is normally an increase in both the frequency and amplitude of GnRH that induces LH–FSH secretion. Patients with AN have a characteristic "hypothalamic amenorrhea syndrome" with a variable reduction in pulsatile hypothalamic GnRH gonadostat signaling to the pituitary gland, resulting in a failure of ovulation.

In patients with AN, 20–25% may actually experience amenorrhea before the onset of significant weight loss, and 50–75% will experience amenorrhea during the course of dieting and weight loss (Katz & Volenhoven, 2000). In some patients with AN, amenorrhea occurs only after more marked weight loss. Menstrual irregularities are also common in BN, albeit much less severe and less prevalent than in AN (Gendall, Bulik, Joyce, McIntosh, & Carter, 2000). Upon restoring weight toward normal in those with AN, many patients will experience a resumption of their normal menstrual cycle. This relationship was more recently confirmed in a study demonstrating that menses can be expected to resume in many patients with AN at a weight approximately 90% of IBW (Golden et al., 1997). Other studies have found the weight requirement for resumption of menses to be more variable and better predicted by the weight at which menstruation ceases (Sweene, 2004). Thus, a critical weight may be necessary, but not sufficient, for menstrual function, and other factors may also be important (Gendall et al., 2006). In terms of treatment, efforts should be directed toward overall treatment of the ED, since there may be little inherent value in the actual administration of female sex hormones to patients with AN.

The thyroid abnormalities in individuals with AN resemble those of the "euthyroid sick syndrome," wherein total thyroxine (T4) and triiodothyronine (T3) levels are low. However, levels of thyroid-stimulating hormone (TSH) usually remain in the normal range (Mehler, 2001). Levels of T3 usually decrease in proportion to the degree of weight loss. Total T4 levels are low because it is preferentially converted to a biologically inactive reverse T3. As is true in the euthyroid sick syndrome, thyroid hormone replacement is not beneficial and is not indicated. Thyroid function is usually normal in those with BN.

Osteoporosis is a disease characterized by low bone mass and deterioration of the microarchitectual structure of bone, resulting in bone fragility and the clinical syndrome of nontraumatic fractures as a direct result of this low bone mass. Osteoporosis is quantitatively defined by bone densitometry measurements, using dual-energy X-ray absorptiometry (DEXA), as a z-score greater than a –2.5 standard deviation decrement from young bone mass. A loss of bone mass with a z-score from –1 to –2.5 standard deviations is classified as osteopenia. Peak bone mass is defined as the highest level of bone mass achieved as a result of normal growth. The majority of skeletal bone growth occurs during childhood and adolescence. The timing of peak bone mass may vary, but generally occurs between ages 17 and 22, a time that unfortunately frequently correlates with the onset of AN. Rapid bone loss, at an annual average rate of 2.5%, occurs in young women with osteoporosis. Osteoporosis is present in almost 40% of patients with AN, and osteopenia is present in 92% of these women (Grinspoon et al.,

2000). Trabecular bone, found in the lumbar spine and hips, is more affected than cortical bone.

There is emerging evidence suggesting that loss of bone mineral density appears to be rapid and occurs relatively early in the disease. Some studies suggest an illness duration longer than 12 months predicts significant loss of bone mineral (Wong, Lewindon, Mortimer, & Shepherd, 2001), but a severe degree of demineralization has been reported in adolescents with just a brief duration of illness. In a study of 73 young women with AN, with a mean age of 17.2 years, 20 months of amenorrhea was found to be the threshold above which the most severe osteopenia was seen (Audi et al., 2002). Therefore, DEXA should be established as an important screening tool for all patients with AN and disease duration greater than 6–12 months to determine the degree of reduction in bone mineral density.

Supplemental estrogen, either in the form of hormonal replacement therapy or as oral contraceptives, is often prescribed in routine practice for patients with AN in an effort to minimize or ameliorate osteopenia or osteoporosis. Recent surveys indicate that this practice is followed 75–80% of the time by practitioners caring for females with AN. In reality, however, there is a distinct paucity of credible evidence supporting this practice.

Another approach is anabolic therapy, in which bone formation is directly stimulated. Dehydroepiandrosterone (DHEA) has not been shown to be effective in improving bone mineral density, even though it is thought to function as an anabolic factor for bone by increasing levels of insulin growth factor (IGF-1) and by stimulation of osteoblast function. There are currently no data from rigorous scientific trials regarding other anabolic agents such as fluoride or the recently released parathyroid hormone medication, teriparatide.

In view of the less than favorable effects of commonly used therapeutic modalities for the bone disease of AN, there has recently been interest in the use of bisphosphonates. Past reticency was predicated on concerns about the safety of these agents in women of reproductive age. Bisphosphonates carry a category C rating for safety in pregnancy because they can persist in the body for many years after the discontinuation of treatment, and there is only anecdotal information about their safety during fetal development; thus the long-term implications for women of childbearing age are of concern.

The first study to demonstrate their potential effectiveness was a closely monitored study of 10 women with AN who received 5 mg of risedronate and had 6- and 9-month bone mineral density measurements. Bone mineral density increased substantially in the spine of those patients who received risedronate (4.1% at 6 months) in contrast with bone loss in the controls, despite weight gain (Miller et al., 2004). A 5% increase in bone mass over a 3-year period is generally deemed clinically significant and is associated with a 25% reduction in fracture risk. The following year a randomized, double-blind, placebo-controlled pilot study of alendronate in 32 osteopenic patients with AN was completed. Although the spine and hip bone mineral density increased in both the treatment and the control groups, percent of increase did not differ significantly between groups.

Currently bisphosphonates should not be used routinely in patients with AN until further research defines their long-term safety and efficacy. However, they might be considered for severe osteoporosis, especially when the disease is unlikely to revert in the near future.

Some research has shown an increased risk for the development of an ED in individuals diagnosed with Type I diabetes mellitus (Crow, Keel, & Kendall, 1989). A recent meta-analysis concluded that the rate of BN was significantly higher than in controls but that the rate of AN, although numerically higher, was not significantly different (Mannucci, Rotella, Ricca, et al., 2005). Affected individuals are characterized as having poor metabolic control. In a study involving 109 patients, Takii, Uchigate, Tokunaga, and colleagues (2008) demonstrated that the duration of insulin omission was the factor most closely associated with the development of retinopathy and nephropathy.

Peveler and colleagues (2005) interviewed 87 patients who had been interviewed at baseline, between ages 11 and 25, who were recontacted after 8–12 years. Thirteen individuals met criteria at baseline for an ED, and 31 (35.6%) misused insulin for weight control purposes. This literature suggests that disordered eating and EDs complicate the management of diabetes significantly.

Neurological Problems

Neurological abnormalities have been described in patients with AN. On computer tomography (CT) or magnetic resonance imaging (MRI) scanning, patients with AN often show evidence of cerebral atrophy with ventricular enlargement (Herholz, 1996), a condition often referred to as "pseudoatrophy." Although extremely rare, there have also been reports of Wernicke's encephalopathy in patients with AN (Peters, Parvin, Petersen, Faircloth, & Levine, 2007).

Renal Problems

Patients with AN may demonstrate a reduction in glomerular filtration rate and problems concentrating their urine (Boag, Weerakoon, Ginsburg, Havard, & Dandona, 1985; Lowinger, Griffiths, Beumont, Scicluna, & Touyz, 1999). Of particular concern, however, is literature suggesting that some patients with AN eventually develop chronic renal disease (Herzog, Deter, Fiehn, & Petzold, 1997). This possibility appears to be particularly likely in patients with long-standing illness (Takakura et al., 2006).

Binge-Eating Disorder

BED has not clearly been associated with medical complications arising directly from binge-eating symptoms. Rather, for the most part the complications of BED are conceived of as relating to the obesity that often accompanies it (Grucza, Przybeck, Thomas, & Cloninger, 2007; Telch & Agras, 1994). On the other hand, it is not clear that this relationship has been adequately explored. Only a limited number of studies has examined the relationship between medical complications and BED, and subjects with various medical problems are commonly excluded from BED treatment studies. Two critically important questions remain unanswered: (1) Does having BED confer risk for medical problems above and beyond that associated with a given level of obesity? (2) When BED is present, and when other medical complications are already present, does having BED impact the outcome of those coexisting medical problems? We address each of these questions in turn.

BED and Risk for Medical Complications

Several studies have examined the association between BED and medical problems. Johnson, Spitzer, and Williams (2001) examined a variety of psychiatric and physical illnesses among approximately 5,000 female subjects in primary care settings in a cross-sectional study. BED became increasingly common in this group as subjects became older. Diabetes mellitus was more commonly reported in those with BED (as well as BN, which was also studied) than in those without BED, and overall levels of health problems were higher in the participants with BED compared to those without.

Two studies have examined the same question using data from twin study registries. In the first (Bulik, Sullivan, Kendler, 2002) participants with obesity were separated by the presence or absence of binge eating (59 with binge eating, 107 without). Those with binge eating reported higher levels of health dissatisfaction (30.5% vs. 15%), and they also reported higher rates of hypertension, visual impairment, asthma or respiratory illness, cardiac problems, osteoporosis, and "any major medical disorder." However, none of these differences reached statistical significance, perhaps due to the limited sample size. A second study examined similar questions in roughly 8,000 Norwegian twin registry participants ages 18–45 (Reichborn-Kjennerud, Bulik, Sullivan, Tambs, & Harris, 2004). This sample identified a relatively high 6-month prevalence of binge-eating behavior (5.2% among women, 3.8% among males). Males with binge eating were more likely to report pain symptoms, including neck and shoulder pain, low back pain, chronic muscular pain, and also were more likely to report impairment due to physical health problems within the last month. Each of these differences was statistically significant after adjusting for body mass index (BMI). Among female participants, rates of these medical problems were similar, but the differences were not significant after adjusting for BMI.

Finally, one study examined gastrointestinal symptoms in people with binge eating (Crowell, Cheskin, & Musial, 1994). This study examined 119 obese subjects and 77 normal-weight control subjects, all female, categorized as those reporting binge eating and those without binge eating. A variety of both upper and lower gastrointestinal symptoms were more common among those reporting binge eating than in those not reporting binge eating, with the highest rates occurring in those who were both obese and reported binge eating.

Thus, in summary, there is some evidence to suggest that a variety of physical health complaints are more common in individuals with BED than in similarly obese individuals without binge eating.

BED and the Course of Other Medical Problems

One can imagine several situations in which having BED could directly impact the course of medical problems. One of the best examples is Type II diabetes mellitus. There is conflicting evidence regarding whether BED increases the risk for Type II diabetes, with evidence for BED prevalence rates in Type II diabetics as high as 25% (Crow, Kendall, Seaquist, Praus, & Thuras, 2001) and as low as 1.4% (Allison et al., 2007). The second of these studies, the largest study to date, examined the rate of BED among participants in the Look AHEAD treatment study of Type II diabetics. It is somewhat unclear why the observed rates were so much lower in this study than in other previous studies. One possible explanation is that the participants in Look AHEAD were substantially older than those in the previous studies, and perhaps individuals without current binge eating in this study might have experienced it at a younger age. Also of note is work indicating that in those with binge eating who have Type II diabetes, the binge eating usually develops earlier (Herpertz et al., 2000, 2001).

Another critical question is whether having BED impacts glycemic control or diabetic complications. There is evidence to suggest this is true for other kinds of disordered eating in those with Type I diabetes (Rydall, Rodin, Olmsted, Devenyi, & Daneman, 1997). In studies comparing hemoglobin A1C in those with Type II diabetes with and without binge eating or BED, however, no differences in glycemic control were found (Crow et al., 2001; Herpertz et al., 2000; Wing, Marcus, Epstein, Blair, & Burton, 1989). Also of relevance is a study by Kenardy, Mensch, Bowen, Green, and Walton (2001) reporting in a randomized trial for binge eating in Type II patients that reduced binge eating results in improved glycemic control.

Two additional factors tend to complicate such relationships. Just as there is evidence to suggest that depression increases risk for developing problems such as heart disease and hypertension, there is now much evidence suggesting that the presence of depression influences outcome in heart disease (e.g., Frasure-Smith & Lésperance, 2008) and perhaps Type I diabetes mellitus as well (Hassan, Loar, Anderson, & Heptulla, 2006; Roy, Roy, & Affouf, 2007). Because depression co-occurs with BED so often, disentangling causal relationships is a challenge. A second complicating factor is the issue of obesity. The impact of obesity on glycemic control in a wide variety of other medical problems is significant, and attempts to examine this relationship will have to control carefully for BMI.

Summary

EDs are frequently complicated by medical abnormalities. Medical assessment is necessary at the onset of the evaluation process, and periodic reassessment is often necessary as well. A clinician knowledgeable about these medical issues should be part of the assessment treatment team.

References

Allison KC, Crow SJ, Reeves RR, West DS, Foreyt JP, Dilillo VG, et al. Binge eating disorder and night eating syndrome in adults with type 2 diabetes. *Obesity (Silver Spring)*, 15:1287–1293.

Attri N, Ravipati M, Agrawal P, Healy C, & Feller A. (2008). Rumination syndrome: An emerging case scenario. *Southern Medical Journal*, 101:432–435.

Audi L, Vargas DM, Gussinye M, Yeste D, Marti G, & Carrascosa A. (2002). Clinical and biochemical determinants of bone metabolism and bone mass in adolescent female patient with anorexia nervosa. *Pediatric Research*, 51:497–504.

Bermudez O, & Beightol S. (2004). What is refeeding syndrome? *Eating Disorders*, 12:251–256.

Boag F, Weerakoon J, Ginsburg J, Havard CW, & Dandona P. (1985). Diminished creatinine clearance in anorexia nervosa: Reversal with weight gain. *Journal of Clinical Pathology*, 38:60–63.

Bulik CM, Sullivan PF, & Kendler KS. (2002). Medical and psychiatric morbidity in obese women with and without binge eating. *International Journal of Eating Disorders*, 32:72–78.

Cooke RA, Chambers JB, Singh R, Todd GJ, Smeeton NC, Treasure J, et al. (1994). QT interval in anorexia nervosa. *British Heart Journal*, 72:69–73.

Crow A, Keel PK, & Kendall D. (1989). Eating disorders and insulin dependent diabetes mellitus: A review. *Psychosomatics*, 39:233–243.

Crow SJ, Kendall K, Seaquist E, Praus B, & Thuras P. (2001). Binge eating and other psychopathology in Type II diabetes mellitus. *Intetnational Journal Eating Disorders*, 30:222–226.

Crowell MD, Cheskin LJ, & Musial F. (1994). Prevalence of gastrointestinal symptoms in obese and normal weight binge eaters. *American Journal of Gastroentrology*, 89:387–391.

Derman T, & Szabo CP. (2006). Why do individuals with anorexia nervosa die?: A case of sudden death. *International Journal of Eating Disorders*, 39:260–262.

Doufas AG, & Mastorakos G. The hypothalamic–pituitary–thyroid axis and the female reproductive system. *Annals of New York Academy Science*, 960:65–76.

Facchini M, Sala L, Malfatt G, Bragato R, Redaelli G, & Invitti C. (2006). Low k+ dependent QT prolongation and risk for ventricular arrhythmias in anorexia nervosa. *International Journal of Cardiology*, 106:170–176.

Frasure-Smith N, & Lespérance F. (2008). Depression and anxiety as predictors of two-year cardiac events in patients with stable coronary artery disease. *Archives of General Psychiatry*, 65(1):62–71.

Galetta F, Franzoni F, Prattichizzo F, Rolla M, Santoro G, & Pentimone F. (2003). Heart rate variability and left ventricular diastolic function in anorexia nervosa. *Journal of Adolescent Health*, 32:416–421.

Gendall KA, Bulik CM, Joyce PR, McIntosh VV, & Carter FA. (2000). Menstrual cycle irregularity in bulimia nervosa. *Journal of Psychosomatic Research*, 49:409–415.

Gendall KA, Joyce PR, Carter FA, McIntosh VV, Jordan J, & Bulik CM. (2006). The psychobiology and diagnostic significance of amenorrhea in patients with anorexia nervosa. *Fertility and Sterility*, 85:1531–1535.

Golden NH, Jacobson MS, Schebendach J, Solanto MV, Hertz SM, & Shenker IR. (1997). Resumption of menses in anorexia nervosa. *Archives of Pediatrics and Adolescent Medicine*, 151:16–21.

Grinspoon S, Thom E, Pitts S, Gross E, Mickley D, Miller K, et al. (2000). Prevalence and predictive factors for regional osteopenia in women with anorexia nervosa. *Annals of Internal Medicine*, 133:790–794.

Grucza RA, Przybeck, Thomas R, & Cloninger CR. (2007). Prevalence and correlates of binge eating disorder in a community sample. *Comparative Psychiatry*, 48:124–131.

Hassan K, Loar R, Anderson BJ, & Heptulla RA. (2006). The role of socioeconomic status, depression, quality of life, and glycemic control in Type 1 diabetes mellitus. *Journal of Pediatrics*, 149:526–531.

Herholz K. (1996). Neuroimaging in anorexia nervosa. *Psychiatry Research*, 62:105–110.

Herpertz S, Albus C, Kielmann R, Hagemann-Patt H, Lichtblau K, Köhle K, et al. (2001). Comorbidity of diabetes mellitus and eating disorders: A follow-up study. *Journal of Psychosomatic Research*, 51:673–678.

Herpertz S, Albus C, Lichtblau K, Kohle K, Mann K, & Senf W. (2000). Relationship of weight and eating disorders in Type 2 diabetic patients: A multicenter study. *International Journal of Eating Disorders*, 28:68–77.

Herzog W, Deter HC, Fiehn W, & Petzold E. (1997). Medical findings and predictors of long-term physical outcome in anorexia nervosa: A prospective, 12-year follow-up study. *Psychological Medicine*, 27:269–279.

Isner JM, Roberts WC, Heymsfield SB, & Yager J. (1985). AN and sudden death. *Annals of Internal Medicine*, 102:49–52.

Johnson GL, Humphries LL, Shirley PB, Mazzoleni A, & Noonan JA. (1986). Mitral valve prolapse in patients with AN and bulimia. *Archives of Internal Medicine*, 146:1525–1529.

Johnson JG, Spitzer RL, & Williams JB. (2001). Health problems, impairment and illnesses associated with bulimia nervosa and binge eating disorder among primary care and obstetric
gynecology patients. *Psychological Medicine*, 31:1455–1466.

Kamel N, Chami T, Andersen A, Rosell FA, Schuster MM, & Whitehead WE. (1991). Delayed gastrointestinal transit times in AN and bulimia nervosa. *Gastroenterology*, 1011:11320–11324.

Katz M, & Volenhoven B. (2000). The reproductive consequences of anorexia nervosa. *BJOG: An
International Journal of Obstetrics and Gynaecology*, 107:707–713.

Kenardy J, Mensch M, Bowen K, Green B, & Walton J. (2002). Group therapy for binge eating in
Type 2 diabetes: A randomized trial. *Diabetic Medicine*, 19:234–239.

Krantz MJ, Donahoo WT, Melanson EL, & Mehler PS. (2005). QT interval dispersion and resting metabolic rate in chronic anorexia nervosa. *International Journal of Eating Disorders*,
37:166–170.

Krantz MJ, & Mehler PS. (2004). Resting tachycardia, a warning sign in anorexia nervosa: case
report. *BMC Cardiovascular Disorders*, 4:10.

Lo Russo L, Campisi G, De Fede O, Di Liberto C, Panzarella V, & Lo Muzio L. (2008). Oral
manifestations of eating disorders: A critical review. *Oral Diseases*, 14:479–484.

Lowinger K, Griffiths RA, Beumont PJ, Scicluna H, & Touyz SW. (1999). Fluid restriction in
anorexia nervosa: A neglected symptom or new phenomenon? *International Journal of Eating
Disorders*, 26:392–396.

Mannucci E, Rotella F, Ricca V, Moretti S, Placidi GF, & Rotella CM. (2005). Eating disorders
in patients with Type 1 diabetes: A meta-analysis. *Journal of Endocrinological Investigation*,
28:417–419.

Mehler PS. (2001). AN in primary care. *Annals of Internal Medicine*, 134:1048–1059.

Melanson EL, Donahoo WT, Krantz MH, Poirier P, & Mehler PS. (2004). Resting and ambu-
latory heart rate variability in chronic anorexia nervosa. *American Journal of Cardiology*,
94:1217–1220.

Merrett ND, Wilson RB, Cosman P, & Biankin AV. (2008). Superior mesenteric artery syndrome:
diagnosis and treatment strategies. *Journal of Gastrointestinal Surgery*, 13(2):287–292.

Miller K, Grieco KA, Mulder J, Grinspoon S, Mickley D, Yehezkel R, et al. (2004). Effects of risedronate on bone density in anorexia nervosa. *Journal of Clinical Endocrinology and Metabolism*, 89:3903–3906.

Milosevic A, Brodie DA, & Slade PD. (1997). Dental erosion, oral hygiene, and nutrition in eating disorders. *International Journal of Eating Disorders*, 21:195–199.

Mont L, Castro J, Herreros B, Pare C, Azqueta M, Magrina J, et al. (2003). Reversibility of cardiac abnormalities in adolescents with anorexia nervosa after weight recovery. *Journal of the
American Academy of Child and Adolescent Psychiatry*, 42:808–813.

Morris LG, Stephenson KE, Herring S, & Marti JL. (2004). Recurrent acute pancreatic in
anorexia and bulimia. *Journal of the Pancreas*, 5:231–234.

Nogou A, & Suter M. (2008). Almost routine prophylactic cholecystectomy during laparoscopic
gastric bypass is safe. *Obesity Surgery*, 18:535–539.

Olivares JL, Vazquez M, Fleta J, Morena LA, Perez-Gonzalez JM, & Bueno M. (2005). Cardiac
findings in adolescents with AN at diagnosis and after weight restoration. *European Journal
of Pediatrics*, 164:383–386.

Overby KJ, & Litt IF. (1988). Mediastinal emphysema in an adolescent with anorexia nervosa
and self-induced emesis. *Pediatrics*, 81:134–136.

Peters TE, Parvin M, Petersen C, Faircloth VC, & Levine RL. (2007). A case report of Wernicke's
encephalopathy in a pediatric patient with anorexia nervosa—restricting type. *Journal of
Adolescent Health*, 40:376–383.

Peveler RC, Bryden KS, Neil HA, Fairburn CG, Mayou RA, Dunger DB, et al. (2005). The relationship of disordered eating habits and attitudes to clinical outcomes in young adult females with Type 1 diabetes. *Diabetes Care*, 28:84–88.

Pomeroy C, Mitchell JE, Roerig J, & Crow S. (2002). *Medical complications of psychiatric illness*. Washington, DC: American Psychiatric Association.

Rechlin T, Weis M, Ott C, Bleichner F, & Joraschky P. (1998). Alterations of autonomic cardiac control in anorexia nervosa. *Biological Psychiatry*, 43:358–363.

Reichborn-Kjennerud T, Bulik CM, Sullivan PF, Tambs K, & Harris JR. (2004). Psychiatric and medical symptoms in binge eating in the absence of compensatory behaviors. *Obesity Research*, 12:1445–1454.

Roche F, Barthelemy JC, Mayaud N, Pichot V, Duverney D, German N, et al. (2005). Refeeding normalizes the QT rate dependence of female anorexic patients. *American Journal of Cardiology*, 95:277–280.

Roy MS, Roy A, & Affouf M. (2007). Depression is a risk factor for poor glycemic control and retinopathy in African-Americans with Type 1 diabetes. *Psychosomatic Medicine*, 69:537–542.

Rydall AC, Rodin GM, Olmsted MP, Devenyi RG, & Daneman D. (1997). Disordered eating behavior and microvascular complications in young women with insulin-dependent diabetes mellitus. *New England Journal of Medicine*, 336:1849–1854.

Shamim T, Golden NH, Arden M, Filiberto L, & Shenker IR. (2003). Resolution of vital sign instability: An objective measure of medical stability in anorexia nervosa. *Journal of Adolescent Health*, 32:73–77.

Solomon SM, & Kirby DF. (1990). The refeeding syndrome: A review. *Journal of Parenteral and Enteral Nutrition*, 14:90–97.

Sweene, I. (2004). Weight requirements for return of menstruation in teenage girls with eating disorders, weight loss and secondary amenorrhea. *Acta Pedatrica*, 93:1449–1455.

Takakura S, Nozaki T, Nomura Y, Koreeda C, Urabe H, Kawai K, et al. (2006). Factors related to renal dysfunction in patients with anorexia nervosa. *Eating and Weight Disorders*, 11:73–77.

Takii M, Uchigata Y, Tokunaga S, Amemiya N, Kinukawa N, Nozaki T, et al. (2008). The duration of severe insulin omission is the factor most closely associated with the microvascular complications of Type 1 diabetic females with clinical eating disorders. *International Journal of Eating Disorders*, 41:259–264.

Telch CF, & Agras WS. (1994). Obesity, binge eating and psychopathology: are they related? *International Journal of Eating Disorders*, 15:53–61.

Weinstein HD, & Halabis JS. (1986). Subconjunctival hemorrhage in bulimia. *Journal of the American Optometric Association*, 57:366–367.

Wing RR, Marcus MD, Epstein LH, Blair EH, & Burton LR. (1989). Binge eating in obese patients with type II diabetes. *International Journal of Eating Disorders*, 8:671–679.

Wong JC, Lewindon P, Mortimer R, & Shepherd R. (2001). Bone mineral density in adolescent females with recently diagnosed anorexia nervosa. *International Journal of Eating Disorders*, 29:11–16.

Yager J, & Andersen AE. (2008). Clinical practice: Anorexia nervosa. *New England Journal of Medicine*, 353:1481–1488.

Yager J, Devlin MJ, Halmi KA, Herzog DB, Mitchell JE, Powers P, et al. (2006). American Psychiatric Association practice guidelines for the treatment of patients with eating disorders. *American Journal of Psychiatry*, 160:1–128.

PART II

Treatment of Anorexia Nervosa

This section of the book details what is known concerning the available treatments for patients with anorexia nervosa (AN). The first four treatment chapters include "mini-manuals," so that the reader can study how the treatments are actually administered in detail and see the specific techniques involved. The remaining chapters cover additional treatment methods (pharmacotherapy), treatment components (nutrition), and intensive multidisciplinary approaches (inpatient and day hospital). This section also includes two chapters devoted to special topics (compulsory treatment and understanding chronicity) that reflect unique challenges posed by severely disturbed patients with AN.

Chapter 5, by Kathleen M. Pike, Jacqueline C. Carter, and Marion P. Olmsted, describes in detail cognitive-behavioral therapy (CBT) for patients with AN. This approach was originally used in a randomized trial at Columbia University to examine its effectiveness as a relapse prevention strategy, compared to nutritional counseling, although some modifications have been made to it since that time. CBT, adapted to varying degrees, is often used as a core component at many specialized treatment centers for AN.

Chapter 6, by Virginia V. W. McIntosh, Jennifer Jordan, and Cynthia M. Bulik, describes a specialist supportive clinical management approach to the treatment of patients with AN. Their initial controlled trial found that this approach was more effective than two comparison treatments (that have demonstrated efficacy for bulimia nervosa) in the short term, although in longer term follow-up the superiority was not maintained. However, the acceptability of this treatment to patients with AN was quite high, and clinicians can profit by studying the mini-manual here in detail for ideas regarding how to engage these challenging patients.

In Chapter 7, Kate Tchanturia and David Hambrook describe an approach to help remediate some of the cognitive abnormalities present in patients with AN. This very interesting new development in our field is based on neuropsychological test findings and follows promising initial applications with other disorders. The details of this approach, which is offered as a method to facilitate or enhance patients' abilities to benefit from other therapies, are explained effectively.

Chapter 8, by Ivan Eisler, James Lock, and Daniel le Grange, describes the theory and methods of a specific family-based approach that is often referred to as the "Maudsley method," because it was originally developed at the Maudsley Hospital in London. Although the data on this approach are still limited, studies using it—and the publication of the manual in book form—have been two of the most exciting developments in the treatment of those with AN in recent years.

Next is a chapter reviewing pharmacotherapy for patients with AN, by Allan S. Kaplan and Andrew Howlett. As will be seen, there are some interesting new developments in this area, but overall pharmacotherapy appears to have a very limited role in the treatment of patients with AN—and the actual resistance of these patients to drug treatment is both surprising and frustrating. This limited role makes AN unusual among psychiatric disorders.

Cheryl L. Rock then reviews nutritional rehabilitation issues in patients with AN. Nutritional rehabilitation represents a central component of treatment for AN. This chapter explores the complexities of effective refeeding and nutritional interventions necessary for safe and healthy weight restoration.

Marion P. Olmsted, Traci L. McFarlane, Jacqueline C. Carter, Kathryn Trottier, D. Blake Woodside, and Gina Dimitropoulos then describe special issues related to treating patients with AN in intensive inpatient and day hospital treatment programs. They describe indications for such intensive treatments and address clinical challenges regarding continuity of care across multidisciplinary treatment teams.

Stephen W. Touyz and Terry Carney provide a clearly reasoned and articulated evaluation of issues surrounding compulsory treatment of patients with AN. These issues are faced by many clinicians who work with these patients, and this chapter authoritatively covers both the clinical and legal literatures.

Part II closes with a chapter by Michael Strober, who reviews clinical issues pertaining to chronic refractory patients with AN. As clinicians know, this is an all-too-common outcome for patients with AN. Working with such chronically ill patients is particularly demanding and raises special challenges that require great skill and expert care. Strober's astute description of the phenomenology and therapeutic considerations for managing the severely ill patient with AN is essential reading for clinicians.

It would be wonderful if this section of the book were longer or contained treatments with stronger evidence bases. Unfortunately, the treatment literature on AN remains surprisingly small, and more treatment research in AN is sorely needed.

CHAPTER 5

Cognitive-Behavioral Therapy for Anorexia Nervosa

Kathleen M. Pike, Jacqueline C. Carter, and Marion P. Olmsted

This chapter describes the cognitive-behavioral approach to the treatment of anorexia nervosa (AN). Originally developed by Aaron T. Beck and colleagues (e.g., Beck, 1976; Beck, Rush, Shaw, & Emery, 1979), cognitive-behavioral therapy (CBT) has become one of the most influential and well-validated models of psychotherapy available. CBT has demonstrated efficacy for a broad range of psychiatric disorders, including depression, anxiety disorders, substance abuse, and eating disorders (EDs) (see Nathan & Gorman, 2002; Wilson, Grilo, & Vitousek, 2007).

CBT for AN has been elaborated in recent years by several authors (Fairburn, Shafran, & Cooper, 1999; Pike, Carter, & Olmsted, 2004; Pike, Devlin, & Loeb, 2004; Pike, Loeb, & Vitousek, 1996). The model has expanded and evolved as our understanding of the psychopathology of AN has progressed. Current CBT models address cognitive and behavioral disturbances linked to the core features of AN as well as more encompassing issues of temperament, character, and motivation. In this chapter we review the empirical support of CBT for AN, describe our view on the cognitive-behavioral formulation of AN, and present an abbreviated version of the most recent CBT treatment manual for AN (Pike et al., 2004).

The Cognitive-Behavioral Formulation of AN

The treatment manual presented in this chapter is based on a CBT model that views overvalued ideas about the significance of control over eating, shape, and weight as the core maintaining mechanism in AN. A central premise of the CBT model of AN is that ED symptoms are maintained by the interaction between *cognitive disturbances* involving overconcern for eating, shape, and weight and *behavioral disturbances* that affect eating and weight control behavior. Certain personality characteristics and temperament, coupled with low self-esteem, appear to predispose some individuals to internalize sociocultural ideals about the importance of thinness and the myth that achieving such ideals will mitigate feelings of low self-esteem and ineffectiveness. A dysfunctional schema that attaches primary value to control over eating, shape, and weight develops as individuals internalize these beliefs. This dysfunctional cognitive schema is expressed behaviorally by extreme weight control behaviors aimed at attaining unrealistic levels of thinness and control. For those individuals who are able to maintain the extreme dietary restriction, severe emaciation follows, resulting in AN-restricting subtype (AN-R). For many individuals, this vigilant dietary restriction is intermittently interrupted with episodes of loss of control, such that subjective overeating occurs. In response to the loss of control and the overeating, many individuals redouble their efforts and engage in various compensatory purging behaviors, resulting in AN-binge–purge subtype (AN-B-P) (or bulimia nervosa [BN]).

As the ED develops, the individual's self-concept and feelings of self-worth increasingly revolve almost exclusively around control over eating, shape, and weight. As the disorder becomes more entrenched, there is often a belief that food restriction and maintaining a low weight are the only way to experience any sense of self-esteem. The physiological and psychological effects of starvation reinforce the cognitive and behavioral disturbances. For example, the food preoccupation associated with starvation is experienced as a threat to maintaining control over eating and results in increased efforts to restrict food intake. Thus, the disorder becomes self-perpetuating.

One of the strengths of the CBT-AN model is its acknowledgment that EDs are multidetermined. Thus, in addition to the core components of the CBT-AN model described above, CBT-AN recognizes that various biological factors may contribute to increased vulnerability for the development of AN, and this possibility is addressed in the psychoeducational component of CBT-AN. Additional factors that can contribute to the etiology and maintenance of AN, such as problems with motivation for recovery, difficulties with emotion regulation, core negative beliefs, and interpersonal problems, are also often incorporated into CBT-AN, as needed.

Empirical Support of CBT for AN

The empirical database on CBT for AN is limited. However, several recent investigations provide preliminary support of the utility of CBT for AN, particularly for weight-restored individuals. Cooper and Fairburn (1984) published the first case-series report of CBT for AN with promising results. Since then only five randomized controlled studies of CBT for acute AN have been published. In the first study Channon and colleagues (1989) randomly assigned 24 adult patients with AN to either CBT, behavior therapy (BT), or an eclectic "treatment-as-usual" control condition. All treatments involved 18 sessions of individual therapy over 6 months, followed by six booster sessions over the next 6 months. Compliance with treatment was significantly better in CBT and BT as compared with the control condition. All randomized subjects were included in the analyses. No significant differences in outcome were found between the three treatment conditions. Overall, significant improvements were found in weight, nutritional status, and menstrual functioning, based on Morgan and Russell (1975) ratings in all three conditions.

In the second study, 35 adult patients with AN were randomized to either CBT or nutritional counseling for 6 months (Serfaty, Turkington, Heap, Ledsham, & Jolley, 1999). Unfortunately, the results of this study were uninterpretable because all of the participants in the nutritional counseling condition dropped out. In contrast, the attrition rate in the CBT condition was low (8%). A small but statistically significant increase in weight was observed among 87% of participants who received CBT (mean change = +1.6 body mass index [BMI] units). CBT participants also reported significant reductions on self-report measures of depression and ED attitudes.

A third study, conducted by Ball and Mitchell (2004), compared individual CBT with behavioral family therapy in a mixed sample of 25 adolescents and young adults (mean age = 18) with AN. Treatment involved 25 sessions over a 12-month period. No between-group differences were found at posttreatment or 6-month follow-up; approximately 78% of patients in both conditions were classified as having a "good outcome" in terms of weight and menstrual functioning at follow-up. "Good outcome" was defined as weight within 10% of average body weight, no bulimic symptoms, and resumption of menses. The relatively high rates of remission in this study may be related to the young age of the participants.

In the fourth study McIntosh and colleagues (2005) compared CBT with interpersonal psychotherapy (IPT) and nonspecific supportive clinical management (NSCM) for AN in 56 adult patients. Treatment involved 20 sessions over 20 weeks. The intent-to-treat results showed that IPT was significantly less effective than NSCM. The effectiveness of CBT fell between IPT and NSCM and was not significantly different from either. The dropout rate and degree of residual eating pathology were both high, and the effect sizes in terms of weight gain were small in all three treatment conditions.

Finally, Gowers and colleagues (2007) randomized 167 adolescent patients with AN to inpatient treatment, 24 sessions of outpatient therapy, or treatment as usual in the community. Treatment lasted up to 6 months. The outpatient therapy condition comprised elements of both CBT and family therapy. Adherence to treatment allocation was 65%. In the inpatient condition, 49% remained in treatment for at least 4 weeks, and the mean length of stay was 15 weeks. In the outpatient condition, 75% attended at least four therapy sessions. In the treatment-as-usual condition, 70% attended the usual first-line treatment appointments in community-based clinics with no additional specialized treatment. At 1-year follow-up, there were no statistically significant differences among the three groups in terms of weight outcome, based on intent-to-treat analyses. It was found that patients in all three conditions had made substantial improvements in terms of weight and ED psychopathology. The researchers concluded that there is no advantage of specialized treatment over treatment as usual and no advantage of inpatient treatment over outpatient treatment for AN. Of note, the attrition rate in this study was substantial (i.e., > 50% in the inpatient condition), and there was a significant rate of treatment nonadherence.

There have also been two studies of CBT for weight-restored patients with AN. Pike, Walsh, Vitousek, Wilson, and Bauer (2003) conducted a year-long posthospital study evaluating CBT for weight-restored adults with AN. In this study 77% of the CBT group (n = 18) reported an intermediate or better outcome according to modified Morgan–Russell criteria. The CBT group achieved a better recovery in terms of overall clinical pathology and dropout and relapse rates, compared to the comparison group that received supportive nutritional counseling (n = 15). Although these findings are promising, the sample size was small. Also, this study established efficacy for CBT compared to supportive nutritional counseling, but it did not compare CBT to another psychotherapy intervention, so we do not know whether the reported efficacy is a CBT-specific effect or a psychotherapy-specific effect. A subsequent study comparing CBT to another psychotherapy intervention is necessary to provide further support and clarification of these findings.

In an attempt to further evaluate the role of CBT for weight-restored individuals, Carter, McFarlane, Bewell, and colleagues (2008) recently conducted a nonrandomized clinical trial comparing CBT (n = 46) and maintenance treatment as usual (MTAU) (n = 42) for weight-restored adults with AN. The MTAU condition was intended to mirror follow-up care as usual in the community. When relapse was defined as a BMI ≤ 17.5 for 3 months or the resumption of regular binge-eating and/or purging behavior for 3 months, time to relapse was significantly longer in the CBT condition as compared with MTAU. At 1 year, 65% of the CBT group and 34% of the MTAU group had not relapsed.

In summary, none of the five published randomized trials on CBT for *acute* AN provides evidence that CBT was superior to comparison treatments. However, these studies were limited by small sample sizes, high rates of attrition, short durations of treatment, and other methodological problems. The two studies of weight-restored patients with AN provide promising preliminary evidence for the effectiveness of CBT in preventing relapse and improving recovery rates following weight restoration.

An Abbreviated CBT Manual for AN

This "mini-manual" represents an abbreviated version of the treatment approach employed in the clinical trial described by Pike and colleagues (2003) and Walsh and colleagues (2007). Originally developed by Pike, Vitousek, and Wilson (1993), it was revised in 1998 by the same authors and subsequently by Pike, Carter, and Olmsted (2004). In addition, this mini-manual draws on the supplemental relapse prevention modules for CBT developed by Carter and colleagues (2006), which focus on preventing early weight loss, enhancing self-efficacy, and addressing body image disturbances and excessive exercise.

Overview of CBT for AN

This treatment program includes four phases. Phase I outlines specific strategies for initiating treatment, orienting patients to CBT and assessing and enhancing motivation with the intent of promoting engagement in treatment. This phase draws on the "transtheoretical model of change" by Prochaska, DiClemente, and Norcross (1992), motivational interviewing strategies described by Miller and Rollnick (1991), and Vitousek, Watson, and Wilson's (1998) discussion of these issues specifically as they relate to treatment for AN. Phase II describes the weight gain protocol and interventions focused on the cognitive distortions and behavioral dysfunction pertaining to the patient's eating habits and weight. Phase III describes a schema-based approach that addresses relevant issues that extend beyond the specific domain of eating and weight.

Phase IV focuses on reviewing the course of treatment to consolidate gains and prepare to continue working independently after the therapy ends. Additionally, during the last phase of treatment, individuals prepare a personalized program of relapse prevention based on the course of therapy.

Clinical trials evaluating CBT-AN for weight-restored individuals with AN utilized treatment programs designed to include approximately 50 sessions over the course of 1 year. The treatment program evaluated in the McIntosh and colleagues (2005) study was comprised of only 20 sessions and targeted individuals with acute AN. As discussed above, the longer duration of treatment for individuals who had already achieved minimal weight restoration shows greater promise in terms of AN treatment than the shorter version of CBT-AN for those with acute AN.

Although the phases of the manual are presented in sequence, in practice, therapy rarely progresses exactly according to the nomothetic course outlined. Typically, interventions from Phases I, II, and III are utilized throughout the course of therapy, as needed, according to the particular issues and challenges of each patient. A hierarchy of symptoms serves to guide the clinician's judgment regarding the appropriate level of intervention. The first order of therapy is to engage patients in treatment and enhance motivation for recovery. Once goals are set, treatment focuses on normalization of eating behavior, achieving a healthy weight, and reducing the level of weight concern using the CBT interventions described in Phase II. However, in those cases when a patient is unable to progress in the work of normalizing her eating and gaining weight using the interventions described in Phase II, the focus of therapy shifts to issues of motivation (Phase I) as well as possible maladaptive schemas that are interfering with treatment (Phase III). Also, if at any point in treatment the patient begins to lose weight, therapy returns to an explicit focus on weight gain in the course of recovery and a review of issues raised and addressed in Phases I and II.

At the outset of treatment, it is important to discuss conditions for terminating outpatient treatment and recommending more intensive inpatient or day hospital programs. Specifically, dangerously low weight, serious medical complications, and suicidality may require termination of outpatient treatment. In addition to reviewing these parameters with the individual with AN, it can be helpful to conduct a session with the individual's family and/or spouse to provide information regarding AN and to discuss how best to support the therapeutic work for the individual with AN.

PHASE I: Getting Started—Orientation to CBT, Engagement, and Motivation

Phase I provides an introduction to the structure and rationale of CBT, assessment of motivation, and enhancing motivation for recovery.

Introduction to the Structure and Rationale of CBT

CBT begins with an explicit introduction to the structure and rationale of the treatment. This overview includes the theoretical underpinnings of CBT, structure of the sessions, therapeutic relationship, collaborative nature of CBT, focus on the here and now, self-monitoring, weight monitoring, and work between sessions.

The theoretical underpinnings of CBT, as described at the beginning of the chapter, are explicitly shared with patients once the initial assessment has been completed, so that an individual case formulation of the theoretical model may be presented using the patient's own experience. This is often a powerful intervention in organizing what has heretofore been chaotic and only partially understood. Tailored to the individual's unique history, this theoretical framework provides the rationale for CBT and guides the remainder of treatment.

The Therapeutic Relationship

As with all forms of psychotherapy, the efficacy of CBT is mediated by the therapeutic relationship, and therapists need to attend to building a trusting therapeutic alliance from the start (Orlinsky, Grawe, & Parks, 1994; Pike, Devlin, & Loeb, 2004). The nonspecific therapist qualities of warmth, empathy, respect, and openness are as essential to CBT as they are to all others forms of psychotherapy (Thompson & Williams, 1987; Truax & Mitchell, 1971). In addition, CBT requires that therapists are comfortable being active in sessions, thinking strategically, and providing structure and direction, especially at the beginning of treatment. Given the higher level of activity from the start, it is important that CBT therapists find a therapeutic balance between this level of activity and suspending their own assumptions and judgments so that they can provide an empathic balance of promoting change and enhancing understanding as patients grapple with recovery (Young, Weinberger, & Beck, 2001).

CBT is a collaborative treatment; that is, therapist and patient work together toward a common goal, jointly articulate the focus of each session, and take responsibility for keeping the treatment session on track. The therapist emphasizes that one of the primary goals of CBT is for the patient to learn the skills necessary for her to become "her own therapist," so that she can continue to make changes after treatment terminates. Establishing personal control and normal eating is expected to take time, and patients are encouraged to anticipate difficulties and be persistent in their efforts.

Structure of the Session

Every CBT session has an explicit internal structure that includes weight assessment and discussion of weight status, review of self-monitoring and between-session work, agenda setting, working on core issues of the agenda, setting goals for between-session work in the upcoming days, and summarizing the session. The structure of the session is maintained collaboratively. Although CBT therapists are active in treatment, this is not a therapist-led treatment; therapist and patient work together jointly on each component of the session.

Getting Started

CBT begins with a focus on the present by specifically targeting current eating pathology and its implications for current functioning. CBT approaches to treatment recognize that EDs are multidetermined and that different factors are involved in the development and maintenance of the disorder. By the time the individual presents for treatment, the ED has often taken on a life of its own. Thus, addressing the current issues and achieving resolution of symptoms are the most powerful starting points because they will bring some immediate relief and increase the patient's sense of self-efficacy about recovering from the ED. Moreover, from a CBT perspective, resolution of the acute issues will bring clarity of vision in analyzing the more distal, developmental factors. Therapists explicitly share this approach to treatment with patients, so the information serves as both an orientation and a therapeutic intervention.

Weight Monitoring

It is important to establish a regular schedule for monitoring weight during treatment. Consistent weight monitoring can be achieved in a variety of ways—at the beginning of each session with the therapist, at home with a parent, at school with a nurse, etc. The essential elements are that the schedule is regular and that someone initially assists the patient in monitoring her weight. After weight gain is completed and the patient's weight is stable, it is healthy for her to assume this responsibility. At the outset of treatment, the concept of an optimal weight range is discussed with the patient, and as she seems ready to commit to a weight gain protocol, the therapist and patient explicitly discuss and design a personalized weight gain plan, as described in Phase II.

Working between Sessions

An essential part of CBT is the work that is done between sessions, and its importance is stressed from the start. Between-session tasks target particular behavior patterns that are problematic and offer the patient the opportunity to experiment with changes in the context of a supportive therapeutic environment. The therapist reviews carefully the patient's experience with doing this work between sessions and builds on it for subsequent steps. The amount of effort that a patient expends on between-session work will be influenced by the attention it receives from the therapist. Therefore, it is crucial that the therapist integrate these efforts into each session. If a patient does not complete between-session tasks, it is essential that the therapist explore with the patient to understand the resistance. Typically, when the therapist and patient set the goals collaboratively, the patient sees the value and is invested in the work, and the likelihood of compliance is much higher.

Self-Monitoring

Self-monitoring, an important component of CBT, is not limited to recording food intake but also includes recording social and emotional experiences and situations that contextualize the ED. Self-monitoring is frequently experienced as tedious by patients with AN, and therapists are encouraged to let patients adapt the self-monitoring procedures in ways that make the task valuable for them so that they actually are motivated to do it. Sometimes highly perfectionistic patients use the self-monitoring to provide obsessional levels of detail. The critical issue is to use the self-monitoring to constructively communicate about the patient's experience between sessions. Thus the clinician and patient need to adapt the procedures and personalize the process according to the specific therapeutic needs of the patient. As noted, in addition to addressing the core issues related to food intake (or lack thereof), therapists use the self-monitoring to help patients begin to reconnect their emotional and interpersonal worlds with their eating by exploring contextual factors. Where does the patient eat? With whom does she eat?

How is she feeling? What was she thinking right before a meal? How did she manage to skip a meal when she was visiting with a friend? What was she thinking and feeling before she binged?

A thorough review of the patient's self-monitoring will help her begin to identify eating situations that range from extremely difficult to extremely manageable. In this way, the therapist and patient can discuss what differentiates these situations and begin to expand the patient's ideas about the range of thoughts, feelings, and behaviors that accompanies eating. The purpose of this portion is to begin to point out the limitation and inaccuracy of labeling oneself solely as "anorexic." Pointing out cognitive distortions, such as "labeling" and "all-or-nothing thinking," lays the groundwork for cognitive work that will follow in subsequent sessions.

Assessing and Enhancing Motivation

One of the essential first steps in treatment is assessing whether and why an individual is motivated for treatment. Such work is the bedrock for establishing a trusting therapeutic alliance and for effectively engaging patients in committing to the difficult work of pursuing recovery. CBT for AN makes use of the "transtheoretical model" (Proschaska & DiClemente, 1983; Prochaska et al., 1992) and motivational interviewing (Miller & Rollnick, 1991) to provide a framework for assessing and enhancing motivation at multiple levels.

Vitousek and colleagues (1998) have addressed the issue of motivation from both a theoretical and practical perspective with specific regard to those with AN. Throughout the course of this treatment, therapists draw on the recommendations provided by Vitousek and colleagues. These authors emphasize the importance of acknowledging the ego-syntonic nature of extreme thinness and self-control and the desperation that is associated with "choosing" AN as a solution. They encourage therapists to explicitly acknowledge the difficulties of making real changes in one's life and remind them not to "attach surplus meaning to resistance." By employing a Socratic style and using the patient's language to conceptualize and collaborate on making change, therapists are able to communicate respect and hope for patients. It is important to remain honest and curious with patients. Although certain aspects of the disorder are universal, it is constructive for therapists to also focus on and validate the individuality of each patient. In fact, recovery is strongly associated with the reemergence of the individuality of each person.

It can be very helpful early in treatment for the therapist to become familiar with the patient's values and life goals. This information provides the context for examining the impact the ED is likely to have on the patient's life and helps to identify competing goals as residing within the patient as opposed to between the patient and the therapist. Consider the following conversation:

THERAPIST: I understand that controlling your weight is very, very important to you, but I'm not sure whether it is more important to you than becoming a lawyer, as you have planned.

PATIENT: Well, I expect to do both.

THERAPIST: You mentioned the other day that you have had trouble concentrating on your work and that you aren't doing very well at school. What are the chances of your getting into law school if you aren't able to study effectively and pull up your grades?

PATIENT: Not very good; you need high grades to get in.

THERAPIST: And as we discussed before, poor concentration and reduced mental capabilities are a side effect of being poorly nourished and underweight.

PATIENT: I know you think I should eat more.

THERAPIST: You are right, that is my bias, but what you think is more important. If you focus on controlling your weight and ignore the impact of being poorly nourished on other areas of your life, there's a good chance you won't get into law school. It's really up to you; the decision is yours. My job is to help you sort through the options and make a thoughtful choice. Will working on your weight be enough to satisfy you for the rest of your life, or do you need other things in your life?

In addition to assessing motivation, psychoeducation is an important component of treatment in the early phase of CBT. This includes reviewing the multiple causes of AN, its associated biological risks and sequelae, the deleterious consequences of semistarvation (illustrated via the case study in the Minnesota Study of Semi-Starvation), the relationship of weight gain to menstrual functioning, normalization of eating behavior, and basic nutritional education regarding the consumption of fat, carbohydrates, and protein in a healthy diet. A summary of core psychoeducational components for AN treatment is provided by Treasure (1997). Therapists and patients are encouraged to make use of the wealth of psychoeducational information available to assist in treatment and recovery.

PHASE II: Core Cognitive and Behavioral Interventions for AN

Phase II employs CBT interventions that focus on identifying, understanding, and changing maladaptive cognitions and behaviors that serve to maintain the ED. The specific focus of Phase II depends on the patient's readiness and motivation for change, and therapists need to use judgment in choosing the most appropriate and effective CBT interventions in relation to the specific issues of each patient. The latitude to tailor treatment to the individual needs of the patient is essential for good therapy; however, therapists can also make use of the Hierarchy of Symptoms Guidelines(Figure 5.1) to help guide the focus of treatment.

Weight Gain Protocol and Meal Planning

During Phase II, it is important to establish a weight gain goal and meal plan. Therapists begin by reviewing the reasons why the patient needs to gain weight to reach a healthy level in order to overcome the ED (see Rock & Curran-Celentano, 1994) and integrate examples from the patient's own history. In addition, therapists present the rationale for thinking in terms of a weight *range* rather than a specific number. In negotiating a preliminary weight gain goal, it is important to take into account the patient's level of readiness to change. Although the ultimate goal is to achieve a healthy weight

Is Patient Motivated for Treatment?

If yes:	If no:
Proceed with core CBT interventions described in Phase II.	Focus on motivational enhancement strategies of Phase I.

Is Patient Participating In Weight Gain Protocol?

If yes:	If no:
Proceed with core CBT interventions described in Phase II and continue to challenge patient with behavioral exercises included in the weight gain protocol.	If she is losing weight but not in medical danger, return to motivational enhancement strategies. If she describes being motivated but is behaviorally unable to implement weight gain strategies, adjust behavioral plans, enlist significant other, consider schema-based approaches. If she is not losing weight but also not gaining weight, utilize specific AN motivational enhancement strategies such as cost–benefit analysis, projecting forward, writing one's own obituary.

Is Patient Binge-Eating and/or Purging?

If yes:	If no:
Review dietary restraint model of binge–purge cycle (Fairburn, Wilson, & Marcus, 1993). Utilize CBT behavioral strategies outlined in Phase II for normalizing eating behaviors. Utilize CBT cognitive interventions for building alternative coping strategies for stressful situations. Discuss the possibility of increasing lab work medical monitoring of patient's clinical status if she is vomiting and/or using laxatives.	Continue to steadily challenge patient to normalize her eating behavior in terms of frequency, variety, and quantity of intake, as described in the weight gain protocol and in Phase II.

Is the Patient's Self-Schema Sabotaging Her Capacity to Successfully Engage in Treatment?

If yes:	If no:
Proceed with schema-based work described in Phase III.	Stick with core cognitive and behavioral interventions described in Phase II.

FIGURE 5.1. Hierarchy of Symptoms Guidelines.

(typically a minimum BMI of 20 kg/m^2), some patients may find this amount to be overwhelming initially. Instead, they may need to set weight gain goals in manageable steps. For example, it may be helpful to suggest an initial 2- to 3-kilogram weight gain goal and progress from there. The aim is to gradually increase caloric intake to achieve a 0.5- to 1.0-kilogram increase in weight per week.

A meal plan is a helpful tool for teaching patients when, what, and how much to eat. In some cases, it can be helpful to engage a nutritionist in establishing a meal plan. The initial focus is on helping patients meet their calorie goal with a subsequent focus on the quality and variety of food intake as weight gain progresses. Self-monitoring is an important tool for establishing normal eating habits and tracking progress.

Behavioral Experimentation

Behavioral experimentation between sessions is one of the pillars of CBT. Initially the behavioral experimentation for those with AN is largely focused on specific areas related to the weight gain protocol and normalization of food intake. As individuals progress in treatment, the behavioral experimentation may be focused more broadly to assist patients in the cognitive work of CBT as well. Stepwise behavioral experimentation in the interpersonal realm is an essential aspect of the integration of cognitive and behavioral interventions. (See Figure 5.2 for a Behavioral Experiment Worksheet.)

With each successive session, the therapist and patient build on the previous session. To the extent that cognitive distortions interfered with the patient's successful completion of the task, these are identified and examined. To the extent that the task was accomplished successfully, the therapist and patient decide on the next logical step in the normalization of the patient's eating patterns and establish that step as the behavioral challenge on which to focus between sessions. This work requires the construction of a hierarchy of behavioral challenges and includes addressing the issue of forbidden foods in a thoughtful manner to establish a stepwise sequence that steadily aids the individual in normalizing her eating.

It is extremely important that therapy focus not only on the elimination of symptoms but also on building strengths. As patients reconnect to strengths that help them function independently of the ED, they gain confidence about engaging in treatment, at which point resolution of the eating disorder usually gains momentum. Skill development might include relaxation training, stress management, problem solving, assertiveness training, social skills with an emphasis on building healthy friendships, and attention to emotional and physical self-care.

Identifying and Challenging Dysfunctional Thoughts

The concept of dysfunctional thoughts or cognitive distortions is a central component of CBT, and in Phase II, treatment focuses on identifying cognitive distortions and understanding their role in perpetuating the ED. Patients are encouraged to engage in testing the validity or evidence of cognitions, and therapists and patients work together to formulate functional or adaptive "challenges" or responses to the dysfunctional thoughts. One of the templates that can be useful in conducting this work is the Dysfunctional Thought Record (Figure 5.3).

PLAN

Data to be collected: _____

What I have to do: _____

_____

Is this task suitable for me at this time? (Or is it too hard?) _____

_____

What can I do if I feel overwhelmed? _____

_____

What maladaptive thoughts can I anticipate? _____

_____

How will I cope with these? _____

_____

Do I expect to have urges for any symptomatic behavior? _____

_____

How will I cope with these? _____

_____

Under what circumstances is it appropriate to delay or cancel the experiment? _____

_____

Prediction or hypothesis: _____

_____

OUTCOME

What happened? _____

_____

What conclusion is supported by the data? _____

_____

Is any follow-up experiment required? _____

_____

FIGURE 5.2. Behavioral Experiment Worksheet.

SITUATION	FEELINGS	DYSFUNCTIONAL THOUGHT(S)	CHALLENGE DYSFUNCTIONAL THOUGHT(S)
Describe the problematic situation (specific situations will be linked to problems with eating; more general problematic situations may also be addressed).	Specify the feelings that you were aware of at this time.	Specify the thought(s) that preceded the problematic eating, response, or general behavior.	1. What is the evidence for and against these thoughts? 2. Is there an alternative way of viewing the event? 3. What is the effect of having this thought?

FIGURE 5.3. Dysfunctional Thought Record.

In practice, CBT often combines self-monitoring, behavioral experimentation, and the challenging of dysfunctional thoughts, as demonstrated in the following examples.

Example 1

THERAPIST: I see [from the patient's self-monitoring food diary] that you have done an excellent job of sticking to the structure of your meal plan and having all your meals and snacks. How do you feel about this?

PATIENT: I'm feeling a lot better physically than I was before, and I know I needed to gain some weight. So I'm glad that I increased my eating even though it has been very difficult.

THERAPIST: What do you think a good next step would be?

PATIENT: If I eat more, I will gain too much weight.

THERAPIST: Is that the reason that you have been using nonfat yogurt and not using butter or salad dressing?

PATIENT: Yes, I know that people eat way too much fat and end up with too much fat on their body.

THERAPIST: If you were going to take your eating up a step, would it be easier to eat more food or to eat food that is more calorie-dense?

PATIENT: I don't want to do either. But theoretically I guess it would be easier to have larger portions at dinner and maybe have a granola bar some days.

THERAPIST: What do you think about making sure that you have a whole portion of chicken or fish for dinner each day and adding a granola bar to your afternoon snack? We will continue to monitor your weight carefully each week and adjust your eating plan if you are gaining weight too quickly. Do you think you could do that for 1 week and see what happens?

Note: The therapist makes a mental note that using added fats is more difficult for the patient and decides to return to this issue in a subsequent session.

Example 2

THERAPIST: I see from your eating diary that you missed dinner on Tuesday, and you noted that you were upset with Jill. What was going on?

PATIENT: Jill called at the last minute and said that she couldn't go to the movie with me because a friend had dropped in, but I'm over it now.

THERAPIST: Oh, how did you get over it?

PATIENT: Well, I just told myself that it isn't worth causing trouble over and that I should just forget it.

THERAPIST: So you don't plan to let Jill know that her behavior bothered you?

PATIENT: No, it's just not worth it to me.

THERAPIST: You've mentioned that before about other situations in which you didn't want to speak to someone you were upset with or someone who borrowed something and didn't give it back. Have you noticed that?

PATIENT: It's true. I don't want to make trouble or push things.

THERAPIST: What is your worry? What might happen if you pushed things?

PATIENT: I don't want people to be mad at me and to dislike me.

Over the next few weeks, the patient and therapist address the patient's belief that people will dislike her if she asserts herself or asks for anything. Eventually they set up a behavioral experiment that involves the patient making a small assertive request to a friend and noting how the friend responds. They also develop strategies for following the meal plan even when the patient is stressed or distressed.

Preventing Weight Loss after Minimum Target Weight Has Been Achieved

For individuals recovering from AN, the transition from eating for weight *gain* to eating for weight *maintenance* is often challenging. Most are terrified that continuing to eat normally will cause further weight gain, and urges to shave calories, miss exchanges/supplements, skimp on portion size, increase exercise, skip added fats, and cut back on high-energy foods may be intense at this stage. Due to the unavoidable repeated pairings between eating and weight gain during early stages of treatment, individuals with AN are scared that if they continue to eat normally, they will continue to gain weight. However, patients typically need to eat a lot more calories than they expect in order to maintain their target weight and prevent weight loss. When people cut back on their eating to avoid further weight gain, weight loss is the inevitable result. A recent research study found that even a small amount of weight loss following achievement of target weight is strongly associated with subsequent relapse in AN. Thus, it is essential that therapists educate patients about these issues. Therapists may find it therapeutic to share with patients the experience of one individual ("The Little Things that Grow," Figure 5.4). This individual had relapsed in the past partially due to early weight loss after discharge from inpatient treatment, and she now knows the importance of maintaining her weight to prevent relapse. The therapist can encourage the patient to take an experimental approach to recovery and gather evidence about what really does happen to her weight if she follows her maintenance meal plan. If necessary, ask her to try the experiment 1 week at a time. In terms of cognitive restructuring, it is useful to identify and challenge beliefs about weight maintenance and relapse.

Addressing Body Image Disturbance

Body dissatisfaction is a core feature of EDs. The repeated checking of body shape or weight ("body checking") and the avoidance of seeing actual body shape or weight ("body avoidance") have been hypothesized to maintain body image disturbance and contribute to increased dietary restraint (Farrell & Lee, 2005; Shafran, Fairburn, Nelson, & Robinson, 2003). There is a strong association between body checking and over-evaluation of shape and weight. One of the goals of CBT is to assess and reduce body checking and body avoidance. The approach described in this regard is based on the work of Roz Shafran and colleagues.

Fighting through intensive treatment is an exhausting journey. Reaching the end of this portion of recovery is an incredible relief. I remember feeling overjoyed that the work was finally complete. After all, the weight had been gained and the meal plan was etched into my mind. I felt ready to face the world with my armor of coping strategies and had no intention of returning to my disordered ways. I have come to realize that there is danger in this time, and that the anorexic voice can sneak in undetected and take over faster than I would have ever believed. The truth is that leaving treatment marks the starting point of a new battle. Transitioning back into the real world is, as we are warned, an equally difficult and dangerous time. I've discovered that the "little things" that seem unimportant are my greatest threats for relapse.

Toward the end of treatment, the concept of maintenance is repeatedly stressed and restressed by professionals. The importance of maintaining above one's low end, maintaining the meal plan, maintaining the food choices and variety, and maintaining the separation from exercise is repeated time and time again. There are graphs, studies, and extensive pieces of data that prove the importance of holding onto all the changes. At the end of my first inpatient stay I remember thinking that all this sounded a bit paranoid. The reentry of the anorexic voice came in the form of a "What's the big deal?" attitude. The accompanying thoughts seemed innocent enough. I remember thinking "Who cares if I am 2 pounds below my goal weight? Why does it matter if I use diet products? Everyone does it! I don't want to go back to my illness, I just want to be healthy and fit!" Although these thoughts don't seem distorted, they represent a shifting definition of healthy that led me back into the throes of my disorder. Something that started as simply as switching to skim milk landed me back in treatment within a matter of months. If there is one thing I have learned, it is that the little things grow.

Straying away from the maintenance meal plan fuels the disorder and keeps it alive and well. I've discovered that feeding the anorexia, whether it's in the form of a couple pounds or skimping on portions, leads me down the slippery path. Soon the little things grow in number and severity. If there is one piece of advice I could give somebody leaving treatment, it would be this: "Don't feed the voice." Maintaining seems arduous and overly cautious at times, but the anorexia only needs a little bit of fuel to start a fire. The shifting view of "healthy" that strays from what we were taught in treatment is likely the disorder trying to worm its way in.

Now having completed my second inpatient stay, I know the "little things" I have to watch out for. I am faced with all the familiar urges and annoying anorexic thoughts. I still find myself doubting and questioning the importance of maintaining all the little things. However, I know from experience that where my eating disorder is concerned, the smallest spark can restart the fire. Although it continues to be a struggle, I know that my path to freedom requires my continued efforts and vigilance. So in the name of recovery, I will continue to fight against all aspects of my disorder, including the "little things."

FIGURE 5.4. "The Little Things That Grow," written by a former patient.

Body checking typically involves excessive behaviors aimed at identifying any signs of weight gain or assessing one's shape (Shafran et al., 2003), whereas body avoidance is just the opposite—that is, refusal to be weighed, avoidance of mirrors or other reflective surfaces, and the wearing of baggy clothes to conceal one's shape. Both of these behaviors contribute to negative thoughts and feelings about body shape and weight. Therapists can make use of the Body Image Avoidance Questionnaire (Rosen, Srebnik, Saltzberg, & Wendt, 1991) and Body Checking Questionnaire (Reas, Whisenhunt, Netemeyer, & Williamson, 2002) to formally assess these aspects of patient functioning and measure progress in terms of body image satisfaction over the course of treatment. Treatment strategies directed at body image include psychoeducation about the negative impact of body checking and body avoidance, exercises that help individuals distance themselves from negative body image thoughts, body image exposure exercises, and cognitive work on developing other aspects of self-identity that enhance self-esteem, as described by Pike and colleagues (1996). In addition, it is useful to encourage patients to get rid of "sick" clothes that are too small for them and support them in obtaining comfortable clothing in an appropriate size. Wearing clothes that are too small draws their attention to their body size and shape. Wearing clothes that are too big or baggy is another form of avoidance and tends to be associated with negative body image.

When addressing body image issues with the patient, it is especially important to validate her feelings and at the same time introduce doubt and distance about the associated beliefs:

> PATIENT: I am really frightened of gaining weight because I already feel so huge and fat.
>
> THERAPIST: I know it really bothers you to feel so fat, and it seems that you feel that way most of the time.
>
> PATIENT: Yes, I do.
>
> THERAPIST: If I recall correctly, your weight has changed over the last year and you have felt fat the whole time at a few different weights. Is that right?
>
> PATIENT: Yes, it is, although I did feel even fatter when my weight was higher.
>
> THERAPIST: What do you make of the fact that other people think your weight is too low?
>
> PATIENT: I can see that too, if I try really hard, but it doesn't match at all with the way I feel.
>
> THERAPIST: I wonder if this very heavy feeling that you have could be about something other than what you weigh. I know you feel very fat, but what if this feeling somehow means that you are distressed and this feeling somehow got tied to your body, and the details about other things that are happening somehow got lost along the way? What do you think about the idea of recording how fat you feel in your self-monitoring diary several times each day and also noting what else is going on at the time and whether you have any other feelings?

Combating Excessive Exercise

Many individuals with AN engage in excessive exercise. Typically, it is therapeutic for patients to refrain from all exercise until related issues have been discussed in therapy and patients have maintained a minimum target weight for at least 1 month. CBT therapists encourage the use of behavioral strategies (e.g., distraction, delay, self-talk), stimulus control (e.g., disassemble exercise equipment, put gym membership on hold, hide running shoes) and thought records to assist patients in resisting urges to exercise. In addition, it is helpful to encourage patients to assume an "experimental approach" to *not* exercising, so that they can gain actual experiential data on what it is like *not* to exercise. It is important to underscore the fact that refraining from exercise at this stage in treatment is a temporary measure, much like wearing a cast on a broken limb.

It can be helpful to encourage physical activity that cannot turn into excessive exercise and that is not aimed primarily at weight control (e.g., some types of yoga, crafts, social activities such as ice skating with friends). If sufficient time has passed during which the patient continues to maintain her weight and has remained symptom-free (e.g., 1 or 2 months), it may be reasonable to gradually implement moderate exercise with careful planning and testing. The emphasis should be placed on having fun, socializing, developing a skill, and improving health rather than controlling weight and shape or burning calories.

PHASE III: Schema-Based Cognitive Therapy and Related Clinical Issues

General Outline of Schema-Based CBT

Vitousek and Hollon (1990) argue that the cognitive schema of AN can contribute to an understanding of both the "choice" and maintenance of the disorder. Unlike most other psychological disorders, one of the hallmark features of AN is the ego-syntonic nature of the disturbance. Individuals with AN choose to maintain an excessively low body weight, at least in part, via the cognitive schema that overvalues weight and thinness. Individuals with AN value and rely on their symptoms to simplify, organize, and manage the stresses and conflicts of life. Once established, this cognitive schema operates automatically. The automatic nature of such cognitive processing can account, at least in part, for the maintenance or stability of the psychopathology and its resistance to change (Bemis, 1983; Striegel-Moore & McAvay, 1986).

At this stage in treatment the therapist works with the patient on diversifying her self-schema to include a wider range of roles and activities that meaningfully enhance her sense of self. Although the exact details of the ED schema will vary, the core of the schema is typically of the form, "I am anorexic and must stay this way because it brings me control, mastery, and somehow makes me special." The therapist helps the patient separate the *goals* of achieving control, mastery, and importance from the *means*. It is essential that the therapist support the patient's needs and desires to have control, mastery, and self-importance in life; these goals are normative and healthy. The therapist emphasizes that the work of therapy is not to alter these goals but to work on how to achieve them more adaptively.

In addition to the ED schema that tends to be fairly explicit and within the patient's conscious awareness, additional maladaptive schemas may contribute significantly to the underlying issues related to the ED and therefore will need to be addressed in the course of treatment. For patients with AN, maladaptive schemas in the interpersonal realm appear to be intricately linked with the more conscious ED schema. Some examples of maladaptive interpersonal schemas include (1) feeling unable to take care of oneself and undeserving of nurturing by others; (2) believing that achieving nurturing, rewarding relationships will not be possible for oneself; (3) feeling worthless and undesirable to others in terms of appearance, social skills, inner worth, etc; (4) believing that to have any worth one must be loved by everyone, and therefore one must avoid conflict at all cost (e.g., "I dare not be rejected by others").

To the extent that patients are unable to participate successfully in the other components of this psychotherapy intervention or remain symptomatic, it can be useful to evaluate whether and which maladaptive schemas or core negative beliefs are interfering with making greater progress in treatment. The therapist and patient can identify the relevant maladaptive schemas that contribute to the core pathology of the ED. Given the rigid nature and chronic course that is characteristic of AN, this level of intervention is designed to address the deeper and probably more historical dysfunctional assumptions that contribute to the ED.

The primary focus of these sessions is to work with the patient on her specific maladaptive schemas with the goal of gaining awareness of the role that such schemas play in the ED and challenging the schemas using the range of CBT techniques. The specific details of these sessions will need to be shaped by the particular maladaptive schemas of a given patient. The therapist remains active, and change techniques are implemented explicitly and systematically. In particular, the therapist continues to emphasize the importance of homework and experimenting with behavioral change. The therapist and patient continue to work collaboratively to evaluate the current data derived from such experimentation, and they continue to utilize an empirical approach to evaluating the validity and functionality of the maladaptive schemas.

Affect Regulation and Interpersonal Effectiveness Skills

Issues of affect regulation and difficulties in interpersonal relationships plague many individuals with AN. It is often the case that resolution of the behavioral symptoms of the ED results in greater clarity regarding these more global problems. This entire CBT intervention is designed to enhance our patients' ability to self-regulate and successfully manage interpersonal situations. In addition to the program outlined here, especially in the later phases of treatment, it may also be useful for therapists to incorporate Linehan's (1993) work, which was designed for individuals with borderline personality disorder. These interventions are based on sound cognitive-behavioral principles and may be effectively adapted for our patients with AN. In particular, Linehan provides clear and useful descriptions of interventions aimed at enhancing interpersonal effectiveness skills and affect regulation.

Treating Individuals with Binge Eating and Purging

A significant percentage of individuals with AN report binge eating and purging, and a significant minority of these individuals will go on to develop BN. Thus, it is important to assess and address these aspects of the eating disturbance carefully and employ CBT interventions that specifically target binge eating and purging, as needed. It is unusual for individuals with AN to report binge eating without purging; however, it is not unusual for individuals to report purging in the absence of binge eating. Treating patients who report binge eating, compared to those who do not, requires first determining the nature of the binge-eating episodes. To the extent that the subjective reports do not meet criteria for an objective bingeing, the primary thrust of the behavioral interventions will be consistent across all patients: The goal is not to alter the specific behavior that the patient describes as a binge but rather to focus on normalizing eating three meals per day, plus snacks, and increasing the variety of food with which the patient is comfortable. The cognitive interventions for these patients focus on identifying and challenging the distortions that make average meals and snacks "binges."

Individuals with AN who purge need to be monitored carefully, given their increased risk for medical complications. Vomiting and any other compensatory behaviors, such as laxative or diuretic abuse, are driven by the same core dysfunctional thoughts as the excessive restraint characteristic of all patients with AN. All of these behaviors are pursued to achieve the central aim of extreme thinness because individuals with AN believe that such efforts will provide a sense of control, mastery, and self-worth. Thus, the cognitive interventions directed at vomiting are the same as those used to address excessive restriction. These cognitive techniques elucidate and challenge the dysfunctional thinking underlying these compensatory behaviors and restriction, since all of these behaviors are motivated by the same underlying core beliefs. Behavioral interventions such as the use of delay strategies and alternatives are designed to inhibit the purging behavior.

Using the Therapeutic Relationship to Address Maladaptive Thoughts and Schemas

The therapist can make use of the therapeutic relationship to explore the patient's general feelings and assumptions about interpersonal relationships. As mentioned above, patients with AN often have significant interpersonal problems. For example, many patients describe problems in balancing attachment and autonomy in relationships, feeling excessively dependent, vulnerable, and mistrustful. Also, many individuals with AN describe feeling worthless and unlovable. CBT therapists stay alert to any indications that the patient holds such dysfunctional schemas and use the Dysfunctional Thought Record (Figure 5.3) to explore and challenge such distortions with the patient. In addition, therapists can use the relationship to make explicit the maladaptive assumptions that the patient may hold regarding interpersonal relationships. In doing so, the goal is to articulate and challenge any maladaptive schemas that are identified.

PHASE IV: Ending Treatment and Relapse Prevention

In preparing for the termination of treatment, the therapist and patient review specific CBT tools and strategies that the patient has found most helpful. It should be emphasized to the patient that the goal of treatment is not to solve all potential problems while in treatment, but to learn the skills necessary to manage such problems adaptively in the future. This stage offers the patient the opportunity to describe an enhanced sense of self-efficacy as a result of the gains she has made in treatment. At this point, the therapist can reiterate that as long as the patient continues to employ what she has learned, she will be acting as her own therapist and thereby decrease her risk of relapse.

The therapist helps the patient think ahead to potentially stressful situations and challenges that lie in the near future. During these sessions, the therapist helps the patient practice and plan for particular challenges. Anticipation and planning are key elements in preventing relapse. However, the therapist also emphasizes that no one stays exactly on course 100% of the time. As much as possible, the therapist helps the patient learn to identify and monitor cues that she is "off course." The more attentive and responsive the patient is to such cues, the less likely she is to relapse. (See Figure 5.5, Self-Therapy Worksheet, and Figure 5.6, Relapse Prevention Plan.)

Specific End-of-Treatment Interventions

As described below, some key factors in making the ending therapeutic include letting up on perfectionism, acceptance, anticipating the loss, and recognizing that successful treatment does not always prevent relapse. A wide range of interventions can be used to assist with the consolidation of therapy and relapse prevention. Table 5.1 highlights some of the most common and useful strategies.

One way to maintain a watchful eye and ensure that you continue to work independently is to provide a time and a structure for regularly checking in with yourself. Consider setting up a very important appointment with yourself to work through items in a structured way. Remember to pick a time when you will have some privacy and be able to focus on yourself.

Date and time of appointment: _____

How is my eating going? Did I restrict at all? Do I need to change anything about my eating?

Have I had any eating-disordered symptoms of any kind? If so, what do I need to do about them?

How am I doing with my body image? Do I need to change anything related to this?

How am I doing with having feelings, being aware of them, and finding appropriate forms of expression?

Is any thought or feeling haunting me? What do I need to do about it?

How am I doing in my relationships? Do I need to address anything related to this area?

How am I doing with my job, schoolwork, or daily activities? Do I need to change anything related to these?

Am I aware of how hard I am working to maintain my recovery? Am I giving myself credit?

What am I most proud of this week?

What challenge am I setting for myself in the week to come?

FIGURE 5.5. Self-Therapy Worksheet.

Relapse can be triggered by any set of circumstances that makes it easy to slide off your meal plan, not eat regular meals, or diet. Examples include being physically ill with the flu or unable to eat for any reason, being very busy or stressed, skipping meals to save time, stressful events, negative emotions, and self-defeating thoughts. One critical strategy is to maintain a high level of vigilance: Be aware of what is going on!

What factors or situations might be likely to lead you to relapse (i.e., what do you need to watch out for)? _____

_____

_____

What do you have in place to keep yourself vigilant? _____

_____

_____

If you start to slip, what do you need to do in terms of your eating behavior and meal plan? _____

_____

_____

Other symptoms that might need attention: _____

_____

What do you need to do about these? _____

_____

What maladaptive thoughts can you expect? _____

_____

What will you do about these? _____

_____

What do you need in terms of social support? _____

_____

_____

What are the chances that your difficulties will go away on their own? _____

_____

_____

FIGURE 5.6. Relapse Prevention Plan.

TABLE 5.1. End-of-Treatment Interventions

Below is a list of possible interventions that may assist in the work around ending treatment.

1. Case summary: Ask your patient to write her own case summary, highlighting what was especially useful, what was difficult, etc.

2. Risks for relapse: Ask your patient to write about the risks that she sees on the horizon. In that regard it is also useful to have her identify cues that will tell her she is off course or at risk for relapsing and have her prepare a plan for how to minimize or avert such risk.

3. Goal Setting: Patients can prepare a list of goals for the coming month, 3 months, 1 year.

4. Encourage patients to review CBT materials from therapy and keep a folder of the materials that seem most relevant.

5. Have your patient project forward to when she is an old woman. As she reflects on the life she imagines, how does she want to be remembered (by the therapist, friends, or family)? What does she want her legacy to be? Throughout this discussion, you can link your patient's desires to the year's work of CBT.

6. Ask your patient to write about past relapses and to be as detailed as possible about the patterns that were central to relapsing; discuss with her how she can handle things differently this time.

7. Review specific processes of CBT interventions, such as food diaries, Dysfunctional Thought Record, and problem solving. Find out how the patient is using these instruments at the end of treatment and discuss how she can maximize their utility for transitioning out of treatment.

8. Role playing: Use this technique to anticipate and work through any anticipated difficult situations.

9. Explore what the patient thinks it would mean if she were to relapse. Does it mean that treatment didn't work? If so, it may make her less likely to seek help when she needs it. It may be useful to use the analogy of a shower here (e.g., "You get dirty after a shower, but that doesn't mean the shower didn't work; moreover, getting dirty isn't so scary when you know how to shower").

10. Emphasize growth potential of slips.

Letting Up on Perfectionism and Acceptance

Therapists' acceptance of patients facilitates patients' self-acceptance. In turn, this self-acceptance relieves the misery of feeling unworthy that many individuals with AN feel. Some individuals with AN will always be vulnerable to reengaging in eating pathology, but if they can accept this susceptibility and pay attention to markers of risk, they can achieve a higher and stabler level of functioning. Sometimes individuals expect too much from treatment, and helping them let go of mythical ideals can facilitate a more constructive ending. Assisting patients to identify ideals that empower and those that defeat their own growth can be very therapeutic—not only beauty ideals but ideals about the way they think they should live. Linking the perfectionism to demoralization and relapse is an important goal of treatment and its termination.

Anticipating the Loss

Throughout the treatment and with increasingly explicit reference, it may be helpful to discuss the possible feelings of loss that are associated with ending treatment. It is useful to help patients plan for how they will take care of themselves in the face of such loss. This aspect of treatment is important because it give patients a clear message of support from the therapist: They have the needed ability to take care of themselves.

Acceptance That a Successful Intervention Does Not Always Prevent Relapse

Many of our patients require multiple treatments. To the extent that the disorder will run its course, a particular intervention may be therapeutic in its capacity to reduce deleterious effects. Also, putting into practice all the components of CBT often takes time. Although a patient may not be able to successfully avert a relapse, she may have learned a lot during the course of treatment that will ultimately contribute to a more complete recovery.

References

Ball J, & Mitchell P. (2004). A randomized controlled study of cognitive behavior therapy and behavioral family therapy for anorexia nervosa patients. *Eating Disorders*, 12:303–314.

Beck AT. (1976). *Cognitive therapy and the emotional disorders.* New York: International Universities Press.

Beck AT, Rush AJ, Shaw BF, & Emery G. (1979). *Cognitive therapy of depression.* New York: Guilford Press.

Bemis KM. (1983). A comparison of functional relationships in anorexia nervosa and phobia. In PL Darby, PE Garfinkel, DM Garner, & DV Coscina (Eds.), *Anorexia nervosa: Recent developments in research* (pp. 403–416). New York: Liss.

Carter JC, McFarlane TL, Bewell CV, Olmsted MP, Woodside DB, Kaplan AS, et al. (2008). Maintenance treatment for anorexia nervosa: A comparison of cognitive behavior therapy and treatment as usual. *International Journal of Eating Disorders*, 42:202–207.

Carter JC, McFarlane TL, Olmsted MP, & Pike KM. (2008). *CBT for weight-restored AN: Supplemental treatment modules.* Unpublished manual.

Channon S, de Silva P, Helmsley D, & Perkins R. (1989). A controlled trial of cognitive behavioral and behavioral treatment of anorexia nervosa. *Behaviour Research and Therapy*, 27:529–535.

Cooper PJ, & Fairburn CG. (1984). Cognitive behaviour therapy for anorexia nervosa: Some preliminary findings. *Journal of Psychosomatic Research*, 28:493–499.

Fairburn CG, Shafran R, & Cooper Z. (1999). A cognitive behavioural theory of anorexia nervosa. *Behaviour Research and Therapy*, 37:1–13.

Farrell C, & Lee M. (2005). Assessment of body size estimation: A review. *European Eating Disorders Review*, 13:75–88.

Gowers SG, Clark A, Roberts C., Griffiths A, Edwards V, Bryan C, et al. (2007). Clinical effectiveness of treatments for anorexia nervosa in adolescents: Randomized controlled trial. *British Journal of Psychiatry*, 191:427–435.

Linehan MM. (1993). *Cognitive-behavioral treatment of borderline personality disorder.* New York: Guilford Press.

McIntosh VVW, Jordan J, Carter FA, Luty SE, McKenzie JM, Bulik CM, et al. (2005). Three psychotherapies for anorexia nervosa: A randomized controlled trial. *American Journal of Psychiatry*, 162:741–747.

Miller WR, & Rollnick S. (1991). *Motivational interviewing: Preparing people for change.* New York: Guilford Press.

Morgan HG, Hayward AE. (1988). Clinical assessment of anorexia nervosa: The Morgan–Russell outcome assessment schedule. *British Journal of Psychiatry*, 152:367–371.

Nathan PE, & Gorman JM. (Eds.). (2002). *A guide to treatments that work* (2nd ed.). New York: Oxford University Press.

Orlinsky DE, Grawe K, & Parks BK. (1994). Process and outcome in psychotherapy: *Noch einmal.*

In A. E. Bergin & S. L. Garfield (Eds.), *Handbook of psychotherapy and behavior change* (4th ed., pp. 270–376). New York: Wiley.

Pike KM, Carter J, & Olmsted M. (2004). *Cognitive behavioral therapy manual for anorexia nervosa.* Unpublished manuscript.

Pike KM, Devlin MJ, & Loeb KL. (2004). Cognitive-behavioral therapy in the treatment of anorexia nervosa, bulimia nervosa, and binge eating disorder. In JK Thompson (Ed.), *Handbook of eating disorders and obesity* (pp. 130–162). Hoboken, NJ: Wiley.

Pike KM, Loeb K, & Vitousek K. (1996). Cognitive-behavioral therapy for anorexia nervosa and bulimia nervosa. In JK Thompson (Ed.), *Body image: Eating disorders and obesity* (pp. 253–302). Washington, DC: American Psychological Association.

Pike KM, Walsh BT, Vitousek K, Wilson GT, & Bauer J. (2003). Cognitive behavioral therapy in the post-hospital treatment of anorexia nervosa. *American Journal of Psychiatry*, 160:2046–2049.

Proschaska J, & DiClemente C. (1983). Stages and processes of self-changing of smoking: Toward an integrative model of change. *Journal of Consulting and Clinical Psychology*, 51:390–395.

Proschaska J, DiClemente C, & Norcross J. (1992). In search of how people change. *American Psychologist*, 49:1102–1114.

Reas DL, Whisenhunt BL, Netemeyer RG, & Williamson, DA. (2002). Development of the Body Checking Questionnaire: A self-report measure of body checking behaviors. *International Journal of Eating Disorders*, 31:324–333.

Rock CL, & Curran-Celentano J. (1994). Nutritional disorder of anorexia nervosa: A review. *International Journal of Eating Disorders*, 15:187–203.

Rosen JC, Srebnik D, Saltzberg E, & Wendt S. (1991). Development of a Body Image Avoidance Questionnaire. *Psychological Assessment: A Journal of Consulting and Clinical Psychology*, 3:32–37.

Serfaty MA, Turkington D, Heap M, Ledsham L, & Jolley E. (1999). Cognitive therapy versus dietary counseling in the outpatient treatment of anorexia nervosa. *European Eating Disorders Review*, 7:334–350.

Shafran R, Fairburn CG, Nelson L, & Robinson PH. (2003). The interpretation of symptoms of severe dietary restraint. *Behaviour Research and Therapy*, 41:887–894.

Striegel-Moore R, & McAvay G. (1986). Psychological and behavioral correlates of feeling fat in women. *International Journal of Eating Disorders*, 5:935–947.

Thompson JK, & Williams DE. (1987). An interpersonally based cognitive behavioral psychotherapy. In M Herson, RM Eisler, & PM Miller (Eds.), *Progress in behavior modification* (Vol. 21, pp. 230–258). New York: Sage.

Treasure J. (1997). *Anorexia nervosa: A survival guide for families, friends and sufferers.* London: Psychology Press.

Truax CB, & Mitchell KM. (1971). Research on certain therapist interpersonal skills in relation to process and outcome. In AE Bergin & SL Garfield (Eds.), *Handbook of psychotherapy and behavior change: An empirical analysis* (pp. 299–344). New York: Wiley.

Vitousek K, & Hollon SD. (1990). The investigation of schematic content and processing in eating disorders. *Cognitive Therapy and Research*, 14:191–214.

Vitousek K, Watson S, & Wilson GT. (1998). Enhancing motivation for change in eating disorders. *Clinical Psychology Review*, 18:476–498.

Wilson GT, Grilo CM, & Vitousek KM. (2007). Psychological treatments for eating disorders. *American Psychologist*, 62:199–216.

Young JE, Weinberger AD, & Beck AT. (2001). Cognitive therapy for depression. In DH Barlow (Ed.), *Clinical handbook of psychological disorders* (3rd ed., pp. 264–308). New York: Guilford Press.

CHAPTER 6

Specialist Supportive Clinical Management for Anorexia Nervosa

Virginia V. W. McIntosh, Jennifer Jordan, and Cynthia M. Bulik

Specialist supportive clinical management (SSCM) for anorexia nervosa (AN) is an outpatient treatment that can be offered to individuals with low weight in usual clinical practice. The treatment was developed for a psychotherapy trial for AN (McIntosh et al., 2005), as a comparison treatment to cognitive-behavioral therapy (CBT) and interpersonal psychotherapy (IPT). It combines features of clinical management (Fawcett, Epstein, Fiester, Elkin, & Autry, 1987) and supportive psychotherapy (Dewald, 1994). SSCM addresses the core symptoms of AN, including low weight, restrictive eating patterns, and inappropriate compensatory behaviors. The therapy focuses on facilitating normal eating and the restoration of weight; providing high-quality education, information, and advice about AN, eating, and weight; and addressing other life issues, as identified by the patient.

Theoretical Models in the Development of SSCM

The theoretical basis of SSCM is the synthesis of two existing treatment models—clinical management and supportive psychotherapy—both with established efficacy in the treatment of some mental health problems.

Clinical Management

"Clinical management" refers to the provision of good quality clinical care from an experienced clinician. In addition, there may or may not be a further specific treatment regimen (Fawcett et al., 1987). Clinical management highlights the generic role of health professionals in ensuring safety; providing care, support, and education; and doing no harm (Joyce, 1995). These prerequisites form the basis of treatment, and within this context the clinician may also choose to use other specific treatments. The evidence is mixed regarding whether more specialized treatments confer added benefit to sound clinical management for diverse clinical problems (Baskin, Tierney, Minami, & Wampold, 2003). For example, a recent randomized controlled trial for patients with major depression who had coronary artery disease found that the combination of a specialized treatment (IPT) and medication was not superior to the combination of clinical management plus medication (Lesperance et al., 2007). It may be that the failure to detect significant effects between treatments is due to the underrecognized impact of nonspecific factors common to all clinical interventions (Ablon & Jones, 1998, 1999). The contribution of nonspecific factors has been estimated to be as great as two-thirds of treatment effects obtained (Roberts, Kewman, Mercier, & Hovell, 1993).

The National Institute of Mental Health Treatment of Depression Collaborative Research Program compared four treatments for depressed outpatients: clinical management plus placebo pill, clinical management plus imipramine, CBT, or IPT (Elkin, Parloff, Hadley, & Autry, 1985). Clinical management included attending to the therapeutic relationship; providing psychological support, instruction, advice, education, and information; and eliciting patients' expressions of thoughts and feelings about their illness; and it proscribed interventions related to specific organized systems of psychotherapy (Fawcett et al., 1987). Overall, little difference was found in outcome between clinical management and the two specialized psychotherapies (Elkin et al., 1989), raising the question of the likely effectiveness of nonspecific psychotherapy factors for the treatment of depression. This study identified one of the main goals of clinical management as fostering and maintaining a therapeutic relationship between patient and clinician that promotes adherence to the treatment regimen.

Clinical management relies on a thorough assessment of the history of the disorder, education about the disorder (symptoms and diagnosis), what causes it (maintaining and associated factors), what will happen if it is left untreated (outcome), and what can be done about it (treatment) (Joyce, 1995). An open discussion of these issues is important because patients may present with ideas that differ from the clinician's, and this incompatibility of views may hinder treatment. Patients may describe fears or prejudices about mental health problems that need to be understood and addressed in order for good clinical management to proceed. Sharing the diagnosis and a working understanding of the problem with the patient in this way enables the clinician to provide, and the patient to receive, care and treatment. Ongoing education about the disorder can be provided in spoken form and augmented with written materials. As well as enhancing the psychoeducation received verbally, providing patients with written materials allows them to share the diagnosis and management of their condition with family members or friends.

Clinical management emphasizes ongoing monitoring and review of the core symptoms of the disorder. This process involves the identification of "core" or "target" symptoms to be agreed upon by the clinician and the patient. Clinical management aims to prevent relapse and includes understanding the warning signs of illness recurrence. The role of changing life events in the patient's improvement should also be considered. Thus, part of clinical management includes the clinician's encouragement and support for coping with these changes.

Clinical management includes the key strategies of supporting the resumption of normal eating and return to a normal weight (National Institute for Health and Clinical Excellence, 2004; Yager et al., 2000). A key feature of AN is the patient's abnormal nutritional status and dietary patterns. Nutritional factors have been identified in both the onset and maintenance of the disorder (Garner, 1993). Dieting is an important trigger of the illness, often initiated as an understandable response to personal or interpersonal concerns, or to major life changes or stressful events (Bruch, 1977; Garner & Garfinkel, 1980). Despite considerable evidence for the efficacy of supervised weight gain in an inpatient setting, there is general agreement the relapse rates are high (Herzog, Zeeck, Hartmann, & Nickel, 2004). It may be that the enforced or institutionalized eating that produces the weight gain during hospitalization may not generalize to everyday life, or to the maintenance of normal weight levels (Wilson, Touyz, O'Connor, & Beumont, 1985). Treatment that facilitates a return to normal weight by encouraging and supporting normal eating in the usual environment through outpatient treatment is likely to be more effective.

In summary, clinical management comprises education, care and support, and the development of a therapeutic relationship that promotes adherence to treatment. Clinical management for AN emphasizes the relearning of normal eating leading to the restoration of weight (McIntosh et al., 2006).

Supportive Psychotherapy

Luborsky (1984) described supportive psychotherapy as including techniques such as demonstrating support, acceptance, and affection toward the patient; working together with the patient to make changes; communicating optimism that goals are achievable; focusing on the patient's strengths and respecting the patient's defenses; and acknowledging the growing ability of the patient to accomplish results without the clinician's help. Supportive psychotherapy uses techniques such as active listening, verbal and nonverbal attending, open questioning, reflection, praise, reassurance, advice, and clinician self-disclosure (Barber, Stratt, Halperin, & Connolly, 2001; Barrowclough et al., 2001; Winston, Pinsker, & McCullough, 1986).

Supportive psychotherapy has been widely practiced in clinical settings, including general practice and other medical settings (Bloch, 2006; Rockland, 1993). Although historically supportive psychotherapy has been held in low regard, when compared with exploratory dynamic therapies (Berlincioni & Barbieri, 2004), there is evidence of its effectiveness with a wide range of clinical problems, including bulimia nervosa (BN), schizophrenia, borderline conditions, anxiety and affective disorders, and dual-diagnosis alcohol and psychiatric problems (Barrowclough et al., 2001; Fairburn, Kirk, O'Connor, & Cooper, 1986; Hellerstein, Pinsker, Rosenthal, & Klee, 1994; Nightingale & McQueeney, 1996). Evidence also exists that patients highly value a supportive therapeutic stance (Richards et al., 2006). Supportive psychotherapy aims to assist patients by providing an encouraging therapeutic context with a warm, optimistic clinician, within which the patient is helped to make changes and explore issues that promote change.

Review of Treatment Literature

There is existing evidence of the effectiveness of each of the two individual components of SSCM: clinical management and supportive psychotherapy.

SSCM as an integrated treatment for AN has been the subject of one published clinical trial to date (McIntosh et al., 2004). The therapy was delivered as a nonspecialized psychotherapy comparison for AN, compared with CBT and IPT in a clinical trial. Both CBT and IPT have established efficacy in the treatment of other eating disorders (EDs), including BN (Wilson, Grilo, & Vitousek, 2007) and binge-eating disorder (BED) (Agras, Walsh, Fairburn, Wilson, & Kraemer, 2000; Wilfley et al., 2002), with strong theoretical and empirical rationales for their application in AN (Garner, Vitousek, & Pike, 1997; McIntosh, Bulik, McKenzie, Luty, & Jordan, 2000).

In this controlled clinical trial, 56 women with AN diagnosed using broad weight criteria, including individuals whose weight was in the "lenient" weight range (i.e., BMI 17.5–19 kg/m^2) (McIntosh et al., 2004), were randomly assigned to one of three therapies (IPT, CBT, or SSCM). Therapy consisted of approximately 20 weekly therapy sessions over 6 months. Over 60% of patients completed therapy, with approximately half of these having a good or very good outcome at the end of treatment. In comparison, of those participants who did not complete the trial, only one had a good outcome. Analyses of all randomized patients revealed significant differences among the therapies on the primary global outcome measure (a 4-point scale ranging from 4 = meets full criteria for the AN spectrum to 1 = no significant features of an eating disorder) (McIntosh et al., 2005). Contrasts of the specific treatments revealed that SSCM was superior to IPT, and that CBT outcomes, which were between those of SSCM and IPT, did not differ significantly from either IPT or SSCM. These findings are contrary to the study's central hypothesis that the specialized psychotherapies (IPT, CBT) would result in superior outcome. Since the study's sample size was small with limited statistical power and the rates of attrition were high, replication of this study and other tests of the effectiveness of SSCM are needed.

Further research is also needed to determine which components of SSCM may contribute to its efficacy. It is possible to speculate about the therapeutically important components of SSCM, particularly within the context of the clinical trial in which the outcome of SSCM was compared with that of CBT and IPT. Key SSCM elements include psychoeducation and the focus on normalizing eating for patients with AN. However, as these are also core strategies in CBT, it is noteworthy that SSCM was more effective than CBT for those completing the trial. CBT included additional strategies, most notably key *cognitive* components—identification and evaluation of automatic thoughts and core beliefs, and cognitive restructuring—whereas SSCM explicitly avoided such techniques. It is possible that the focus on normalizing eating and psychoeducation are key effective components of both SSCM and CBT. If this is the case, extensive focus on cognitions within CBT would result in reduced time spent on other elements of therapy. Although studies of pure psychoeducation are lacking, there is some support for the efficacy of psychoeducation as a treatment for problematic eating patterns and EDs (Geist, Heinmaa, Stephens, Davis, & Katzman, 2000; Ricca et al., 1997; Stice, Orjada, & Tristan, 2006; Strachan & Cash, 2002), and there is evidence of a relation between high levels of information and advice giving and a strong therapeutic alliance with anxious patients (Sexton, Hembre, & Kvarme, 1996).

Treatment component analyses suggest that specific cognitive interventions may add little to the treatment outcome in depression. Rapid response within CBT often occurs prior to the introduction of cognitive interventions for depression (Longmore & Worrell, 2007), and in BN outcome is predicted by response early in CBT, at which stage therapy is focused on psychoeducation, building a therapeutic alliance, and the introduction of normal eating habits (Fairburn, Marcus, & Wilson, 1993). In cognitive therapy for depression, symptom reduction has been found to relate to the more concrete cognitive strategies (e.g., examination of evidence for beliefs, practicing rational responses, and identifying cognitive errors) rather than more abstract CBT strategies (i.e., exploring underlying assumptions, the personal meaning of thoughts, the adaptive value of beliefs, the relation of thoughts and feelings, and encouraging the distancing of beliefs) (DeRubeis & Feeley, 1990). Behavioral activation has been found to be more effective than full CBT in the treatment of depression (Dimidjian et al., 2006).

It is also possible that SSCM's psychotherapeutic context, in which the patient determines the additional focus of the therapy session, and an encouraging therapeutic stance that respects, rather than challenges, the patient's defenses may be key mechanisms in its effectiveness.

Treatment Manual for SSCM

Orienting the Patient to SSCM

Early in therapy, a key task is to discuss aspects of therapy explicitly, including the patient's expectations, the patient's and clinician's roles and responsibilities during therapy, and practical matters related to the frequency and timing of sessions. Overall, therapy consists of two strands that run simultaneously throughout the sessions. The first is the gradual return to normal eating in order to restore weight to within a healthy range. The second involves attending to other life issues that may relate directly or indirectly to restrictive eating and low weight, or may be unrelated. The clinician's role is to support and encourage the patient as she makes changes in her eating and in other areas. The clinician will also give good quality information about food, eating, body shape, weight, and AN, and advice about strategies that may be helpful. The orientation to therapy includes discussion of a model of the development of AN (see Figure 6.1).

Establishing and Reviewing Target Symptoms

Early in therapy the clinician works with the patient to identify the symptoms of AN, including those "target symptoms" that will be monitored within SSCM. Figure 6.2 lists symptoms to be reviewed. Together the clinician and patient decide which of the patient's current symptoms play a key role in the disorder and will become major foci of treatment, establishing the Target Symptom Checklist (see Figure 6.3). These target symptoms are then reviewed at each session.

The purpose of the review of target symptoms is threefold: (1) to identify those key behaviors or problems that are part of the illness of AN for the patient; (2) to reassure the patient that her problems are understood by the clinician and are part of the clinical syndrome of AN; and (3) to establish the symptom focus as an essential part of each therapy session and to prompt monitoring of specific aspects of the patient's progress.

The clinician is explicit about the improvements expected in the target symptoms of AN (weight gain, normalized eating, and the elimination of compensatory behaviors). Whenever possible, the clinician enhances expectancies of a positive outcome by identifying strengths in the patient's presentation. It is also desirable to enhance the

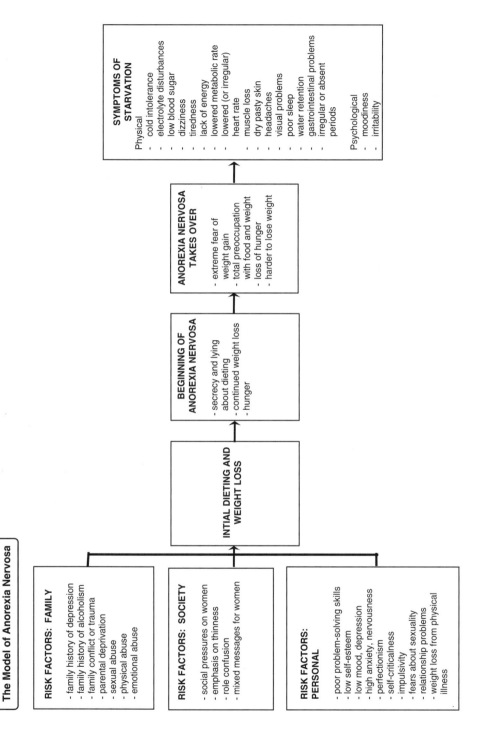

The Model of Anorexia Nervosa

RISK FACTORS: FAMILY

- family history of depression
- family history of alcoholism
- family conflict or trauma
- parental deprivation
- sexual abuse
- physical abuse
- emotional abuse

RISK FACTORS: SOCIETY

- social pressures on women
- emphasis on thinness
- role confusion
- mixed messages for women

RISK FACTORS: PERSONAL

- poor problem-solving skills
- low self-esteem
- low mood, depression
- high anxiety, nervousness
- perfectionism
- self-criticalness
- impulsivity
- fears about sexuality
- relationship problems
- weight loss from physical illness

INITIAL DIETING AND WEIGHT LOSS

BEGINNING OF ANOREXIA NERVOSA

- secrecy and lying about dieting
- continued weight loss
- hunger

ANOREXIA NERVOSA TAKES OVER

- extreme fear of weight gain
- total preoccupation with food and weight
- loss of hunger
- harder to lose weight

SYMPTOMS OF STARVATION

Physical
- cold intolerance
- electrolyte disturbances
- low blood sugar
- dizziness
- tiredness
- lack of energy
- lowered metabolic rate
- lowered (or irregular) heart rate
- muscle loss
- dry pasty skin
- headaches
- visual problems
- poor sleep
- water retention
- gastrointestinal problems
- irregular or absent periods

Psychological
- moodiness
- irritability

FIGURE 6.1. SSCM model of AN.

Eating disorder behaviors	Physical/emotional consequences	Related issues
Dietary restriction	Constipation	Alcohol/drug problems
Binge eating	Cold intolerance	Suicidality
Vomiting	Body image disturbance	Self-mutilation
Diuretic use	Body dissatisfaction	Obsessionality
Laxative use	Changes in sexual interest/behavior	Low self-esteem
Appetite suppressant use	Amenorrhea	Social withdrawal
Use of diet pills/amphetamines	Low energy	Social eating problems
Emetic use	Fatigue	
Excessive fluid intake	Irritability	
	Hyperactivity	
	Low motivation	
	Low mood	
	Level of insight	

FIGURE 6.2. Symptoms to be reviewed.

patient's motivation for therapy by reviewing the disadvantages and discomfort associated with having AN and gathering sufficient information to identify how things will be different when the ED improves. Once improvements are noted in eating patterns, clinical considerations dictate the content, extent, and frequency of the target symptom enquiry, but this review continues throughout the course of therapy, to a greater or lesser degree.

Nutritional Education and Advice

The primary goals for normalizing eating include establishing a pattern of regular eating from a variety of food groups, eating sufficient food for good health, restoring normal weight, and the resumption of reproductive functioning to the extent that it is disturbed. Other goals include being able to engage in food-related social activities, normalizing food-related activities such as shopping and food preparation, and eliminating idiosyncratic food-related activities such as unhealthy compensatory behaviors (vomiting, overexercising, laxative abuse), calorie counting, and rituals and obsessions around food and eating.

When assessing the patient's current pattern of eating, it is important to gain detailed information about food-related activities, including food shopping, cooking, and preparation. Gathering information about other aspects of eating, such as eating with other people, will help to establish the broad goals of normalizing eating. Normal

NAME _____   SESSION # _____   Date _____

Changes since last session:
Note frequency/severity where appropriate.

Weight: _____ kg   Change since last session: _____ kg

No. of meals eaten per day _____

No. of days of regular eating _____

Exercise _____

Vomiting _____

Laxatives _____

Other compensatory behaviors _____

_____

_____

Menstruation   Y/N

Other target symptoms _____

_____

_____

_____

_____

_____

_____

_____

_____

_____

_____

_____

_____

_____

FIGURE 6.3. SSCM Target Symptom Checklist.

eating generally involves eating three meals and two or three snacks per day, eating a wide variety of foods to provide nutritionally adequate food intake, and eating a sufficient amount of food to prevent the symptoms of starvation and to maintain weight in the normal range. It is normal to have food preferences, and the patient is encouraged to think about the foods she prefers. However it is not normal or desirable to eliminate food groups or food types from one's diet in order to control weight or shape, and it is not normal or desirable for underweight individuals to avoid eating foods they like. Many women with AN are fearful that once they begin to eat more normally, they will be unable to stop and will become very fat. The clinician reassures the patient that normal eating also involves knowing when to stop eating, and explains that learning when she has eaten enough is part of normal eating.

Early in therapy, a description of the goals for normal eating and the rationale behind them are provided. Evaluation of the patient's current eating and encouragement to eat regular meals and snacks also occur. Once this pattern is established, the clinician ensures that the patient is eating adequate quantities of food and encourages eating a broader range of foods. The clinician gives instructions for eating normal meals, increasing the variety of foods eaten, normalizing the eating rate, and introducing feared or "forbidden" foods into the diet (Beumont, O'Connor, Touyz, & Williams, 1987; Hsu, Holben, & West, 1990; Huse & Lucas, 1985). In addition, the clinician reviews the patient's progress at each session, being alert to her achievements, acknowledging and praising accordingly, and encouraging her to tackle progressively more. The patient is encouraged to begin by incorporating less difficult foods into her diet initially, only gradually working toward more difficult eating practices. The clinician helps the patient to decide how to do this and how to cope with the anxiety that normal eating invariably provokes. Education is given about good nutrition (Treasure et al., 1995), including individual nutritional needs, metabolism, the relationship between dieting and binge eating, how to choose nutritious foods, planning food shopping, eating out, and the discussion of menu options. Because a major content area of SSCM is the resumption of normal eating, the therapy includes detailed discussion of how to increase the regularity, variety, and quantity of food with the aim of gaining weight. The clinician gives the same message repeatedly and employs multiple ways of helping the patient to eat more.

If the patient resists focusing on eating or is unwilling to increase food choices, the clinician acknowledges the patient's anxiety about making these changes, tries to understand the particular problems that the patient is experiencing, and takes these into account. The clinician gently reminds the patient that normalizing eating is the only way we know to recover from AN. It may be helpful to revisit options, be creative, and ask the patient what things she thinks she *could* do, such as discussing increasing the quantity of safe foods if she feels unable to increase food variety immediately. If the patient feels completely unable to make a change, the clinician may simply accept that perhaps this week the patient is unable to introduce something new into her diet, thus making the task for the week to consolidate changes so far. The clinician may reframe the patient's feeling of being unable to make a further change as a sign that the pace of change was faster than ideal. The clinician may ask the patient if there are any other problems or pressures in her life that may be making it hard to focus on making changes in eating. Therapy then focuses on assisting with these areas.

Psychoeducation about Food, Eating, Body Shape, Weight, and AN

SSCM includes a substantial psychoeducational component, with verbal and written information and advice about AN and other areas relevant to the ED (Garner, Rockert, Olmsted, Johnson, & Coscina, 1985). Psychoeducational materials are made available on a wide variety of topics and may include a definition of AN, sociocultural influences on eating disorders, effects of starvation, ineffectiveness of dieting, ineffectiveness of purging, theories of biological and genetic contributions to weight status and body shape, exercise as weight control, healthy exercise, consequences of eating disorders, the cycle of disordered eating, society's fat phobia, what the scales are really telling the patient, nutrition and recovery from EDs, fertility and EDs, and bone health. The clinician is responsible for providing the patient with good quality information about AN, including its symptoms.

Dealing with Unhelpful Body Focus

SSCM uses this psychoeducational information-giving approach to combat the unhelpful body focus in AN. Several written handouts address the sociocultural context in which thinness is prized and the "fat phobia" inherent in Western societies. In addition, the clinician may recommend reading related to body acceptance that encourages a more positive appraisal of a range of body shapes and sizes. In addition, the patient may be encouraged to stop dwelling on body dissatisfaction by shifting focus onto other attributes about which she feels more positively. Similarly, if the patient is engaging in body checking, she may be encouraged to "notice" the effect of obsessing or ruminating about body and weight, recognizing that undue focus on body shape and weight has deleterious effects and leads to abnormal eating and self-starvation. This new understanding may prompt the clinician to give advice about reducing this unhelpful focus by interrupting the pattern and distracting herself by increasing more constructive activities (i.e., keeping busy).

Monitoring Physical Status

Regular weighing during the early states of therapy is important for monitoring weight status, either at each session or at home between less frequent sessions, and helps to address and regulate behavioral extremes related to the fear of weight gain: both the avoidance of weighing or excessive weighing. Once eating patterns and weight have stabilized, weighing may be needed less frequently. Other physical measures taken at the beginning of treatment, and thereafter as clinically indicated, include blood pressure, body temperature, electrocardiogram (EKG), heart rate, and blood screen (including routine biochemistry, lipid screen, vitamin assays, thyroid function, iron studies, and hematology count). Close regular monitoring of health status may be arranged with the patient's general medical practitioner.

Establishing a Weight Range Goal

The expectation of weight gain during treatment is an essential aspect of the clinical management of AN. The specifics of a weight range goal are best discussed toward the end of the initial phase of treatment, when sufficient information has been imparted to the patient and a therapeutic relationship has been established. Discussing goals for weight gain is perhaps the most anxiety-provoking aspect of treatment and has the potential to increase resistance if broached in detail too early in treatment. Figure 6.4 is a chart designed to summarize the patient's weight history and key symptoms of AN (a blank chart is provided in Figure 6.5). The patient's target weight range is an individually determined healthy body weight range that takes into account her own premorbid and family weight history. In general, in outpatient settings, a slow, steady rate of weight gain is the goal, approximately 0.5 kg/week (Herzog et al., 2004). The clinician reviews with the patient what the physical consequences of being within this target weight range are likely to be for her, such as the return of regular menstruation (in individuals with amenorrhea or dysmenorrhea), improved sleep, and increased energy and concentration.

The clinician acknowledges with the patient the distress she may feel at the prospect of weight gain, empathizing without entering into bargaining regarding weight goals. Information about goals and guidelines for weight gain are presented from the stance of promoting patient well-being.

If the patient resists weight gain, the clinician can explore the patient's reasons and fears and acknowledge her distress. Furthermore, the clinician can encourage the patient to review the model of the onset of AN, revisit psychoeducational material related to the effects of starvation and the need for weight restoration, and renegotiate the goal for the week. If the patient does not like being weighed or wants to avoid knowing her current weight, the clinician can assess the reasons for the patient's anxiety and desire to avoid weighing and normalize this response, noting that many patients share this fear.

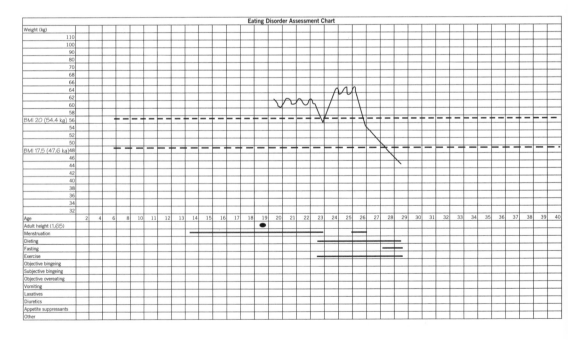

FIGURE 6.4. Weight and symptom chart example.

Eating Disorder Assessment Chart

Weight (kg): 110, 100, 90, 80, 70, 68, 66, 64, 62, 60, 58, 56, 54, 52, 50, 48, 46, 44, 42, 40, 38, 36, 34, 32

Age	2	4	6	8	10	11	12	13	14	15	16	17	18	19	20	21	22	23	24	25	26	27	28	29	30	31	32	33	34	35	36	37	38	39	40
Adult height ( )																																			
Menstruation																																			
Dieting																																			
Fasting																																			
Exercise																																			
Objective bingeing																																			
Subjective bingeing																																			
Objective overeating																																			
Vomiting																																			
Laxatives																																			
Diuretics																																			
Appetite suppressants																																			
Other																																			

FIGURE 6.5. Weight and symptom chart.

The patient could be given a handout on "what the scales are really telling us," which discusses the range of issues associated with overvaluing weight information. The clinician reminds the patient that weight is charted weekly as a way of monitoring progress toward weight restoration. The clinician recommends that the patient review the information with the clinician because "it's probably better to know than to fear the worst," and that although it might be distressing sometimes, keeping a quiet eye on her weight, without attending too much or overinterpreting it, is also likely to be reassuring in the long run. The potential risk of the patient's avoiding knowing her weight and then finding out inadvertently and having to deal with a feeling of shock can also be mentioned. If the patient remains insistent that she does not wish to know her current weight, the clinician could agree to this in the short term but revisit the issue at a later session.

Support with Life Issues or Problems

A key task of SSCM is to provide support, including understanding, giving advice, and encouraging change, in other areas of the patient's life in which she identifies that she has concerns. Although such issues may appear to relate to the development of, or may be sequelae to, the problems with eating and low weight, it may be unclear whether they are in fact related directly, or in any way, to her current illness. However, a key task of SSCM therapy is to explore these issues within a supportive psychotherapy model, even in the absence of a theoretical link between the life issues and the ED.

If the patient does not raise other issues for discussion or support or there are no other problems of note outside the ED, the clinician can ask in general how things are going in different spheres of the patient's life. If no difficulties are present or reported, the clinician can inquire about the patient's future life plans. If there is nothing else to discuss, this can be acknowledged explicitly and the session can be terminated early by agreement. If the patient is responding well in terms of the ED symptoms but is not yet within the healthy weight range and all other areas of her life are going smoothly, the clinician could discuss with the patient if she would like to space out the sessions or meet for shorter sessions routinely unless issues arise that need more time.

If the clinician believes that the patient has problems, but the patient does not seem to be aware of them or does not raise them in therapy, the clinician can inquire from time to time how things are going in other areas of the patient's life (including this area of possible difficulty) and remind the patient that she can discuss any issues she wishes. It may be helpful for the clinician to note an issue or area that appears to be important. However, if the patient does not express any concern and there are no harm issues, in keeping with the nonconfrontational stance of SSCM the clinician may leave such an issue unaddressed until the patient chooses to raise it for discussion.

Finally, if the patient wants to talk predominantly about other life issues, the clinician can negotiate to schedule this discussion for later in the session, after the systematic review of normalized eating and target symptoms.

Phases of Intervention

SSCM is divided into three phases of therapy. Although the division between these phases is not firmly fixed, the major tasks of each phase are different, and therapy usually follows the pattern described here.

First Sessions

Therapy begins with the clinician conducting a thorough assessment, including a full history of the course of the present episode, of previous episodes of AN, and of past treatments for the ED, including her response to these. The clinician obtains sufficient information about the detail of the patient's eating to establish what changes must be made for her to implement normal eating patterns.

Following the initial assessment, the patient is oriented to SSCM, the target symptoms are identified, and the goals for weight gain and normal eating are identified and agreed upon. In the initial phase of SSCM, the clinician's role is active, with assessment and psychoeducation being prominent tasks. The clinician has an important role in fostering positive expectations regarding the outcome of therapy. This may involve providing reassurance and encouragement to continue despite difficulties.

Midphase

Most of the "work" of SSCM occurs during the middle phase. This phase involves ongoing monitoring of target symptoms and the provision of support and encouragement in attaining the goals of normal eating and the restoration of weight. Regular weekly weighing continues until the target weight has been achieved and maintained. The frequency of weighing can be reduced as the target weight is approached. In the middle and final phases, the clinician is likely to be somewhat less active, while still maintaining the focus on eating and weight issues in each session. For the remainder of the session, it is left to the patient to raise issues in other areas of her life, such as family, school or work, and social life.

Concluding Phase

The final phase includes discussion of issues related to the end of therapy, including making plans for the future and appropriately marking the end of the therapeutic relationship. Toward the end of therapy the patient is encouraged to express her reactions to the therapy and her attitude toward the clinician, and the clinician acknowledges and addresses the patient's concerns about having to deal with future issues on her own without therapy or the clinician. Progress and changes the patient has made are reviewed, with a focus on how to maintain these.

Case Illustration

"Susannah," a composite case, is used to illustrate the tasks of therapy across the phases and sessions of therapy. Susannah is a 27-year-old woman working full time as a secretary. She is married with no children. At presentation for SSCM, she met criteria for AN—binge–purge subtype. Her current weight was 47.5 kg (BMI 17.3) and ED symptoms included restricting, intermittent binges, and overexercising behaviors. She also met current criteria for major depressive disorder and social phobia and had a past history of BN and self-harm. AN developed 3 years previously after Susannah had lost weight following a relationship breakup. Table 6.1 below details the session-by-session content of her 20 sessions of therapy.

TABLE 6.1. Session-by-Session Content for Susannah's Therapy

	Clinician focus and SSCM strategies	Other content and patient-initiated focus
Session 1	Oriented to SSCM, roles, expectations, logistics. Presented SSCM model of AN and individualized for Susannah. Reviewed symptoms to establish target symptom checklist. Discussed need for weight gain in a general sense. Asked to self-monitor food intake and note binges for a few weeks. Noted strengths and previous achievements and positive prognostic aspects to convey hopeful expectations. *Handouts*: SSCM Model of AN; What Is AN?	Target symptoms agreed and Target Symptom Checklist established: restrictive eating, bingeing, preoccupation with food, excessive exercise, eating and body image (weight and shape). Initial focus to be on restricting and bingeing. *Issues raised by Susannah*: Other concerns included low mood, insecure job, financial stress, strained marriage.
Session 2	*Review Target Symptom Checklist (restrictive eating, bingeing, preoccupation, excessive exercise)* Overview of normal eating principles (regular meals, variety and sufficient quantity) but reassured that these would be established gradually at her pace. Set goal for normalizing eating: to introduce a small safe snack at afternoon tea. *Handouts*: What Is Normal Eating?	Symptoms unchanged except no binges since Session 1. Weight ↓ 0.5 kg Eating three small meals but no snacks. *Issues raised by Susannah*: None.
Session 3	*Review Target Symptom Checklist (restrictive eating, bingeing, preoccupation, excessive exercise)* Prescribed normal eating: regular meals and snacks. Prepared for Christmas: idea of keeping to relatively safe foods, limiting alcohol, but taking a flexible approach. Formalized target weight range based on premorbid weight. *Handouts*: Effects of Dieting; Effects of Starvation—Keyes Study (highlight preoccupation)	Introduced an apple most days as a snack but binged on two occasions due to increased availability of special foods at Christmas parties. Weight unchanged. *Issues raised by Susannah*: Stress management: Plans to limit contact with difficult people.
Session 4	*Review Target Symptom Checklist (restrictive eating, bingeing, preoccupation, excessive exercise)* Reviewed progress with meals and snacks and praised achievements. Introduced anti-binge strategies: Increase flexibility of eating—"loose planning." Discussed trajectory of weight restoration. Reassured her that the big increase this week is likely to be due to fluid changes and other metabolic adjustments. Acknowledged her discomfort about weight gain. Reminded of the cost in maintaining underweight status with reference to symptoms such as preoccupation, low mood, reduced social life, etc., and how these are likely to improve once she approaches a healthy weight. Asked what other people value most about her. Gave feedback on pleasant aspects of personality witnessed in session (warmth, sense of humor, smart). *Handouts*: Meals and Snacks (3 + 3); What Are the Scales Telling You?	Eating is less restrictive, one binge. Weight ↑ 2.1 kg *Issues raised by Susannah*: "I don't have a great personality, so I need to be slim."

(cont.)

TABLE 6.1. *(cont.)*

	Clinician focus and SSCM strategies	Other content and patient-initiated focus
Session 5	*Review Target Symptom Checklist* (*restrictive eating, bingeing, preoccupation, excessive exercise*) Reviewed weight—reframed as speedy return to normal weight but pace will slow down. Discussed increased hunger as body tries to reestablish healthy weight so strategy is to try to channel rather than fighting it. Increase to three snacks and ensure that she is eating sufficient quantity. Discussed ways of managing eating in the evening so that she eats a large enough meal, then does other activities to keep busy until suppertime when she can eat a snack, as she requires. Focused on managing guilt after eating; reviewed positive changes—in physical improvement, concentration, sense of humor, libido. Discussed ways of improving self-esteem; encouraged to stop dwelling on perceived faults and increase activities at which she is good. Discussed need to say no sometimes. *Handouts:* Symptoms of Starvation (draw attention to erratic eating during recovery); Assertiveness	One binge Some overeating emerging. Is eating three meals and two snacks. Weight ↑ 1.1 kg Feels guilty after eating but feeling better physically and emotionally. *Issues raised by Susannah:* Poor boundaries with colleagues and house guests. Need to increase self-esteem.
Session 6	*Review Target Symptom Checklist* (*restrictive eating, bingeing, preoccupation, excessive exercise*) Encouraged to see subjective binges as a sign that she needs to do something about the situation at work and to develop her coping skills. Discussed ways of managing stress at work: talk to boss about difficulties and getting help she needs; confide in workmates and family to get support. Discussed the possibility of her taking a short holiday with supportive friend or husband; attend to need for sleep, lifestyle balance, and resuming yoga classes. *Handouts:* Emotional Self-Care	No binges Two subjective binges Eating more regularly—less "junk" food. Weight ↑ 0.6 kg Less preoccupation with food and eating. *Issues raised by Susannah:* Stress at work (feeling unsupported leads to subjective binges).
Session 7	*Review Target Symptom Checklist* (*restrictive eating, bingeing, preoccupation, excessive exercise*) Reviewed overexercise symptom. Commended on reducing excessive amount of exercise to recommended levels. Discussed need to increase flexibility in types of exercise, reintroduce fun as motivation, adjust to circumstances. Reviewed body image/weight concerns Empathized about discomfort over weight change; encouraged to buy some new clothes; reassured and encouraged to reduce focus and use distraction. *Handouts:* Sociocultural Influences on Eating Disorders	No binges More regular eating. Exercise is no longer excessive but is still rigidly adhered to. Weight ↑ 0.5 kg Increasingly self-conscious about weight gain; clothes no longer fit well. *Issues raised by Susannah:* Considering resigning from her job.

(cont.)

TABLE 6.1. *(cont.)*

	Clinician focus and SSCM strategies	Other content and patient-initiated focus
Session 8	*Review Target Symptom Checklist* *(restrictive eating, bingeing, preoccupation, excessive exercise)* Encouraged more variety. Noted that weight is now in the healthy range but still short of premorbid weight. Praised adjusting to reality of attaining healthy weight range by buying new clothes. Reviewed body dissatisfaction; encouraged to (1) work on accepting normal weight, (2) remind herself of health and psychological benefits of being healthy weight, (3) refrain from dwelling on weight issues, and (4) distract herself from negative weight focus by engaging in more constructive activity that makes her feel better. *Handouts*: Food Variety; Food Pyramid	No binges Regular eating but little variety in breakfast or lunch. Weight ↑ 1.2 kg (BMI 21.8) Has bought new clothes that fit her current size. *Issues raised by Susannah*: Reported that her continued worrying about weight gain was annoying her husband.
Session 9	*Review Target Symptom Checklist* *(restrictive eating, bingeing, preoccupation, excessive exercise)* Addressed body image dissatisfaction issue again as per last session. Encouraged to shop in places that have appropriate size/styles that suit her. Encourage to do self-care and activities that feel good for her body. *Handouts*: Body Image	No binges Eating regular meals/snacks. No longer preoccupied with eating and food. Weight ↑ 0.2 kg Still very bothered by weight and shape issues. *Issues raised by Susannah*: None
Session 10	*Review Target Symptom Checklist* *(restrictive eating, bingeing, preoccupation, excessive exercise)* Cautioned her that erratic eating or undereating can lead to binge eating. Focused on eating sufficient quantity and reestablishing regularity of meals. Listened to her concerns about work. *Handouts*: Cycle of Disordered Eating: Restrict–Binge	No binges More erratic eating (busy) Hunger ↑ this week Weight ↑ 0.5 kg *Issues raised by Susannah*: Anxiety about work
Session 11	*Review Target Symptom Checklist* *(restrictive eating, bingeing, preoccupation, excessive exercise)* Encouraged her to increase size of snack at afternoon tea time. Encouraged her to ask husband to help out with, or to cook, dinner. Discussed easy, quickly prepared nutritious meals and the need to change purchasing practices to have healthy easy options on hand. Noted more gradual, steady weight increase. Encouraged self-soothing (using more social support, relaxing activities, getting enough sleep and rest). *Handouts*: Pleasurable Activities	No binges Very tired after work, less motivated to cook meal. Weight ↑ 0.7 kg *Issues raised by Susannah*: Less social contact because busy at work.

(cont.)

TABLE 6.1. *(cont.)*

	Clinician focus and SSCM strategies	Other content and patient-initiated focus
Session 12	*Review Target Symptom Checklist* *(restrictive eating, bingeing, preoccupation, excessive exercise)* Reminded that for optimal functioning, she needs to cover basic nutritional needs regarding food groups; encouraged to increase fruit, vegetables. Reassured that recovery is not just about weight restoration but about the need to consolidate normal eating patterns for long-term health. Reassured that it is entirely appropriate for her to continue attending sessions and of the good progress she has made to date. *Handouts*: refer to Food Pyramid again	No binges Unbalanced food pyramid—too many cookies, sweets (comfort eating). Weight ↑ 0.6 kg *Issues raised by Susannah*: "I shouldn't need to come to therapy because I don't have AN anymore."
Session 13	*Review Target Symptom Checklist* *(restrictive eating, bingeing, preoccupation, excessive exercise)* Noted improvements in eating and exercise. *Handouts*: Mood Management	No binges Eating regularly, better variety, less "comfort eating"; has substituted healthier foods at snack times rather than cookies. Weight ↑ 0.6 kg Exercise less rigid. *Issues raised by Susannah*: Feeling a bit blue in mood again lately.
Session 14	*Review Target Symptom Checklist* *(restrictive eating, bingeing, preoccupation, excessive exercise)* Congratulated on efforts and progress to date. Reiterated desirability of making food choices in line with food pyramid with regard to the balance of treat food versus core nutritional elements. Reassured about weight changes and that it is likely to slow down as she gets closer to premorbid weight. Discussed ways of comforting herself other than using food if feeling low. Discussed trying to behave "as if" she feels confident and attractive, as she felt the last time she was at this weight. Stressed importance of maintaining same level of care for appearance (grooming and nice clothes) as when thinner. *Handouts*: Ineffectiveness of Dieting	No binges Regular eating; Susannah notes that she no longer feels that she is dieting. Still eating a few two many sweets and chocolates, but less comfort eating. Weight ↑ 1.0 kg Exercise within normal limits; not driven. *Issues raised by Susannah*: "I feel less confident, less attractive." Starts new job next week.
Session 15	*Review Target Symptom Checklist* *(restrictive eating, bingeing, preoccupation, excessive exercise)* Normalized increase in stress to do with starting new job. Reminded to look after herself physically and emotionally, including using family/social support. Listened to marital issues. *Handouts*: None	No binges Eating regularly; reasonable variety and quantity. Regular exercise, not excessive. Weight ↓ 0.8 kg *Issues raised by Susannah*: New job issues; mood a bit low, anxious. Reported some success with "as if" exercise. Discussed marital tension.

(cont.)

TABLE 6.1. *(cont.)*

	Clinician focus and SSCM strategies	Other content and patient-initiated focus
Session 16	*Review Target Symptom Checklist* *(restrictive eating, bingeing, preoccupation, excessive exercise)* Reassured again about process of settling into new job and commended for using social support well. *Handouts*: None	No eating disorder symptoms. Eating normally. Weight ↑ 0.3 kg *Issues raised by Susannah*: Anxiety reducing in new job.
Session 17	*Review Target Symptom Checklist* *(restrictive eating, bingeing, preoccupation, excessive exercise)* Reviewed coping at work as per last session. Reassured re her strengths and ability to perform in work role; reminded of past pattern of forming good friendships in the workplace after feeling uncomfortable initially. *Handouts*: None	No eating disorder symptoms Regular eating No change in weight *Issues raised by Susannah*: Still some anxiety but feeling more comfortable with coworkers and with task requirements of new job; marital situation more settled this week.
Session 18	*Review Target Symptom Checklist* *(restrictive eating, bingeing, preoccupation, excessive exercise)* Normalized lack of appetite with illness but reminded to get back on track with normal eating as soon as she is able. Reminded of anxiety management strategies discussed earlier. *Handouts*: Dealing with Anxiety	No binges Ate less due to illness. No overexercising. Weight ↓ 0.5 kg *Issues raised by Susannah*: Anxiety at work.
Session 19	*Review Target Symptom Checklist* *(restrictive eating, bingeing, preoccupation, excessive exercise)* Discussed rebound hunger and the need to eat what the body needs. Discussed normalization of weight and normal fluctuations around a stable weight. Prepared for end of therapy. *Handouts: None*	No binges Overall normalized eating but a little comfort eating again. Weight ↑ 0.4 kg *Issues raised by Susannah*: A little anxious about ending therapy.
Session 20	*Review Target Symptom Checklist* *(restrictive eating, bingeing, preoccupation, excessive exercise)* Reviewed changes in target symptoms over therapy. Focused on significant improvements. Reiterated key/useful strategies, especially importance of maintaining normalized eating and ways of dealing with situations where she comfort eats. Reviewed outstanding problems and issues. Normalized anxiety about ending therapy. Noted strengths and affirmed her capacity to cope without therapy and clinician. Discussed where and how she could access future assistance if necessary. Exchanged goodbyes.	Stable weight; BMI 23 (around premorbid level) Eating normally mostly, but still some mild comfort eating on occasion. Exercise more flexible and at normal levels. No preoccupation with food/eating. Still dissatisfied with weight but more resigned to this and no wish to embark on dieting again. Appreciates her improved overall health. Still has mood and anxiety issues at times but overall is coping better at this stage. *Issues raised by Susannah*: Anxiety about coping on her own without therapy/clinician.

Summary

SSCM is a nonspecific therapy combining clinical management of AN with supportive psychotherapy principles, designed to be delivered by clinicians experienced in the treatment of individuals with EDs. Although there is evidence for the efficacy of both clinical management and supportive psychotherapy, the combined treatment, as elaborated here, is still relatively novel in the treatment of AN. The results of one clinical trial were promising, but this study requires replication with a larger sample and further research to determine the most effective components of SSCM.

References

Ablon JS, & Jones EE. (1998). How expert clinicians' prototypes of an ideal treatment correlate with outcome in psychodynamic and cognitive-behavior therapy. *Psychotherapy Research*, 8:71–83.

Ablon JS, & Jones EE. (1999). Psychotherapy process in the National Institute of Mental Health Treatment of Depression Collaborative Research Program. *Journal of Consulting and Clinical Psychology*, 67:64–75.

Agras WS, Walsh T, Fairburn CG, Wilson GT, & Kraemer HC. (2000). A multicenter comparison of cognitive-behavioral therapy and interpersonal psychotherapy for bulimia nervosa. *Archives of General Psychiatry*, 57:459–466.

Barber JP, Stratt R, Halperin G, & Connolly MB. (2001). Supportive techniques: Are they found in different therapies? *Journal of Psychotherapy Practice and Research*, 10:165–172.

Barrowclough C, King P, Colville J, Russell E, Burns A, & Tarrier N. (2001). A randomized trial of the effectiveness of cognitive-behavioral therapy and supportive counseling for anxiety symptoms in older adults. *Journal of Consulting and Clinical Psychology*, 69:756–762.

Baskin TW, Tierney SC, Minami T, & Wampold BE. (2003). Establishing specificity in psychotherapy: A meta-analysis of structural equivalence of placebo controls. *Journal of Consulting and Clinical Psychology*, 71:973–979.

Berlincioni V, & Barbieri S. (2004). Support and psychotherapy. *American Journal of Psychotherapy*, 58:321–334.

Beumont PJV, O'Connor M, Touyz SW, & Williams H. (1987). Nutritional counselling in the treatment of anorexia and bulimia nervosa. In PJV Beumont, GD Burrows, & RC Casper (Eds.), *The handbook of eating disorders, Part 1: Anorexia and bulimia nervosa* (pp. 349–360). Amsterdam: Elsevier.

Bloch S. (2006). Supportive psychotherapy. In S. Bloch (Ed.), *An introduction to the psychotherapies* (4th ed., pp. 215–235). Oxford, UK: Oxford University Press.

Bruch H. (1977). Psychological antecedents of anorexia nervosa. In RA Vigersky (Ed.), *Anorexia nervosa* (pp. 1–10). New York: Raven Press.

DeRubeis RJ, & Feeley M. (1990). Determinants of change in cognitive therapy for depression. *Cognitive Therapy and Research*, 14:469–482.

Dewald PA. (1994). Principles of supportive psychotherapy. *American Journal of Psychotherapy*, 48:505–518.

Dimidjian S, Hollon SD, Dobson KS, Schmaling KB, Kohlenberg RJ, Addis ME, et al. (2006). Randomized trial of behavioral activation, cognitive therapy, and antidepressant medication in the acute treatment of adults with major depression. *Journal of Consulting and Clinical Psychology*, 74:658–670.

Elkin E, Parloff MB, Hadley SW, & Autry JH. (1985). NIMH Treatment of Depression Collaborative Research Program: Background and research plan. *Archives of General Psychiatry,* 42:305–316.

Elkin I, Shea MT, Watkins JT, Imber SD, Sotsky SM, Collins JF, et al. (1989). NIMH Treatment of Depression Collaborative Research Program: General effectiveness of treatments. *Archives of General Psychiatry,* 46:971–982.

Fairburn CG, Kirk J, O'Connor M, & Cooper PJ. (1986). A comparison of two psychological treatments for bulimia nervosa. *Behaviour Research and Therapy,* 24:629–643.

Fairburn CG, Marcus MD, & Wilson GT. (1993). Cognitive-behavioral therapy for binge eating and bulimia nervosa: A comprehensive treatment manual. In CG Fairburn & GT Wilson (Eds.), *Binge eating: Nature, assessment, and treatment* (pp. 361–404). New York: Guilford Press.

Fawcett J, Epstein P, Fiester SJ, Elkin E, & Autry JH. (1987). Clinical management: Imipramine/placebo administration manual. *Psychopharmacology Bulletin,* 23:309–321.

Garner DM. (1993). Pathogenesis of anorexia nervosa. *Lancet,* 341:1631–1635.

Garner DM, & Garfinkel PE. (1980). Socio-cultural factors in the development of anorexia nervosa. *Psychological Medicine,* 10:647–656.

Garner DM, Rockert W, Olmsted MP, Johnson CL, & Coscina DV. (1985). Psychoeducational principles in the treatment of bulimia and anorexia nervosa. In DM Garner & PE Garfinkel (Eds.), *Handbook of psychotherapy for anorexia nervosa and bulimia* (pp. 147–177). New York: Guilford Press.

Garner DM, Vitousek KM, & Pike KM. (1997). Cognitive-behavioral therapy for anorexia nervosa. In DM Garner & PE Garfinkel (Eds.), *Handbook of treatment for eating disorders* (2nd ed., pp. 94–144). New York: Guilford Press.

Geist R, Heinmaa M, Stephens D, Davis R, & Katzman DK. (2000). Comparison of family therapy and family group psychoeducation in adolescents with anorexia nervosa. *Canadian Journal of Psychiatry,* 45:173–178.

Hellerstein DJ, Pinsker H, Rosenthal RN, & Klee S. (1994). Supportive therapy as the treatment model of choice. *Journal of Psychotherapy Practice and Research,* 3:300–306.

Herzog T, Zeeck A, Hartmann A, & Nickel T. (2004). Lower targets for weekly weight gain lead to better results in inpatient treatment of anorexia nervosa: A pilot study. *European Eating Disorders Review,* 12:164–168.

Hsu GLK, Holben B, & West S. (1990). Nutritional counseling in bulimia nervosa. *International Journal of Eating Disorders,* 11:55–62.

Huse DM, & Lucas AR. (1985). Treatment of anorexia nervosa: Dietary considerations. In RT Frankle, J Dwyer, L Moragne, & A Owen (Eds.), *Dietary treatment and prevention of obesity* (pp. 201–210). London: Libbey.

Joyce PR. (1995). The clinical management of depression. In PR Joyce, SE Romans, PM Ellis, & TS Silverstone (Eds.), *Affective disorders* (pp. 35–46). Christchurch, NZ: Christchurch School of Medicine.

Lesperance F, Frasure-Smith N, Koszycki D, Laliberte MA, van Zyl LT, Baker B, et al. (2007). Effects of citalopram and interpersonal psychotherapy on depression in patients with coronary artery disease: The Canadian Cardiac Randomized Evaluation of Antidepressant and Psychotherapy Efficacy (CREATE) trial. *Journal of the American Medical Association,* 297:367–379.

Longmore RJ, & Worrell M. (2007). Do we need to challenge thoughts in cognitive behavior therapy? *Clinical Psychology Review,* 27:173–187.

Luborsky L. (1984). *Principles of psychoanalytic psychotherapy.* New York: Basic Books.

McIntosh VV, Bulik CM, McKenzie JM, Luty SE, & Jordan J. (2000). Interpersonal psychotherapy for anorexia nervosa. *International Journal of Eating Disorders,* 27:125–139.

McIntosh VVW, Jordan J, Carter FA, Luty SE, McKenzie JM, Bulik CM, et al. (2005). Three psychotherapies for anorexia nervosa: A randomized controlled trial. *American Journal of Psychiatry*, 162:741–747.

McIntosh VVW, Jordan J, Carter FA, McKenzie JM, Luty SE, Bulik CM, et al. (2004). Strict versus lenient weight criterion in anorexia nervosa. *European Eating Disorders Review*, 12:51–60.

McIntosh VVW, Jordan J, Luty SE, Carter FA, McKenzie JM, Bulik CM, et al. (2006). Specialist supportive clinical management for anorexia nervosa. *International Journal of Eating Disorders*, 39:625–632.

National Institute for Health and Clinical Excellence (NICE). (2004). *Eating disorders: Core interventions in the treatment and management of anorexia nervosa, bulimia nervosa and related eating disorders*. London: Author.

Nightingale LC, & McQueeney DA. (1996). Group therapy for schizophrenia: Combining and expanding the psychoeducational model with supportive psychotherapy. *International Journal of Group Psychotherapy*, 46:517–533.

Ricca V, Mannucci E, Mezzani B, Di Bernardo M, Barciulli E, Moretti S, et al. (1997). Cognitive-behavioral therapy versus combined treatment with group psychoeducation and fluoxetine in bulimic outpatients. *Eating and Weight Disorders*, 2:94–99.

Richards DA, Lankshear AJ, Fletcher J, Rogers A, Barkham M, Bower P, et al. (2006). Developing a UK protocol for collaborative care: A qualitative study. *General Hospital Psychiatry*, 28:296–305.

Roberts AH, Kewman DG, Mercier L, & Hovell M. (1993). The power of nonspecific effects in healing: Implications for psychosocial and biological treatments. *Clinical Psychology Review*, 13:375–391.

Rockland LH. (1993). A review of supportive psychotherapy, 1986–1992. *Hospital and Community Psychiatry*, 44:1053–1060.

Sexton HC, Hembre K, & Kvarme G. (1996). The interaction of the alliance and therapy microprocess: A sequential analysis. *Journal of Consulting and Clinical Psychology*, 64:471–480.

Stice E, Orjada K, & Tristan J. (2006). Trial of a psychoeducational eating disturbance intervention for college women: A replication and extension. *International Journal of Eating Disorders*, 39:233–239.

Strachan MD, & Cash TF. (2002). Self-help for a negative body image: A comparison of components of a cognitive-behavioral program. *Behavior Therapy*, 33:235–251.

Treasure J, Todd G, Brolly M, Tiller J, Nehmed A, & Denman F. (1995). A pilot study of a randomised trial of cognitive analytical therapy vs. educational behavioral therapy for adult anorexia nervosa. *Behaviour Research and Therapy*, 33:363–367.

Wilfley DE, Welch RR, Stein RI, Spurrell EB, Cohen LR, Saelens BE, et al. (2002). A randomized comparison of group cognitive-behavioral therapy and group interpersonal psychotherapy for the treatment of overweight individuals with binge-eating disorder. *Archives of General Psychiatry*, 59:713–721.

Wilson AJ, Touyz SW, O'Connor M, & Beumont PJV. (1985). Correcting the eating disorder in anorexia nervosa. *Journal of Psychiatric Research*, 19:449–451.

Wilson GT, Grilo CM, & Vitousek KM. (2007). Psychological treatment of eating disorders. *American Psychologist*, 62:199–216.

Winston A, Pinsker H, & McCullough L. (1986). A review of supportive psychotherapy. *Hospital and Community Psychiatry*, 37:1105–1114.

Yager J, Andersen AE, Devlin M, Egger H, Herzog D, Mitchell J, et al. (2000). Practice guidelines for the treatment of patients with eating disorders (Rev. ed.). American Psychiatric Association Working Group on Eating Disorders. *American Journal of Psychiatry*, 157:1–39.

CHAPTER 7

Cognitive Remediation Therapy for Anorexia Nervosa

Kate Tchanturia and David Hambrook

There is currently limited evidence to support psychological or pharmacological treatments for anorexia nervosa (AN) (Bulik, Berkman, Brownley, Sedway, & Lohr, 2007; Claudino et al., 2007), and there is no established first-choice treatment for adults suffering from this illness (National Institute for Health and Clinical Excellence [NICE], 2004; Wilson, Grilo, & Vitousek, 2007). Indeed, a recent review suggests that outcomes for AN have not improved in the past 50 years (Steinhausen, 2002). The reasons for the limited efficacy of existing psychological interventions for AN are multifarious and include such factors as high dropout rates, the ego-syntonic nature of AN, patients' inability or unwillingness to confront personal and emotional issues, and the negative influence of low body weight and malnourishment on cognitive processing and stamina. All of these factors make meaningful engagement in the therapeutic process difficult for patients. Given the limited evidence base of existing therapies for AN, it is important that clinicians and researchers are innovative in the development of new approaches to the treatment of this condition. This chapter outlines the rationale and development of a form of cognitive remediation therapy (CRT) that has been specifically tailored to meet the needs of the AN population.

Foundations of CRT for AN

CRT was originally conceptualized and developed as an intervention for patients with brain lesions with the aim of rehabilitating a wide range neuropsychological difficulties often experienced by this patient group (e.g., Goldberg, 2001). In this context cognitive remediation is concerned with the rehabilitation of neurological insults through the implementation of simple cognitive and behavioral exercises that can affect and improve function in specific brain regions that have been damaged or surrounding regions that might be useful in compensating for injuries (e.g., Parentâe & Herrmann,

2003; Sohlberg & Mateer, 2001). Cognitive remediation identifies impaired cognitive functions and brain regions through neuropsychological assessment and neuroimaging, and then repetitive cognitive and behavioral exercises are employed to strengthen or bolster these cognitive domains, such as working memory or response inhibition.

Siegle, Ghinassi, and Thase (2007) suggest that CRT can be subsumed under the class of "neurobehavioral therapies"—that is, an emerging category of psychological intervention that addresses the biological mechanisms thought to underlie psychological disorders, in the same sense that pharmacological and surgical treatments address such mechanisms. These new neurobehavioral interventions, however, use behavioral rather than somatic methods to affect mechanisms. Following successful applications in brain-injury-derived psychological disorders, CRT has been modified and developed to address impaired cognitive functions seen in other mental health problems, such as psychosis (e.g., Bark et al., 2003; Greig, Zito, Wexler, Fiszdon, & Bell, 2007; Wykes & Reeder, 2005), obsessive–compulsive disorder (Park et al., 2006), age-related mental health problems (Goldberg, 2005), attention-deficit/hyperactivity disorder (ADHD) (Stevenson, Whitmont, Bornholt, Livesey, & Stevenson, 2002), and depression (Siegle et al., 2007).

Cognitive remediation techniques developed out of a tradition of neuropsychological assessment and neuroimaging that have documented deficits in specific cognitive functions across different psychiatric conditions. CRT aims to bolster whatever cognitive capacities are weak and also to develop compensatory strategies. The CRT program for AN described here is tailored for the difficulties experienced by patients with AN. Indeed, the current package is derived from systematic neuropsychological research documenting that patients with AN exhibit impaired functioning across several cognitive domains (Southgate, Tchanturia, & Treasure, 2009; Tchanturia, Campbell, Morris, & Treasure, 2005). This hypothesis-driven experimental research has directly informed the current CRT package for AN. Two of the most important findings emerging from this research are that patients with AN tend to exhibit cognitive inflexibility (poor set shifting), and an excessively detailed information-processing style at the expense of thinking holistically (i.e., weak central coherence). Each of these characteristics is discussed in turn.

Cognitive Inflexibility in AN

Several studies have reported that patients with AN display a trait of cognitive inflexibility (poor set shifting) (Roberts, Tchanturia, Stahl, Southgate, & Treasure, 2007; Tchanturia et al., 2005). Set shifting involves the ability to move flexibly back and forth between tasks, operations, or mental sets (Lezak, 2004), and allows for the adaptation of behavior in response to changing demands within the environment. Problems with set shifting may underlie cognitive inflexibility that manifests itself in concrete and rigid approaches to problem solving and in rule-bound behaviors. Performance on experimental set-shifting tasks is often used as a measure of mental flexibility; these require the inhibition of previous stimulus–response associations (i.e., suppressing activation of no-longer relevant information) in order to change to newly defined ones.

Patients with AN perform significantly worse than individuals without eating disorders (EDs) on experimental assessments of set shifting (Roberts et al., 2007; Southgate et al., 2009). Although starvation may intensify these difficulties, they are not simply the result of malnourishment and low body weight, because weight gain alone does not improve cognitive performance (Tchanturia et al., 2004). Indeed, broad set-shifting difficulties have been documented in individuals with AN both during the acute phase of the illness and after weight restoration (Green, Elliman, Wakeling, & Rogers, 1996; Kingston, Szmukler, Andrews, Tress, & Desmond, 1996; Tchanturia et al., 2004).

Patients with AN frequently show problematic set-shifting capacities outside of the laboratory as well. Indeed, people with AN tend to be highly rigid in many aspects of their day-to-day lives, and this inflexibility is especially evident in multitasking situations. For example, trying to cook a meal and attend to one's children at the same time or sitting down and having a meal with one's family while simultaneously trying to engage in meaningful social conversation both involve the ability to multitask. In both of these scenarios, several "sets" need to be maintained simultaneously and responses must shift continuously between them. Clinical experience with patients with AN suggests that these types of task are especially challenging for this patient group, who much prefer to have just one task on which to focus at a time. Whereas some individuals with AN are fully aware of their behavioral and cognitive inflexibility (Treasure, Lopez, & Roberts, 2007), others do not readily recognize this feature and may feel criticized when people comment on it.

This characteristic rigidity or inflexible way of thinking and behaving can act as a real hindrance to those who exhibit it. For example, an inflexible thinking style is likely to mean that an individual relies on strict habits and rules to order his/her life. This rule-bound way of living can impede the individual's involvement in new opportunities and experiences, monopolize time that could be used more productively, and result in relationship difficulties if the rules become extremely rigid. Schmidt and Treasure (2006) have proposed that this cognitive rigidity is one of four important maintaining factors in AN, and research has found that such inflexibility predicts negative treatment outcomes in AN (Crane, Roberts, & Treasure, 2007; Lilenfeld, Wonderlich, Riso, Crosby, & Mitchell, 2006). For all of these reasons, one of the targets for treatment in AN should be improving the patient's ability to think in a flexible manner.

Weak Central Coherence in AN

The term "central coherence" has been used to refer to the natural tendency to process incoming information in context, integrating features to derive a gestalt (Frith, 1989). "Weak central coherence," therefore, refers to a cognitive style in which information remains fragmented as opposed to integrated, with processing occurring at the level of *detail* as opposed to the *whole*. In the context of AN, central coherence has been measured using various neuropsychological assessment tools, including the Rey–Osterrieth Complex Figure Test (Osterrieth, 1944), the Matching Familiar Figures Test (Kagan, 1966), and the Embedded Figure Test (EFT; Witkin, Oltman, Raskin, & Karp, 1971). Such tasks measure the tendency to focus on details as opposed to the gestalt. There is now growing evidence to suggest that people with AN exhibit this detail-focused information-processing style. In particular, they excel at tasks that require a piecemeal processing style, but perform less well in tasks that require global information processing (Gillberg, Råstam, Wentz, & Gillberg, 2007; Lopez, Tchanturia, et al., 2008; Southgate, Tchanturia, & Treasure, 2008; Tokley & Kemps, 2007).

Although in some contexts a detail-focused processing style may provide an advantage, having an *extreme* tendency to focus on the minutia at the expense of processing information in a global fashion can soon become problematic. Because an extreme detail focus makes it difficult for some patients with AN to "see the forest for the trees," they can become extremely preoccupied with details, order, and symmetry. This way of thinking is evident particularly in relation to food and eating; many patients with AN express excessive preoccupation with details such as calorie content, where the food is positioned on the plate, counting items on the plate, etc., all at the expense of comprehending overall nutritional value or enjoying the taste.

Furthermore, individuals with AN demonstrate a preoccupation with details in many other areas of their lives, such as work and school. For example, it is not uncommon to hear that people with AN will persevere with homework until it is absolutely perfect or stay late at the office to make absolutely sure that their work is of the highest standard and that all tasks have been completed. The ability to process information as a function of context and therefore to respond appropriately to the task at hand is, like cognitive flexibility, an important skill in everyday life. Both in the workplace and at school, one must continually assess the degree of detail that is required to make a particular assignment fit for purpose. The ability to step back and assess a particular assignment in global terms allows one to prioritize one's workload—which should, in turn, enable a healthy balance between feeling overwhelmed and feeling satisfied. This seems to be a skill that is particularly problematic for individuals with AN.

Translating Experimental Research into Clinical Practice

The cognitive characteristics described above are not explicitly targeted in most psychological interventions for AN. However, the findings outlined have recently been integrated into etiological (Southgate, Tchanturia, & Treasure, 2005) and maintenance models of AN (Schmidt & Treasure, 2006). Consequently, these have facilitated their translation into clinical practice, namely the Maudsley model of treatment for AN (Treasure, Tchanturia, & Schmidt, 2005). This method of working with adult patients with AN integrates research from the neurosciences along with clinical and empirical evidence regarding cognitive and socioemotional functioning in AN. Utilizing a motivational and reflective framework, the Maudsley model aims to help patients with AN work toward positive changes in *how* they think and behave, rather than focusing on *what* they are thinking and doing, per se. This model argues that the early stages of treatment for AN should focus primarily on the process of thinking and reflection on thinking styles ("metacognition"), with the intention that this foundation will make it easier to work with the content of thoughts later in therapy.

Mechanisms of Change in CRT

CRT operates on the assumption that practice (i.e., learning) within a safe and playful environment will improve performance and increase confidence in using a particular skill. CRT therefore provides patients with AN with a "laboratory" wherein they can actively discover new, perhaps more helpful, thinking strategies. The primary function of CRT is to improve thinking *processes*, rather than thought *content*. Thought content, and how this might maintain AN, is something that should be addressed in other psychological interventions.

As well as giving individuals an opportunity to practice new thinking skills, this intervention is very much about encouraging metacognition—that is, reflection on cognitive style—particularly focusing on strengths and weaknesses of thinking strategies, challenging anxieties relating to thinking style, and building confidence. Focusing on simple material that is not related to the core AN symptomatology (e.g., eating, weight, emotions) allows patients to create and develop collaborative, trustful relationships with their therapist, which might help to prepare these individuals for more challenging psychological therapy.

What Does CRT for AN Involve?

CRT is an intensive training component of the Maudsley model and specifically encourages people to reflect on and try to modify the way they think, with a particular focus on improving cognitive flexibility. It is a manualized clinician-led intervention consisting of multiple versions of a variety of tasks and mental exercises that address the difficulties in flexibility and holistic processing described in this chapter (Baldock & Tchanturia, 2007; Pretorious & Tchanturia, 2007). Specifically, CRT for AN consists of a 10-session module, wherein clinician and patient meet twice a week for 30–45 minutes each, to work collaboratively to complete simple cognitive tasks and reflect on these. The overall aim of these sessions is to encourage patients to reflect on their information-processing styles and behaviors, and to help patients apply new, more adaptive strategies in their day-to-day lives by implementing small behavioral changes.

Cognitive Flexibility Tasks

The Stroop task is one example of how set-shifting ability can be practiced in CRT. This task requires participants to read across a line of words by saying aloud the color in which each word is printed, while ignoring what the word actually says. After a few trials, the participant is then asked to switch to saying what the word actually says while ignoring the color. Throughout the task, patients are asked to "switch" back and forth from one set to the other, thus practicing flexible thinking (e.g., Figure 7.1). Other examples of cognitive flexibility tasks include going through the alphabet and alternating between generating girls and boys name for each letter; building a tower using plastic tokens of different shapes, sizes, and colors and switching between these dimensions as sorting principles ("token towers" task); circling place names while underlining animal words from a list of different words ("embedded words" task); and reversing the order of a string of letters or numbers ("manipulation" task).

Holistic Processing Tasks

These tasks are primarily used to increase patients' ability to begin to be able to "see the forest for the trees." The focus is therefore on increasing the use of global strategies when approaching different tasks as opposed to paying extreme attention to detail. These exercises involve developing a "bigger picture" approach in the verbal and visual

Ask the participant to say the opposite compass direction to where the arrow is pointing.

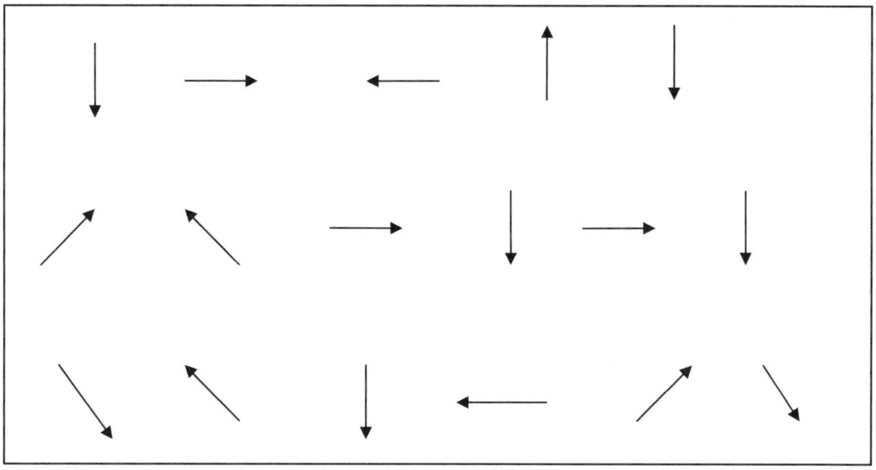

FIGURE 7.1. Switching task.

domains. An example of one of the tasks used in CRT to improve holistic thinking is the "geometric figures" task. This task requires participants to describe a geometric figure (presented to them on a piece of paper; see example in Figure 7.2) for the clinician to draw. When asked to do this task, patients with AN tend to identify details instead of the global features of the figure. This strategy is suboptimal because focusing heavily on the details of the shape makes it difficult for the person drawing to produce an accurate representation of the figure.

Another example of an exercise designed to improve holistic processing is the "main idea" task. This task requires the patient to (1) summarize a body of text (e.g., a letter, e-mail, newspaper article) into a few main bullet points or (2) generate a catchy title. Again, this task encourages patients to think holistically rather than becoming overconcerned with details.

Reflection on Thinking Styles

Practicing the tasks described above is one of the components of the CRT package; however, reflection on these tasks and exploring thinking styles are also essential. The purpose of this reflection is to help patients become aware of their cognitive strategies, particularly inflexible thinking patterns and their tendency to focus on details. Clinician-directed open-ended (or Socratic) questioning is useful in eliciting this reflection, especially in the early stages of therapy. Several question prompts might prove useful in helping patients reflect on their thinking, for example;

- "What strategies have you made use of while doing this task?"
- "Do you often use this strategy?"
- "Does it differ from the way you usually think about things?"
- "Can you think of an example from real life when you might have used a similar strategy?"

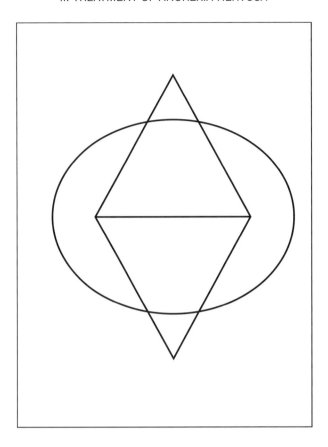

FIGURE 7.2. Geometric figures task.

Identifying Strengths and Weaknesses and Relating to Real Life

Once patients have identified the strategies they have used in the tasks, it is important that they begin to identify strengths and weaknesses in these thinking styles by relating them to situations and strategies in their own lives. For example, after having identified their thinking styles in a particular task, patients might be asked, "Can you think of a situation where this way of thinking might be helpful/unhelpful in real life?" At first, some patients will find it difficult to generate real-life examples. If so, the clinician can provide some examples. However, it is preferable to encourage patients to generate their own examples that have personal meaning and salience.

As patients begin to generate their own examples of when and where their particular style of thinking might be helpful or hindering, strengths and weaknesses in information-processing styles can be identified through guided discovery. For example, a patient might say that he/she is actually quite good at being able to do many things at once (multitasking), such as preparing a meal, looking after children, and doing the laundry. This information-processing style should be noted as a strength and acknowledged as such. Alternatively, the patient might observe that he/she is not particularly good at multitasking and becomes anxious and frustrated when he/she has to do many things at once. In such a case, this problem with flexibility should be identified as a potential weakness in information processing that should become an area for further discussion and planning of specific strategies that will help the patient to cope with it.

Learning New Strategies

Once patients have started to think about their thinking, it is important for clinicians and patients to collaboratively explore new strategies, first by having patients practice them in the in-session tasks and then in their day-to-day lives. After identifying unhelpful strategies in the sessions, patients are encouraged to think about and try out possible new strategies that might be more effective in processing and responding to information. For example, if a patient seems to focus excessively on detail in the aforementioned geometric figures task, he/she could be asked, "What might have been a more effective way of completing this task?" This form of Socratic questioning facilitates discussion about possible alternative strategies that might make it easier for the clinician to draw the figure. It is important to note that because of the relative simplicity of the cognitive exercises and the interactive nature of treatment sessions, clinicians should aim to ensure that sessions are playful, enjoyable, and motivational as much as possible. In particular, it is important for clinicians to express praise for their patients' strengths and the efforts they make. Patients must also be reminded that any mistakes that they make will not be judged in any way.

From Therapy Sessions to Real Life: Behavioral Experiments

After new strategies have been explored and practiced in the sessions, patients are encouraged to start applying their newly learned strategies to real-life situations. Patients might be able to think about applying a shifting strategy when they are at work: having to pay attention to one stimulus or task, but then switch and respond to possibly several other tasks all at the same time (e.g., typing an e-mail, answering a phone call, thinking about what will be on the agenda in an upcoming meeting, preparing a report). As well as *thinking* about how they might successfully transfer their newly learned strategies to real life, in the later sessions, patients are encouraged to *carry out small behavioral experiments* between sessions where they can actually practice implementing their new strategies in real-life situations.

This component of CRT relies on clinicians' ability to illicit personally relevant information from their patients. That is, clinicians should have a good idea about how patients are able to cope with their cognitive difficulties and how they are able to find ways to compensate for them in everyday life. Such information provides clinicians with knowledge of their patients' natural coping strategies and, coupled with information about their interests and hobbies, can be used to collaboratively design personally relevant behavioral experiments. For instance, a patient might practice "bigger picture" processing by watching a film and then explaining to a friend what it was about, without going into the minute details of what happened from scene to scene. This skill could be practiced by summarizing the film's plot in the space of a single text message to a friend. Simple and undemanding behavioral tasks such as these help patients put into practice what they have been learning in their sessions and promote direct transfer to their day-to-day functioning. Overall, CRT focuses on skills rather than the illness and aims to help individuals consider the bigger, more comprehensive picture of how cognition relates to daily functioning. For cognitive remediation to be effective, improved cognition on specific tasks done during treatment needs to generalize to daily life.

The Structure of CRT for AN

CRT in its current form is structured and primarily protocol-driven. In order to gauge the clinical benefit of the intervention, patients undergo a baseline neuropsychological assessment before they start CRT, taking tests that measure set-shifting ability and central coherence. Where possible, patients are also assessed after completing 10 sessions of CRT, and at 6- and 12-month follow-ups. After patients have completed their baseline assessment, they are assigned a therapist who works with them on a one-to-one basis for the duration of the CRT intervention. As previously mentioned, our current CRT package comprises ten 30- to 45-minute sessions, which are generally organized in the following way (see Table 7.1 for summary):

• Sessions 1–3 are dedicated to building up a collaborative therapeutic relationship, which involves the clinician clearly explaining the rationale of CRT to patients. Some, but not all, patients will be aware of the cognitive styles they employ in everyday life and how these might exacerbate their problems. An open discussion focusing on the common cognitive problems experienced by people with AN can help to elucidate for patients how these might manifest in their own lives. Such discussions offer not only

TABLE 7.1. CRT Structure Outline

Sessions	Main components
Sessions 1–3	• Building up a collaborative therapeutic alliance • Explaining the rationale of CRT for AN • Introducing and practicing exercises to identify the predominant cognitive style • Making links between cognitive exercises and behaviors out of session
Sessions 4–6	• Mainly practicing cognitive exercises • Reflecting on strengths and weaknesses of predominant cognitive style • Designing behavioral experiments in session • Practicing behavioral experiments between sessions • Reflecting on the results and strategies learned in the behavioral experiments and how to overcome obstacles • Encouraging transferring skills to daily life
Sessions 6–8	• Practicing cognitive exercises • Greater emphasis on designing, practicing, and discussing behavioral experiments than in earlier sessions • Making links between behavioral experiments and behaviors in real life
Session 9	• Same as sessions 6–8 • Reflecting on and discussing strategies to maintain changes after CRT • Reflecting on and discussing difficulties that might arise after CRT and how they could be overcome • Introducing "goodbye letter" exchange for next session
Session 10	• Exchanging and discussing goodbye letters • Ending CRT

the opportunity to normalize their own cognitive style (strengths and weaknesses), but also allow the clinician to respond sensitively and empathetically to these issues, thus helping to build rapport. Several of the exercises used in CRT encourage a playful interaction between clinician and patient. For example, in the geometric figures task patients choose a shape and describe it for the clinician to draw. Similarly, the token towers task involves a game-like dynamic, with clinician and patient taking turns to choose the sorting rule. Patients are also encouraged to make links between what they are observing about themselves in sessions and how this fits with their thinking and behavior in their everyday experiences.

- Sessions 4–6 continue practice with the tasks but also include designing and practicing small behavioral experiments outside sessions. The aim of these tasks is to reinforce strategies that have been discussed using the exercises and increase behavioral generalization after CRT has ended. Feedback on homework is discussed at the beginning of each session.

- Sessions 6–8 are also usually spent practicing the cognitive exercises, but more time is allocated to discussing and designing behavioral experiments. Patients are encouraged again to make links between the strategies and behaviors they have been practicing in sessions with their real-life experience.

- Session 9 follows the same format as sessions 6–8; however, time is also given to a discussion of ways in which patients might carry forward what they have learned in therapy to their lives post-CRT. Specific strategies are discussed and designed that will help patients maintain their increased flexibility. In addition, the idea of the "goodbye letter" is introduced (see below).

- Session 10 involves patient feedback from previously set homework, a summary and overview of what has been achieved so far, and an exchange of goodbye letters.

In session 9 the idea of goodbye letters is discussed between clinician and patient. Patients are encouraged to write a short letter to their therapist reflecting on:

- What was useful about CRT.
- What was not useful.
- If and how the intervention was applicable to everyday life.
- How the experience can be maintained after completing the 10 sessions of CRT.
- How the intervention could be improved.

Clinicians also write a letter to their patients, focusing on their key strengths and how their thinking style and behaviors have changed during the course of CRT. The tone of these letters is always positive and motivational. The goodbye letters serve several aims. First, they provide an identifiable end to the CRT pretreatment module and summarize for patients what has been achieved so far and how their newly acquired strategies might be used in the future. Second, letters from patients to clinicians are also very helpful for the clinical team more widely, as they provide insight into aspects of CRT that are subjectively useful for patients and can suggest ways in which the intervention might be improved in its future development.

In addition to writing goodbye letters to patients, clinicians are encouraged to "evaluate as they go": That is, after each session clinicians keep a record of their and their patients' key observations and objectives (see Figure 7.3).

Session Number:				
Task	Patient's reflections: What did you learn from these tasks?	Patient's reflections: What did the task show you about your thinking style?	Patient's reflections: Real-life examples?	Therapist comment
Geometric figures				
Stroop				
Behavioral task				

FIGURE 7.3. Clinician record of patient's progress.

The model of CRT presented here is based on an individual or one-to-one format. There are two reasons why this approach has been adopted. First, one-to-one meetings between clinicians and patients provide the opportunity to establish healthy therapeutic relationships. Second, one-to-one sessions allow clinicians to continuously assess and formulate their patients' strengths and weaknesses in processing and thereby tailor the structure and content of their treatment in line with this idiosyncratic formulation.

Preliminary Outcome Data

Preliminary evidence regarding the efficacy of CRT for AN is limited but encouraging. Four small studies by our group are currently published or in press. The first (Davies & Tchanturia, 2005) is a descriptive case report outlining the clinical benefits of CRT for a single inpatient with AN. Baseline tests of set shifting and executive function were administered prior to commencing CRT, and follow-up assessments were made at the end of a 10-session package of CRT, at 2 months follow-up, and at 6 months follow-up. This patient demonstrated a marked improvement in cognitive set-shifting skills after 10 sessions of CRT. A second case study (Tchanturia, Whitney, & Treasure, 2006) replicated these findings and reported marked improvements on several measures of cognitive flexibility after just 10 sessions of CRT. The third study (Tchanturia, Davies, & Campbell, 2007) reports the findings of a case series of four patients with AN who received 10 sessions of CRT.

More recently our group has completed a pilot case series evaluating cognitive changes after CRT in a severe inpatient AN sample (Tchanturia et al., 2008). Twenty-three patients with AN completed a neuropsychological test battery (including measures of cognitive flexibility and central coherence) and several self-report clinical measures before and after 10 sessions of CRT. Results indicated the following:

1. Compared to baseline, after CRT there were significant improvements in the majority of the neuropsychological measures (Tchanturia et al., 2008).
2. Self-reported cognitive flexibility and global information processing significantly improved (Genders et al., 2008).
3. Patients viewed the intervention as subjectively useful, as assessed by a qualitative evaluation of their goodbye letters (Whitney, Easter, & Tchanturia, 2008).
4. Clinicians found that the intervention was easy to deliver and that CRT was a valuable new addition to the treatment of AN (Easter & Tchanturia, in press).

The observations mentioned here, although encouraging, need further investigation and replication. CRT for AN is a new intervention and is currently undergoing evaluation in a number of clinical centers in Europe and the United States.

CRT and Other Interventions

The structure and content of CRT for AN draws on that of cognitive remediation approaches for other psychological disorders (e.g., Park et al., 2006; Wykes & Reeder,

2005). Having said this, CRT for AN was designed specifically to remediate the characteristics of cognitive inflexibility and weak central coherence displayed by many patients with AN. In addition to this specific focus on targeting subtle information-processing biases, CRT for AN also incorporates a nondirective motivational approach wherein patient's strengths are praised and weaknesses in processing styles are discussed in a cost–benefit manner. Indeed, CRT incorporates three of the central components of motivational interviewing, as described by Rollnick and Miller (1995) and Treasure (2004):

- Clinicians are encouraged to express empathy by using reflective listening to convey understanding of the patient's point of view.
- CRT helps to support and build self-efficacy by building the patient's confidence that change is possible and by praising achievements and progress. Clinicians adopt a warm and positive stance, offering frequent encouragement. CRT clinicians aim for equality between themselves and the patient, which is particularly easy in CRT, as the tasks can be directed both by the patient and clinician.
- Because of the specificity of the material covered in CRT and its affectively neutral nature, the intervention provides a safe and unthreatening environment for patients to engage in the therapeutic process.

CRT also provides the opportunity to experience a positive therapeutic environment at a time when many patients may not be physically or cognitively well enough to manage the complexities and intensity of other psychotherapeutic approaches. Having said this, we do not suggest that CRT should be considered a stand-alone treatment. Instead, it can be seen as an integral part of patients' package of care, from their initial admission to the program to discharge and follow-up. In practice, this can be achieved in a number of steps involving different members of a multidisciplinary team. In our pilot study of CRT for AN (Tchanturia et al., 2008) the treatment was implemented in the following way. Soon after admission to the inpatient unit, each patient was administered a neuropsychological assessment, including some of the set-shifting and central coherence assessments mentioned above. After their assessment, patients were assigned a CRT therapist and met weekly on the ward to complete their 10 sessions. Through clinical supervision and sharing of patient information among clinicians, key information about patients' neuropsychological profiles and progress can be shared within the team. Different members of the team are then able to integrate this information into the patients' overall formulation and care plan.

As has already been suggested, CRT is not an alternative to other therapeutic interventions. We propose that CRT is a promising pretreatment for, and/or adjunct to, other standard psychological interventions, for example, cognitive-behavioral therapy (CBT). Of course, there are many different "types" of CBT that have been designed to target the cognitive and behavioral maintaining factors that are specific to AN and EDs more generally. Despite the diversity of the foci of the various cognitive-behavioral models and therapies that have been advanced for AN (for a review, see Wilson et al., 2007), a number of general principles unite them. In particular, CBT models of development, maintenance, and treatment are generally unified in the view that in order to achieve change, maladaptive cognitive and behavioral aspects of the phenomenology of AN must be targeted and in some sense restructured. In AN, the cognitive aspects that might be addressed include (but are not limited to) negative self-evaluation; body image disturbance; preoccupation with eating, weight, and shape; perfectionism; lack of motivation for change; and the ego-syntonicity of the disorder. Behaviors that might be addressed primarily include dietary restriction and compensatory behaviors, but also other maintaining behaviors such as binge eating and social withdrawal or avoidance.

CBT approaches provide a general heuristic for understanding how and why AN has developed and is maintained. As noted elsewhere (e.g., NICE, 2004; Wilson et al., 2007) there is a relatively limited evidence base for the efficacy of CBT for AN, and it remains unclear whether CBT is any more effective than alternative less-symptom-focused psychotherapies (McIntosh et al., 2005). The reasons as to why CBT has so far achieved limited success in the treatment of AN are many. Shafran and Segal (1990) have suggested several client characteristics that are necessary for meaningful engagement in therapy. These include an ability to access relevant cognitions; an awareness of, and ability to differentiate, different emotional states; acceptance of the cognitive rationale for treatment; and the ability to accept personal responsibility for change. For a variety of reasons, not the least of which are severe malnourishment and low body weight, many patients with AN do not possess these characteristics, which means that they may not be physically and psychologically able to engage meaningfully in CBT. This is true particularly for those individuals at the most severe end of the AN spectrum. In such cases, Baldock and Tchanturia (2007) provide a rationale as to how and why CRT and CBT might be mutually compatible, with CRT being seen as a platform into more complex psychological therapy. One reason might be due to the nonemotive nature of CRT and its objective to remediate cognitive functioning rather than tackle core beliefs, affective states, or ED psychopathology. Patients with AN are often avoidant of emotions (e.g., Geller, Cockell, & Goldner, 2000), and CRT may therefore be appealing because it provides a structured, unthreatening therapeutic environment. Furthermore, the tasks involved in CRT are viewed by many of our patients as fun and engaging and can therefore provide respite from their preoccupation with food, exercise, and weight.

CRT may also lay the foundations for meaningful and effective engagement in other psychological therapies in a number of ways. CRT improves awareness of cognitive strategies, including cognitive inflexibility and extreme detail focus, both of which may contribute to obsessive–compulsive-type symptoms. This finding is relevant for other psychological interventions that focus on cognition; a recent systematic review of randomized controlled trials (RCTs) for AN found that obsessive–compulsive-type traits seem to negatively moderate treatment outcome (Crane et al., 2007). That is, patients who exhibit more of these traits are likely to do less well in therapy, particularly in terms of treatment dropout. If CRT is effective in reducing these obsessional and perfectionistic traits and in teaching patients to adapt more flexibly and efficiently to novel situations, then (in theory) their outcomes are likely to improve in other therapies. This hypothesis has yet to be tested formally, however.

Implementing CRT prior to starting other psychological interventions may also be beneficial for patients with AN because CRT actively targets the basic thought processes that are necessary for meaningful engagement in more complex cognitive therapy. For example, the ability to hold multiple perspectives in mind and move back and forth between these perspectives (a form of set shifting) is very important in CBT. The "Theory A, Theory B" technique that is often used in designing behavioral experiments in CBT requires one to consider two separate perspectives, generate evidence for both, and then make decisions regarding which "theory" is closer to reality. Equally important in CBT is the ability to adopt a global perspective on a problem or situation. If someone considers him/herself to be personally responsible for some dreaded consequence, for example, then a global view would be essential in trying to generate a list of other contributing factors with which to challenge the original belief. One can see from these two examples that the contents of many maladaptive thoughts, which are the target for CBT, are underpinned by the basic thought processes that are the target of CRT.

Although there are fundamental differences between CRT and CBT, there are also a number of underlying similarities. These include the nonspecific aspects of therapy, such as unconditional positive regard and the motivational stance described above. Furthermore, the behavioral tasks of CRT are similar to classic CBT behavioral experiments. Behavioral tasks carried out by the patient as homework are a useful way not only of ensuring behavioral generalization and direct transfer, they also aim to alleviate patients' anxieties about the consequences of implementing their newly acquired strategies in everyday life, and furthermore provide them with positive experiences regarding the consequences of change.

Table 7.2 highlights some of the similarities and differences between CRT and CBT. While emphasizing that CRT and CBT are not the same, our experience suggests that they are indeed compatible, and CRT works well as a pretreatment step toward engagement in CBT.

CRT in Different Clinical Settings

In the previous sections of this chapter CRT has been discussed primarily in terms of our experience of implementing this intervention in a severely affected inpatient context. In such settings CRT may be an effective first step in engaging patients in therapy before they can benefit from more complex psychological therapies. A great advantage of CRT in residential contexts is that it does not necessarily require expert involvement from clinical psychologists or psychiatrists. CRT is manualized and requires relatively basic training before being administered. The practical and financial benefits of this

TABLE 7.2. Comparing CRT with CBT

CRT	CBT
Targets basic thought processes	Targets thought content
Does not focus on core eating disorder symptomatology	Core eating disorder symptomatology target of treatment
Affectively neutral material	High emotional salience
Behavioral tasks to test out and practice new strategies	Behavioral experiments to test out specific thoughts or beliefs
Nondirective and motivational	Directive and motivational

are obvious, as it means that CRT can be effectively delivered by nurses, psychology assistants, and trainees. Having said this, all therapists delivering CRT should receive supervision from a suitably qualified and experienced clinician (e.g., clinical psychologist, therapist, psychiatrist).

In inpatient settings where we see the most severely ill clients, it is likely that some patients may find it particularly difficult to learn new strategies and recognize the advantages of flexible and holistic thinking styles. These individuals are likely to be those who benefit most from practicing and reflecting on the cognitive tasks, if only to enhance their chances of understanding the importance of set shifting and global processing. In outpatient services, where the clinical severity of patients with AN is likely to be less dire, CRT might more usefully be implemented in a briefer, less intense format.

A recent report (Lopez, Roberts, Tchanturia, & Treasure, 2008) described the pilot testing of a form of neuropsychological feedback similar to CRT in an outpatient setting. Here patients were assessed using a neuropsychological test battery, and if information-processing biases were present (i.e., if scores were one standard deviation above or below that of the healthy population in two or more of the administered tasks), patients attended a further session for feedback and formulation. The feedback involved presenting patients with the results of their neuropsychological assessment in a motivational interviewing format. Results were presented in the form of charts and in the context of scores of other people with AN and a healthy comparison population. Feedback and formulation were personalized, encouraging patients to reflect on where their information-processing biases emerge in general aspects of their life and in relationship to food and shape/weight, and then consider strategies they might use to overcome these biases.

Preliminary feedback from patients who have received these forms of CRT or neuropsychological feedback interventions suggest that they are well accepted and perceived as personally relevant (Lopez, Roberts, et al., 2008). In particular, the focus on the thinking process rather than the content of the ED psychopathology helps individuals with AN to reflect upon and understand why they are trapped within their illness. The neuropsychological feedback used by Lopez, Roberts, and colleagues (2008) is briefer than CRT and works on the basis of information sharing and reflection, whereas CRT is based on cognitive training, reflection, and behavioral experiments. Nevertheless, the briefer approach described above is one example of how CRT might be adapted to a particular service or context. Indeed, CRT as outlined in this chapter may not be relevant for all cases of AN, as approximately 20% of patients presenting for treatment do not exhibit significantly impaired set shifting or weak central coherence (Lopez, Roberts, et al., 2008). In some cases, patients may experience problems in one domain and not the other. Due to this heterogeneity, hybrid versions of intense and brief forms of CRT could be adapted in relation to the particular cognitive and neuropsychological profile of patients and the context of the service in which the intervention is used.

Future Directions

CRT for AN is a potentially interesting novel intervention, particularly for those individuals who present at the more severe end of the AN spectrum. Indeed, CRT may be an effective new tool for clinicians treating those with EDs because it has been developed specifically to address underlying thinking styles that may represent obstacles to recovery in traditional therapies. Targeting these subtle neuropsychological deficits early on, and in conjunction with more complex therapies, could potentially lead to improved therapeutic outcomes for this difficult-to-treat illness, which has been associated with a negative outlook for a long time.

Preliminary data from our group show neuropsychological and clinical improvements following CRT, as well as positive attributions regarding these changes. The evidence base for CRT in AN is limited at the present time, but it is growing. At the time of writing, CRT for AN is being studied in various treatment centers in small-scale case series and RCTs. In addition to this work, much still needs to be achieved in terms of our understanding of the underlying biological substrates of AN and how these map onto the neuropsychological impairments in individuals with AN. Siegle and colleagues (2007) suggest that cognitive remediation techniques are one of the burgeoning neurobehavioral therapies—that is, those therapies that aim to target neurobiological and neurocognitive mechanisms thought to underlie psychological disorders. Although there is solid neuropsychological evidence demonstrating neurocognitive dysfunction in AN, and preliminary evidence suggesting that CRT may improve functionality, we still know very little about the links between CRT and changes in neurobiological parameters. It is clear that more basic science research is necessary before we can fully understand the specific brain mechanisms underlying AN. We still know less than researchers in other mental health fields (e.g., schizophrenia) about the neurobiological correlates of AN, and even less about the specific neural processes underlying the cognitive impairments seen in this population and how these might be affected by treatment. In the psychosis field, for example, several well-designed studies have already documented cognitive and functional brain changes as a result of cognitive remediation therapy (e.g., Penades et al., 2002; Wykes et al., 2002). Fortunately, the number of neuroimaging studies involving patients with EDs is growing. Ideally, future studies in AN will follow the lead of the psychosis researchers and combine neuropsychology with neuroimaging methods to help elucidate and delineate the neural mechanisms that are susceptible to intervention and bring about clinically significant improvement.

Acknowledgments

We would like to thank H. Davies, C. Lopez, J. Whitney, C. Reeder, O. Kyriacou, A. Easter, E. Baldock, N. Pretorius, L. Southgate, L. St. Louis, K. Schulze, M. Roberts, T. Wykes, J. Treasure, U. Schmidt, and I. Campbell for their contributions to the development of CRT for AN.

References

Baldock E, & Tchanturia K. (2007). Translating laboratory research into practice: Foundations, functions, and future of cognitive remediation therapy for anorexia nervosa. *Therapy*, 4:285–292.
Bark N, Revheim N, Huq F, Khalderov V, Ganz ZW, & Medalia A. (2003). The impact of cognitive remediation on psychiatric symptoms of schizophrenia. *Schizophrenia Research*, 63:229–235.

Bulik CM, Berkman ND, Brownley KA, Sedway JA, & Lohr KN. (2007). Anorexia nervosa treatment: A systematic review of randomized controlled trials. *International Journal of Eating Disorders*, 40:310–320.

Claudino AM, Hay PJ, Lima MS, Schmidt U, Bacaltchuk J, & Treasure JL. (2007). Antipsychotic drugs for anorexia nervosa [Protocol]. *Cochrane Database of Systematic Reviews*, Issue 4 (Article No. CD006816), DOI: 10.1002/14651858.CD006816.

Crane AM, Roberts ME, & Treasure J. (2007). Are obsessive–compulsive personality traits associated with a poor outcome in anorexia nervosa?: A systematic review of randomized controlled trials and naturalistic outcome studies. *International Journal of Eating Disorders*, 40:581–588.

Davies H, & Tchanturia K. (2005). Cognitive remediation therapy as an intervention for acute anorexia nervosa: A case report. *European Eating Disorders Review*, 13:311–316.

Easter A, & Tchanturia K. (in press). Cognitive remediation therapy for anorexia nervosa: A qualitative analysis of therapists' end of treatment letters. *Journal of Child Clinical Psychiatry*.

Geller J, Cockell S, & Goldner E. (2000). Inhibited expression of negative emotions and interpersonal orientation in anorexia nervosa. *International Journal of Eating Disorders*, 28:8–19.

Genders R, Davies H, St Louis L, Kyrnacau O, Hambrook D, & Tchanturia K. (2008). Long-term benefits of CRT for anorexia. *British Journal of Healthcare Management*, 14(12):105–109.

Gillberg I, Råstam M, Wentz E, & Gillberg C. (2007). Cognitive and executive functions in anorexia nervosa ten years after onset of eating disorder. *Journal of Clinical and Experimental Neuropsychology*, 29:170–178.

Goldberg E. (2001). *The executive brain frontal lobes and the civilized mind*. Oxford, UK: Oxford University Press.

Goldberg E. (2005). The *wisdom paradox: How your mind can grow stronger as your brain grows older*. Bath, UK: Simon, & Schuster.

Green MW, Elliman NA, Wakeling A, & Rogers PJ. (1996). Cognitive functioning, weight change, and therapy in anorexia nervosa. *Journal of Psychiatric Research*, 30:401–410.

Greig TC, Zito W, Wexler BE, Fiszdon J, & Bell MD. (2007). Improved cognitive function in schizophrenia after one year of cognitive training and vocational services. *Schizophrenia Research*, 96:156–161.

Kagan J. (1966). Reflection–impulsivity: The generality and dynamics of conceptual tempo. *Journal of Abnormal Psychology*, 1:17–24.

Kingston K, Szmukler G, Andrews D, Tress B, & Desmond P. (1996). Neuropsychological and structural brain changes in anorexia nervosa before and after refeeding. *Psychological Medicine*, 26:15–28.

Lezak MD. (Ed.). (2004). *Neuropsychological assessment* (3rd ed.). New York: Oxford University Press.

Lilenfeld L, Wonderlich S, Riso L, Crosby R, & Mitchell J. (2006). Eating disorders and personality: A methodological and empirical review. *Clinical Psychology Review*, 26:299–320.

Lopez C, Roberts R, Tchanturia K, & Treasure J. (2008). Using neuropsychological feedback therapeutically in treatment for anorexia nervosa: Two illustrative case reports. *European Eating Disorders Review*, 16(6):411–420.

Lopez C, Tchanturia K, Stahl D, Booth R, Holliday J, & Treasure J. (2008). An examination of the concept of central coherence in women with anorexia nervosa. *International Journal of Eating Disorders*, 41:143–152.

McIntosh V, Jordan J, Carter FA, Luty SE, McKenzie JM, Bulik CM, et al. (2005). Three psychotherapies for anorexia nervosa: A randomized, controlled trial. *American Journal of Psychiatry*, 162:741–747.

National Institute for Clinical Excellence. (2004). *Eating disorders: Core interventions in the treat-*

ment and management of anorexia nervosa, bulimia nervosa and related eating disorders. Clinical Guideline 9. London: Author.

Osterrieth P. (1944). *Le test de copie d'une figure complex: Contribution à l'étude de la perception et de la memoire* [Test of copying a complex figure: A contribution to the study of perception and memory]. *Archives de Psychologie,* 30:286–350.

Parentâe R, & Herrmann DJ. (2003). *Retraining cognition: Techniques and applications* (2nd ed.). Austin, TX: Pro-Ed.

Park HS, Shin YW, Ha TH, Kim YY, Lee YH, & Kwon JS. (2006). Effect of cognitive training focusing on organizational strategies in patients with obsessive–compulsive disorder. *Psychiatry and Clinical Neurosciences,* 60:718–726.

Penades R, Boget T, Lomena F, Mateos JJ, Catalan R, Gasto C, et al. (2002). Could the hypofrontality pattern in schizophrenia be modified through neuropsychological rehabilitation? *Acta Psychiatrica Scandinavica,* 105:202–208.

Pretorious N, & Tchanturia K. (2007). Anorexia nervosa: How people think and how we address it in cognitive remediation therapy. *Therapy,* 4:423–431.

Roberts M, Tchanturia K, Stahl D, Southgate L, & Treasure J. (2007). A systematic review and meta-analysis of set-shifting ability in eating disorders. *Psychological Medicine,* 37:1075–1084.

Rollnick S, & Miller WR. (1995). What is motivational interviewing? *Behavioural and Cognitive Psychotherapy,* 23:325–335.

Schmidt U, & Treasure J. (2006). Anorexia nervosa: Valued and visible. A cognitive–interpersonal maintenance model and its implications for research and practice. *British Journal of Clinical Psychology,* 45:343–366.

Shafran JD, & Segal ZV. (1990). *Interpersonal processes in cognitive therapy.* New York: Basic Books.

Siegle GJ, Ghinassi F, & Thase ME. (2007). Neurobehavioral therapies in the 21st century: Summary of an emerging field and an extended example of cognitive control training for depression. *Cognitive Therapy and Research,* 31:235–262.

Sohlberg MM, & Mateer CA. (2001). *Cognitive rehabilitation: An integrative neuropsychological approach.* New York: Guilford Press.

Southgate L, Tchanturia K, & Treasure J. (2005b). Building a model of the aetiology of eating disorders by translating experimental neuroscience into clinical practice. *Journal of Mental Health,* 14:553–566.

Southgate L, Tchanturia K, & Treasure J. (2008). Information processing bias in anorexia nervosa. *Psychiatry Research,* 160:221–227.

Southgate L, Tchanturia K, & Treasure J. (2009). Neuropsychological studies in eating disorders: A review. In PI Swain (Ed.), *Eating disorders: New research* (pp. 1–69). New York: Nova Science.

Steinhausen H. (2002). The outcome of anorexia nervosa in the 20th century. *American Journal of Psychiatry,* 159:1284–1293.

Stevenson CS, Whitmont S, Bornholt L, Livesey D, & Stevenson RJ. (2002). A cognitive remediation programme for adults with attention deficit hyperactivity disorder. *Australian and New Zealand Journal of Psychiatry,* 36:610–616.

Tchanturia K, Brecelj M, Sanchez P, Morris R, Rabe-Hesketh S, & Treasure J. (2004). An examination of cognitive flexibility in eating disorders. *Journal of International Neuropsychological Society,* 10:513–520.

Tchanturia K, Campbell IC, Morris R, & Treasure J. (2005). Neuropsychological studies in anorexia nervosa. *International Journal of Eating Disorders,* 37:S72–S76.

Tchanturia K, Davies H, Lopez C, Schmidt U, Treasure J, & Wykes T. (2008). Neuropsychological task performance before and after cognitive remediation in anorexia nervosa: A pilot case series. *Psychological Medicine,* 38:1371–1373.

Tchanturia K, Whitney J, & Treasure J. (2006). Can cognitive exercises help treat anorexia nervosa? *Eating and Weight Disorders*, 11:e112–e116.

Tokley M, & Kemps E. (2007). Preoccupation with detail contributes to poor abstraction in women with anorexia nervosa. *Journal of Clinical and Experimental Neuropsychology*, 29:734–741.

Treasure J. (2004). Motivational interviewing. *Advances in Psychiatric Treatment*, 10:331–337.

Treasure J, Lopez C, & Roberts M. (2007). Endophenotypes in eating disorders: Moving towards etiologically based diagnosis and treatment based on pathophysiology. *Pediatric Health*, 1:171–181.

Treasure J, Tchanturia K, & Schmidt U. (2005). Developing a model of the treatment for eating disorder: Using neuroscience research to examine the how rather than the what of change. *Counselling and Psychotherapy Research*, 5:1–12.

Whitney J, Easter A, & Tchanturia K. (2008). Service users' feedback on cognitive training in the treatment of anorexia nervosa: A qualitative study. *International Journal of Eating Disorders*, 41:542–550.

Wilson GT, Grilo CM, & Vitousek KM. (2007). Psychological treatment of eating disorders. *American Psychologist*, 62:199–216.

Witkin HA, Oltman P, Raskin E, & Karp SA. (1971). *A manual for the Embedded Figures Test.* Palo Alto, CA: Consulting Psychologists Press.

Wykes T, Brammer M, Mellers J, Bray P, Reeder C, Williams C. et al. (2002). Effects on the brain of a psychological treatment: Cognitive remediation therapy. Functional magnetic resonance imaging in schizophrenia. *British Journal of Psychiatry*, 181:144–152.

Wykes T, & Reeder C. (2005). *Cognitive remediation therapy for schizophrenia: Theory and practice.* New York: Routledge Taylor & Francis Group.

CHAPTER 8

Family-Based Treatments for Adolescents with Anorexia Nervosa

Single-Family and Multifamily Approaches

Ivan Eisler, James Lock, and Daniel le Grange

Despite the admonition by the earliest clinicians to describe and treat anorexia nervosa (AN) that families were the "worst attendants" (Gull, 1874) and likely to be "pernicious influences" (Laseque, 1873) on their children with the disease, family therapy for the disorder, at least for adolescents, has been a common clinical strategy used for more than 40 years. Although family therapy is sometimes also advocated for adult sufferers with AN (Dare, Eisler, Russell, Treasure, & Dodge, 2001), its principal use has been in the treatment of younger patients with AN. A range of family therapy models has been proposed and used clinically, including structural (Minuchin, Rosman, & Baker, 1978), behavioral (Robin & Foster, 1989), Milan systemic (Selvini-Palazzoli, 1974), strategic (Madanes, 1981), feminist (Luepnitz, 1988; Schwartz & Barrett, 1988), attachment (Dallos, 2004), solution-focused (Jacob, 2001), and—most notably in recent years—narrative (Madigan & Goldner, 1998; White, 1989) approaches. However, only a few have been systematically studied to date, and these generally all have a similar conceptual framework. This approach is exemplified by the treatment model described in this chapter, which was developed at the Maudsley Hospital in the 1980s and is now manualized as family-based treatment for AN (FBT-AN; Lock, Le Grange, Agras, & Dare, 2001). The National Institute for Health and Clinical Excellence (NICE; 2004) guidelines indicated that such specific family interventions directly targeting the AN or restrictive eating disorders (EDs) should be offered to young patients. This NICE recommendation was made with a "grade of B," reflecting the general lack of research in this area; all other suggested treatment guidelines for AN were given a "grade of C." Thus, FBT-AN is currently the best-established treatment for adolescents with AN; recent modifications of this approach include a separated version to assist families with high levels of criticism, and FBT-multifamily group to address isolation and provide additional support to families using FBT-AN.

The central feature of this approach to family therapy can be characterized as helping parents to learn the types of behavioral and psychological strategies that are implemented by nurses who are in charge of an inpatient hospital weight restoration plan. However, instead of professionals undertaking this task in a hospital, FBT-AN aims to empower parents to do this at home with the consultant expertise of the therapist to help them. Thus, FBT-AN leverages parental love and understanding of their child and family in the service of promoting behavioral change around eating and weight in the outpatient community, where these skills must ultimately be mastered. The strategy minimizes professional resources while maximizing family ownership of the dilemmas and their solutions. This approach leads to a treatment whose effects are more generalizable and where the skills to promote change and prevent relapse are located in the family.

Theoretical Model and Its Historical Origins

Early theories informing family therapy for those with an ED (Minuchin et al., 1975; Selvini-Palazzoli, 1974) assumed that a specific type of family organization or pattern of family interaction existed that explained the development of an ED in a particular individual. This assumption was in keeping with the prevailing approach to family therapy at the time, with explanatory models (e.g., the "psychosomatic family" model of AN; Minuchin, Rosman, & Baker, 1978) playing a central role in the development of family treatments such as structural family therapy or behavioral family therapy (Robin et al., 1989). Many of the intervention techniques that we use today are derived directly from these approaches, even though our conceptual understanding of how such interventions lead to change has evolved considerably.

There are two main reasons for the conceptual shift in understanding family therapy for AN. The first involves general developments in the field of family therapy in the past 20 years; the field has moved away from understanding family therapy as a treatment *of* families (with the implication that the family was problematic or dysfunctional) to a treatment *with* families. Accordingly, the meetings with families provide the *context* for change rather than the *target* of change, leading to more collaborative approaches and an emphasis on mobilizing family resources rather than aiming to change the family (Eisler & Lask, 2008). Exploring the dynamics of family processes thus moves away from an etiological framework to one of understanding possible maintenance mechanisms, many of which may have had an adaptive role that lost its functionality in the process of the family adjusting to living with a persistent and all-pervasive difficulty such as AN (Whitney & Eisler, 2005).

The second reason for the conceptual shift is determined by the lack of any convincing evidence for the existence of a link between a particular type of family functioning and AN. Although some studies have reported poorer family functioning in AN (e.g., Steiger, Liquornik, Chapman, & Hussain, 1991; Waller, Calam, & Slade, 1989), these studies had considerable methodological limitations. Most come from self-report studies, often based on samples of chronically ill patients, making it difficult to distinguish between cause and effect. Community-based studies (Råstam & Gillberg, 1991) or studies of student samples (McNamara & Loveman, 1990) have generally found much smaller effects, some of which may be accounted for by factors such as depression

(Blouin, Zuro, & Blouin, 1990). Observational studies, which overcome some of the limitations of self-report research, have provided contradictory findings. Although a number have reported differences between AN and control families, the findings differ from study to study (Humphrey, 1989; Kog & Vandereycken, 1989; Røijen, 1992) and even when significant differences are found in mean scores, the majority of families' scores are within a "normal" range (Ravi, Foresberg, Fitzpatrick, & Lock, 2009; Røijen, 1992). Overall, at best, one can conclude that while there may be some family risk factors, these do not have the force of an explanatory mechanism that identifies necessary conditions for the development of the disorder. Moreover, if such risk factors exist, they are probably nonspecific, increasing the risk of developing a range of disorders rather than being specific to AN (for more detailed reviews, see Eisler, 1995, in press; Vandereycken, 2002).

The lack of an obvious family etiology means that we need a different way of thinking about the family dynamics that we observe when working with families. Illness family models (Rolland, 1994; Steinglass, Bennett, Wolin, & Reiss, 1987) offer a perspective for understanding the processes through which families accommodate to serious and enduring problems. As clinicians we may observe unusual, strange, or even bizarre interactions in families, but often these become readily understandable when viewed in the context of the impact of the disorder on the family (Nielsen & Bara-Carril, 2003). Steinglass (1998) described in some detail the process of such family reorganization as an increasing disruption of family routines and family regulatory mechanisms, whereby day-to-day decision making becomes more difficult, to the point where the problem becomes the central organizing principle of family life. Family responses vary depending on the nature of the illness, the type of family organization and interactional style, and their particular life-cycle stage when the illness occurs. What may be less variable is the way in which the centrality of the ED magnifies certain aspects of the family's dynamics and narrows its range of adaptive behaviors. We have suggested (Eisler, 2005) the following as some of the ways in which families become reorganized around AN:

1. *The central role of the symptom in family life.* The high levels of preoccupation with thoughts of food and weight in an individual with AN is paralleled by the way that issues around food and eating take center stage in the family. Much of the interaction between family members focuses on food, eating, or weight to the point that all relationships in the family seem to become defined by them. Just as the young woman may judge her self-worth by whether she is able to resist eating, so interpersonal relationship feelings and emotions in the family become moderated by food- and weight-related behaviors.

2. *Narrowing of time focus to the here and now.* An alteration of the perception of time and a change in the salience of past, present, and future time frames is a well-documented phenomenon associated with a range psychological disturbances (Cutting, 1997; Keough, Zimbardo, & Boyd, 1999; Wyllie, 2005). We have observed a similar phenomenon affecting the whole family (Whitney & Eisler, 2005). The anxiety engendered by the intensity of mealtimes results in the family gradually being unable to focus on anything other than the present. This narrowing of the family's time frame makes it difficult to tolerate uncertainty and take any risks. Trying anything new may feel impossible because nothing beyond any initial negative response seems to matter. This attitude tends to lead to an avoidance of difficult circumstances or a failure to challenge illness behaviors that become increasingly entrenched. Families often comment that they feel that time has come to a standstill.

3. *Inflexibility in daily life patterns.* When asked to describe what they have tried to do to help their daughter, families typically describe having tried a range of different approaches with an increasing experience of ineffectiveness, resulting in an ever-narrowing repertoire of behaviors among all family members. Their patterns of interaction can become ever more predictable and the roles that each person takes on more fixed. To the clinician, the limited patterns of interaction may appear as rigidity, but they may simply reflect the narrowing of the family routines in response to the illness.

4. *The amplification of aspects of family function.* As a result of family adjustment to living with AN, preillness patterns of family functioning may become more pronounced and may then be perceived as part of the problem. For instance, if one member of the family tends to take on the role of peacemaker when differences of opinion appear, this role may become more pronounced with increasing attempts "not to make things worse." Similarly, preexisting differences in closeness and distance between family members may become more pronounced. It is probably this process that gives rise, above all, to the assumption that what we are observing is a manifestation of family dysfunction rather than the family's adjustment to the problem.

5. *Diminishing ability to meet family life-cycle needs.* As the AN takes hold on daily life, the expected developmental changes in the family, such as moving toward increasing autonomy of their adolescent child and the gradual evolution to a more adult–adult relationship, seem impossible and, if anything, family members may feel that they are regressing to an earlier stage in the family life cycle. Meeting the varied needs of different family members—be it siblings, parents, or the family as a whole—becomes ever more difficult, and this difficulty is often accompanied by strong feelings of guilt on the part of the parents (Perkins, Winn, Murray, Murphy, & Schmidt, 2004). Paradoxically, the sufferers themselves may feel guilty about the extra attention they are receiving and about the additional burden they are imposing on the family—and, at the same time, often experience the extra attention as intrusive rather than caring.

6. *The loss of a sense of agency (helplessness).* When first meeting a family seeking help for the daughter, often the most striking aspect is the sense of helplessness and despair. This is generally as true of the parents as it is of the young person. Although winning the battle with hunger may give the young person a brief sense of mastery and control, the battles around food at mealtimes have the opposite effect, regardless of how successful she may be in resisting her parents' exhortations to eat. Parents will similarly recount that they feel helpless and have no control over what their daughter does and indeed that they have lost control over their lives as a whole (Cottee-Lane, Pistrang, & Bryant-Waugh, 2004).

A General Treatment Framework for FBT-AN

FBT-AN is an integrative treatment approach that draws on a number of earlier models of family therapy, including structural family therapy, strategic family therapy, narrative family therapy, and Milan systemic family therapy (cf. Dare & Eisler, 1995). We have previously described how this approach has evolved over a number of years in the context of a series of treatment trials (Dare, Eisler, Colahan, & Crowther, 1995; Eisler, 2005; Lock et al., 2001). Here we outline a general framework under three conceptual headings: (1) maintenance, (2) influencing, and (3) meaning creation. These headings are, of course, not mutually exclusive, and most interventions will include elements of all three. Describing basic interventions under these headings is, however, more useful than focusing on distinct models of family therapy, which would provide a much more artificial categorization and would not reflect day-to-day practice particularly well.

Maintenance Frameworks

Much of the early theoretical work informing family therapy was concerned with the idea of the family as a self-regulating social system (Jackson, 1957) and the way in which family interactions and family structures maintain problems. Two influential strands of family therapy (structural and behavioral) have drawn heavily on these notions, although arguably they tended to confound descriptions of maintenance interactional patterns with etiological explanatory accounts. While we have argued that the family explanatory models, such as the psychosomatic family model, lack empirical validity, the exploration of family interactional patterns that may have a role in maintaining the difficulty (either because they are reinforcing problem behaviors or because they interfere with effective adaptive family mechanisms such as positive parenting) remains a legitimate task for therapists to undertake, and structural or behavioral interventions are useful tools for this purpose.

    An important distinction needs to be made here. Unlike etiological mechanisms that we would expect to find fairly universally in our target population, maintenance mechanisms may not necessarily be so ubiquitous and indeed may sometimes be quite specific to a particular family. This difference has implications for the way in which we conduct our therapeutic inquiry. For instance, the psychosomatic family model assumes that an inability to deal with conflicts is one of the important factors underlying the development of AN. Although the empirical evidence shows that this is not the case, in general, there are clearly individual families for whom conflict avoidance has become a problem and may need to be addressed as part of treatment. The clinician, however, needs to be clear that this is not a surreptitious inquiry about "causes" by saying, for instance: *"There is nothing wrong with disliking arguments. In fact, most of the time it is a good thing. Sometimes, however, this position can get in the way of dealing with difficult issues. Has that been true for you? How has this position changed since your daughter started developing anorexia?"* If family members agree that they avoid conflict more than is useful right now, the therapist can begin to highlight when this behavior occurs. For example, the therapist may ask hypothetical questions, such as, *"What would happen if your mother hadn't intervened when you were beginning to argue with your dad?"*

    At some point most families will inquire about possible causes of AN in their child. This questioning provides an opportunity to make a clear distinction between a general understanding of the different factors that may contribute to the development of the disorder, the impossibility of knowing how these may have combined in the case of their child, and emphasizing that having an answer to the "why" question seldom tells us what to do so that their daughter can start the process of recovery.

    Structural intervention techniques were developed by Minuchin and colleagues (Minuchin & Fishman, 1981) originally for clinical work with deprived families of delinquent boys and were later applied to AN (Minuchin et al., 1975, 1978). The here-and-now focus of structural interventions is of particular relevance for understanding and intervening in possible maintenance mechanisms of this disorder. Inquiring about the usual way in which the family operates—family rules, roles, and boundaries—and how these have changed around the eating problems will illuminate family strengths as well as potential areas of difficulties. Often it is helpful to use structural interventions that encourage parents to work together to find a way of jointly managing the difficulty. For the therapist this includes actively intervening with encouraging language, highlighting family successes, and framing the role of the parents as responsible and "in charge" of the children. Therapists may include enactments in which families are encouraged to demonstrate their usual family processes and interactions within the therapeutic session to provide an opportunity for therapists to help families to "do it differently" and to assess the impact of following a different pattern. The family meal, described in the FBT-AN mini-manual included in this chapter, is a good example, as is the use of role plays in multifamily group (MFG) treatment. For the most part, such enactments are aimed at (1) clarifying the degree of flexibility that is still available to family members to change the way they are currently interacting, and (2) reinforcing areas of strength and resilience that may have gotten buried by the sense of hopelessness and despair that accompanies AN.

Influencing Frameworks

All therapies are concerned with bringing about change. The interventions that we discuss here are primarily characterized by their purposive nature and the fact that they focus primarily on *how change* is brought about while remaining "agnostic" regarding the question of how any problems might have arisen. Historically, two groups of family therapy approaches are most clearly defined by an influencing framework: strategic therapies (Haley, 1963) and brief therapies (Watzlawick, Weakland, & Fisch, 1974), both types developed by the group at the Mental Research Institute (MRI) in Palo Alto, California, the latter eventually developing into what is now known as solution-focused therapy (de Shazer, 1985; Jacob, 2001). The Palo Alto group was particularly interested in the way in which symptoms became part of the family regulatory system through repeated, ineffective, attempts at solutions, which then became part of what was blocking change. When using a strategic intervention, the therapist takes responsibility for influencing the family in a particular direction.

Therapists are often uncomfortable in accepting the role of expert, preferring to adopt a more collaborative stance. This less directive stance stems partly from a recognition that the therapist is not, in fact, an outside observer of the family process who could use his/her "metaposition" to gain an understanding of the family dynamic and then simply intervene to bring about change (Hoffman, 1985; von Foerster, 1979). Being in the position of expert can skew the therapeutic relationship, partly because of issues of power and control, thereby undermining the family and reinforcing a sense of dependence on professionals. As the designated expert, the therapist is more obviously allied with the parents, making it more difficult to engage the young person. While it is important to be aware of these pitfalls, clinicians should not assume that they can be avoided by simply adopting a more neutral position. These pitfalls are as much a product of the nature of the problem as they are of the position adopted by the therapist. An awareness of these issues and a willingness to address them openly with the family is more effective than attempting to avoid their ever occurring. Feedback from families about their experiences of treatment shows consistently that such expertise is valued and, when used wisely, can promote desired change. Being aware of how and when to use our authority is key, as is acknowledging the limitations of our knowledge.

A good example of some of these principles is the use of the initial assessment, which includes medical and nutritional evaluation. A detailed medical and risk assessment of the young person is important both to ensure the physical safety that is required for outpatient treatment to be possible and also as an important strategic element in the process of engagement that shapes the therapeutic relationship with the therapist. The initial assessment contributes to the creation of an environment in which the family feels supported and has a sufficient sense of safety to be able to accept responsibility to look for alternative ways of managing the problem of AN.

Meaning-Creating Frameworks

A central idea in all family therapy approaches is that individual problems are embedded in, and shaped by, their social context and in turn contribute to shape this context. Understanding the interpersonal nature of problems requires that we become concerned with language, beliefs, cognitions, and narratives because these are central to social interaction. The ideas about the importance of beliefs in shaping behavior have been developed by a number of authors in the family therapy field. In the early 1980s Boscolo and Cecchin (who had been part of the original Milan team with Mara Selvini-Palazzoli and Guliana Pratta), started developing a style of work that abandoned much of the early strategic components and focused instead on the process of the interview and the way it could bring forward new perceptions, unexplored stories, and hidden meanings (Bertrando, 2006; Boscolo, Cecchin, Hoffman, & Penn, 1987). More recent developments have placed language and narratives center stage for several influential therapy approaches, in particular narrative therapy (Madigan & Goldner, 1998; White & Epston, 1989) and collaborative language systems therapy (Anderson & Goolishian, 1988). These approaches emphasize the relativity of observed reality and see language and narratives as the vehicle through which people acquire their definitions of self. Individual problems are understood to be, at least in part, the result of the filtering of experiences through narratives that people construct about themselves. These individual narratives are seen as being embedded in wider systems narratives via cultural, political, and educational contexts (Pare, 1995).

Although the narrative and language approaches are theoretically distinct, there is a clear overlap with cognitive therapies both at a conceptual level (i.e., in seeing beliefs and meanings attached to problems as central targets of treatment) and at the level of intervention techniques (e.g., the use of behavioral scaling techniques by narrative therapists; the use of externalization of the problem in some cognitive-behavioral therapy [CBT] approaches). Exploring narratives and meanings are particularly useful in the later stages of treatment when addressing issues of adolescent development, but this approach may also be important early—for example, when trying to engage an "uninvolved" father through exploring alternative narratives about his absence (*"Is your father not here because he does not care or because he does not believe that he can help?"; "If he believed that you would want him to help, would he come?"*). Exploring beliefs is also useful if the treatment is "stuck," and it is necessary to understand the origins of the sense of helplessness and beliefs about the impossibility of parental action.

An important contribution from narrative approaches is the idea of externalizing the problem through the use of "externalizing conversations" (White & Epston, 1989) in which, for example, AN is labeled as separate from the young person. This requires the use of language and phrases that make sense to the family and are appropriate to the child/adolescent's age. Often, AN will be described as having a "voice." Most young people and their families respond positively to such conversations. Some, however, do not, particularly if they feel that this technique is being imposed or if the young person feels that it may give the parents a license to take control. It is therefore important to start by inquiring if the technique makes sense. Providing information about AN and the effects of starvation is also a powerful way of labeling the disorder problem as a quasi-external force taking over the young person's life, which is difficult to resist without help. This perspective gives new meaning to some behaviors and experiences accompanying the eating problems. For instance, describing the effects on healthy volunteers of being starved (Allen, 1991; Keys, Brozek, Henschel, Mickelsen, & Taylor, 1950) and the many parallels with someone suffering from AN (low mood, preoccupation with food, fear of losing control) can change the perception of the anorexic behaviors as being willful and under the young person's control to something that has taken over and requires the combined efforts of the family to resist. When working in MFG-FBT, a staff member may take on the role of speaking the voice of AN, to considerable effect, for the families present.

Treatment Literature
with Emphasis on Randomized Controlled Trials

Family therapy derived from the original work of the Maudsley group for adolescent AN has been subjected to five randomized controlled trials. A total of 220 adolescent subjects has received treatment in these comparisons. The studies' subject pools have ranged in size from 18 to 86 subjects and utilized a range of entry criteria, outcome measures, and follow-up intervals; hence, many aspects of these studies are not directly comparable. However, despite this limitation, it is clear from these studies, taken as a whole, that adolescents with short-duration AN who received this form of family therapy tended to experience substantial benefits.

The first study to examine family therapy for AN was published by Russell and colleagues at the Maudsley hospital in London (Russell, Szmukler, Dare, & Eisler, 1987). This study compared family therapy to a supportive individual therapy and encompassed four subgroups of patients: adolescents with short-duration AN (less than 3 years), adolescents with long-duration AN, patients with adult-onset AN, and patients (mainly adults) with bulimia nervosa (BN). Patients were randomized to either treatment arm following an inpatient weight restoration program lasting about 3 months that brought patients to about 90% of expected body weight for height. The aim of the study was to determine if family or individual therapy would help patients maintain the weight gained in the hospital and make additional gains posthospitalization. The main finding was that only the adolescent subgroup with a short duration of AN demonstrated a differential treatment effect that favored family treatment. At 5-year follow-up (Eisler et al., 1997), family therapy remained superior in the adolescent subgroup with short-duration AN.

The next study to appear, also from the Maudsley group, was a pilot study by Le Grange, Eisler, Dare, and Russell (1992) comparing two forms of FBT: a separated or conjoint format offered over a period of 6 months. The conjoint form, which was used in the Russell and colleagues (1987) study, called for all family members to be present for all sessions; however, it was noted that in some instances, parental criticism (or expressed emotion) of the daughter or son with AN was elevated to such an extent that it conceivably interfered with the effectiveness of the approach. Given that expressed emotion had been shown to be relevant to outcomes in depression and schizophrenia as well as in subject retention in AN studies (Szmukler, Eisler, Russell, & Dare, 1985), it was hypothesized that families with higher levels of expressed emotion (or criticism) might have better results if the parents were seen separately from their child. The study found no overall differences between groups, but subjects from families with higher levels of expressed emotion did better in separated family treatment, with 80% of subjects achieving a good or intermediate outcome (using Morgan–Russell outcome categories). Eisler and colleagues (2000) published a study examining the same hypothesis with a larger sample and a full year of treatment. Again, there were few overall differences between the groups except for those who had high levels of expressed emotion—where, once again, separated FBT seemed to be more beneficial in reducing AN symptoms. In this study 63% achieved good or intermediate outcome (using Morgan–Russell outcome categories) at the end of treatment. However, the conjoint treatment was more effective in bringing about individual psychological change in symptoms of depression and obsessionality, for example. At a 5-year follow-up (Eisler, Simic, Russell, & Dare, 2007) the effects of raised levels of parental criticism were still detectable: This group of patients did less well, as shown in the relative lack of weight gain since the end of outpatient treatment.

Robin and colleagues (1999; Robin, Siegal, & Moye, 1995) published a small study comparing a form of family treatment similar to the Maudsley form of family therapy, called behavioral family systems therapy (BFST), to a developmentally targeted individual therapy, ego-oriented individual therapy (EOIT). BFST included an initial focus on parentally mediated weight restoration, which was followed by a systems type of family therapy aimed at family processes, combined with cognitive restructuring techniques directed at distorted cognitions about food and weight. The comparison treatment (EOIT) was an active, specific, and focused therapy targeting adolescent developmental issues of self-mastery and autonomy. Hence, it was designed to be a more rigorous comparison individual treatment for family therapy than the supportive therapy used in the Russell and colleagues (1987) study. BFST was designed to include the whole family (conjoint), whereas EOIT had both individual sessions with the patient and collateral parental sessions that were used to support the parents in working on adolescent themes. Furthermore, a dietician was part of the treatment team to provide nutritional counseling to the adolescent. At the end of treatment (mean length of treatment was 15.9 months) BFST was significantly more effective at weight restoration and menstrual return than EOIT. The authors concluded that both BFST and EOIT are useful treatments for adolescents with AN, but that BFST is more efficient and effective in early weight and menstrual return.

These trials suggested that family treatment aimed at weight restoration was likely an effective treatment for adolescent AN, but there were a number of questions about the specifics of the treatment approach and its application that required further study. First, because manuals had not been used in the Maudsley studies, the consistency and fidelity of the family therapy depended on standard supervisory processes. It was also uncertain how much family therapy was needed to be effective. Russell and colleagues (1987) and Eisler and colleagues (2007) both employed an approximately year-long version of FBT, composed of about 20 sessions, whereas Le Grange and colleagues (1992) had employed a 6-month version of FBT that included about 10 sessions. Outcomes did not appear to differ related to dose. Finally, although the results of these studies were promising, the numbers of subjects remained small, so there was a need for a larger study demonstrating the usefulness of the approach.

In order to address these dilemmas, Lock and colleagues (2001) wrote a treatment manual that provided a detailed program for FBT-AN. This manual was designed to be an accurate representation of the form of family therapy used in the Maudsley studies. Furthermore, the manual for FBT-AN was designed to be used in a study addressing the question of optimal therapeutic dose of family therapy by comparing a 6-month–10-session dose to a 12-month–20-session dose (Lock, Agras, Bryson, & Kraemer, 2005). In this study 86 adolescents with AN (mean body mass index [BMI] 15.9) were randomized to one of these two doses. At the end of treatment, no differences were found between the groups on weight, eating-related psychopathology, or general psychopathology. Furthermore, 67% had a BMI of 20 or more and scores on the Eating Disorder Examination (Cooper & Fairburn, 1987) within two standard deviations of published norms. At follow-up about 4 years later, these results were maintained (Lock, Couturier, & Agras, 2006). The authors concluded that this study added additional substantive evidence to the database supporting the effectiveness of FBT-AN by having demonstrated its usefulness in a detailed manualized format applied to a relatively large cohort of patients.

In addition to these treatment studies, several authors have examined questions about patient attrition, patient and family satisfaction, and therapeutic alliance in FBT-AN (Lock, Couturier, Bryson, & Agras, 2006; Pereira, Lock, & Oggins, 2006). It is noteworthy that attrition from treatment is a major obstacle to both clinical treatment and research studies of AN (Halmi et al., 2005). In adult studies, where attrition rates average 50%, there is as yet no clear strategy on how best to address this problem. However, adolescent family treatment studies appear to have attrition rates in the range of 10–15% (Le Grange & Lock, 2005). This lower rate is likely due to the fact that parents can compel their children to attend treatment as well as the likelihood that this less chronically ill population is more amenable to considering treatment. It remains unclear how important the form of treatment is relative to attrition; however, one recently published large study of adolescents with AN that did not include a family therapy arm had an attrition rate of 35% (Gowers et al., 2007). Another feature of the family therapy studies worthy of note is the low rate of relapse—less than 10%—once recovery has been achieved (Eisler et al., 1997, 2007; Lock, Couturier, & Agras, 2006). This is considerably lower than reported rates of relapse following weight restoration in the hospital, typically 25–30% following an initial admission, rising to as high as 60–75% following second and subsequent admissions (Lay, Jennen-Steinmetz, Reinhard, & Schmidt, 2002; Steinhausen, Seidel, & Winkler Metzke, 2000; Strober, Freeman, & Morrell, 1997).

From the outset, the demanding nature of FBT-AN was a concern. Families were required to bring all family members, which necessitated taking time away from work, disruption of sibling schedules, and complicated travel arrangements. In addition, weight restoration in FBT-AN requires commitment, energy, time, and patience on the part of parents. In spite of these concerns, two studies have been published that suggest that both adolescents and parents find FBT an acceptable treatment, and satisfaction with the process and outcome appear to be high (Krautter & Lock, 2004; Le Grange &

Gelman, 1998). In addition, studies of therapeutic alliance suggest that adolescents and parents make strong bonds with their therapists and that these bonds are important in staying in treatment and making early progress in terms of weight (Pereira et al., 2006). However, over time, behavioral change (i.e., weight progress) becomes the more important mediator of outcome for both improvements in eating-related psychopathology as well as in maintaining a good therapeutic alliance.

Despite the positive finding supporting the usefulness of FBT-AN, the empirical base of support for the approach remains both small and complicated by a range of important limitations on the generalizability of findings. Relatively few adolescents have been enrolled in the five RCTs of FBT-AN, with an average cell size of about 20 per group. Thus only one study is likely to have an adequate cell size for confidence in comparative outcomes, and this study was related to dose rather than an alternative treatment (Lock et al., 2005). In addition, three of the trials were conducted at the same site, and only two studies employed manualized versions of treatment (Lock et al., 2005; Robin et al., 1999). Perhaps most important, though, entry criteria (including strategies for the calculation of weight thresholds) as well as outcome measures were extremely variable, making it problematic to compare results (Couturier & Lock, 2006a, 2006b). As a result, at this point it is most accurate to say that FBT-AN, in a range of formats, is acceptable, feasible, and leads to generally good outcomes in adolescents with short-duration AN. How FBT-AN compares to other treatments for AN in this population remains unclear. Nonetheless, FBT-AN has the best evidence for effectiveness of available treatments and as a result is the first choice option at this time (Bulik et al., 2007; NICE, 2004).

Mini-Manual of FBT-AN

In FBT-AN parents are the main resource in the treatment of their adolescent children with AN. Mobilizing parents and family members to take action to change behaviors related to AN differentiates this approach from other family and individual therapies for AN. Treatment takes place over three defined phases. The first phase aims to reinvigorate parents in their roles to make behavioral changes within the family system, specifically in regard to their child's eating behaviors. Therapy is almost entirely focused on AN and its symptoms in this phase. In order to strengthen parental efforts, the therapist promotes a strong parental alliance. At the same time siblings are encouraged to support one another. To promote empowerment, families are encouraged to work out for themselves the best way to achieve weight restoration, though the therapist provides expert consultation, feedback, and guidance.

The second phase begins after the parents have successfully facilitated normalized eating and weight gain in their child, and there is significantly less struggle over these dilemmas. The aim of this second phase is to help the adolescent with AN to take over eating on her own under the guidance of her parents. Usually, this transition is tapered and gradual and is accompanied by an examination of adolescent issues that are commonly associated with food and weight (e.g., parties, sleepovers, dating, clothes shopping).

Once the adolescent is eating independently at an age-appropriate level, the third phase begins. This is a brief phase that focuses on general adolescent developmental concerns around autonomy, parental roles, and related themes. The aim of this phase is to make sure that the adolescent is back on a normal adolescent developmental trajectory and that the family is prepared to manage these concerns without the ED interfering.

FBT-AN differs from other treatments of adolescent AN in a number of important ways. First, the adolescent is seen as having a severe psychiatric disease that has led to life-threatening distortions in her physical health, thinking, and behavior. As a result, the adolescent is seen as not functioning on an adolescent level, but because of AN, in need of definitive help from parents around eating. Thus, rather than focusing initially on helping the adolescent to manage eating and weight on her own, FBT-AN encourages parental control over the adolescent's eating; however, from the start it is emphasized that this control is temporary and that the ultimate aim is for the adolescent to be able to achieve age-appropriate independence. In this way this approach is starkly contrasted to therapies for AN that suggest that the disease is a struggle for control from intrusive and domineering parents. It is also agnostic as to the cause of AN and does not blame the patient or parents for its development. Parents often struggle with taking control of weight restoration because of the confusing nature of AN symptoms, bewilderment over the change that has occurred in their child's temperament, and the fear that they caused AN.

FBT-AN is also highly focused on the task of weight restoration, particularly in the first two phases of treatment, as opposed to focusing on general family processes, adolescent problems, or past history of problematic behaviors. Any difficulties in the way that the family functions are always seen as being due, at least in part, to the way in which the family has accommodated to the illness. This does not mean that families with a child with AN are never dysfunctional. In our clinical practice we meet the full range of families whose functioning falls along a continuum from good to bad. However, even when we meet a family that is clearly functioning very poorly, we do not assume that this dysfunctionality provides us with an explanation of the ED, and we do assume that some of what we observe is likely to have been exacerbated by the presence of AN.

Phase I: Outpatient Weight Restoration under Parental Control

In the first phase FBT-AN is almost entirely focused on AN and includes a family meal. This intervention provides the therapist with an opportunity to directly observe the familial interaction patterns around eating. The therapist makes careful and persistent requests for united parental action directed toward changing patterns of eating and exercise in their child to promote weight restoration, which is the primary concern at this point of the treatment. This perspective permits the therapist to disclaim the notion that the parents have caused AN and instead to express sympathy for the parents' plight. In addition, the therapist directs the discussion in such a way as to create and reinforce a strong parental alliance around their efforts at weight restoration in their child, on the one hand, and to align the patient with the sibling subsystem, on the other. This phase is particularly characterized by attempts to absolve the parents from the responsibility of causing the illness and by complimenting them, as much as possible, on the positive aspects of their parenting of their children. The families are encouraged to work out for themselves how best to refeed their anorexic child. While acknowledging the expertise of the therapist, together with the rest of the team, in AN, this is always contrasted with the fact that they do not have the answer as to what *any individual family* will need to do to overcome the problem. When asked directly for advice on how to manage AN-associated difficulties, the therapist may offer examples of what other families have found helpful.

Prior to starting the treatment, the therapist, along with the medical team, will have already determined that the patient has AN and is medically stable for outpatient treatment. The entire family is invited and strongly encouraged to attend all sessions of FBT-AN. The main goals for the first session are to begin to engage the family in treatment and to obtain a specific history of how members see AN as developing within their family. Before beginning each family session, the therapist weighs the patient, thereby also monitoring and addressing the patient's response to any weight change in sessions. Initially the patient may be silent, passive, or angry, but over time, as the therapist encourages her to discuss how she feels, their relationship generally improves (Pereira et al., 2006). This brief time without the family serves to build trust that becomes increasingly important when the adolescent is taking back control over eating in the later phases of FBT, but at no point does this visit become a directed individual psychotherapy session. The therapist records the weight on a weight chart and shares this information with the family at the outset of each session. Thus, the weight chart provides immediate and specific feedback to the family about how things are going in their focused efforts to restore their child's health.

The first session is important in setting the tone of the overall therapy. The therapist intends to activate the family to take action while, at the same time, assuring them that he/she will help them with the problems they will certainly face. The initial meeting is similar in many ways to any other engagement of a family in therapy. The therapist makes contact with each family member and identifies the focus for the work ahead. These introductions are followed by an exploration of family perceptions of the problem and its development and a discussion of the effects of the ED on the family as a whole. The therapist also tries to make connections with all family members by listening to their descriptions of their interests and activities and exploring their various narratives about their experience of the problem, particularly ones that are not at the forefront of the family's presentation, and asks questions that may enable or highlight alternative narratives or meanings to the ones that the family automatically presents. Throughout the session, the therapist is simultaneously warm and supportive, but also worried and alarmed at the state of their child's health as a result of starvation and AN. The therapist assures each family member of his/her importance in the treatment.

Following the initial engagement the therapist quickly moves to a focused interview of each family member's perception of how the ED developed and what the family has tried thus far to help. The therapist uses circular questioning to help facilitate the elaboration of a rich family narrative about how the ED developed, past attempts to treat it, and current dilemmas the family is facing in trying to help. Techniques such as circular questioning draw on the assumption that individual problems are connected or embedded in patterns of relationships, and aim to illuminate or make visible what these patterns are; so instead of simply asking, "*What is the problem?*", one might ask, "*How would different people in the family describe your problem?*", "*Who worries about it?*", or "*When people get worried how ill you are, does it make it more or less likely that you will eat?*" (Eisler & Lask, 2008; Tomm, 1988). The process of taking a focused history on the development of

AN allows the therapist to identify major changes in behavior, thoughts, and relationships that result from the disorder. The problem-focused orientation fits with the here-and-now focus of the family. Unlike the family, though, the therapist holds a broader time frame (based on the experience of having been through the process of therapy with other people) that extends to the future and includes an expectation of change. The therapist conveys this perspective by describing the nature of the treatment being offered and the part that families generally play in this, emphasizing that, like they themselves, most families at this stage of treatment do not believe that they can help their child and that the task of the therapist and the rest of the team is to help *them* through this difficult time.

The therapist uses this information to stress that the patient has a disease, has changed dramatically, and has little control over the disorder. "Externalizing conversations" provide information about the effects of starvation and reinforce the notion of a separation of the child from AN. Although this separation may seem artificial, it often allows family members to address the self-starvation as a disease rather than an oppositional and willful act of a rebellious adolescent, as noted previously. At the same time, externalization of this type also helps the patient feel less responsible and guilty about causing the family problems associated with AN. This strategy is central to maintaining a therapeutic relationship with the adolescent while attacking AN.

Once the therapist has successfully helped the family achieve some degree of acceptance that AN is a disease, he/she emphasizes the seriousness of the disorder to raise parents' anxiety and concern to a level that they feel compelled to take definitive action to combat the maintaining behaviors of AN. Intensifying parental anxiety around the gravity of the illness is aimed at mobilizing family resources to enable the parents to use their sense of responsibility, knowledge, and skills to restore their child's weight. To counteract their concern that this will make their child unhappy and lead to undesirable conflicts, the therapist emphasizes the mortality rate of AN, the morbidity associated with it, including osteoporosis, infertility, and brain matter loss, as well as the psychological and social problems, including school failure, depression, anxiety, and suicide (Rome & Ammerman, 2003).

These discussions often result in an intense and frequently emotional experience, to which the therapist should respond with sympathy but without in any way minimizing the gravity of the situation. This mindset sets the larger stage for the therapist to ask the parents to take on the challenging behaviors of their child that are leading to severe weight loss. The therapist argues that the family is the best resource to help the child recover. Other treatments may help in the short term with weight gain (e.g., hospitalization, residential treatment), but it is difficult to generalize learning mastered in those settings to home. Furthermore, parents know and love their children and can thereby be particularly committed to, and knowledgeable about, their needs. Although the therapist leaves decisions about refeeding to the parents, ideas about how to proceed are sometimes offered (e.g., organizing meals so that parents can monitor them more effectively). In addition, the therapist warns the parents to minimize "anorexic debate" and to avoid fruitless discussion about diet foods, amount to eat, and exercise. The therapist may suggest that for the first few weeks of treatment, it may be necessary for the patient to be absent from school and be under parental supervision 24 hours a day. Similarly, the therapist may advise the parents that one or both of them might need to take a leave of absence from work for 2–3 weeks in order to get things started as a team.

The therapist should end the session by acknowledging the burden that has been placed upon the parents, while also generating a sense of optimism that the parents will be able to work out a way to save their child's life. At this point, the therapist asks the parents to bring a meal for the next session that they believe will help restore their child's health.

The second session in Phase I involves a family meal, as noted. The therapist uses the family meal to evaluate current mealtime processes (when the family eats, who is present, who prepares the meals) in order to understand better the family resources available to assist with mealtime monitoring. In addition, the meal the parents bring provides information about what they believe will help their child gain weight or reveals their hesitancies about confronting the problems of self-starvation (e.g., when they bring a meal that clearly placates anorexic behaviors). The therapist uses this information to provide direct coaching to the parents in helping their child eat a little more than she planned. This is accomplished by encouraging parents to (1) agree on what should be eaten, (2) support each other in the effort to get their child to eat, and (3) be a united front in making demands about eating more. The meal is not an opportunity to bully, physically force consumption, or to heckle the child. Instead, the therapist encourages supportive and understanding comments, while insisting that food be eaten. Most of the time parents succeed in this effort and experience increased hope and confidence in their abilities. Even when they are not successful, the therapist frames the mealtime session as a first step and a learning experience and encourages the parents to take the learning home and keep trying. While the therapist is encouraging the parents, efforts are simultaneously made to help the child understand that no one is blaming her for how hard it is to eat; instead, this difficulty is a result of what AN does to her thinking and behavior. This externalization process continues to promote parental action while not blaming either the parents or the child for the difficult struggle. To reinforce this notion, siblings are asked to support their sister or brother with AN, not by helping the parents with weight restoration, but by saying or doing supportive things to help with the patient's distress during this process, which is often considerable during this session.

The remainder of Phase I consists of sessions that begin with a review of the progress (or lack of progress), according to the weight chart, along with detailed discussion of what the parents have done to promote weight restoration, the obstacles they are facing, and a review of possible solutions. The therapy is highly focused on behavioral change in Phase I and avoids exploring issues not closely linked to the process of weight restoration. This stance is taken to make sure that the therapy stays with AN rather than veering into other psychological or developmental issues that might distract the family from the main task of Phase I. Although these sessions can be taxing because of this exclusive focus, they send a clear message about the central importance of symptom disruption in the FBT-AN model.

At the same time, attention to family criticism of the patient, when it is present, must also be a part of the therapist's treatment. It has been shown that parental criticism can make it harder for the patient to respond to parental demands for weight restoration. Parental criticism may originate in parental guilt about causing AN, as a reaction to what appears to be defiant behavior but is really AN, or simply indicate poor parenting style or a poor relationship between the adolescent and parents. Depending on the origin of the problem, different foci are used by the therapist. In some instances it may be necessary to change the therapy to a separated form, wherein parents meet separately with the therapist, rather than subject the patient to the ongoing criticism. We have already described the importance of continuing to absolve the parents from the responsibility of causing the illness, reinforcing positive aspects of parental behavior, and emphasizing that most of the patient's behavior around eating is, in fact, outside of the patient's control—all of which ultimately helps to foster more sympathy for the patient's dilemmas and difficulties and thereby diminish criticism. It is often also helpful to explore some of the interpersonal dynamics and meanings around critical behaviors, although this needs to be done in a way that does not simply end up criticizing the critical parent. For instance, the daughter might be asked if she is more aware of the tone of her parent's voice or the raised level of anxiety, and to which of the two she tends to respond. If the therapeutic relationship with the parents is strong, it is possible to ask them if they know when they sound critical and if they can differentiate when this is driven by anxiety and when by frustration. This inquiry may lead to a conversation about the way in which caring can be experienced as control and concern as nagging. All such discussions are highly focused to address these issues solely insofar as they interfere with efforts at weight restoration, rather than suggest either familial or parental psychopathology.

If there are difficulties in establishing systematic progress, it may be necessary to explore the role that AN has acquired in the dealing with emotions, feelings, and interpersonal relationships. It is important that such explorations again stress the question of how these dynamics have developed around the AN rather than what role they may have played in its development. It is often effective to use an example of a situation in which healthy, adaptive responses, over time, became unhelpful or even perpetuated a problem (e.g., a parent who becomes more involved in looking after his/her child in the aftermath of a car accident, who later finds it difficult to step back, in turn making it more difficult for the child to develop his/her own coping strategies).

Phase II: Helping the Adolescent Eat on Her Own

Once the patient has achieved a body weight close to normal and is eating without too much struggle with parental supervision, it is time to begin the process of handing back control over eating and exercise to the adolescent in an age-appropriate manner. For the most part, the parents now feel confident in their ability to help their child and experience overall decreased anxiety. However, the therapist reminds the parents that it is ultimately the goal for their child to eat without their monitoring and control of this process to the extent required during the period of weight restoration. In short, the goal for this phase is for the child to eat in an age-appropriate way. Parents are encouraged to "test the water" of their child's readiness to take this on by decreasing their monitoring and allowing more independence about food choices and meal processes. Most often parents are quite happy to do this, but at times, the worry that AN behaviors and thinking will become stronger again makes some parents hesitant. In all cases, the therapist consults with the parents, but leaves decision making up to them. In this way expert opinion is available for consideration, but power remains with the parents. Weight graphs are continued throughout this phase to assure parents that as they relinquish control over eating, their child continues to make weight progress (or alert parents and therapist if the reverse occurs).

Toward the end of Phase II, themes of eating with others become more pronounced. In this way, developmental issues become the subject of sessions, though confined to those related to eating. Topics such as eating on sleepovers, dates, dances, and parties are common topics that need to be addressed during Phase II. In addition, clothes and shopping may become a theme as the patient requires new clothing to fit a healthier body or for other social purposes now that there is more involvement with peers. Often, siblings play an increasingly important role in sessions during this phase. Older siblings are often models for normative adolescent development and provide relevant information to the topics under discussion. Furthermore, as the child with AN becomes healthier, there are more opportunities to engage siblings in age-appropriate and normative ways.

Phase III: Normal Adolescence and Termination

The third phase of FBT is a short period of treatment that aims to assess overall progress and to try to help the adolescent reclaim a normal path of adolescent development. As a result of having had AN, the adolescent has often missed school, experienced social isolation, been dependent on parents and family, and experienced psychological distress, all of which may have negatively affected adolescent development. However, at the same time, because many adolescents with AN have not been ill for long, this off-the-mark trajectory can be more easily righted. The therapist begins this phase by describing the three main stages of adolescence: pubertal change, social identity development, and intimacy and vocational themes. The therapist wishes to help parents develop an empathic stance toward the dilemmas these issues raise for adolescents by asking them to remember their own struggles during adolescence. This approach "turns the tables" on the parents a bit and is usually a delight for the patient and siblings. At the same time, though, it helps the parents to frame their concerns about parenting an adolescent (especially if the child with AN is their first attempt). The process leads to an identification of any concerns about adolescent development for the child with AN. Some patients may relate continuing concerns about pubertal development (menstruation, height, and body shape), whereas for most reentering the social world of peers, beginning dating, and for older adolescents, preparing to separate from their parents as they leave for college or work are the issues of interest. Parents are also urged to evaluate their own needs as a couple as their children are entering adolescence or may be preparing to leave home.

Because for some time AN has acted as a mediator of relationships in the family, the parents may find it difficult to deal with normal adolescent issues. If they have disagreements or clashes with their daughter, they may find it difficult to differentiate between adolescent and anorexic behavior, continuing the process of externalization and labeling everything as due to AN. Parents in such situations may tolerate behavior such as bad language or aggressive or even violent behavior (e.g., "*She wouldn't normally behave like that—it is the anorexia that makes her do that*") that they would normally find unacceptable. Or they may dismiss their daughter's dissatisfaction, irritation, or complaints as just being due to AN. The earlier process of externalization needs to be replaced with "de-externalization," insofar as normal adolescent processes of seeking autonomy and increasing capacities for self-assertion are not confused with the irrational and distorted preoccupations and behaviors of AN that seem to share some of these feature.

Ending treatment is a highly variable process. For some families little more is required than a reflection on how far they have come and what they have learned about themselves. For other families the process of ending therapy highlights the parallels between the difficulty that parents may have had in handing back control of eating to their adolescent and the process of growing up and becoming independent. Ending may become protracted when these processes bring forward the therapist's own wishes to see things through until "all problems have been resolved." Discussions of whose responsibility it would be to do something if eating problems resurfaced and returning to themes of safety and uncertainty may be important at this stage.

Multifamily Group Program (MFG-FBT)

MFG-FBT therapy for AN shares both the conceptual framework and much of the structure and intervention techniques used in the single-family FBT-AN approach described above. Here we focus on the additional features that distinguish multifamily work. The main additional therapeutic ingredient of MFG is that it builds on the shared experiences of families and uses the group dynamics to maximize the resources and adaptive mechanisms of each family. Bringing together different families having to deal with a similar problem and connecting them with each other to harness their strengths and resources reshape all relationships in the group, including the relationships with the therapists. The MFG format helps to dilute the potency of the relationships and some of the potentially negative dynamics and helps the families overcome a sense of isolation and the feeling that no one can really understand what they are up against.

Observing others struggling with similar problems has the additional benefit of serving as a mirror, allowing family members to see areas of poor functioning ("*Are we like that as well?*") as well as strengths that may have become hidden. The context of multifamily day treatment creates an intensity that is unusual in work with individual families. The shared group experience quickly helps to create a group cohesion and a supportive atmosphere in which difficulties can be tackled and new things tried without the usual paralyzing fear that "doing something different could make things worse." Although the families mainly remain here-and-now oriented, they soon realize that each of the other families is in a somewhat different phase. Hearing how other families have overcome problems helps currently struggling families to broaden their own time frame and consider trying out new things.

The Structure and Phases of MFG-FBT

The overall structure of the MFG program has a similar phased approach to the one described earlier for single-family FBT-AN. It too begins with a clear problem-focused phase wherein the parents are encouraged to find ways of helping their daughters overcome their weight and food fears and then later moving to adolescent- and relational-focused work. The overall MFG program is offered for 1 year and combines work with the MFG (typically six families) and single-family FBT-AN treatment with the intent to enhance and boost the effectiveness of the single-family approach.

The initial engagement is the same as in single-family FBT-AN, with at least one, and sometimes more, family meetings before families are invited to join the group. This allows a good working relationship with the family to be established and the nature of the group program to be explained. Families, often skeptical at first, are invited to attend an *introductory evening* to learn more about the group before making a final decision about joining.

Introductory Evening

Families come to an informal meeting where the details of the group are presented with an opportunity to meet staff and also a "graduate" family from a previous group. A short psychoeducational talk is given about the effects of starvation and the prognosis and sequelae of AN. The rest of the meeting is given over to talking with members of the graduate family about their experience of the group. This is usually a crucial component of the evening. The young person will generally be doing quite well and yet will say that a year ago, she was just like all the other young people in the room, feeling hopeless, miserable, and not believing that life could be any different. Seeing this living embodiment of success has a strong effect, particularly on the parents, whose sense of hope is also strengthened by listening to her parents talk about their often grueling yet ultimately positive experiences.

The 4-Day Workshop

The week following the introductory evening the families take part in a 4-day intensive workshop that provides the core intervention of the MFG program. Figure 8.1 shows an example of the structure of a typical workshop day. During the 4 days a range of activities is implemented, including multifamily discussion groups, separate groups for parents and adolescents addressing a variety of topics, such as living with AN and the effect on family life, practical issues around managing mealtimes (parent group), and motivational issues (adolescent group). A variety of creative and nonverbal techniques is used, including role plays, family sculpts, and drawing. Some of the tasks can be completed by families individually (e.g., genograms or drawing a timeline of how things might change over the course of the year) and then discussed in the larger group.

Joint family meals are an important part of the program and again have many similar features described in the earlier section on the family meal. In addition to the joint

9:00–9:30	Multifamily feedback from previous day
9:30–10:15	Parents: What works, what does not work around meals
	Adolescents: Food magazines, paper plates; "the meal I would prepare for my parent"
10:15–10:45	Morning snack
10:45–12:15	Meal role play (adolescents and parent role-playing each other)
12:15–1:30	Multifamily lunch
1:30–2:00	Break
2:00–3:30	"Internalized other" interview (adolescents interviewed in role as a parent while parents observe through one-way screen)
3:45–4:15	Afternoon snack
4:15–5:00	Extensive feedback of all families to each other and to staff

FIGURE 8.1. An example of the structure of the MFG workshop program: Day 2.

(multi) family meals supported by staff, other activities help to promote change in the eating patterns, including role plays of mealtimes, with parents and young people swapping roles; "foster meals" where the adolescent is joined by a mother and father from a different family in the group; and parent group discussions of "tricks that AN plays."

The 4-day block that forms the early part of the intensive multifamily program has a major impact on the families' sense of agency (Salaminiou, 2005). Having mostly started the program with a sense of helplessness and an expectation that it is up to the professionals to find solutions, they leave with a determination and a renewed belief in their ability to find their own solution. When working with families individually, this shift is equally important but is usually less striking and is generally slower to occur.

Follow-Up Group Meetings

Following the initial 4-day workshop the group meets again for six to seven meetings over the course of 9–12 months. The initial meeting takes place after 2 weeks with the gaps between sessions gradually lengthening. Between group meetings families meet individually with their therapist with a frequency that is determined by their need. Some families require very few additional meetings, whereas others seem to need more ongoing support, although in general the number of individual family sessions is relatively low and diminishes as the year progresses.

Compared to single-family FBT-AN, the focus is somewhat broader, even at an early stage. While there is continued emphasis on tackling the eating problems, there are additional activities around family coping styles, body image and its social and cultural context, and many others. As the group meetings continue, it is useful to include activities that broaden family members' time frame, which, as noted above, has tended to become overly foreshortened because of the crisis that AN perpetuates in the family. For instance, the adolescents may be asked to imagine that they are in a time period 20 years on and are writing an article (or making a video film) about how they recovered from AN and how their lives and their relationships changed. Useful discussions can be generated in the group, doing sculpts of the family with and without anorexia present, doing a timeline showing how different family members will be affected by the gradual disappearance of AN and how their needs will be met, and so on. Another technique is to interview the adolescents as a group in role as one of their parents, while the parents observe (with their daughters' knowledge) from behind a one-way screen, and then asking the parents to reflect on what they heard.

Ending the Group

Ending the MFG is not coterminous with ending therapy and addresses different issues. For the group it is useful to reinforce the central idea of the program: that it is the families rather than the professionals who hold the responsibility for what happens in their lives. The family group may devise a ritual to mark the ending of the group, or the parents and adolescents may each do this separately. For some families treatment may come to an end with just a final goodbye session following the ending of the group, whereas other families may need to continue for some further time on an individual basis.

Conclusions

There is a fairly wide consensus that family therapy that focuses on the mobilizing of family resources to tackle eating problems is currently the treatment of choice for young adolescents with AN, although this consensus is based on a small literature with limited evidence. Unfortunately, at present we do not know whether other approaches might work equally well or differently. In clinical practice both individual approaches and other family-oriented treatments are used, but little is known about how these compare with FBT. There are several large ongoing multicenter studies, both in the United States and in the United Kingdom, that should add to our knowledge of how FBT-AN compares with other treatments. We know little about the mechanisms of change underpinning FBT-AN and even less about factors that might impede effective treatment. Comorbid problems such as persistent depression or obsessive–compulsive disorder (OCD) (perhaps particularly if they predate the AN) and family factors may moderate outcome. Would adding a targeted intervention for these problems help the 15–20% of patients that do not respond to FBT? However, these limitations in our knowledge should not obscure the fact that most adolescents get better with FBT, particularly if the treatment is undertaken early in the course of the disorder before the negative effects of living with an eating problem have taken too great a toll.

Additional Resources

Manuals

- Lock J, & Le Grange D. (2005). *Help your child beat an eating disorder.* New York: Guilford Press.
- Lock J, Le Grange D, Agras WS, & Dare C. (2001). *Treatment manual for anorexia nervosa: A family-based approach.* New York: Guilford Press.

Training

- *Maudsley Hospital Training*: The Child and Adolescent Eating Disorder team at the Maudsley hospital in London provides training in single-family and multi-family therapy for adolescent AN, including 1- to 2-day workshops or intensive training in London and extended, outreach site-based team training. For further details, contact Ivan Eisler (*i.eisler@iop.kc.ac.uk*) or Pennie Fairbairn (*pennie.fairbairn@slam.nhs.uk*) in London.
- *Stanford University and University of Chicago Based Training*: Contact James Lock (*jimlock@stanford.edu*) or Daniel le Grange (*legrange@uchicago.edu*) for information on training in manualized FBT-AN or FBT-BN at either university site and visit *train2treat4ed.com* for local site-based training.

References

Allen, J. (1991). *Biosphere 2: The human experiment.* New York: Viking.

Anderson H, & Goolishian, H. (1988). Human systems as linguistic systems: Evolving ideas for the implications in theory and practice. *Family Processes*, 27:371–393.

Bertrando P. (2006). The evolution of family intervention for schizophrenia: A tribute to Gianfranco Cecchin. *Journal of Family Therapy*, 28:4–22.

Blouin AG, Zuro C, & Blouin J. (1990). Family environment in bulimia nervosa: The role of depression. *International Journal of Eating Disorders*, 9:649–658.

Boscolo L, Cecchin G, Hoffman L, & Penn P. (1987). *Milan system family therapy: Conversations in theory and practice.* New York: Basic Books.

Bulik CM, Berkman N, Kimberly A, Brownly JS, Sedway JA, & Lohr KA. (2007). Anorexia nervosa: A systematic review of randomized clinical trials. *International Journal of Eating Disorders*, 40:310–320.

Cooper Z, & Fairburn CG. (1987). The Eating Disorder Examination: A semi-structured interview for the assessment of the specific psychopathology of eating disorders. *International Journal of Eating Disorders*, 6:1–8.

Cottee-Lane D, Pistrang N, & Bryant-Waugh R. (2004). Childhood onset anorexia nervosa: The experience of parents. *European Eating Disorders Review*, 12:177.

Couturier J, & Lock J. (2006a). What constitutes remission in adolescent anorexia nervosa?: A review of various conceptualizations and a quantitative analysis. *International Journal of Eating Disorders*, 39:183.

Couturier J, & Lock J. (2006b). What is recovery in adolescent anorexia nervosa? *International Journal of Eating Disorders*, 39:559–555.

Cutting J. (1997). *Principles of psychopathology: Two worlds—two minds—two hemispheres.* Oxford, UK: Oxford University Press.

Dallos R. (2004). Attachment narrative therapy: Integrating ideas from narrative and attachment theory in systemic family therapy with eating disorders. *Journal of Family Therapy*, 26:65.

Dare C, & Eisler I. (1995). Family therapy. In GI Szmukler, C Dare, & J Treasure (Eds.), *Handbook of eating disorders: Theory, treatment and research* (pp. 334–349). Chichester, UK: Wiley.

Dare C, Eisler I, Colahan M, & Crowther C. (1995). The listening heart and the chi square: Clinical and empirical perceptions in the family therapy of anorexia nervosa. *Journal of Family Therapy*, 17:57.

Dare C, Eisler I, Russell GFM, Treasure J, & Dodge E. (2001). Psychological therapies for adult patients with anorexia nervosa: A randomised controlled trial of out-patient treatments. *British Journal of Psychiatry*, 178:216–221.

de Shazer S. (1985). *Keys to solutions in brief therapy.* New York: Norton.

Eisler I. (1995). Family models of eating disorders. In GI Szmukler, C Dare, & J Treasure (Eds.), *Handbook of eating disorders: Theory, treatment and research* (pp. 155–176). Chichester, UK: Wiley.

Eisler I. (2005). The empirical and theoretical base of family therapy and multiple family day therapy for adolescent anorexia nervosa. *Journal of Family Therapy*, 27:104–131.

Eisler I. (in press). Anorexia nervosa and the family. In JH Bray & M Stanton (Eds.), *Wiley-Blackwell handbook of family psychology.* Oxford, UK: Wiley-Blackwell.

Eisler I, Dare C, Hodes M, Russell GFM, Dodge E, & Le Grange D. (2000). Family therapy for adolescent anorexia nervosa: The results of a controlled comparison of two family interventions. *Journal of Child Psychology and Psychiatry*, 41:727–736.

Eisler I, Dare C, Russell GFM, Szmukler GI, le Grange D, Dodge, E. (1997). Family and individual therapy in anorexia nervosa: A five-year follow-up. *Archives of General Psychiatry*, 54:1025–1030.

Eisler I, & Lask J. (2008). Family interviewing and family therapy. In M Rutter et al. (Eds.), *Rutter's child and adolescent psychiatry* (5th ed., pp. 1062–1078). Oxford, UK: Wiley-Blackwell.

Eisler I, Simic M, Russell GFM, & Dare C. (2007). A Randomised controlled treatment trial of two forms of family therapy in adolescent anorexia nervosa: A five year follow up. *Journal of Child Psychology and Psychiatry*, 48:552–560.

Gowers S, Clark A, Roberts C, Griffiths A, Edwards V, Bryan C., et al. (2007). Clinical effectiveness of treatments for anorexia nervosa in adolescents: Randomised controlled trial. *British Journal of Psychiatry*, 191:427–435.

Gull W. (1874). Anorexia nervosa (apepsia hysteria, anorexia hysteria). *Transactions of the Clinical Society of London*, 7:222–228.

Haley J. (1963). *Strategies of psychotherapy*. New York: Grune & Stratton.

Halmi CA, Agras WS, Crow SJ, Mitchell J, Wilson GT, Bryson SW, et al. (2005). Predictors of treatment acceptance and completion in anorexia nervosa: Implications for future study designs. *Archives of General Psychiatry*, 62:776–781.

Hoffman L. (1985). Beyond power and control: Towards a "second order" family systems therapy. *Family Systems Medicine*, 3:381–396.

Humphrey L. (1989). Observed family interactions among subtypes of eating disorders using structural analysis of social behavior. *Journal of Consulting and Clinical Psychology*, 57:206–214.

Jackson D. (1957). The question of family homeostasis. *Psychiatric Quarterly*, 79–90.

Jacob F. (2001). *Solution focused recovery from eating distress*. London: BT Press.

Keough KA, Zimbardo PG, & Boyd JN. (1999). Who's smoking, drinking, and using drugs?: Time perspective as a predictor of substance use. *Basic Applied Sociology and Psychology*, 21:149–164.

Keys A, Brozek J, Henschel A, Mickelsen O, & Taylor HL. (1950). *The biology of human starvation*. Minneapolis: University of Minnesota Press.

Kog E, & Vandereycken W. (1989). Family interaction in eating disordered patients and normal controls. *International Journal of Eating Disorders*, 8:11–23.

Krautter T, & Lock J. (2004). Is manualized family-based treatment for adolescent anorexia nervosa acceptable to patients?: Patient satisfaction at end of treatment. *Journal of Family Therapy*, 26:65–81.

Laseque E. (1873). De L'anorexie hysterique. *Archives Generales De Medecine*, 21:384–403.

Lay B, Jennen-Steinmetz C, Reinhard I, & Schmidt M. (2002). Characteristics of inpatient weight gain in adolescent anorexia nervosa: Relation to speed of relapse and re-admission. *European Eating Disorders Review*, 10:22–40.

Le Grange D, Eisler I, Dare C, & Russell GFM. (1992). Evaluation of family treatments in adolescent anorexia nervosa: A pilot study. *International Journal of Eating Disorders*, 12:347–358.

Le Grange D, & Gelman T. (1998). The patient's perspective of treatment in eating disorders: A preliminary study. *South African Journal of Psychology*, 28:182–186.

Le Grange D, & Lock J. (2005). The dearth of psychological treatment studies for anorexia nervosa. *International Journal of Eating Disorders*, 37:79–81.

Lock J, Agras WS, Bryson S, & Kraemer HC. (2005). A comparison of short and long term family therapy for adolescent anorexia nervosa. *Journal of the American Academy of Child and Adolescent Psychiatry*, 44:632–639.

Lock J, Couturier J, & Agras WS. (2006). Comparison of long term outcomes in adolescents with anorexia nervosa treated with family therapy. *Journal of the American Academy of Child and Adolescent Psychiatry*, 46:666–672.

Lock J, Couturier J, Bryson S, & Agras WS. (2006). Predictors of dropout and remission in family therapy for adolescent anorexia nervosa in a randomized clinical trial. *International Journal of Eating Disorders*, 39:639–647.

Lock J, Le Grange D, Agras WS, & Dare C. (2001). *Treatment manual for anorexia nervosa: A family-based approach*. New York: Guilford Press.

Luepnitz DA. (1988). *The family interpreted: Psychoanalysis, feminism and family therapy*. New York: Basic Books.

Madanes C. (1981). *Strategic family therapy*. San Francisco: Jossey-Bass.

Madigan SP, & Goldner EM. (1998). A narrative approach to anorexia: Discourse, reflexivity and questions. In MF Hoyt (Ed.), *The handbook of constructive therapies* (pp. 380–400). San Francisco: Jossey-Bass.

McNamara K, & Loveman C. (1990). Differences in family functioning among bulimics, repeat dieters, and non-dieters. *Journal of Clinical Psychology*, 46:518–523.

Minuchin S, Baker L, Rosman BL, Liebman R, Milman L, & Todd TC. (1975). A conceptual model of psychosomatic illness in children: Family organization and family therapy. *Archives of General Psychiatry*, 32:1031–1038.

Minuchin S, & Fishman HC. (1981). *Family therapy techniques*. Cambridge, MA: Harvard University Press.

Minuchin S, Rosman BL, & Baker L. (1978). *Psychosomatic families: Anorexia nervosa in context*. Cambridge: Harvard University Press.

National Institute for Health and Clinical Excellence. (2004). *Eating disorders: Core interventions in the treatment and management of anorexia nervosa, bulimia nervosa and related eating disorders*. London: Author.

Nielsen S, & Bara-Carril N. (2003). Family, burden of care and social consequences. In J Treasure, U Schmidt, & E Vanfurth (Eds.), *Handbook of eating disorders* (pp. 75–90). London: Wiley.

Pare DA. (1995). Of families and other cultures: The shifting paradigm of family therapy. *Family Processes*, 34:1–19.

Pereira T, Lock J, & Oggins J. (2006). The role of therapeutic alliance in family therapy for adolescent anorexia nervosa. *International Journal of Eating Disorders*, 39:677–684.

Perkins S, Winn S, Murray J, Murphy R, & Schmidt U. (2004). A qualitative study of the experience of caring for someone with bulimia nervosa. Part 1: The emotional impact of caring. *International Journal of Eating Disorders*, 36:268.

Råstam M, & Gillberg C. (1991). The family background in anorexia nervosa: A population based study. *Journal of the American Academy of Child and Adolescent Psychiatry*, 30:283–289.

Ravi S, Foresberg S, Fitzpatrick K, & Lock J. (2009). Is there a relationship between parental self-reported psychopathology and symptom severity in adolescents with anorexia nervosa. *Eating Disorders*, 17:63–71.

Robin AL, & Foster SL. (1989). *Negotiating parent–adolescent conflict: A behavioral–family systems approach*. New York: Guilford Press.

Robin AL, Siegal PT, & Moye A. (1995). Family versus individual therapy for anorexia: Impact on family conflict. *International Journal of Eating Disorders*, 4:313–322.

Robin AL, Siegal PT, Moye A, Gilroy M, Dennis AB, & Sikand A. (1999). A controlled comparison of family versus individual therapy for adolescents with anorexia nervosa. *Journal of the American Academy of Child and Adolescent Psychiatry*, 38:1482–1489.

Røijen S. (1992). Anorexia nervosa families a homogeneous group?: A case record study. *Acta Psychiatrica Scandinavica*, 85:196–200.

Rolland JS. (1994). *Families, illness and disability: An integrative treatment model*. New York: Basic Books.

Rome E, & Ammerman S. (2003). Medical complications of eating disorders: An update. *Journal of Adolescent Health*, 33:418–426.

Russell GFM, Szmukler GI, Dare C, & Eisler I. (1987). An evaluation of family therapy in anorexia nervosa and bulimia nervosa. *Archives of General Psychiatry*, 44:1047–1056.

Salaminiou EE. (2005). *Families in multiple family therapy for adolescent anorexia nervosa: Response to treatment, treatment experience and family and individual change.* PhD thesis, Kings College, University of London.

Schwartz RC, & Barrett MJ. (1988). Women and eating disorders. *Journal of Psychotherapy and the Family,* 3:131–144.

Selvini-Palazzoli M. (1974). *Self Starvation: From the intrapsychic to the transpersonal approach to anorexia nervosa.* London: Chaucer.

Steiger H, Liquornik K, Chapman J, & Hussain N. (1991). Personality and family disturbances in eating-disorder patients: Comparison of "restricters" and "bingers" to normal controls. *International Journal of Eating Disorders,* 10:501–512.

Steinglass P. (1998). Multiple family discussion groups for practice with chronic medical illness. *Family Systems and Health,* 16:55–70.

Steinglass P, Bennett LA, Wolin SJ, & Reiss D. (1987). *The alcoholic family.* New York: Basic Books.

Steinhausen HC, Seidel R, & Winkler Metzke C. (2000). Evaluation of treatment and intermediate and long-term outcome of adolescent eating disorders. *Psychological Medicine,* 30:1089–1098.

Strober M, Freeman R, & Morrell W. (1997). The long-term course of severe anorexia nervosa in adolescents: Survival analysis of recovery, relapse, and outcome predictors over 10–15 years in a prospective study. *International Journal of Eating Disorders,* 22:339–360.

Szmukler GI, Eisler I, Russell GFM, & Dare C. (1985). Anorexia nervosa, parental "expressed emotion" and dropping out of treatment. *British Journal of Psychiatry,* 147:265–271.

Tomm K. (1988). Interventive interviewing: Part III. Intending to ask lineal, circular, strategic or reflexive questions? *Family Process,* 27:1–15.

Vandereycken W. (2002). Families of patients with eating disorders. In CG Fairburn & KD Brownell (Eds.), *Eating disorders and obesity: A comprehensive handbook* (2nd ed., pp. 215–220). New York: Guilford Press.

von Foerster H. (1979). Cybernetics of cybernetics. In KK Krippendorff (Ed.), *Communication and control in society* (pp. 5–8). New York: Gordon & Breach.

Waller G, Calam R, & Slade P. (1989). Eating disorders and family interaction. *British Journal of Clinical Psychology,* 28:286.

Watzlawick P, Weakland J, & Fisch R. (1974). *Change: Principles of problem formation and problem resolution.* New York: Norton.

White M. (1989). Anorexia nervosa: A cybernetic perspective. *Family Therapy Collections,* 20:117–129.

White M, & Epston D. (1989). *Literate means to therapeutic ends.* Adelaide, Australia: Dulwich Centre.

Whitney J, & Eisler I. (2005). Theoretical and empirical models around caring for someone with an eating disorder: The reorganization of family life and interpersonal maintenance factors. *Journal of Mental Health,* 14:575–585.

Wyllie M. (2005). Lived time and psychopathology. *Philosophy, Psychiatry, and Psychology,* 12:173–185.

CHAPTER 9

Pharmacotherapy for Anorexia Nervosa

Allan S. Kaplan and Andrew Howlett

The treatment of anorexia nervosa (AN) is frequently long term and highly challenging. Outcome studies have shown that AN is often a chronic illness, with only half of the patients achieving full recovery in long-term follow-up studies (Steinhausen, 2002). Currently, recommended treatments for AN rely on a multidisciplinary approach, reflecting the multidimensional nature of the illness that was first elucidated over two decades ago (Garfinkel & Garner, 1982). However, there is limited empirical support for the range of treatments used (Fairburn & Harrison, 2003). Pharmacological interventions have always been seen as an adjunct to this multidiscipilinary approach.

Neurobiological studies suggest that multiple systems of neurotransmitters and neurohormones are involved in the control of appetite and eating and do not work in isolation (Kaye, Frank, Bailer, & Henry, 2005). Disturbances of serotonin activity as well as altered dopaminergic function have been reported in AN (Bosanac, Norman, Burrows, & Beumont, 2005). Abnormalities in these monoamines occur both centrally and peripherally and are known to be involved in the regulation of feeding, mood, and cognition. These abnormalities are particularly obvious in the acute underweight state and, for the most part, appear to normalize with weight restoration, although some abnormalities have been found to persist. This persistence raises the possibility that they may play a role in the underlying pathophysiology of this disorder (Claudino et al., 2007).

Different classes of drugs have been utilized in the treatment of AN, usually with the aim of improving appetite or weight, time to recovery, or reducing the core symptoms of AN and its associated psychopathology. Empirical evidence for the efficacy of medications for AN, however, is lacking for the most part and regulatory agencies in the United Kingdom (Medicine and Health Care Regulatory Agency [MHRA]) and the United States (Food and Drug Administration [FDA]) have not approved any specific medication for AN treatment. As a result, pharmacological approaches to AN recommended in recognized treatment guidelines, such as those published by the American Psychiatric Association (APA) and National Institute for Health and Clinical Excellence (NICE) rely on uncontrolled trials and accepted clinical practice. Despite the absence of evidence for their efficacy, in clinical practice the majority of patients with AN are treated with psychotropic medications to treat comorbid disorders, to facilitate eating through the anxiolytic properties, or to effect appetite and/or weight (Rossi et al., 2007).

This chapter reviews the evidence-based research on the use of pharmacotherapies, including antidepressants, antipsychotics, and other less common agents, that have been used to treat AN. Information is provided from published case reports, open-label studies and randomized controlled trials (RCTs), as well as published international clinical guidelines. Wherever possible, we have attempted to differentiate between outpatient and inpatient settings and the phase of the disorder, including the acute weight restoration phase as well as the maintenance phase. We also briefly discuss potential new pharmacological approaches to AN.

Antidepressants

Antidepressants are the first-line agents for the treatment of a number of psychiatric disorders, including depression, obsessive–compulsive disorder (OCD), and bulimia nervosa (BN). Considering that many patients with AN also suffer from these comorbid conditions, it is not surprising that antidepressants have been tested during both the acute and maintenance phase of this disorder. A meta-analysis evaluating the efficacy and acceptability of antidepressant treatment in the acute phase of AN concluded that the lack of quality data precludes any firm conclusions or clinical recommendations (Claudino et al., 2006). Claudino and colleagues (2006) noted that four placebo-controlled trials that meet quality criteria for inclusion in the meta-analysis did not find significant evidence for the superiority of antidepressant treatment versus placebo for improving weight gain, eating disorder (ED) psychopathology, or associated functioning.

Fluoxetine

Fluoxetine has been studied in RCTs in both the acute phase as well as the maintenance phase of AN in an attempt to prevent relapse. Attia, Haiman, Walsh, and Flater (1998) evaluated the effectiveness of fluoxetine in underweight patients being treated in an inpatient setting and determined that there was no difference between fluoxetine and placebo in facilitating weight gain. Fluoxetine was also compared in an unblinded fashion to other antidepressants: nortriptyline and amineptine (Brambilla, Draisci, Peirone, & Brunetta, 1995a, 1995b). Both studies reported no statistically significant differences between the different antidepressants in body mass index (BMI) or depression levels at posttreatment.

Fluoxetine as an agent to maintain recovery and prevent relapse was studied in two separate double-blinded RCTs of outpatients after weight recovery from an inpatient stay (Kaye et al., 2001; Walsh et al., 2006). Kaye and colleagues (2001) reported on 35 weight-restored patients randomized to placebo or up to 60 mg/day of fluoxetine for 1 year. Those (10 of the 16 subjects) who remained on fluoxetine showed a significant difference between baseline and end of study in terms of increase in weight and reductions in depression, anxiety, obsessions and compulsions, and core ED symptoms. In a larger multisite RCT, conducted at Columbia University and the University of Toronto (Walsh et al., 2006), investigators compared fluoxetine to placebo in 93 weight-restored patients with AN followed for 1 year, all of whom who were receiving concomitant cognitive-behavioral therapy (CBT). All subjects initially gained weight to a BMI of at least 19 in an inpatient or day hospital setting and were then randomly assigned in a double-blind fashion to receive either placebo or fluoxetine up to 80 mg/day for 1 year. Subjects were seen weekly for manualized CBT and assessed monthly on a variety of psychometric measures. In contrast to the earlier Kaye and colleagues study, this larger RCT failed to observe any benefit of adding fluoxetine versus placebo to CBT, in terms of reducing time to relapse and in maintaining weight. In addition, there was no advantage for fluoxetine over placebo on any clinical variable other than anxiety, including depression, or on ED-specific psychopathology. There were significant differences in the methodology of these two studies, which likely account for their different findings, including the fact that subjects in the Kaye and colleagues study were not limited to trial-specific or standardized outpatient treatment, which may explain the high relapse rate in the placebo group in this study. In addition, the Kaye and colleagues study included a smaller number of subjects and excluded individuals with the binge–purge subtype of AN, which may have inflated the possibility of a false-positive result.

Other Selective Serotonin Reuptake Inhibitors: Sertraline, Citalopram

Open studies have also examined the efficacy of sertraline (Santonastaso, Friederici, & Favaro, 2001) and citalopram (Fassino et al., 2002). Neither study, however, found any drug effect on weight gain in outpatients with AN.

Bupropion

Bupropion is another antidepressant worth mentioning because it is unusual among the antidepressants in having both noradrenergic and dopaminergic reuptake inhibiting effects. Even though one study showed quite a dramatic response to bupropion in terms of a reduction in binge eating and purging for patients with BN (Horne et al., 1988), it also reported an unacceptably high rate of seizures (4 of 55 subjects) in these patients. Subsequently, the FDA issued a black box warning concerning the use of bupropion in patients with EDs because of the increased risk of seizures in these patients, especially those who are binge-eating and purging (American Psychiatric Association, 2006). Generally, bupropion is avoided in those with AN as well.

Clinical Application, Dosages, and Adverse Effects of Antidepressants

There is a lack of evidence to support the use of antidepressants in underweight patients with AN. There are many methodological limitations in the published trials, including small sample sizes, short duration of treatment, the presence of concomitant treatments, and high attrition rates, all which make it difficult to ascertain the efficacy of antidepressants alone. In addition, secondary outcomes such as the effect on the core psychopathological symptoms of AN and associated comorbididity are not reported. Most antidepressants, however, continue to be used to treat comorbid conditions such as major depression or OCD when they occur in patients with AN; however, the efficacy of antidepressants for these conditions may be mitigated by the effects of starvation on neurotransmitter functioning. Finally, the use of antidepressants in children, adolescents, and young adults for the treatment of EDs as well as depression and OCD needs to be closely monitored, given the warning on increased suicidal risk in these populations while using these agents.

First-Generation Antipsychotics

Reports of the use of first-generation antipsychotics (FGAs) in cases of AN date back to the 1960s. The first trials of FGAs tested chlorpromazine against standardized inpatient treatment without drugs. Although higher weight gain occurred in the short term, in the chlorpromazine group patients suffered serious side effects, including grand mal seizures. In the end no difference was observed in terms of weight gain between groups (Dally & Sargant, 1966). Other small trials of FGAs for AN examined pimozide versus placebo (Vandereycken & Pierloot, 1982) and also versus behavioral therapy (Weizman, Tyano, Wijsenbeek, & Ben David, 1985) but failed to find any clear benefit for pimozide. Also, no benefit for sulpiride versus placebo was found (Vandereycken, 1984). An open trial of haloperidol reported significant changes from baseline to 6 months on three EDI subscales and in BMI (Cassano et al., 2003); interpretation of these findings is unclear because patients also received additional treatments.

Second-Generation Antipsychotics

In more recent years there has been renewed interest in using antipsychotics to treat AN with the second-generation antipsychotics (SGAs), given their broader range of targeted symptoms and different spectrum of side effects. The rationale for using SGAs is based on their effects on cognition, affect, and activity—core disturbances in patients with AN—which are all mediated, in part, by dopamine. With regard to cognitions, individuals with AN demonstrate a cognitive disturbance best characterized as "aberrant salience to internal stimuli," a concept that has been described in schizophrenia with regard to external stimuli (Kapur, 2003). Patients with AN misinterpret internal sensations, such as postprandial fullness or bloating, as a feeling of fatness. Many consider the body image disturbance so prominent in AN to be of near delusional proportions, often presenting as a fixed, false belief that the patient is obese in the presence of severe emaciation. Some patients also report hearing internal "voices," described by some as hallucinatory in nature, telling them not to eat. The consensus in the field, however, is that the preoccupation with weight and shape is best conceptualized phenomenologically as an overvalued idea and that the voices are best understood as pseudo-hallucinations (Claudino et al., 2007). Nevertheless, an argument could be made that SGAs may be helpful with the cognitive disturbances described by patients with AN.

Similarly, patients with AN also experience intense dysphoria and anxiety, which could very well respond to the anxiolytic and mood stabilization properties of SGAs. Finally, some patients with AN demonstrate abnormal levels of hyperactivity in the face of decreasing energy supply—another symptom that (theoretically) could respond to

SGA dopamine-blocking drugs. Given less preoccupation with weight and shape, less anxiety and less drive to exercise, patients with AN who respond to SGAs may be able to eat more and then gain weight, not necessarily as a side effect of these drugs but as a direct salutary effect on the psychopathology of AN. In addition to these psychopathological symptoms that provide a rationale for using SGA to treat AN, the side effect profile of these agents, related to their propensity to stimulate weight gain, provides a rationale for evaluating these medications in patients with AN (Claudino et al., 2007).

Olanzapine

Olanzapine is the SGA most commonly reported in the literature in the treatment of AN. Case reports have noted some overall improvement in weight gain and cognition as well as improved body image (Boachie, Goldfield, & Spettigue, 2003; Dunican & Del-Dotto, 2007; Jensen & Mejlhede, 2000; La Via, Gray, & Kaye, 2000; Malina et al., 2003; Mehler et al., 2001). Olanzapine has also been studied in three open-label trials. Mondraty and colleagues (2005) compared olanzapine to chlorpromazine, examining for reductions in anorexic rumination (i.e., intrusive cognitions and rituals) in inpatients with AN. The olanzapine group had a significant reduction in degree of ruminations and were noted to be calmer, better able to participate in the inpatient program, and reported being less preoccupied with body image and their usual eating-related concerns compared to the chlorpromazine group. There were no significant differences in the average amount of weight gained. Barbarich and colleagues (2004) studied 17 hospitalized patients with AN using a 6-week trial of olanzapine and detected significant reduction in depression, anxiety, and core ED symptoms and a significant increase in weight (Barbarich et al., 2004). Powers, Santana, and Bannon (2002) conducted an open trial to determine if olanzapine was effective in producing weight gain. With weekly monitoring sessions and group psychoeducation sessions, the majority of subjects gained some weight, but few achieved ideal body weight, and some lost weight.

Finally, three recent double-blind RCTs have evaluated the effectiveness of olanzapine in patients with AN (Attia, Kaplan, Haynos, Yilmaz, & Musante, 2008; Bissada, Tasca, Barber, & Bradwejn, 2008; Brambilla et al., 2007). Bissada and colleagues (2008) found that, compared to placebo, the addition of olanzapine to intensive day hospital treatment led to more rapid weight gain, but overall the same amount of weight gain was achieved. Brambilla and colleagues (2007) tested olanzapine versus placebo in a group of subjects that was also all receiving CBT and found that those treated with olanzapine showed greater improvement in some of the EDI subscales but no difference in weight, compared to those subjects who were treated with placebo. A just-completed unpublished RCT of olanzapine in underweight outpatients with AN who were not on any other treatment showed that patients on olanzapine gained weight more rapidly than those on placebo over 8 weeks of treatment (Attia et al., 2008).

Quetiapine

There is a report of five cases treated with quetiapine in adolescents with severe, treatment-refractory AN. The results showed positive psychopathological effects and good tolerability (Mehler-Wex, Romanos, Kirchheiner, & Schulze, 2008). There are also two open trials using quetiapine (Bosanac et al., 2007; Powers, Bannon, Eubanks,

& McCormick, 2007). In an outpatient setting, Powers et al. studied the effects of quetiapine on a group of 19 adolescents and adults with AN and showed that the Positive and Negative Syndrome Scale (PANSS) scores declined significantly and there were some improvements in measures of anxiety, depression, and obsession–compulsive symptoms. However, there was no difference in the mean weight from baseline to 10 weeks.

Bosanac and colleagues (2007) studied individuals with AN admitted to a specialized unit because of disease severity and comorbid depression. In this trial quetiapine doses were much higher, at an average of 800 mg per day, than those previously reported. There was significant difference in the Eating Disorder Examination—12th edition (EDE-12) restraint score at 4 weeks and significant change in the EDE-12 and BMI at 8 weeks, although only one patient reached a BMI of 17.5.

Amisulpride, Risperidone, and Aripiprazole

In one RCT the SGA agent amisulpride (available in Europe but not the United States) was compared to fluoxetine and clomipramine, without a placebo arm (Ruggiero et al., 2001). There were no statistical differences between groups on end-of-treatment mean weight gain or core AN symptoms.

Other SGAs such as risperidone and aripiprazole have been found to be less likely to cause significant weight gain in patients with schizophrenia and therefore may be more acceptable to patients with AN. Risperidone was reported to have some benefit in a case study of an adolescent girl with both AN and autism (Fisman, Steele, Short, Byrne, & Lavallee, 1996). A clinical report of two adolescents with AN noted that risperidone appeared to improve thoughts related to food and body image (Newman-Toker, 2000). Similarly, aripiprazole was used in a patient with chronic AN with psychotic symptoms, comorbid with epilepsy, and chronic renal failure (Aragona, 2007). Aragona reported improvement in the Scale for the Assessment of Negative Symptoms (SANS) and the Scale for the Assessment of Positive Symptoms (SAPS), specifically on scores for hallucinations and delusions, although the patient's weight remained stable. Attia et al. reported an open-label trial of aripiprazole in outpatients with AN and found no significant effect on weight gain, mood, or anxiety (Attia, Kaplan, Schroeder, Federici, & Staab, 2005).

Clinical Application and Side Effects of SGAs

Currently SGAs remain experimental drugs used off label in more severe cases of AN characterized by unremitting resistance to gaining weight (American Psychiatric Association, 2006). European guidelines (NICE) are less clear regarding the clinical utility of these drugs (National Collaborating Centre for Mental Health, 2004). Individuals with AN who may benefit from SGAs need to be informed of the indications, risks, and potential benefits of these agents. Adherence is a significant obstacle to the use of these drugs in this patient group; patients with AN are reluctant to take any medications, especially those that have weight gain as an established side effect. Olanzapine remains the only atypical agent for which there is some evidence of efficacy in RCTs. All of the currently published trials are limited by their small sample sizes and high attrition rates, and their results are confounded with those of concurrent treatments. Definitive evidence to support their use generally is lacking and awaits larger RCTs that should also attempt to determine, through pharmacogenetics, which patients may be more likely to respond to these drugs.

If SGAs are being used, these medications should be titrated slowly. Most SGA dosages used in case reports, open trials, and RCTs have been low to moderate compared to their approved primary use in schizophrenia and bipolar disorder. Dosages for olanzapine ranged from 2.5 to 10 mg; quetiapine, 150–800 mg; risperidone, 1 mg; and aripiprazole, 30 mg. It is important to be aware of adverse events and side effects in this population, since these patients can be medically unstable, vulnerable to side effects, and, not surprisingly, concerned about any changes to their body. Despite the propensity of SGAs to cause clinically significant side effects in patients with schizophrenia and bipolar illness taking higher doses, especially weight gain and the metabolic syndrome, these drugs appear to be surprisingly well tolerated. The lower doses used in patients with AN and the relatively short period of time in the trials minimize the risks. However, when using any of the SGAs, basic medical laboratory tests (e.g., electrocardiogram [EKG], serum fasting glucose and lipids, liver enzymes, serum prolactin levels) should be conducted, and any evidence of akathesia and extrapyramidal symptoms (EPS) should be ascertained at baseline and at regular intervals. Specific concern about QTc prolongation with some of the SGAs dictates the need for regular cardiac monitoring with EKGs.

Other Agents

A number of other agents has been used experimentally in the treatment of AN. These include lithium, zinc, cyproheptedine, prokinetic agents such as cisapride, and appetite-stimulating agents such as tetrahydrocannabinol (THC). RCTs using zinc (Birmingham, Goldner, & Bakan, 1994; Katz et al., 1987; Lask, Fosson, Rolfe, & Thomas, 1993), cyproheptedine (a serotonin antagonist) (Halmi, Eckert, LaDu, & Cohen, 1986), and cisapride (a prokinetic agent used to accelerate gastric emptying) (Szmukler, Young, Miller, Lichtenstein, & Binns, 1995) as well as THC (Gross et al., 1983) have not proven to be helpful in improving appetite, achieving weight gain, or reducing psychological symptoms. One RCT of lithium in the acute treatment of AN (Gross et al., 1981) found a small increase in weight in patients with AN compared to placebo. However, the use of a drug such as lithium in patients with AN, in whom fluid and electrolyte status can be compromised, presents potential safety issues. None of these agents is currently recommended for the treatment of AN.

Potential New Compounds

With the absence of any definitive evidence-based drug treatments for AN, investigators need to think "outside the box" in developing new psychopharmacological approaches to treatment. There are some intriguing compounds that may prove useful in the future treatment of AN. These include corticotropin-releasing hormone (CRH) antagonists, D-Cycloserine, and a number of orexigenic and anorectic antagonist peptides.

It has been well described that patients with AN have elevated cortisol levels associated with elevated secretion of CRH. Elevated levels of CRH are associated with increased anxiety and depression and decreased eating (Owens & Nemeroff, 1991).

Several CRH antagonists have been developed and are in clinical trials to treat depression and may be useful in the treatment of AN. D-Cycloserine, a cognitive enhancer, is a partial agonist at the *N*-methyl-D-aspartate (NMDA) receptor and a drug that has been utilized successfully to improve extinction of fear in patients with phobias undergoing behavioral exposure (Ressler et al., 2004). If AN is associated with an abnormal sensitivity to fear conditioning, then D-Cycloserine may be useful as an adjunctive treatment to enhance the effects of exposure therapy in AN. D-Cycloserine has recently been studied in a small sample of subjects with AN, with no demonstrable effect; however, studies in a larger sample of patients are nonetheless warranted (Steinglass et al., 2007).

Peptides that either increase or decrease feeding could play a role in the pathophysiology and future pharmacological treatment of AN. Orexigenic peptides include opioids, neuropeptide Y, ghrelin, and galanin; anorectic peptides include leptin, agouti relate peptide (AGRP), and bombesin-like peptides (gastrin-releasing peptides). There is some evidence to suggest that there is dysregulation of these peptides in AN. Agonists of orexigenic peptides and antagonists of anorectic peptides could play a role in the future pharmacological treatment of AN (Roerig, Mitchell, & Steffen, 2005).

Adherence to Treatment and Meaningful Outcomes

AN remains one of the most difficult psychiatric disorders to treat, partly because of the lack of motivation for recovery in most patients. One of the major obstacles has been adherence to treatment in both the acute and relapse prevention phases of the illness (Halmi et al., 2005; Walsh et al., 2006). When used, pharmacotherapy should always be combined with psychotherapy in the treatment of AN. In addition to establishing rapport and trust with patients, compliance enhancement and motivational strategies (Feld, Woodside, Kaplan, Olmsted, & Carter, 2001) should be part of any psychotherapeutic approach.

AN is a disorder with psychopathological disturbances of an enduring nature and with a typically slow course of recovery. Knowing what works best for patients requires that clinical trials of sufficient duration be conducted to measure meaningful outcomes, both nutritional and psychopathological. Even when weight is a primary outcome measure, studies have reported this figure in a variety of ways, including the number of patients achieving target weight or weight within the normal range, the mean rate of weight gain, and the time to achieve target weight. In future trials it would be useful to systematically report the number of patients achieving normal weight at the end of the trial, as full weight restoration to a statistically normal range is associated with better outcomes (Claudino et al., 2006). Moreover, clinically significant, as opposed to statistically significant, changes in measures of characteristic psychopathology should be reported in future treatment studies, since normalization of such measures is the ultimate goal of treatment. Finally, the impact of any intervention, including pharmacotherapy, needs to address quality-of-life is issues for patients with AN.

Summary

More than any other psychiatric disorder, AN remains largely resistant to pharmacological interventions. As such, the treatment of AN requires a multidisciplinary approach and, in the absence of evidence for the efficacy of pharmacotherapy, individual psychotherapy remains the cornerstone of treatment for the disorder. The initial priority should always be medical stabilization and nutritional rehabilitation in addition to the treatment of core psychopathological symptoms and any comorbid psychiatric conditions. At this point in time the decision as to whether to use psychotropic medication and, if so, which medications, needs to be based on the patient's clinical presentation and the severity of illness.

Finally, a significant percentage of patients with AN are resistant to any interventions, chronically ill, and psychosocially and medically disabled. The needs of these individuals, in particular, have been largely neglected by the field and deserve our compassionate clinical support and focused research attention, especially in developing new drugs that may be helpful in improving the quality of their lives (Kaplan, Rockert, Viera-Morlock, Rais, & Whiteside, 2007).

References

American Psychiatric Association. (2006). Treatment of patients with eating disorders, third edition. *American Journal of Psychiatry*, 163:4–54.

Aragona M. (2007). Tolerability and efficacy of aripiprazole in a case of psychotic anorexia nervosa comorbid with epilepsy and chronic renal failure. *Eating and Weight Disorders*, 12:54–57.

Attia E, Haiman C, Walsh BT, & Flater SR. (1998). Does fluoxetine augment the inpatient treatment of anorexia nervosa? *American Journal of Psychiatry*, 155:548–551.

Attia E, Kaplan AS, Haynos A, Yilmaz Z, Musante D. (2008, September). *Olanzapine vs. placebo for outpatients with anorexia nervosa.* Paper presented at the annual meeting of the Eating Disorder Research Society, Montreal.

Attia E, Kaplan AS, Schroeder L, Federici A, & Staab R. (2005, September). *Atypical antipsychotic medication in anorexia nervosa.* Paper presented at the annual meeting of the Eating Disorders Research Society, Toronto.

Barbarich NC, McConaha CW, Gaskill J, La Via M, Frank GK, Achenbach S, et al. (2004). An open trial of olanzapine in anorexia nervosa. *Journal of Clinical Psychiatry*, 65:1480–1482.

Birmingham CL, Goldner EM, & Bakan R. (1994). Controlled trial of zinc supplementation in anorexia nervosa. *International Journal of Eating Disorders*, 15:251–255.

Bissada H, Tasca GA, Barber AM, & Bradwejn J. (2008). Olanzapine in the treatment of low body weight and obsessive thinking in women with anorexia nervosa: A randomized, double-blind, placebo-controlled trial. *American Journal of Psychiatry*, 165:1281–1288.

Boachie A, Goldfield GS, & Spettigue W. (2003). Olanzapine use as an adjunctive treatment for hospitalized children with anorexia nervosa: Case reports. *International Journal of Eating Disorders*, 33:98–103.

Bosanac P, Kurlender S, Norman T, Hallam K, Wesnes K, Manktelow T, et al. (2007). An open-label study of quetiapine in anorexia nervosa. *Human Psychopharmacology*, 22:223–230.

Bosanac P, Norman T, Burrows G, & Beumont P. (2005). Serotonergic and dopaminergic systems in anorexia nervosa: A role for atypical antipsychotics? *Australia and New Zealand Journal of Psychiatry*, 39:146–153.

Brambilla F, Draisci A, Peirone A, & Brunetta M. (1995a). Combined cognitive-behavioral, psychopharmacological and nutritional therapy in eating disorders: 1. Anorexia nervosa, restricting subtype. *Neuropsychobiology*, 32:59–63.

Brambilla F, Draisci A, Peirone A, & Brunetta M. (1995b). Combined cognitive-behavioral, psychopharmacological and nutritional therapy in eating disorders: 2. Anorexia nervosa—binge-eating/purging type. *Neuropsychobiology*, 32:64–67.

Brambilla F, Garcia CS, Fassino S, Daga GA, Favaro A, Santonastaso P, et al. (2007). Olanzapine therapy in anorexia nervosa: Psychobiological effects. *International Clinical Psychopharmacology*, 22:197–204.

Cassano GB, Miniati M, Pini S, Rotondo A, Banti S, Borri C, et al. (2003). Six-month open trial of haloperidol as an adjunctive treatment for anorexia nervosa: A preliminary report. *International Journal of Eating Disorders*, 33:172–177.

Claudino AM, Hay PJ, Silva de Lima M, Schmidt U, Bacaltchuk J, & Treasure JL. (2007). Antipsychotic drugs for anorexia nervosa [Protocol]. *Cochrane Database of Systematic Reviews*, Issue 4 (Article No. CD006816), DOI: 10.1002/14651858.CD006816.

Claudino AM, Silva de Lima M, Hay PJ, Bacaltchuk J, Schmidt U, & Treasure JL. (2006). Antidepressants for anorexia nervosa. *Cochrane Database of Systematic Reviews*, Issue 1 (Article No. CD004365), DOI: 10.1002/14651858.CD004365.pub2.

Dally P, & Sargant W. (1966). Treatment and outcome of anorexia nervosa. *British Medical Journal*, 2:793–795.

Dunican KC, & DelDotto D. (2007). The role of olanzapine in the treatment of anorexia nervosa. *Annals of Pharmacotherapy*, 41:111–115.

Fairburn CG, & Harrison PJ. (2003). Eating disorders. *Lancet*, 361:407–416.

Fassino S, Leombruni P, Daga G, Brustolin A, Migliaretti G, Cavallo F, et al. (2002). Efficacy of citalopram in anorexia nervosa: A pilot study. *European Neuropsychopharmacology: Journal of European College of Neuropsychopharmacology*, 12:453–459.

Feld R, Woodside DB, Kaplan AS, Olmsted MP, Carter JC, (2001). Pretreatment motivational enhancement therapy for eating disorders: A pilot study. *International Journal of Eating Disorders*, 29:393–400.

Fisman S, Steele M, Short J, Byrne T, & Lavallee C. (1996). Case study: Anorexia nervosa and autistic disorder in an adolescent girl. *Journal of the American Academy of Child and Adolescent Psychiatry*, 35:937–940.

Garfinkel PE, & Garner DM. (Eds.). (1982). *Anorexia nervosa: A multidimensional perspective*. New York: Brunner/Mazel.

Gross HA, Ebert M, Faden V, Goldberg S, Kaye W, Caine E, et al. (1983). A double-blind trial of delta 9-tetrahydrocannabinol in primary anorexia nervosa. *Journal of Clinical Psychopharmacology*, 3:165–171.

Gross HA, Ebert MH, Faden V, Goldberg S, Nee L, & Kaye W. (1981). A double-blind controlled trial of lithium carbonate primary anorexia nervosa. *Journal of Clinical Psychopharmacology*, 1:376–381.

Halmi K, Agras S, Crow S, Mitchel J, Wilson T, Bryson S, et al. (2005). Predictors of treatment acceptance and completion in anorexia nervosa: Implications for future study designs. *Archives of General Psychiatry*, 62:776–781.

Halmi K, Eckert E, LaDu T, & Cohen J. (1986). Anorexia nervosa: Treatment efficacy of cyproheptadine and amitriptyline. *Archives of General Psychiatry*, 43:177–181.

Horne R, Ferguson J, Pope H, Hudson J, Lineberry L, Ascher J, et al. (1988) Treatment of bulimia with bupropion: A multicenter controlled trial. *Journal of Clinical Psychiatry*, 49:262–266.

Jensen VS, & Mejlhede A. (2000). Anorexia nervosa: Treatment with olanzapine. *British Journal of Psychiatry*, 177:87.

Kaplan A, Rockert W, Viera-Morlock R, Rais H, & Whiteside L. (2007, October). *Assertive community treatment for eating disorders*. Poster session presented at the annual meeting of the Eating Disorder Research Society, Pittsburgh, PA.

Kapur S. (2003). Psychosis as a state of aberrant salience: A framework linking biology, phenomenology, and pharmacology in schizophrenia. *American Journal of Psychiatry*, 160:13–23.

Katz RL, Keen CL, Litt IF, Hurley LS, Kellams-Harrison KM, & Glader LJ. (1987). Zinc deficiency in anorexia nervosa. *Journal of Adolescent Health*, 8:400–406.

Kaye WH, Frank GK, Bailer UF, & Henry SE. (2005). Neurobiology of anorexia nervosa: Clinical implications of alterations of the function of serotonin and other neuronal systems. *International Journal of Eating Disorders*, 37:15–19; discussion 20–21.

Kaye WH, Nagata T, Weltzin TE, Hsu LK, Sokol MS, McConaha C, et al. (2001). Double-blind placebo-controlled administration of fluoxetine in restricting- and restricting–purging-type anorexia nervosa. *Biological Psychiatry*, 49:644–652.

Lask B, Fosson A, Rolfe U, & Thomas S. (1993). Zinc deficiency and childhood-onset anorexia nervosa. *Journal of Clinical Psychiatry*, 54:63–66.

La Via MC, Gray N, & Kaye WH. (2000). Case reports of olanzapine treatment of anorexia nervosa. *International Journal of Eating Disorders*, 27:363–366.

Malina A, Gaskill J, McConaha C, Frank GK, La Via M, Scholar L, et al. (2003). Olanzapine treatment of anorexia nervosa: A retrospective study. *International Journal of Eating Disorders*, 33:234–237.

Mehler-Wex C, Romanos M, Kirchheiner J, & Schulze UM. (2008). Atypical antipsychotics in severe anorexia nervosa in children and adolescents: Review and case reports. *European Eating Disorders Review*, 16:100–108.

Mondraty N, Birmingham CL, Touyz S, Sundakov V, Chapman L, & Beumont P. (2005). Randomized controlled trial of olanzapine in the treatment of cognitions in anorexia nervosa. *Australian Psychiatry*, 13:72–75.

National Collaborating Centre for Mental Health. (2004). Core interventions in the treatment and management of anorexia nervosa, bulimia nervosa and related eating disorders. *National Institute for Clinical Excellence*, 3:261–234.

Newman-Toker J. (2000). Risperidone in anorexia nervosa. *Journal of the American Academy of Child and Adolescent Psychiatry*, 39:941–942.

Owens M, & Nemeroff C. (1991). Physiology and pharmacology of corticotropin-releasing factor. *Pharmacological Review*, 43:425–473.

Powers PS, Bannon Y, Eubanks R, & McCormick T. (2007). Quetiapine in anorexia nervosa patients: An open label outpatient pilot study. *International Journal of Eating Disorders*, 41:21–26.

Powers PS, Santana CA, & Bannon YS. (2002). Olanzapine in the treatment of anorexia nervosa: An open label trial. *International Journal of Eating Disorders*, 32:146–154.

Ressler KJ, Rothbaum BO, Tannenbaum L, Anderson P, Graap K, Zimand E, et al. (2004). Cognitive enhancers as adjuncts to psychotherapy: Use of D-Cycloserine in phobic individuals to facilitate extinction of fear. *Archives of General Psychiatry*, 61:1136–1144.

Roerig J, Mitchell J, & Steffen K. (2005). New targets in the treatment of anorexia nervosa. *Expert Opinion on Therapeutic Targets*, 9:135–151.

Rossi G, Balottin U, Rossi M, Chiappedi M, Fazzi E, & Lanzi G. (2007). Pharmacological treatment of anorexia nervosa: A retrospective study in preadolescents and adolescents. *Clinical Pediatrics*, 46:806–811.

Ruggiero GM, Laini V, Mauri MC, Ferrari VM, Clemente A, Lugo F, et al. (2001). A single blind comparison of amisulpride, fluoxetine and clomipramine in the treatment of restricting anorectics. *Progress in Neuropsychopharmacology and Biological Psychiatry*, 25:1049–1059.

Santonastaso P, Friederici S, & Favaro A. (2001). Sertraline in the treatment of restricting anorexia nervosa: An open controlled trial. *Journal of Child and Adolescent Psychopharmacology*, 11:143–150.

Steinglass J, Sysko R, Schebendach J, Broft A, Strober M, & Walsh B. (2007). The application of exposure therapy and D-Cycloserine to the treatment of anorexia nervosa: A preliminary trial. *Journal of Psychiatric Practice*, 13:238–245.

Steinhausen HC. (2002). The outcome of anorexia nervosa in the 20th century. *American Journal of Psychiatry*, 159:1284–1293.

Szmukler G, Young G, Miller G, Lichtenstein M, & Binns D. (1995). A controlled trial of cisapride in anorexia nervosa. *International Journal of Eating Disorders*, 17:347–357.

Vandereycken W. (1984). Neuroleptics in the short-term treatment of anorexia nervosa: A double-blind placebo-controlled study with sulpiride. *British Journal of Psychiatry*, 144:288–292.

Vandereycken W, & Pierloot R. (1982). Pimozide combined with behavior therapy in the short-term treatment of anorexia nervosa: A double-blind placebo-controlled cross-over study. *Acta Psychiatrica Scandinavica*, 66:445–450.

Walsh BT, Kaplan AS, Attia E, Olmsted M, Parides M, Carter JC, et al. (2006). Fluoxetine after weight restoration in anorexia nervosa: A randomized controlled trial. *Journal of the American Medical Association*, 295:2605–2612.

Weizman A, Tyano S, Wijsenbeek H, & Ben David M. (1985). Behavior therapy, pimozide treatment, and prolactin secretion in anorexia nervosa. *Psychotherapy and Psychosomatics*, 43:136–140.

CHAPTER 10

Nutritional Rehabilitation for Anorexia Nervosa

Cheryl L. Rock

The goals of nutritional rehabilitation in the treatment of anorexia nervosa (AN) are weight restoration and an improvement in nutritional status. This rehabilitative effort is a critical component of treatment. Although weight restoration alone does not indicate recovery, nutritional rehabilitation promotes the normalization of metabolic problems and medical complications associated with the disorder. Importantly, nutritional rehabilitation also enables the patient to achieve a level of cognitive functioning necessary to understand and respond to psychological counseling and behavioral interventions. A starving individual simply does not have the mental ability to focus on the problems, issues, and solutions that must be addressed in individual and group counseling sessions to promote recovery from the illness.

Nutritional rehabilitation of the patient with AN also poses some risks for these patients. In contrast with the patient who is underweight due to a condition such as infection or other physical illness, low body weight in the patient with AN is typically achieved over a period of months as the result of limiting energy intake and/or increasing energy expenditure. This pattern of weight loss enables metabolic adaptations that affect the interpretation of biochemical and other indicators of malnutrition. In this state of metabolic and physiological adaptation, overly aggressive refeeding, in addition to inadequate monitoring of response, can have dire consequences.

Nutritional rehabilitation also must be approached with sensitivity to the psychological features of the eating disorder (ED). Most patients with AN are initially very conflicted about their involvement in treatment programs, because maintaining a low body weight and other aspects of the ED serve as coping mechanisms, and the eating attitudes are thus tenaciously held. Rather than perceiving the patient as being manipulative and treatment-resistant when problems arise with nutritional rehabilitation, it should be communicated that consuming more food and achieving nutritional rehabilitation are necessary for recovery and that thinking patterns will change in association with improvement. Typically, the patient is terrified of weight gain and is struggling with hunger and urges to eat, yet the food choices deemed acceptable by the patient are too limited to allow sufficient energy intake and normal mental function. Rapport and a trusting relationship with a nutritional counselor can be reassuring to patients as they gain weight, because they will feel that the process is occurring with guidance and oversight, and that eating and consequent weight gain are not out of control.

Energy Requirements and the Refeeding Regimen

Prior to presenting for treatment, the primary feature of the diets of patients with AN is a deficit of energy intake relative to expenditure. Early studies of energy intake in patients with AN suggested an average intake of 800–1,200 kilocalories per day (kcal/day) in stable but low-weight patients. Actual intake, however, varies with stage of illness; greater dietary restriction becomes necessary to promote continued weight loss. Substantial overreporting of energy intake occurs in this patient population (Hadigan et al., 1999), which affects interpretation of data. In response to this severe, sustained energy imbalance, resting energy expenditure (REE) and energy requirements are initially substantially reduced, mediated by changes in thyroid hormone status and physiological changes (Van Wymelbeke, Brondel, Bron, & Rigaud, 2004).

Thus, the initial stage of nutritional rehabilitation, as it is implemented in most structured treatment programs, begins at a level of 1,200–1,800 kcal/day, which is gradually increased by 200–300 kcal/day every 2–4 days, to ultimately achieve 3,000–3,500 kcal/day (Rock, 1997; Treat et al., 2005) or a maximum of 70–100 kcal/kg body weight. The goal is to promote a weight gain of ≥ 1.0 kg/week; however, in the outpatient setting in which medical monitoring is more limited, a smaller rate of weight gain (0.5–0.9 kg/week) is often a more realistic goal and poses less risk for complications.

This relatively high level of energy intake has usually been found to be necessary to achieve weight restoration in both adult and adolescent patients with AN. During the refeeding process, REE increases dramatically, compared to normal subjects who are not eating high-energy diets (Forman-Hoffman, Ruffin, & Schultz, 2006; Van Wymelbeke et al., 2004), presumably as a result of the metabolic effects of the refeeding regimen. In a clinical study of the determinants of REE during the refeeding of low-weight patients with AN, level of energy intake was observed to be the strongest correlate and predictor of REE, although anxiety level, abdominal pain, and cigarette smoking also were observed to be directly related and thus may contribute to resistance to weight gain (Van Wymelbeke et al., 2004). In studies that have examined the potential usefulness of standard equations to predict REE and thus to guide the level of energy intake to prescribe in clinical practice, the formulas have been found to overestimate REE at the initiation of rehabilitation and to underestimate requirements during the refeeding process (Forman-Hoffman et al., 2006; Krahn, Rock, Dechert, Nairn, & Hasse, 1993). Very high levels of physical activity can also explain apparent resistance to weight gain in patients who are being managed as outpatients who use that strategy to achieve and maintain a low body weight (Casper, Schoeler, Kushner, Hnilicka, & Gold, 1991). Patients with AN are significantly more likely than patients with other types of EDs to exercise in excess to control weight, and importantly, level of exercise and degree of dietary restriction tend to be significantly inversely related (Dalle Grave, Calugi, & Marchesini, 2008).

In most circumstances, the level of energy intake necessary to promote weight res-toration can be achieved with regular food at meals and snacks. Energy-dense liquid nutritional supplements are sometimes prescribed if the patient cannot meet the goals with food alone. This approach is a relatively low-risk strategy that does not supplant a primary reliance on food to promote weight gain. Enteral supplementation via tube feeding is an alternative approach to supplementing the diet (Van Wymelbeke et al., 2004), used by some treatment units as an adjunct to the prescribed meals and snacks via nocturnal pump. Compared to oral nutritional supplements, tube feeding is more uncomfortable for patients and has somewhat greater risk for adverse effects of overly aggressive refeeding. Relying on regular food to promote weight restoration is associ-ated with lower risk for medical complications during refeeding. Also, ultimately the patient is going to have to address and learn to cope with the anxiety of eating regular meals and normal food to achieve recovery. Working through this process during the period of the most intensive contact and support that is typical of the initial treatment phase is a strategy that may improve the long-term outcome for the patient.

Parenteral or total parenteral nutrition, in which nutrients and energy sources (carbohydrate, amino acids, lipids) are delivered via peripheral or central vascular access, has also been used to promote weight restoration in patients with AN (Diamanti et al., 2008). The amount of energy that can be provided by peripheral access is limited because nutrition solutions delivered this way cannot exceed 800–900 milliosmoles per kilogram (mOsm/kg), and veins must be in good condition. Thus, parenteral nutrition using central access, via a catheter that is subcutaneously tunneled into the subclavian vein and fed into the superior vena cava, is the usual way that this feeding route is uti-lized. Although there are instances when this feeding route may be lifesaving (Mehler & Weiner, 2007), there are several compelling reasons why this is not recommended as a routine strategy (Silber, 2008). In contrast to parenteral nutrition, even liquid oral supplements or tube feeding via nocturnal pump provide the advantage of promoting the normalization of gastrointestinal function while supplementing the diet without the additional medical risks associated with parenteral nutrition, such as infection.

An overly aggressive refeeding regimen can result in the complication character-ized as the "refeeding syndrome." This syndrome is a recognized risk of the nutritional rehabilitation of patients with AN, particularly during the first few weeks when energy intake is being markedly increased. The condition occurs more often in chronically malnourished individuals, and when the enteral or parenteral feeding routes are used (Miller, 2008), although it has been observed secondary to high-calorie oral refeed-ing in AN (Fisher, Simpser, & Schneider, 2000). A primary feature of this syndrome is hypophosphatemia, with other abnormalities such as hypokalemia, hypomagnesemia, and hyperglycemia, usually accompanied by fluid and sodium retention. As a result of hypophosphatemia and the electrolyte abnormalities, cardiac arrhythmias, respiratory failure, congestive heart failure, hematological abnormalities, and neurological compli-cations may occur (Miller, 2008), although the cardiac atrophy that is often present in patients with AN may independently contribute to the cardiovascular changes that are observed during the initial phase of refeeding.

In addition to initiating treatment at a modest level of energy intake and increas-ing energy intake progressively, as described above, clinical monitoring of response, especially during the first 2 weeks of refeeding, can prevent the development of a full-blown refeeding syndrome. Clinical monitoring should include regular weighing and examination for marked edema, as well as monitoring appropriate blood chemistries, as described in detail elsewhere in this volume (Mehler, Birmingham, Crow, & Jahraus, Chapter 4). The rate at which energy intake is progressively increased should be adjusted if clinical or biochemical abnormalities are noted.

Micronutrients: Vitamins and Minerals

Results from clinical studies and case series reports suggest that vitamin deficiencies occur in up to one-third of patients with AN (Phillipp et al., 1988; Rock & Vasantharajan, 1995; Van Binsbergen, Okink, Van Den Berg, Koppeschaar, & Bennink, 1988). Generally, inadequate dietary intake explains these findings, although evidence suggests that thyroid hormone abnormalities that result from severe dietary restriction may adversely affect riboflavin status by causing an impaired metabolism of this vitamin to the active coenzyme forms (Capo-chichi et al., 1999). The latter finding may be of clinical importance because this suggests that an improvement in energy balance, and thus overall nutritional status (rather than simply providing the vitamin), may be necessary to correct the problem.

Hypercarotenemia is often present in these patients due to the consumption of high-carotenoid foods (i.e., deeply pigmented vegetables and fruits) (Rock & Swendseid, 1993) and is innocuous. Carotenoid absorption is inefficient but unregulated, so peripheral tissue concentrations are largely determined by intake versus relative body mass and tissue capacity: An individual with a smaller body mass has a higher tissue concentration than an individual with greater body mass, at a given dose of carotenoid intake. The conversion of provitamin A carotenoids to vitamin A is very well-regulated, so hypercarotenemia does not cause hypervitaminosis A.

If the nutritional rehabilitation and weight restoration are being accomplished with a balanced, micronutrient-rich diet, sufficient amounts of vitamins to restore good nutritional status are likely to be provided from food sources during refeeding. However, persistently low red blood cell folate concentration, which is a good measure of folate status, has been observed in adolescent patients following a short-term refeeding regimen (Castro, Deulofeu, Gila, Puig, & Toro, 2004). Prescribing a daily multivitamin with recommended (but not excessive) levels of essential vitamins and minerals is advised and does not pose a risk for toxicities or other adverse effects. Amounts of micronutrients in the product prescribed should not exceed 100% Daily Value, which is described on the dietary supplement label.

Calcium and vitamin D intakes are important in the nutritional rehabilitation of both adolescent and adult patients with AN. Osteopenia is a serious and possibly irreversible medical complication of AN, with at least one-half of patients having bone density measurements greater than two standard deviations below age- and gender-matched controls in clinical series reports (Grinspoon, Herzog, & Klibanski, 1997). Results from several studies indicate that some recovery of trabecular bone may be possible with weight restoration and recovery, but compromised bone density and deficits in bone mineral are evident after 11 years of follow-up after weight restoration and recovery (Bachrach, Katzman, Litt, Guido, & Marcus, 1991; Herzog et al., 1993; Ward & Treasure, 1997). Several causative factors have been identified, including hypoestrogenemia, elevated cortisol levels, decreased calcium intake, deficiency of insulin-like growth factor I (a nonspecific result of compromised nutritional status), and excessive physical activity (Grinspoon et al., 1997). Unlike other conditions in which low circulating estrogen concentrations are associated with bone loss (e.g., perimenopause), providing exogenous estrogen has not been shown to preserve or restore bone mass in the majority of patients with AN (Klibanski, Biller, Schoenfeld, Herzog, & Saxe, 1995). Calcium supplementation alone, even at a level of 1,500 mg/day, has also not been found to promote increased bone density in these patients (Klibanski et al., 1995). Sufficient amounts of both calcium and vitamin D are necessary to facilitate restoration of bone mass as hormonal factors normalize during treatment and recovery. Requirements for these nutrients, which are 1,000–1,300 mg/day for calcium and 400 IU/day for vitamin D, can be met by consuming three to four servings of dairy foods, calcium- and vitamin-D-fortified cereal, juice, or soy milk each day. One serving is one cup of milk or yogurt or one ounce of cheese, whether nonfat, low-fat, or regular products.

Zinc has also been suggested to be a micronutrient of particular importance in promoting recovery from AN, because zinc deficiency is associated with reduced food intake and altered taste thresholds. However, zinc balance has been shown to occur even at very low levels of intake (i.e., < 5.5 mg/day), due to compensatory mechanisms that occur at the level of absorption (King, 1990). In a 6-month double-blind clinical trial, Katz and colleagues (1987) found 50 mg/day supplemental zinc to be associated with greater improvement in psychological test scores in adolescent patients with AN, although significant differences in weight gain and taste function were not observed. In a 1-month placebo-controlled trial, 14 mg/day supplemental zinc was found to be associated with an increased rate of gain in body mass index (BMI) but not weight gain in hospitalized patients with AN (Birmingham, Goldner, & Bakan, 1994). Notably, the Daily Value for zinc is 15 mg/day, so a standard multiple vitamin with minerals that contains 100% Daily Value would provide that amount in addition to that provided by the diet.

Response to Nutritional Rehabilitation

Circulating concentrations of secretory proteins that are often used as clinical laboratory markers of overall nutritional status, such as serum albumin, are sometimes (but not always) reduced in the low-weight patient with AN, depending in part on the state of hydration of the patient when the blood sample was collected and the rate of weight loss (due to the adaptive mechanisms during weight loss). Thus, a change in these concentrations is often not observed in response to nutritional rehabilitation. Notably, clinical laboratory data must be interpreted within the context of the neuroendocrinal and other physiological abnormalities that are present in starvation. For example, hypercholesterolemia, if present, is a consequence of thyroid abnormalities in response to dietary restriction, and a high-energy diet that results in weight restoration (rather than a low-saturated fat, low-cholesterol diet) is the strategy that will normalize lipid levels.

Water retention during refeeding should be anticipated, due to shifts in the secretion of aldosterone in response to changes in dietary intake and other hormonal changes. Thus, change in weight or BMI does not necessarily predict change in lean tissue or fat mass, and a meaningful change in fat mass or fat-free mass may occur without a change in BMI or weight (Trocki & Shepherd, 2000). This is a clinically relevant issue because weight gain is sometimes used as evidence of adherence to the diet plan and therefore can be an inaccurate basis for expanded privileges and rewards in behavioral treatment programs.

With continued refeeding and weight restoration, delayed gastric emptying and related gastrointestinal complaints (e.g., bloating) will generally resolve. Normalization of plasma tryptophan (Attia, Wolk, Cooper, Glasofer, & Walsh, 2005) and adiponectin and leptin (Modan-Moses et al., 2007) concentrations occur in response to nutritional rehabilitation and weight restoration.

Results from several clinical studies provide some insight about changes in body composition that may be anticipated to occur in the patient with AN during weight restoration. Studies of low-weight patients using dual-energy X-ray absorptiometry, underwater weighing, and skinfold measurements to monitor body composition and fat distribution found that increased energy intake to promote weight restoration was associated with significant increases in all major body compartments (e.g., body fat, lean body mass, bone mineral content) (Orphanidou, McCarger, Birmingham, & Belzberg, 1997; Probst, Goris, Vandereycken, & Van Coppenolli, 2000). Although fat comprised the largest amount of the weight gained in the study by Orphanidou and colleagues (1997), results from the skinfold measurements did not suggest preferential fat deposition in any area. In contrast, a disproportionate central adipose tissue deposition (compared to normal-weight subjects) was observed in response to short-term normalization of weight in a study that used both dual-energy X-ray absorptiometry and whole-body magnetic resonance imaging (MRI) to assess body composition (Mayer et al., 2005). A perception of increased abdominal fat can be disturbing to a patient during nutritional rehabilitation, and that concern needs to be addressed. Notably, there are very few studies of body composition in long-term recovered individuals. Even though a greater net gain of body fat typically results from weight restoration in these patients, their body fat usually remains considerably lower than that of healthy control subjects.

Nutritional Counseling and Practical Considerations

Nutritional rehabilitation can be accomplished in various treatment settings, and choice of setting is determined by the presence or absence of metabolic abnormalities, medical complications, and other factors. Hospitalization is indicated for refeeding if the patient is severely nutritionally compromised (e.g., < 75% of recommended weight for height). Weight restoration can also be achieved through outpatient medical care and counseling, although as noted above, a slower rate of weight gain should be expected with that approach. Importantly, two small clinical trials have reported that nutritional counseling without concurrent psychotherapy and multimodal management is unlikely to promote recovery from AN (Pike, Walsh, Vitousek, Wilson, & Bauer, 2008; Serfaty, Turkington, Heap, Ledsham, & Jolley, 1999). Nutritional counseling, even when it includes the specific strategies of dietary guidance and nutritional education described in this chapter, does not support this aspect of care to be used as a stand-alone intervention, although it is a very important component of treatment.

In structured behavioral treatment programs, patients are usually allowed to make at least some of their own food choices from the hospital or psychiatric unit menu within 2–4 weeks of admission, with guidance from a dietitian to ensure that the energy prescription and nutrient needs are met. In most inpatient treatment programs, certain dietary rules about food choices and goals for energy intake must be agreed upon and followed in order for patients to normalize meals and eating patterns. Typically, patients are permitted to select a limited number of foods (i.e., three to five) that they may refuse to eat during the pre-self-select phase, and some personal preferences can be accommodated. For example, a lactovegetarian diet can be nutritionally adequate and sufficiently dense in energy to enable weight restoration, whereas more extreme diets (i.e., one that excludes all animal products) present more problems because of difficulty in achieving adequate energy and nutrient intakes. The meal plan provided typically consists of three meals plus one or two planned snacks each day, with total energy intake distributed to meet current recommendations for general health (20–35% from fat, 45–65% from carbohydrate, and 10–35% from protein).

Inpatient programs typically forbid the inclusion of reduced- or calorie-free products in meals and snacks, as well as food choices and behaviors that patients may have adopted to control hunger. These behaviors include excessive consumption of calorie-free beverages (e.g., coffee, tea, diet soft drinks) and chewing gum. When patients are being managed as outpatients, it is more difficult to mandate and control these behaviors. However, they need to be addressed in nutritional counseling, and recommending some limits is an aspect of guidance that will help to promote recovery.

The nutritional counseling process consists of establishing and monitoring dietary and behavioral goals in a stepwise manner, with the application of cognitive-behavioral counseling strategies to help the patient expand his/her diet (Henry & Ozier, 2006). Individualized guidance and a meal plan that provides a framework for meals and food choices is the usual strategy implemented to ensure a healthy diet that promotes weight restoration. The tool most often used for meal planning is a food group or exchange system. In an exchange system, individual foods are grouped into categories with described portion equivalents based mainly on energy and macronutrient content (Byrd-Bredbenner, Moe, Beshgetoor, & Berning, 2009). This tool allows for the planning of daily menus that consist of a variety of foods and is flexible, but it also can ensure consistent energy and macronutrient intakes that achieve the dietary targets. For example, a breakfast meal for a 3,200 kcal/day diet might consist of the following exchanges: 1 milk, 2 fruit, 4 starch, 2 meat, and 4 fat. One translation would be 1 cup yogurt, 1 cup orange juice, 1 cup cooked cereal with 8 walnut halves, 2 slices toast with 2 teaspoons margarine, and 2 eggs. Alternatively, soy milk could replace the yogurt, a bagel could replace the cereal or toast, cream cheese could replace the margarine, and Canadian bacon could replace the eggs, and the same levels of energy, carbohydrate, protein, and fat would result. Having an assigned number of servings across the food groups for each meal and snack provides a structure that can be translated into a variety of food choices as patients progress from inpatient or partial hospitalization programs into planning and eating meals at home.

The U.S. Department of Agriculture's MyPyramid Food Guidance System (www. mypyramid.gov), which is based on the current U.S. Dietary Guidelines, provides a similar approach to structuring meal planning, using food group servings that can be used to achieve consistent energy and macronutrient intakes. However, this tool is not designed for weight restoration, so the suggested number of food group servings for a given individual must be adjusted to achieve an energy level that will promote weight gain during the initial phase of nutritional rehabilitation. For weight maintenance, this tool is a good resource for translating general guidance into a healthy diet.

Patients also benefit from guidance as to how to begin to include formerly forbidden foods in the diet. One example is to start by including foods in the diet that have both positive health attributes (e.g., a good source of protein or fiber) in addition to the negative attributes (containing sugar or fat). Fear of overeating when exposed to formerly forbidden foods can be managed by planning the meal environment or portion exposure so that the risk for overeating is reduced. Planning meals and snacks with prepackaged prepared foods also can be helpful for some patients during early phases of meal planning in outpatient management. The energy and nutrient content values are provided on the food label, reinforcing factual information, and the portion exposure is limited, which may reduce anxiety in patients fighting the urge to binge-eat. An additional element of structure is provided, offering further reassurance for some patients.

Notably, weight-restored women with AN who choose a diet characterized by low-energy density and limited variety are at greater risk of poor outcome during follow-up (Schebendach et al., 2008). In both observational and clinical studies, energy density of the diet has emerged as a critical factor that affects the likelihood of weight gain during adulthood and weight loss in overweight or obese individuals (Ledikwe et al., 2007; Savage, Marini, & Birch, 2008). A diet comprised of a preponderance of food choices that are low in fat and high in fiber and water promotes greater satiety at a lower level of energy intake, so the observation that this type of dietary pattern would be associated with treatment failure in AN is not surprising. Thus, nutritional counseling should specifically discourage an inordinate emphasis on vegetables and other low-energy density foods, and avoidance of fat, which would facilitate tolerance of a reduced energy diet and thus promote weight loss. Also, limited food choices or lower variety across meals and daily menus has been observed to facilitate weight loss in obesity (Raynor, Jeffery, Tate, & Wing, 2004), so a diet characterized by a variety of foods within and across food groups should be encouraged for the recovering patient with AN.

In the long term, patients usually benefit by continuing a pattern of regular meals and snacks, planning food choices in advance, and monitoring dietary intake via food records or computer dietary analysis software programs that calculate energy intake and nutritional adequacy. Regular follow-up sessions with a nutritional counselor over the time frame necessary for resolution of the psychological issues will help the patient attain and maintain a healthy body weight and true recovery.

In addition to guidance with meal planning, an important component of nutritional counseling is cognitive restructuring focused on deeply held beliefs and thought patterns relating to foods. Nutritional education is a part of this counseling, which involves providing factual information about dieting, nutrition, food content, and the relationship between starvation and physical symptoms. This information can help patients develop more accurate and healthy perceptions and to reframe interpretations. For example, visualizing the restoration of muscle and bone mass that is occurring when eating sufficient amounts of food to promote weight regain, rather than the negative thoughts associated with body fat and adiposity, can help to modify thought patterns that arise during weight restoration.

Nutritional rehabilitation in the adolescent patient must involve parents or caretakers. This means communicating the goals and providing nutrition education to parents, who also may need to modify beliefs and behaviors relating to diet, nutrition, and weight, as well as the patient, so that the family environment involving food supports recovery.

In the initial phase of nutritional rehabilitation, physical activity almost always must be limited due to risk of injury and to create a positive energy balance that permits weight gain. Later counseling efforts should communicate that in the healthy state, exercise is an activity that should be undertaken for enjoyment and fitness (rather than a strategy to simply expend energy and promote weight loss), and that excessive exercise is often a common component of the ED itself. Supervised low-weight strength training is less likely to impede weight gain than other forms of activity and can be psychologically helpful for patients, even during weight restoration.

Other Supportive Activities

In addition to meals and planned snacks provided under supervision, most inpatient and partial hospitalization programs include group activities such as meal preparation, in which patients engage in grocery shopping and preparing a meal with staff guidance and support. Events such as a restaurant meal, followed by a discussion of emotional reactions and attitudinal responses, with a nutritional counselor or other staff can help patients recognize and modify these reactions and responses. Experiencing these food- and eating-related situations while being supported by a reassuring and knowledgeable counselor reinforces the patient's efforts to return to more normal eating behavior as treatment and recovery progress. These types of food-related activities can also be conducted as a component of nutritional counseling in the outpatient setting.

Summary and Conclusions

Nutritional rehabilitation is an important component of the treatment of AN. Metabolic and psychological challenges to weight restoration and normalized eating patterns are present and should be anticipated. However, numerous specific strategies and evidence-based approaches can be useful in achieving the goals of nutritional rehabilitation in these patients. The approach to weight restoration can affect short-term outcome and also can set the stage for successful weight maintenance and normalization of eating behaviors. Nutritional counseling and education using various tools and strategies that focus on the food-related issues and eating behavior provide a unique contribution to the overall treatment of AN.

References

Attia E, Wolk S, Cooper T, Glasofer D, & Walsh BT. (2005). Plasma tryptophan during weight restoration in patients with anorexia nervosa. *Biological Psychiatry*, 57:674–678.

Bachrach LK, Katzman DK, Litt IF, Guido D, & Marcus R. (1991). Recovery from osteopenia in adolescent girls with anorexia nervosa. *Journal of Clinical Endocrinology and Metabolism*, 72:602–606.

Birmingham CL, Goldner EM, & Bakan R. (1994). Controlled trial of zinc supplementation in anorexia nervosa. *International Journal of Eating Disorders*, 15:252–255.

Byrd-Bredbenner C, Moe G, Beshgetoor D, & Berning J. (2009). *Perspectives in nutrition* (8th ed.). New York: McGraw-Hill.

Capo-chichi CD, Gueant JL, Lefebvre E, Bennani N, Lorentz E, Vidailhet C, et al. (1999). Riboflavin and riboflavin-derived cofactors in adolescent girls with anorexia nervosa. *American Journal of Clinical Nutrition*, 69:672–678.

Casper RC, Schoeller DA, Kushner R, Hnilicka J, & Gold ST. (1991). Total daily energy expenditure and activity level in anorexia nervosa. *American Journal of Clinical Nutrition*, 53:1143–1150.

Castro J, Deulofeu R, Gila A, Puig J, & Toro J. (2004). Persistence of nutritional deficiencies after short-term weight recovery in adolescents with anorexia nervosa. *International Journal of Eating Disorders*, 35:169–178.

Dalle Grave R, Calugi S, & Marchesini G. (2008). Compulsive exercise to control shape or weight in eating disorders: Prevalence, associated features, and treatment outcome. *Comprehensive Psychiatry*, 49:346–352.

Diamanti A, Basso MS, Castro M, Bianco G, Ciacco E, Calce A, et al. (2008). Clinical efficacy and safety of parenteral nutrition in adolescent girls with anorexia nervosa. *Journal of Adolescent Health*, 42:111–118.

Fisher M, Simpser E, & Schneider M. (2000). Hypophosphatemia secondary to oral refeeding in anorexia nervosa. *International Journal of Eating Disorders*, 28:181–187.

Forman-Hoffman VL, Ruffin T, & Schultz SK. (2006). Basal metabolic rate in anorexia nervosa patients: Using appropriate predictive equations during the refeeding process. *Annals of Clinical Psychiatry*, 18:123–127.

Grinspoon S, Herzog D, & Klibanski A. (1997). Mechanisms and treatment options for bone loss in anorexia nervosa. *Psychopharmacology Bulletin*, 33:399–404.

Hadigan CM, Anderson EJ, Miller KK, Hubbard JL, Herzog DB, Klibanski A, et al. (1999). Assessment of macronutrient and micronutrient intake in women with anorexia nervosa. *International Journal of Eating Disorders*, 28:284–292.

Henry BW, & Ozier AD. (2006). Position of the American Dietetic Association: Nutrition intervention in the treatment of anorexia nervosa, bulimia nervosa, and other eating disorders. *Journal of the American Dietetic Association*, 106:2073–2082.

Herzog W, Minne H, Deter C, Leidig G, Schellberg D, Wuster C, et al. (1993). Outcome of bone mineral density in anorexia nervosa patients 11.7 years after first admission. *Journal of Bone Mineral Research*, 8:597–605.

Katz RL, Keen CL, Litt IF, Hurley LS, Lellams-Harrison KM, & Glader LJ. (1987). Zinc deficiency in anorexia nervosa. *Journal of Adolescent Health Care*, 8:400–406.

King JC. (1990). Assessment of zinc status. *Journal of Nutrition*, 120:1474–1479.

Klibanski A, Biller BMK, Schoenfeld DA, Herzog DB, & Saxe VC. (1995). The effects of estrogen administration on trabecular bone loss in young women with anorexia nervosa. *Journal of Clinical Endocrinology and Metabolism*, 89:898–904.

Krahn DD, Rock CL, Dechert RE, Nairn KK, & Hasse SA. (1993). Changes in resting energy expenditure in anorexia nervosa patients during refeeding. *Journal of the American Dietetic Association*, 98:434–438.

Ledikwe JH, Rolls BJ, Smiciklas-Write H, Mitchell DC, Ard JD, et al. (2007). Reductions in dietary energy density are associated with weight loss in overweight and obese participants in the PREMIER trial. *American Journal of Clinical Nutrition*, 85:1212–1221.

Mayer L, Walsh BT, Pierson RN, Heymsfield SB, Gallagher D, Wang J, et al. (2005). Body fat redistribution after weight gain in women with anorexia nervosa. *American Journal of Clinical Nutrition*, 81:1286–1291.

Mehler PS, & Weiner KL. (2007). Use of total parenteral nutrition in the refeeding of selected patients with severe anorexia nervosa. *International Journal of Eating Disorders*, 40:285–287.

Miller SJ. (2008). Death resulting from overzealous total parenteral nutrition: The refeeding syndrome revisited. *Nutrition in Clinical Practice*, 23:166–171.

Orphanidou CI, McCargar LJ, Birmingham CL, & Belzberg AS. (1997). Changes in body composition and fat distribution after short-term weight gain in patients with anorexia nervosa. *American Journal of Clinical Nutrition*, 65:1034–1041.

Phillipp E, Pirke KM, Seidl M, Tuschl RJ, Fichter MM, Eckert M, et al. (1988). Vitamin status in patients with anorexia nervosa and bulimia nervosa. *International Journal of Eating Disorders*, 8:209–218.

Pike KM, Walsh BT, Vitousek K, Wilson GT, & Bauer J. (2003). Cognitive behavior therapy in the posthospitalization treatment of anorexia nervosa. *American Journal of Psychiatry*, 160:2046–2049.

Probst M, Goris M, Vandereycken W, & Van Coppenolli H. (2001). Body composition of anorexia nervosa patients assessed by underwater weighing and skinfold-thickness measurements before and after weight gain. *American Journal of Clinical Nutrition*, 73:190–197.

Raynor HA, Jeffery RW, Tate DF, & Wing R. (2004). Relationship between changes in food group variety, dietary intake, and weight during obesity treatment. *International Journal of Obesity and Related Metabolic Disorders*, 28:813–820.

Rock CL. (1997). Nutrition in anorexia and bulimia nervosa. *Baillere's Clinical Psychiatry*, 3:259–273.

Rock CL, & Swendseid ME. (1993). Plasma carotenoid levels in anorexia nervosa and in obese patients. *Methods in Enzymology*, 214:116–123.

Rock CL, & Vasantharajan S. (1995). Vitamin status of eating disorder patients: Relationship to clinical indices and effect of treatment. *International Journal of Eating Disorders*, 18:257–262.

Savage JS, Marini M, & Birch LL. (2008) Dietary energy density predicts women's weight change over 6 y. *American Journal of Clinical Nutrition* 88:677–684.

Schebendach JE, Mayer LES, Devlin MJ, Attia E, Contento IR, Wolf RL, et al. (2008). Dietary energy density and diet variety as predictors of outcome in anorexia nervosa. *American Journal of Clinical Nutrition* 87:810–816.

Serfaty MA, Turkington D, Heap M, Ledsham L, & Jolley E. (1999). Cognitive therapy versus dietary counseling in the outpatient treatment of anorexia nervosa: Effects of the treatment phase. *European Eating Disorders Review*, 7:334–350.

Silber TJ. (2008). A change in the treatment of anorexia nervosa?: Not to soon. *Journal of Adolescent Health*, 42:109–110.

Treat TA, Gaskill JA, McCabe EB, Ghinassi FA, Luczak AD, & Marcus MD. (2005). Short-term outcome of psychiatric inpatients with anorexia nervosa in the current care environment. *International Journal of Eating Disorders*, 38:123–133.

Trocki O, & Shepherd RW. (2000). Change in body mass index does not predict change in body composition in adolescent girls with anorexia nervosa. *Journal of the American Dietetic Association*, 100:457–459.

U.S. Department of Agriculture. (2009). *MyPyramid food guidance system*. Available online at *www.mypyramid.gov*.

Van Binsbergen CJM, Okink J, Van Den Berg H, Koppeschaar H, & Bennink HJTC. (1988). Nutritional status in anorexia nervosa: clinical chemistry, vitamins, iron and zinc. *European Journal of Clinical Nutrition*, 42:929–937.

Van Wymelbeke V, Brondel L, Brun JM, & Rigaud D. (2004). Factors associated with the increase in resting energy expenditure during refeeding in malnourished anorexia nervosa patients. *American Journal of Clinical Nutrition*, 80:1469–1477.

Ward A, Brown N, & Treasure J. (1997). Persistent osteopenia after recovery from anorexia nervosa. *International Journal of Eating Disorders*, 22:71–75.

CHAPTER 11

Inpatient and Day Hospital Treatment for Anorexia Nervosa

Marion P. Olmsted, Traci L. McFarlane, Jacqueline C. Carter, Kathryn Trottier, D. Blake Woodside, and Gina Dimitropoulos

Inpatient (IP) and day hospital (DH) treatment are essential components of comprehensive treatment for patients with moderate to severe anorexia nervosa (AN). Most programs are multimodal and based on a biopsychosocial model. In this chapter we briefly summarize the evidence related to the effectiveness of intensive treatment, and describe the goals and structure of intensive treatment and commonly used therapeutic modalities. Strategies for preparing patients for treatment, enhancing motivation, treating comorbid conditions, providing follow-up treatment, and working with families and caregivers are also considered. Currently, there is no consensus or clear criteria for identifying patients suitable for such intensive treatment; the need for IP or DH interventions is generally based on clinical judgment and indicators related to medical stability, weight and severity of symptoms, rapid decline in weight or food intake, and failure to improve with specialized outpatient care.

The Efficacy of IP and DH Treatment

There is very little research into the efficacy of inpatient and day hospital treatments for eating disorders (EDs). With a few notable exceptions, most of the available evidence is derived from small, uncontrolled studies. This literature has been reviewed elsewhere (Olmsted et al., 2007; Treat, McCabe, Gaskill, & Marcus, 2008; Zipfel et al., 2002) and is summarized briefly here. The three primary dimensions of intensive treatment efficacy are (1) engagement and participation rates, (2) effectiveness for participants, and (3) maintenance of improvement over time.

Engagement with Treatment

A significant number of individuals with severe EDs refuses to participate in intensive treatment whereas another number initiates treatment but leaves prematurely. Reported dropout rates range from 20 to 51% for IP treatment and from 13 to 19% for DH treatment; the available evidence suggests that patients who drop out of intensive treatments appear to be among the more severely ill (Olmsted et al., 2007). This finding highlights one of the most significant treatment challenges in this area.

Treatment Effectiveness for Participants

Results of case series studies of IP treatment for AN have consistently shown that IP treatment is effective at achieving weight restoration. Data from our own center, based on 183 patients admitted to the IP program between 2000 and 2005, are illustrative. The mean body mass index (BMI) at admission was 14.9. Seventy-one patients (39.3%) achieved a BMI of at least 20, 35 (19.1%) achieved a BMI between 18.5 and 20, and 77 (42.1%) had a BMI below 18.5 at discharge. Among the 106 patients (57.9%) who achieved a BMI of at least 18.5, the mean length of stay was 15.1 weeks, the mean weight gain was 13.7 kilograms (kg), and the mean rate of weight gain was 0.95 kg/week. Patients were completely hospitalized at the beginning of treatment, gradually had more passes out of the hospital over time, and most were day attendees for the last 5–6 weeks of treatment. There were also significant improvements on measures of both ED psychopathology and general psychopathology, including depression, anxiety, and self-esteem. In terms of bulimic symptoms, 92.5% were free from binge eating and 88.7% were free from purging symptoms over the 4 weeks preceding the end of IP treatment (Carter, Woodside, & Kaplan, 2000).

Similar short-term outcome has been described for a specialty care continuum in Pittsburgh, in which patients with AN initially receive IP treatment and are then transferred to DH (Treat et al., 2008). After a mean of 5 weeks of IP and 3 weeks of DH treatment, 35.2% of a sample of 71 patients with AN had an excellent outcome, 26.8% had a good outcome, 14.1% were below average, and 23.9% had a poor outcome (Treat et al., 2008).

To date, there have been two published randomized controlled trials of IP treatment for AN (Crisp, Norton, Gowers et al., 1991; Gowers et al., 2007). The first study compared inpatient with two types of outpatient treatment for adults with AN. There was a higher rate of refusal to participate following randomization among patients assigned to inpatient treatment, but there were no significant differences between IP and outpatient treatments in terms of weight gain or Morgan–Russell outcome indices (Morgan & Russell, 1975) at follow-up. In the second study, Gowers and colleagues (2007) compared inpatient treatment, 6 months of specialized outpatient therapy, and 6 months of treatment as usual in the community for 167 adolescents with AN. The outpatient therapy included elements of both cognitive-behavioral therapy (CBT) and family therapy. At 1 year follow-up there were no statistically significant differences between the three groups in terms of weight outcome or Morgan–Russell outcome indices, based on intention-to-treat analysis. Together these two studies provide converging evidence that inpatient treatment provides no long-term advantage over outpatient treatment for patients with sufficient medical stability to be treated as outpatients.

Case series reports of DH treatments that are multimodal and incorporate a cognitive-behavioral focus consistently report significant increases in weight and decreases in binge eating and purging behaviors in patients with AN (see Olmsted et al., 2007; Zipfel et al., 2002). Data from our own center, based on 192 patients with AN admitted to the DH program between 1995 and 2006, are illustrative. Patients were admitted to the DH at a mean BMI of 16.8. In terms of weight outcome, 62 patients (32.3%) achieved a BMI of at least 20, 75 (39.1%) achieved a BMI between 18.5 and 20, and 55 (28.6%) had a BMI below 18.5 at discharge. Among the 137 patients (71.4%) who achieved a BMI of at least 18.5, the mean length of stay was 10.8 weeks, the mean weight gain was 8.0 kg, and the mean rate of weight gain was 0.75 kg/week. There were also significant improvements on measures of ED psychopathology, depression, and self-esteem. In terms of bulimic symptoms, 73.1% were free from binge eating and 59.2% were free from purging symptoms over the 4 weeks preceding the discharge from DH treatment. Similar results have generally been found with DH treatment at other centers, suggesting that DH treatment may be a cost-effective stand-alone or step-down approach for patients with AN (Treat et al., 2008; Zipfel et al., 2002).

The optimal intensity of DH treatment required for effectiveness is unknown. Programs with published outcome data have ranged from 4 or 5 days to 7 days weekly, with no clear trends related to intensity (Olmsted et al., 2007; Zipfel et al., 2002).

Relapse Following Intensive Treatment

Published relapse rates following IP treatment range from 9 to 42%, with an average of 30% for adults and 9% for adolescents. The period of highest risk for relapse appears to be in the first year after discharge (Olmsted et al., 2007). In a study conducted at our center, excessive exercise and residual concern about weight and shape at the end of IP treatment correlated with risk of relapse over the following 15 months (Carter, Blackmore, Sutandar-Pinnock, & Woodside, 2004). Although IP treatment has an essential role to play, this research underscores the need for additional treatment after hospitalization and a definition of wellness that is broader than weight restoration. To our knowledge, there are no published relapse rates for AN following DH treatment.

Goals

Although there are different ways to operationalize treatment based on a biopsychosocial model of EDs, the goals generally include (1) medical stabilization; (2) weight gain; (3) the cessation of binge eating, vomiting, laxative use, overexercise, and other unhealthy behaviors used to control weight; (4) normalization of eating through a balanced and sufficient meal plan; (5) therapeutic exploration of underlying issues and skill development related to affect regulation and interpersonal relationships; and (6) the initiation of a process of comprehensive social and vocational rehabilitation, which is generally not completed during the intensive treatment. Ideally patients are able to reach their target weight and stop binge-eating and purging during intensive treatment and then have several more weeks to consolidate their new patterns and practice normalized eating. Follow-up treatment is critical to support the behavioral changes and to continue work on body image and psychological and vocational rehabilitation. Intensive treatment should be viewed as but one step on a longer journey toward recovery.

Medical Stabilization

The physical safety of the patient is an important priority for any intensive treatment. All patients require a physical examination. We suggest a complete blood count; liver function tests; serum creatinine level; measurement of electrolytes, calcium, magnesium, and phosphate; and an electrocardiogram (EKG) for all patients beginning intensive treatment, given the high frequency of abnormalities secondary to both malnutrition and purging behavior. Assessment of bone mineral density is indicated in all those with AN admitted to intensive treatment. The routine performance of radiological examinations, such as computed tomography (CT) or magnetic resonance imaging (MRI) scans of the head, are not normally indicated for such patients. Regular assessment of blood glucose and lipids are indicated if atypical antipsychotics have been, or are to be, used during treatment.

Medical management of AN is addressed in detail in Chapter 4 of this book. Physicians treating EDs should be familiar with the potential problems that are likely to arise in patients with AN.

Weight Gain

Patients need to be informed about the expectations regarding rate of weight gain and the protocol for increasing calories. Calories beyond the normal maintenance level may be provided as food supplements to increase patients' familiarity with their maintenance meal plan. Activity levels at first are best kept to a minimum to promote weight gain, and asking patients to record all activity can be a helpful tool. There is a paucity of research on what constitutes an optimal rate of weight gain for underweight patients during intensive treatment. The usual considerations relate to the length of treatment versus the likely longer-term outcome after weight restoration. Weight gain targets of about 1 kg per week are common for IP and DH treatment settings. One study found that setting lower weekly weight gain requirements (i.e., 0.5 kg vs. 0.75 kg per week) during IP treatment was associated with better weight maintenance after discharge (Herzog, Zeeck, Hartmann, & Nickel, 2004). Another study showed that faster weight gain during IP treatment was associated with subsequent rehospitalization (Willer, Thuras, & Crow, 2005). Rapid weight gain may make it more difficult for patients to achieve the psychological accommodations needed to support this change. Alternatively, rapid weight gain may mean that patients want to hurry the process so that they can complete the IP treatment and get back to their ED.

Regardless of the expectations of treatment providers about the ideal rate of weight gain, there is growing evidence that the rate and trajectory of a patient's weight gain during treatment have significant predictive value related to treatment response. Hartmann, Wirth, and Zeeck (2007) have reviewed this literature and demonstrated that higher BMI at intake and lower weight gain in the first 4 weeks of IP treatment are associated with failure to gain weight during IP treatment. Converging evidence was provided in another study that showed that patients with smaller weekly weight gains and larger weight losses were more likely to drop out of treatment (Mewes, Tagay, & Senf,

2008). Similarly, a recent study showed that weight gain at a rate of 0.8 kg or more per week during hospitalization was significantly associated with better clinical outcome 12 months later (Lund et al., 2009). Rate and consistency of weight gain are likely behavioral indicators of psychological readiness to work toward recovery. As such, these two indices may provide a very useful flag that specific types of psychological support and intervention are needed.

There is some controversy about what represents an appropriate weight target for patients with AN, and no empirical data to support a specific choice. Most clinicians suggest that a useful guideline is a weight at which normal menstruation occurs, although the resumption of menses is often delayed in patients with AN. Suggested target weights are in the range of 85–95% of chart average, or a BMI of 19–21. In practice, it is essential to have a rationale for setting the target weight and to anticipate that patients will challenge the rationale. Patients are also likely to view the target weight as the "maximum allowable," whereas care providers may see it as a minimum expectation. Setting a target range for weight, with an upper and a lower limit, can be helpful in managing the patient's competing concerns.

In a managed care environment or when treatment resources are limited, the allowed length of stay may determine the designation of a target weight. Two studies based on an IP-DH care continuum have shown that lower weight at the point of discharge from IP and transfer to DH is associated with poorer treatment outcome (Howard, Evans, Quintero-Howard, Bowers, & Andersen, 1999; Treat et al., 2008). In these two studies longer duration of illness and lower admission weights were also associated with poor response to treatment. Lower weight at discharge from IP treatment has also been associated with rehospitalization (Steinhausen, Grigoroiu-Serbanescu, Boyadjieva, Neumarker, & Metzke, 2008). These studies did not specify whether lower transfer and discharge weights indicated that insufficient treatment time was available or that patients were reluctant to gain more weight. However, weight loss immediately after transfer to DH (Treat et al., 2008) or toward the end of intensive treatment (Kaplan et al., 2008) has been associated with worse outcome 6 months later.

Nasogastric feeding and extensive use of supplements are both common in some settings. Nocturnal nasogastric feeding that is voluntary and supplements oral food intake has been associated with higher and faster weight gain than oral refeeding alone and did not result in reduced ratings of patient satisfaction with treatment (Robb, Silber, Orrell-Valente et al., 2002; Zuercher, Cumella, Woods, Eberly, & Carr, 2003). Clinically there is general agreement that supplements should be used in addition to, and not instead of, food and that it is important for procedures such as nasogastric feeding to be noncoercive.

Symptom Control

The therapeutic environment is designed to inhibit symptoms. Whereas traditionally this has meant physical containment, increasingly the importance of psychological containment via support from staff and other patients is recognized. This is as true for patients who are living in the hospital as it is for those who are living at home. Cognitive-behavioral strategies are recommended to control symptoms outside of program hours.

Normalized Eating

Patients should be provided with an individualized, balanced meal plan and educated about the degree of variety required, expectations about including phobic foods (e.g., how many, how soon), the role of food supplements, and the methods for establishing caloric levels as well as changes in them. Most programs expect patients to tackle increasingly difficult eating tasks as they progress through treatment.

Meals within an intensive program are an important component of treatment. When patients eat together as a group, by engaging in a challenging task together, they feel supported. With guidelines and time limits clearly established in advance, staff are able to supervise, support, and coach patients who are having difficulty eating. Staff can also encourage light social conversation around the table as part of normalizing eating and as a means of distraction. In general, patients appreciate a staff approach that is friendly, supportive, and engaged but not blatantly focused on observation and supervision; staff can cultivate a style of being observant while maintaining a more social interactive style. When an individual occasionally requires more intensive coaching, a staff member may need to move closer to her and use a quiet voice to avoid embarrassment (for the patient) and minimize the disruption (for others). In some programs, "eating with the group" occurs from the first day, whereas in others it is a step that occurs after the patient has demonstrated that she is ready. One of the challenges is to balance the need for prorecovery behavior in the group with the potential for individuals who are struggling to be inspired and carried along by the group momentum. Occasionally, unhelpful group dynamics related to "anorexic competition" develop; these may center on speed of eating (i.e., slow), being the last to finish, or needing the most attention from staff. It is helpful to discuss these dynamics openly in the group and to encourage every patient to speak of her experience at meals. This approach can be combined with individually tailored therapeutic challenges such as asking a patient who appears to be caught up in a competition to "do the opposite" by finding herself a more distracting seat at the table and finishing her meal 5 minutes early.

When patients are not in the hospital, either because they are enrolled in a DH program or are on a pass from an IP program, work toward the goal of normalizing eating must continue. Considerable group time may be devoted to planning meals outside of the program, developing strategies to facilitate symptom control and adherence to the meal plan, and reporting back after evenings and weekends away. Patients can be encouraged to share strategies and offer feedback to one another.

Even patients who are in the hospital will need to work together outside of scheduled programming hours to remain free of symptoms and to structure free time. It is generally much more difficult than it might appear to make a hospital ward a guaranteed "symptom-free zone." Patients admitted to the hospital can be allowed some freedom within the institution and will benefit from planning and reviewing excursions.

Underlying Therapeutic Issues

Underlying issues and stressors that maintain the ED can be identified and processed in group, family, and individual therapy formats. The schedule for therapy groups should acknowledge the central importance of body image concerns as well as relationship issues related to autonomy, intimacy and caring, past abuse, ambivalence about recovery, and the function served by the ED. Skill development focused on practical aspects of affect regulation and interpersonal relationships is also very important.

Social and Vocational Rehabilitation

Although it is not practical to undertake comprehensive social and vocational rehabilitation during IP or DH treatment, it is essential to start this work and to develop plans for it to continue after intensive treatment. Social contact, the development of fulfilling relationships, and a means of engaging with the world outside of the ED are needed to help fill the vacuum that may otherwise beckon the return of the ED.

Preparation for Intensive Treatment

Prior to admission, it is helpful to meet with patients at least once to share information about what they can expect from the program and what will be expected of them during their stay. At this step, engagement with the treatment is fostered by open, honest communication, a positive, encouraging attitude, and the informed empathy that experienced staff are able to provide. In our experience, it is important to provide enough detail about the program guidelines that patients have a general awareness of what to expect at this stage but not so much detail that they become overwhelmed.

Patients can be given a written description of the program that they can share with family members and other people involved in their care. At the preparation session, the goals and general structure of the program can be reviewed, including a brief overview of how time in the hospital will be spent and expected length of stay. It is helpful for patients to be aware of the system for determining privilege level (e.g., off-ward passes) and level of independence in terms of eating (e.g., unsupervised meals). In addition, the program expectations for behavior change and weight gain can be discussed. For example, it might be made clear that the treatment unit is to remain a symptom-free area. Depending on the philosophy of the program, rapid abstinence from binge eating and purging might be emphasized. The criteria for premature discharge should also be discussed.

Not surprisingly, patients are often quite interested in finding out about the details of the meal plan requirements at this time. In our experience, it is important to provide enough detail about the meal plan that patients have a good idea of what to expect when they first arrive, without feeling overwhelmed with too much detail about more advanced food risks they will be expected to take later in the program.

For patients who have had prior unsuccessful experiences with intensive treatment, it is helpful to discuss the obstacles to recovery encountered during previous admissions and/or what contributed to relapse. It can also be constructive to discuss how the patient might be able to make better use of the treatment program this time. In addition, it is helpful to educate patients about the process of recovery, including the possibility that they may feel worse, both emotionally and physically, before they feel better.

Structuring Intensive Treatment

In recent years the contents of intensive treatments—the specific psychosocial and nutritional interventions—have become increasingly similar in IP and DH settings, so that the primary differences between the two include the number of treatment hours and the level of external containment provided (Zipfel et al, 2002). Program structures generally include a weekly schedule of activities as well as expectations about attendance, punctuality, and length of stay. The goals of the treatment program and the methods for working toward those goals should be clearly articulated and fully understood by patients and staff members. The philosophy and attitudes of the care providers create the atmosphere of the treatment program and may have a significant impact on efficacy. One important parameter relates to setting "appropriate" expectations; the challenge is to expect enough without expecting so much that patients are too frightened or overwhelmed to begin. Another decision relates to the balance between program requirements and patient responsibility. Some patients will aspire to only the minimum required level of performance. Wherever this line is drawn, some patients may feel that they are being coerced in an unhelpful manner, whereas others may (eventually) appreciate the pressure to face a task that they would not have chosen.

The treatment model should provide guiding principles for staff members, a rationale for their decision-making process, and the structure to provide a consistent, predictable environment for patients. Consistent care can be fostered by encouraging staff members to function as a team and reserving adequate team meeting time to allow for collaborative decision making.

Therapeutic Modalities

Most IP and DH programs are multimodal, incorporating a cognitive-behavioral framework and a group approach with some or all of the following: motivational enhancement, interpersonal therapy, body image therapy, dialectical behavior therapy, family therapy, expressive arts therapy, and some form of experiential therapy. Many of these modalities are described in detail in other chapters of this book. The distinguishing features of IP and DH treatment are the therapeutic milieu and the intensity of the psychosocial treatment. Patients are together for at least 30–40 hours weekly, which creates an intensive therapeutic arena well beyond the scope of outpatient therapy. In this environment various modalities are combined to create a synergistic effect that is much more than the sum of its parts. For example, exposure and response prevention occurs several times daily as patients have meals and refrain from ED symptoms. They may also be exposed to interpersonal conflict, the experience of affect and its expression, and other triggers for symptomatic behavior. Patients who might otherwise feel that they cannot eat or control their symptoms when they are stressed may be motivated by their commitment to the group and inspired by the behavior of other group members. The same synergy is evident when cognitive-behavioral strategies related to planning risky homework activities are bolstered by committing to the group that the homework will be completed.

The principle of graded task assignment is one of the foundations of intensive treatment. In the early stages patients are provided with maximum support and the lowest level of task difficulty. This may mean eating smaller amounts and being confined to an IP unit 24 hours per day. Over time patients are encouraged to eat larger amounts, order more phobic foods in the program and on meal outings (i.e., increased task difficulty), and to "take home" what they have accomplished in the program (i.e., reduce the level of support). In the patient's first attempts to normalize eating out of the hospital, having an easy (less phobic) snack with a friend is good planning. Later in treatment the same patient may be able to have a moderately risky snack at home alone and avoid acting on any subsequent urges. It is important to help the patient correctly identify her level of coping, so that she can make plans that match her needs and abilities. Patients often become adept at helping one another with this. In our experience, a "levels" system that acknowledges progress with an increase in patient autonomy (e.g., time off the unit or having an unsupervised meal) works well in combination with a therapeutic focus on gradually increasing task difficulty.

Enhancing Motivation

It is important to address the ego-syntonic nature of AN (Vitousek, Watson, & Wilson, 1998) throughout intensive treatment. Borrowed from work with addictions, motivational enhancement aims to increase intrinsic motivation in an attempt to increase the probability of permanent behavioral change (Miller & Rollnick, 2002). Although most clients and clinicians are aware of the negative consequences of AN, the benefits are often overlooked. To facilitate change it is useful to acknowledge that the AN likely has benefits for the patient and may be serving an important function (e.g., protection from failure, distraction from painful memories or emotions, provision of a unique identity). Once these functions have been identified, clinicians can address them in treatment. It is helpful to validate certain values and needs ("It makes sense that you want to feel cared for/feel in charge of your life/be distracted") and to help patients find other, more adaptive ways to fulfill these needs.

It is a mistake to assume that patients are ready to relinquish their ED when they accept an admission to IP or DH. There may be significant pressure from frightened friends, family, and health care providers to accept treatment even if the patient is not ready to make changes. Some patients are too undernourished to reflect meaningfully on change before starting weight restoration. Even patients who enter treatment highly motivated are likely to question what they are doing at some point. Ambivalence about change is a normal part of the recovery process and needs to be addressed in an ongoing way.

One way to encourage patients to consider change despite continued ambivalence is to frame treatment as an experiment. The patient's right to choose how to spend her life can be acknowledged directly, along with the importance of conducting a fair experiment over a reasonable length of time to collect good information relevant to her decision. Data from other group members' experiments may bolster the patient's faith or courage. Perceiving intensive treatment as tentative and experimental often gives an ambivalent patient the freedom and the ability to make and maintain changes. Framing the experiment to include the decision to accept intensive treatment, to accept the level of support needed at each step, and to assume progressively more responsibility for recovery-oriented behavior may help the patient retain a sense of control and ownership of the recovery process.

Discharge Planning and Follow-Up Treatment

Upon discharge from intensive treatment, patients are faced with a difficult transition from an environment that offers high levels of support and, in most cases, containment, to one in which they are solely responsible for feeding themselves appropriately and not acting on urges for symptoms. Ideally, this transition should represent one manageable step midway through a series of steps in which the patient takes progressively more responsibility for recovery-oriented behavior. Following discharge from intensive treatment, structured, step-down, follow-up care typically takes 3–6 months with subsequent outpatient support continuing thereafter. There is little research related to follow-up treatment, and one of the challenges is the significant rate of relapse following weight restoration.

The multimodal approach and cognitive-behavioral framework that are well suited to the intensive treatment phase are also typically employed during follow-up. Research suggests that individual CBT may be better than nutritional counseling alone (Pike, Walsh, Vitousek, Wilson, & Bauer, 2003) and also better than multimodal group-based follow-up (Carter et al., 2009) in preventing relapse. For adolescents with shorter durations of illness, family therapy during follow-up may result in a better outcome (Eisler et al., 1997). At our center, a cognitive-behavioral follow-up treatment that specifically addresses previously identified predictors of relapse in AN is being developed (Carter et al., 2004). This intervention focuses on preventing early weight loss, enhancing the importance of recovery, increasing confidence in recovery, and reducing residual weight and shape concerns and excessive exercise. It is also important that follow-up care include a focus on social and vocational rehabilitation.

Discharge planning may involve arranging for services above and beyond those offered by the treatment program in order to meet the patient's individual needs, as well as helping the patient make plans to return to life outside of the intensive treatment program. For some patients this involves developing interests and creating a life that does not center on the ED. In other cases, the challenge is for the patient to return to work, school, and/or a social network and develop new patterns that support continued wellness.

Medical Care

The typical medical complications of AN are covered in Chapter 4. Medical problems that arise while patients are receiving intensive treatment should be treated without interrupting the program, whenever possible.

Treatment of Comorbidities

Most individuals in intensive treatment experience psychiatric comorbidity of one type or another. Depression, anxiety disorders (especially obsessive–compulsive disorder [OCD] and posttraumatic stress disorder [PTSD]) and substance use are all very common areas of comorbidity affecting individuals with EDs. In a general way it is appropriate to provide the usual treatment for such comorbid conditions. For individuals with

AN, diagnosing some conditions, such as depression, can be complex, and the response to treatments such as antidepressant medication may be attenuated. It is useful to reassess both diagnosis and response to treatment once a patient has gained weight and has been eating fairly regularly for about 6 weeks.

The management of comorbid substance use or PTSD presents special problems. Both conditions may become activated as the patient begins to eat more normally and experiences fewer eating symptoms. Ideally, treatment for these comorbid conditions should be integrated into the treatment for the ED. However, some treatment centers do not have expert resources available to provide contemporaneous treatment, and in these cases treatment may need to be either staggered or sequenced. Such an approach can produce significant difficulties when patients are unable, for example, to achieve sufficient progress in their PTSD to tolerate eating more normally, which in itself may be a requirement to benefit from the treatment for PTSD.

Involvement of Family and Caregivers

Families are seen as an important source of support to individuals with the ED, especially when they are receiving treatment in an IP or DH. In adult programs the degree of family involvement in treatment and the recovery process is dictated by the patient. The patient defines what constitutes a family for her, and this definition may vary widely from person to person. The patient determines how much family involvement can occur, with some patients requesting a single meeting and others preferring more frequent and intensive family therapy. Patients often find it helpful to invite their families to treatment as they are moving through transitional phases, such as the onset of intensive treatment and during discharge planning. In contrast to family-based treatments for adolescents with EDs (Lock, Le Grange, Agras, & Dare, 2001; see also Eisler, Lock, & Le Grange, Chapter 8, this volume), families of adult patients are discouraged from having any direct involvement in the restoration of weight and normalized eating, including meal preparation and supervision. Families may play a vital role in assisting patients with social and vocational rehabilitation, however. For instance, families may support patients to reconnect with their peers and form new friendships to strengthen their social network.

Patients with adolescent-onset EDs may face additional challenges when transferring from a pediatric program to an adult IP or DH treatment, and careful advance planning is essential to support families in making this transition. In pediatric programs, much of the responsibility for weight restoration, refeeding, and meal supervision lies with the parents (Lock et al., 2001), whereas adult patients are held responsible for managing their own treatment and recovery process (Woodside & Shekter-Wolfson, 1993). Therefore, during transition from adolescent to adult care a psychoeducational intervention that highlights the fundamental differences between treatment philosophies, policies, and degree of familial involvement may be helpful.

During IP or DH treatment, a family assessment can be arranged at the request of the patient. In this assessment the initial task is to listen empathically to the family's concerns and elicit treatment goals of each family member. The patient is given a major role in defining the agenda and directing the therapeutic process. The focus of family therapy may include ways to improve and enhance the patient's and family members' communication patterns, decision-making processes, problem-solving abilities, and the establishment of healthy boundaries. For example, an important aspect of communication often addressed in family sessions relates to appropriate verbal responses to questions regarding weight gain and body image.

Often patients request additional family sessions when approaching discharge from treatment. In family sessions during the latter phase of treatment, patients may solicit the support of family members to facilitate the transition from hospital to home and the community. It is at this point in the recovery process that patients often express concerns that their family members and peers will decrease their level of involvement and support because the emaciation and eating symptoms that had previously served to elicit caring responses are now under control. Patients may need to inform their families that they continue to require their assistance to effectively cope and manage body and self-image difficulties and the significant uncertainty they may experience when contemplating their future free of the illness.

Treatment of BN

This chapter has described IP and DH treatment for AN, but the treatment for BN is very similar. In practice, DH is often the intensive treatment of choice for BN unless the patient is extremely symptomatic (e.g., frequent and high doses of laxatives or binge eating and vomiting throughout the day), medically unstable, or has uncontrolled Type 1 diabetes. When needed, the IP component of treatment can be relatively short and focused on the goal of breaking the pattern of symptomatic behavior by keeping the patient in a contained environment. DH treatment provides the patient with the opportunity to develop detailed strategies for symptom control, try them out, and revise them, as needed, the next day.

Summary

Intensive therapies are generally effective for patients who are willing to accept this type of treatment. However, significant refusal, dropout, and relapse rates indicate that intensive treatment is not a panacea. We have described the goals, structure, and primary therapeutic modalities commonly included in intensive treatments and presented some strategies to help prepare patients to start this type of intervention, enhance motivation for change, and prepare for discharge following intensive treatment. We have also briefly acknowledged the importance of medical care, treatment of comorbid conditions, and involvement of family members and caregivers. It is important to view intensive treatment as one step in the comprehensive treatment of EDs. Effective interventions focused on increasing motivation for recovery and willingness to participate in intensive treatment along with maintenance therapies to maintain changes and continue the process of psychological, social, and vocational rehabilitation are needed to complete the continuum of care. This approach is especially important in the context of managed care, which has been associated with shorter lengths of stay, faster weight gain, and increased rates of readmission (Willer et al., 2005), and given the preliminary findings that at the end of a year, patients treated with a multimodal outpatient treatment fared just as well as those who received inpatient treatment (Crisp et al., 1991; Gowers et al., 2007).

References

Carter JC, Blackmore E, Sutandar-Pinnock K, & Woodside DB. (2004). Relapse in anorexia nervosa: A survival analysis. *Psychological Medicine*, 34:671–679.

Carter JC, McFarlane T, Bewell C, Olmsted MP, Woodside DB, Kaplan AS, et al. (2009). Maintenance treatment for anorexia nervosa: A comparison of cognitive behavior therapy versus treatment as usual. *International Journal of Eating Disorders*, 42:202–207.

Carter JC, Woodside DB, & Kaplan AS. (2000, May). *Inpatient treatment for anorexia nervosa: Response and predictors of outcome.* Paper presented at the Ninth International Conference on Eating Disorders, New York.

Crisp AH, Norton K, Gowers S, Halek C, Bowyer C, Yeldham D, et al. (1991). A controlled study of the effects of therapies aimed at adolescent and family psychopathology in anorexia nervosa. *British Journal of Psychiatry*, 159:325–333.

Eisler I, Dare C, Russell GFM, Szmukler G, Le Grange D, & Dodge E. (1997). Family and individual therapy in anorexia nervosa: A 5-year follow-up. *Archives of General Psychiatry*, 54:1025–1030.

Gowers S, Clark A, Roberts C, Griffiths A, Edwards V, Bryan C, et al. (2007). Clinical effectiveness of treatments for anorexia nervosa in adolescents. *British Journal of Psychiatry*, 191:427–435.

Hartmann A, Wirth C, & Zeeck A. (2007). Prediction of failure of inpatient treatment of anorexia nervosa from early weight gain. *Psychotherapy Research*, 17:218–229.

Herzog T, Zeeck A, Hartmann A, & Nickel T. (2004). Lower targets for weekly weight gain lead to better results in inpatient treatment of anorexia nervosa: A pilot study. *European Eating Disorders Review*, 12:164–168.

Howard WT, Evans KK, Quintero-Howard CV, Bowers WA, & Andersen AE. (1999). Predictors of success or failure of transition to day hospital treatment for inpatients with anorexia nervosa. *American Journal of Psychiatry*, 156:1697–1702.

Kaplan A, Walsh BT, Olmsted MP, Attia E, Carter J, Devlin M, et al. (2009). The slippery slope: Prediction of weight maintenance in anorexia nervosa. *Psychological Medicine*, 39:1037–1045.

Lock J, Le Grange D, Agras WS, & Dare C. (2001). *Treatment manual for anorexia nervosa: A family-based approach.* New York: Guilford Press.

Lund BC, Hernandez ER, Yates WR, Mitchell JR, McKee PA, & Johnson CL. (2009). Rate of inpatient weight restoration predicts outcome in anorexia nervousa. *International Journal of Eating Disorders*, 42:301–305.

Mewes R, Tagay S, & Senf W. (2008). Weight curves as predictors of short-term outcome in anorexia nervosa inpatients. *European Eating Disorders Review*, 16:37–43.

Miller WR, & Rollnick S. (2002). *Motivational interviewing: Preparing people for change* (2nd ed.). New York: Guilford Press.

Morgan HG, & Russell GFM. (1975). Value of family background and clinical features as predictors of long-term outcome in anorexia nervosa: Four-year follow-up study of 41 patients. *Psychological Medicine*, 5:355–371.

Olmsted MP, Woodside DB, Carter JC, McFarlane TL, Staab R, Colton PA, et al. (2007). Intensive treatments for eating disorders. In GO Gabbard (Ed.), *Treatments of psychiatric disorders* (4th ed., pp. 709–722). Washington, DC: American Psychiatric Association.

Pike KM, Walsh BT, Vitousek K, Wilson GT, & Bauer J. (2003). Cognitive behavior therapy in the posthospitalization treatment of anorexia nervosa. *American Journal of Psychiatry*, 160:2046–2049.

Robb AS, Silber TJ, Orrell-Valente JK, Valadez-Meltzer A, Ellis N, Dadson MJ, et al. (2002). Supplemental nocturnal nasogastric refeeding for better short-term outcome in hospitalized adolescent girls with anorexia nervosa. *American Journal of Psychiatry*, 159:1347–1353.

Steinhausen H, Grigoroiu-Serbanescu M, Boyadjieva S, Neumarker K, & Metzke CW. (2008). Course and predictors of rehospitalization in adolescent anorexia nervosa in a multisite study. *International Journal of Eating Disorders*, 41:29–36.

Treat TA, McCabe EB, Gaskill JA, & Marcus MD. (2008). Treatment of anorexia nervosa in a specialty care continuum. *International Journal of Eating Disorders*, 41:564–572.

Vitousek K, Watson S, & Wilson GT. (1998). Enhancing motivation for change in treatment-resistant eating disorders. *Clinical Psychology Review*, 18:391–420.

Willer MG, Thuras P, & Crow SJ. (2005). Implications of the changing use of hospitalization to treat anorexia nervosa. *American Journal of Psychiatry*, 162:2374–2376.

Woodside B, & Shekter-Wolfson, L. (1993). *Family approach in treatment of eating disorders*. Washington, DC: American Psychiatric Association.

Zipfel S, Reas DL, Thornton CE, Olmsted MP, Williamson DA, Gerlinghoff M, et al. (2002). Day hospitalization programs for eating disorders: A systematic review of the literature. *International Journal of Eating Disorders*, 31:105–117.

Zuercher JN, Cumella EJ, Woods BK, Eberly M, & Carr JK. (2003). Efficacy of voluntary nasogastric tube feeding in female inpatients with anorexia nervosa. *Journal of Parenteral and Enteral Nutrition*, 27:268–276.

CHAPTER 12

Compulsory (Involuntary) Treatment for Anorexia Nervosa

Stephen W. Touyz and Terry Carney

Medicine and ethics, rather than the law, are the dominant players in deciding if and when coercion is appropriately deployed within clinical management of a condition. The same is true of anorexia nervosa (AN), where the medical and ethical debates are arguably even more contested than in the case of involuntary mental health treatment, which itself generates very lively debate (Sjöstrand & Helgesson, 2008). As we have written:

> Decisions about detention for the purposes of treatment; about authorization of medical treatment; and about provision of consent to treatment—all three of these decisions involve the exercise of, and potentially infringement of, fundamental individual liberties. These decisions also represent the intersection of law and medicine, the sites at which the caring responsibilities of medicine brush up against the protective constraints of the law. (Carney et al., 2006, p. 7)

Of course these challenges are not unique to a discussion of AN—many are shared in mental health generally (Carney, 2008).

This chapter concentrates on the medical and ethical turbulence at that intersection between law and medicine. While not overlooking the emerging literature on when and why clinicians actually invoke whatever powers the law permits (Carney, Tait, Richardson, & Touyz, 2008), the emphasis here is on principles at stake.

First, we review the diverse pattern of laws (if any) that may be used in aid of involuntary treatment of AN sufferers in different jurisdictions. Second, we outline some of the ethical principles informing the use of involuntary treatment. Third, and the main section of the chapter, we examine the clinical practice and therapeutic role of coercion within the overall treatment options for dealing with a condition whose chronicity, morbidity, and mortality rates understandably put pressure on clinicians to find "solutions." Fourth, we summarize our conclusion that coercion into treatment has a very limited, but potentially vital, role to play in dealing with patients with AN presenting with life-threateningly low body mass indices (BMIs) or equivalent compromise of their current or future health status.

The Legal Position about Coercion in Aid of Treatment

The law sets its face against the use of coercion (or involuntary treatment) other than with express legal authority. As we discuss below, in practice the law is invoked very conservatively, if at all, by clinicians. For this "bit part" on the clinical stage, however, the law is incredibly *varied* from one part of the world to another (Griffiths, Beumont, Russell, Touyz, & Moore, 1997; Griffiths & Russell, 1998), or even between the constituent states/provinces of federal systems of government (Carney, 2002; Carney, Tait, Saunders, Touyz, & Beumont, 2003). Similar variance exists in Europe (Carney, 2001; Griffiths et al., 1997; Serfaty & McCluskey, 1998).

Outside the United States, mental health "civil committal" laws provide a convenient route for involuntary treatment of patients with severe AN. This is also the case in England and Wales (Griffiths, 1996), Australia (Carney et al., 2006), and parts of Canada (Dolan, 1998; Griffiths & Russell, 1998; Tiller, Schmidt, & Treasure, 1993). In the United States, civil committal for patients with AN is rarely used (Appelbaum & Rumpf, 1998; Griffiths, 1996; Rumpf, Gans, & Bemporad, 1998), partly due to financial complications posed by "managed care" (Andersen, 1998).

Differences can also be found in the approach taken for children compared to adults with AN. In Ontario, Canada, for instance, coercive treatment is permitted for minors but not for adults suffering from AN (Geist, Katzman, & Colangelo, 1996). Within the United States, consent to health care of minors is largely the prerogative of parent(s) or guardian(s), whereas elsewhere in the common law world a "mature minor" rule empowers older adolescents with autonomous choice unless the legislature provides otherwise (Bartholomew & Paxton, 2003; Braverman, 1996; de Cruz, 1999; Devereux, Jones, & Dickenson, 1993). The U.S. Supreme Court's 1979 decision in *Parham* set few limits on *parental* capacity to consent to mental health care of minors (Hartman, 2000; Schmidt, 1985), reading the Fourteenth Amendment as protecting parental or "family" liberty to decide in such cases (Traugott & Alpers, 1997). Although courts do occasionally override parental decision making on "best interests" and other grounds, this is done by *exception* (Penkower, 1996; Sigman & O'Connor, 1991) and usually for minors approaching majority (Meisel, 1995).

In North America, if and when the law *does* authorize coercion, which authority may variously be found in state or provincial laws about mental health, guardianship, or parental consent to health care by minors (Dresser, 1984)? This is because neither the U.S. nor the Canadian constitution entrusts law-making powers in the relevant areas to the national level of government. Other sources of such authority, as found in various jurisdictions, include reliance on the "parens patriae" or inherent "ward of court" powers, child neglect/protection laws, general laws about medical consent, or even common law principles of "consent" to treatment (risking the uncertainty entailed in granting and then withdrawing consent: Dresser, 1984, p. 320).

This is significant in legal terms because each of these branches of law has its own distinctive logic or policy stance (Carney, 2002). The law does not speak with a single voice when the authority to coerce is extended by these laws. Thus, mental health laws are mainly concerned with the potential degree of harm to the patient or others. Adult guardianship provides a "substitute" decision maker when functional capacity is compromised, and child protection focuses on "risk" and impacts on the "best interests" or welfare of the child or young person.

Sometimes such variance is of little consequence. For all practical purposes, equivalent levels of "heavy" coercion can be exercised de facto, entirely *outside* the framework of law (Carney, Tait, & Touyz, 2007). Studies of the "law in action" frequently uncover wide gaps between what the legislature (or court) intended to achieve and what actually occurs in the field. However, in AN treatment there is evidence that differences in the law are of consequence. In the state of New South Wales (NSW), Australia, of two available legal avenues of coercion, adult guardianship (the appointment of a substitute decision maker) was preferred to aid treatment of resistant and at-risk patients in earlier stages of the illness cycle, whereas mental health committal (also authorizing compulsory *treatment* in that jurisdiction) was mainly reserved for more chronic/severe cases (Carney et al., 2003). The mere existence of a legal avenue does not necessarily mean it will be utilized, of course. Identical adult guardianship laws in the state of Victoria (the sister state to NSW) are never used in AN treatment because the tribunal (Victorian Civil and Administrative Tribunal's "civil list") does not entertain such applications as a matter of *policy*.

Understandably this variance gives rise to debate in medicine, as in law, about what (if any) avenue of legal intervention to use (Melamed, Mester, Margolin, & Kalian, 2003) and whether those laws/avenues are adequate (Mitrany & Melamed, 2005). However, an understanding of competing bioethical principles is an important precursor to consideration of the role of coercion in clinical practice.

Ethical Principles Applicable to Coercion in Treatment

The ethical challenges regarding the use of coercion in the treatment of AN also vary somewhat, depending on the ethical framework used for the analysis.

In North America and other parts of the developed Western world, the individualist ethic of "informed consent" is the dominant frame. This elevation of Western human rights traditions of the law, privileging values of individual autonomy (or choice) and participation in medical decision making is not shared by Confucian, Islamic, or other value systems in Asian countries (Lee, 2007). Nor is it, by any means, unchallenged within Western bioethics, where Greco-Roman Hippocratic traditions of the medical imperatives to "do good" (beneficence) and "do no harm" (nonmaleficience) carry considerable weight in debates about compulsory enteral feeding in treatment of AN, or indeed generally (Körner et al., 2006). Compulsory enteral feeding or other involuntary treatment of patients with AN is not ever self-evident. Both Dresser and Draper argue that clinicians should respect decisions made by chronic sufferers, provided the decision maker is "competent" at law (i.e., grasps, retains, weighs, and rationally processes information) even when that decision is irrational or unpopular (Draper, 2000, p. 126; Dresser, 1984, pp. 357, 373).

Sjöstrand and Helgesson (2008, p. 114) argue that there are three main ethical foundations for the use of coercion in mental health care: in the interests of others, to advance the patient's health interests, and lack of autonomy. They question the utilitarian liberal principle (famously enunciated by J.S. Mill) of "harm to others" as a sufficient warrant for *treatment*, drawing support from the European Council's Convention on Human Rights and Biomedicine (1997), and the World Psychiatric Association's insistence on a "best interest" test of the Madrid Declaration on Ethical Standards for Psychiatric Practice (1997). While dubious about "harm to self" in the context of a health interest (because physical illness does not warrant equivalent overriding of objections to beneficial treatments), these authors accept that restoration of autonomy is a valid basis for intervention (p. 115), a premise that leads them to support what may be termed "emergency room" treatment. Such emergency room interventions are based on the "reasonably presumed" intent of the patient to receive treatments that restore the capacity to make autonomous choices, whether due to loss of consciousness (in the case of somatic illnesses) or loss of "insight" into their condition (in the case of nonsomatic illnesses such as mental illness) (p. 116). Coercive treatment serves a "lifesaving" function (Werth, Wright, Archambault, & Bardash, 2003).

By intervening on the basis of a presumed wish to proceed in this fashion, the expectation is that a postrecovery "retrospective consent" will be forthcoming in most cases, thus attracting the ethical defense of so-called "soft paternalism" (the belated, retrospective "thank-you" justification of involuntary action; Fost, 1984, p. 383). This is sometimes expressed as "volitional paternalism," where the higher-order goal (in this case, restoration of the ability to choose) subsumes lower-order goals such as acting on "objections" to treatment (Rothstein, 1998). Alternatively, such interventions can be grounded in the "necessity principle" that authorizes emergency lifesaving surgery absent patient consent, the stomach pumping of apparent drug overdose patients, or, as previously argued, brief involuntary treatment of severe cases of AN (Beumont & Carney, 2003, 2004).

These ethical rationales resonate in clinical decision making about involuntary treatment for AN. Lack of "imminent" risk of death combined with retention of apparently sound reasoning capacity partially explain why U.S. clinicians rarely utilize mental health committal for patients suffering from AN (Appelbaum & Rumpf, 1998, pp. 225–226). And when interventions are contemplated, it is often on the basis that voluntary treatment is doomed to failure and the clinician's "duty of care" necessitates action to preserve life (Griffiths & Russell, 1998).

Where the ethical waters become muddied is in deciding whether the power of autonomous choice has yet been lost or sufficiently compromised as to warrant overriding objections to treatment. This distinction is particularly fraught in the case of AN, where typically patients remain quite articulate and rational in discussing or deciding most aspects of their lives, other than one isolated "pocket" of inability: that is, their inability to accept the gravity of the threat to their life or of the need to accept treatment (Beumont & Carney, 2003). Known as "anosognosia," this condition is also found in people with schizophrenia and bipolar disorder, as well as in conditions such as Alzheimer's disease and Huntington's disease (Torrey & Kress, 2004, p. 40).

In a similar vein to Simona Giordano's (2005, Chapter 3) plea not to fall into the trap of assuming that intervention is warranted on the basis of a presumed incapacity stemming from the making of a *diagnosis* of AN, Sjöstrand and Helgesson argue for close scrutiny to ascertain the *authentic values* or authentic "self" as the guide to whether or not to intervene (2008, pp. 116–118). As Giordano proposes, the assessment should involve close consideration of the *actual* capacities that the patient does or does not display, including the social context in which the patient is operating (2005, Chapter 3).

Of course, it could be contended that the psychiatric proxy of the presence/absence of "insight" as a basis for respecting or overriding patient choice to accept/reject treatments serves as an equally sound basis for engaging the "authenticity" of such value choices. Values certainly do deeply infuse this concept (Freckelton, 2003, pp. 327–329; Vine, 2003, pp. 122–123) but to resort to it effectively *hides* rather than renders explicit those value choices.

So, although coercion may ethically be defensible in high-risk emergency situations, on the basis of necessity or presumed higher goals of patient survival or restoration of capacity for choice, this action should be validated by some transparent and *explicit* canvassing of the values of the patient. There may be legitimate debate about the merits of the various ways of doing so, ranging from external court or tribunal authorization hearings, reliance on "advance directives," consideration by hospital ethics committees or case conferences, or family/career consultation (the "family as commons"). From an ethical standpoint, it is the *openness* of the airing of these issues that is the key ingredient. Medical or clinical practice, however, is the dominant consideration, and it is this topic to which we now turn.

Clinical Practice Regarding Coercion in Treatment

Neither neophytes nor experienced clinicians treating severely ill patients with AN can escape the immutable facts that they will one day be confronted by a resistant or recalcitrant patient who categorically refuses all treatment. It is not difficult to understand how such a scenario rapidly escalates into a full-blown, emotionally charged crisis, especially when the patient is in a life-threatening situation. Patients with AN often insist that they have the right to determine their own fate, even if this determination ultimately leads to untimely death (Touyz, Polivy, & Hay, 2008). We can think of no other place in medicine where the forces of clinical imperativeness and the law collide so strongly as when treating the severely ill patient with AN who steadfastly refuses treatment despite being gravely ill. Should such decisions be left in the hands of capable clinicians to decide and become part of accepted clinical practice incorporated into clinical practice guidelines? If not, are such matters best decided within a legal context in the setting of a courtroom with barristers, lawyers, and finally the magistrate or judge determining what treatment should be carried out and in which setting (Carney et al., 2006)?

Why do patients with AN so strongly resist treatment and what are the psychological reasons for doing so? Goldner (1989) documents this answer well (Table 12.1). Noting the reasons in the table, how does the clinician engage a treatment-resistant patient with AN in therapy? Over recent years, researchers have turned their attention to other disorders such as substance abuse, where motivational factors play a permanent role and techniques such as motivational interviewing (MI) have shown promise (Touyz et al., 2008). The underlying assumption in MI is that motivation cannot be imposed by the clinician but rather rests with the patient, who can be encouraged to take advantage of it by means of a collaborative and empathic approval of treatment. This perspective has resulted in the development of motivational enhancement therapy (MET), which enables the clinician to work with patients so that their "change focused" objectives are realized (Touyz et al., 2008). However, despite the best interests of clinicians, they may

TABLE 12.1. Reasons Why Patients with AN So Often Refuse Treatment

- Patients with AN have a strong sense of self-determination that they are reluctant to abandon.
- Their strong sense of self-determination is characterized by asceticism and rigid inflexibility.
- They experience a marked sense of vulnerability to an outsider's perceived reality, skills, and value judgments.
- They feel humiliated at not being able to address their own difficulties.
- As with so many other patients with mental illness, they fear stigmatization.
- They are adversely influenced by the often less than optimistic view regarding the long-term outcome of the disorder.
- They often have a mistrust of interpersonal relationships.
- They are extremely apprehensive about a perceived loss of control.
- They constantly strive to overcome a pervasive feeling of ineffectiveness.
- They are strongly perfectionistic.
- They have distortions in their thinking, which have an adverse impact on their conceptual, perceptual, and decision-making abilities.
- They often report a mood disturbance that may be exacerbated by the physiological and metabolic imbalances that accompany starvation and malnutrition.

Note. Based on Anderson and Stewart (1983) and Goldner (1989).

well find themselves in a situation where they really have no choice but to insist upon treatment, irrespective of the patient's decision. The following case vignette illustrates the challenges facing the clinician when dealing with a resistant patient.

Mary,[1] who comes from a small rural community, is a 19-year-old second-year university student living at a large urban university. A high academic achiever, she had turned down an opportunity to board at a prestigious private girls' school in the city in order to be closer to her family. She adored her mother and envied her pretty and petite physique. Whereas her sister was thin like her mother, she had inherited her father's larger-framed physique. At the university Mary began exercising regularly, eating salads, and avoiding energy-dense foods. Proud of her weight loss and the complimentary comments about her appearance, her self-esteem rose. She fell in love for the first time, but, as a strict Catholic, was conflicted about engaging in a sexual relationship. She reluctantly agreed, but soon became pregnant. Ashamed to tell her mother, she confided in her boyfriend, but he advised a termination instead of the support she expected. The relationship ended, and Mary was devastated. She decided to terminate her pregnancy. Her studies fell away. By the time she consulted a counselor, she was restricting her eating, exercising strenuously, and inducing vomiting if she felt that she had eaten too much. Her weight was in a free-fall. Tests by her physician revealed that her serum potassium was dangerously low and she had an abnormal electrocardiogram (EKG) characterized by a prolonged QTc interval. This could prove fatal, especially since she was exercising so strenuously.

MARY: Did you get the results of my blood tests and EKG?

CLINICIAN: Yes, and I am afraid to say they are of extreme concern. I have spoken to the doctor, who says that you should be admitted to an eating disorders treat-

---

[1]A pseudonym.

ment program immediately. He is of the opinion that your life is in danger and expressed his clinical concern for your well-being.

MARY: No way! My parents would find out and they would be devastated. My mother would never forgive me. I can't be away from classes because I have my examinations soon and if I don't maintain a high average, I could jeopardize my scholarship. My parents can't afford to pay for my fees. Sorry, hospital is simply out of the question. Don't worry, I'm sure things will work out fine.

CLINICIAN: Don't you think it would be a good idea to involve your parents? I'm sure from all you have told me about them that they would be understanding. You would be able to get the treatment you need and then be able to resume your studies. Isn't that what you really want?

MARY: I couldn't do this to my mother. There is no way whatsoever that I can go into hospital. Couldn't we continue with our sessions as an outpatient? I promise to try harder to eat better and to stop vomiting. Please, listen to me! Why doesn't anyone ever believe me? You have my word!

CLINICIAN: Mary, you don't seem to realize that you are in medical danger and there is a risk that you could die. We simply can't ignore these test results. We need to formulate a treatment strategy that allows your medical concerns to be addressed. Don't you think so?

MARY: If I died, I would be spared the embarrassment of all that has happened. My mother has always regarded me as such a competent daughter. (*Gets particularly distressed.*) Don't you understand? I won't go into hospital. I would rather die. (*Starts sobbing uncontrollably.*) (*Stands up and walks toward the door.*) I can't stand this anymore. I'm going back to my dorm. Please don't be angry with me. It's not your fault. I appreciate your concern, but there is no way I will involve my parents or go into hospital.

CLINICIAN: Mary, if you walk out of my office now, I will institute action to declare you a danger to yourself, and you will be required by law to be admitted to hospital. I am not going to take a risk with your life. You are leaving me with little option.

MARY: How can you betray me like this? I am a law student, what about *my* rights? I guess it was a mistake to have seen you in the first place. If you go ahead with this, you must realize that you will be responsible for destroying the rest of my life and that of my parents—go ahead and destroy it. I will be so ashamed that I will run away from hospital and kill myself and, remember, it will be *your* fault. Do you really want to lose a patient?

CLINICIAN: Mary, I promise you that it is my intention to assist you in overcoming the current crisis, but for now you need to accept urgent medical attention. I am going to initiate the compulsory hospitalization action because I am sufficiently concerned about your well-being. Your doctor asked a cardiologist to review your EKG, and he is extremely worried. I will ask the cardiologist to speak with you and involve the doctor as well. If you give me permission to do so, I really think we should speak to your parents, too.

MARY: How long will I need to stay if I accept going into hospital?

CLINICIAN: Only as long as it takes for your condition to stop threatening your health. I promise.

MARY: (*sobbing*) Would you mind calling my mother? Here is her number.

There may be little option but to contemplate compulsory treatment or guardianship. Griffiths and colleagues (1997) have formulated the following essential guidelines to make this somewhat foreboding task more palatable, especially for the less-experienced clinician.

- The decision to embark upon the involuntary treatment of a patient with AN should be made only once due diligence has been given to the risks and perceived benefits to the patient.
- Consultation with all significant stakeholders should take place, including the patient, the patient's family, and the entire treatment team. Those involved should be provided with support and cognizance given to divergent viewpoints before, during, and after implementation. If these steps are not taken initially, then the differences of opinion often produce a conflicted state of affairs wherein the fragile therapeutic alliance is severely undermined. The golden rule here is *painstaking consultation*.
- The family has the right to know, and should be fully notified as to the reasons, why treatment has been implemented against the patient's will, including the nature of the illness, the purported risks of not intervening, as well as the proposed treatment.
- Where adult guardianship legislation exists, a parent may elect to act as the patient's guardian. However, this course of action can be fraught with difficulty (and contraindicated) when the patient is highly manipulative of parents. If this is the case, it is much more prudent to have a public guardian appointed.
- Because there are several different parties involved in involuntary treatment, it is essential that both a good rapport and open channel of communication are established between the treatment team, the guardian, and the immediate family. This becomes an even greater imperative when restrictive measures (e.g., parenteral or enteral nutrition) are indicated. It is usually invaluable to enlist the support of all parties concerned by discussing the lack of alternative options in what is often a somewhat desperate situation.
- What needs to be kept in mind here is that this is a lengthy journey toward recovery, in which the involuntary treatment could be merely one of several episodes. In the end, successful cooperation by all concerned will be one of the essential components of resolving the impasse. It is therefore especially important to address fears, anxieties and guilt, not only just prior to the implementation of treatment, but throughout.[2]

What Do the Data Tell Us about Those Who Are Formally Coerced?

We recently extracted data from the records of a major Australian specialist AN treatment facility covering over a period of nearly 5 years (Carney, Tait, Wakefield, Ingvarson, & Touyz, 2005). Of the 96 admissions (some multiple, to a maximum of five) by

---

[2]Based on Touyz, Polivy, and Hay (2008).

75 patients with AN, 4 were requested by adult guardians and 11 involved combinations of adult guardianship, mental health civil committal, or community treatment orders. Seven cases wherein coercion proceedings were launched resulted in patients later agreeing to an informal admission. Approximately 40% of admissions was for less than 3 weeks, with a mean stay of 49 days; 36% of the patients was under the age of 20 years.

Some of the patients were given the sole diagnoses of AN. However, nearly three-quarters were diagnosed with other comorbid mental illnesses, and one-third had two or more such diagnoses. The number of previous inpatient hospitalizations was significantly greater for the coerced participants, and they had a lower BMI upon admission (13.2, SD 1.67 kg/m^2 vs. 14.03, SD 1.84 kg/m^2) for the voluntary patients. It probably comes as no surprise that the potentially fatal refeeding syndrome was diagnosed in 10/16 versus 12/58 cases, patients were kept in a secure facility (11/15 versus 1/69), and the need for nasogastric feeding was greater for the coerced patients (12/14 versus 11/59). The salient finding to emerge from this study was that the history of the patients, as measured by their number of previous admissions, is a relevant factor when considering whether to implement legal coercive powers. Comorbidities contribute significantly to the decision-making progress, as does BMI and a past history of refeeding syndrome. Finally, two forms of coercion (i.e., the insertion of a nasogastric tube and being placed in a secure facility) were closely associated with the use of legal coercion. However, these measures were likely to be the result of a legal order rather than the reason for seeking one.

More recently, Thiels (2008) reported a German study in which 25 female patients between the ages of 16 and 39 were admitted to the hospital "with life threatening anorexia nervosa" and "no motivation for treatment." Of these patients, five were voluntary and seven had guardianship orders. Eleven patients were extremely oppositional and refused treatment, demanding discharge, whereas two legal minors were admitted involuntarily using family law procedures.

Following admission, those patients who were in a dire medical state were transferred to the intensive care unit (ICU). Nineteen patients were prescribed antidepressant medication, and all patients were placed on individualized contracts requiring a weight gain of 0.7–1.0 kg per week. Patients commenced their refeeding in a secure facility by eating independently or consuming high-caloric fluids. If this regimen was not successful (i.e., patients failed to gain weight), a feeding tube was inserted with either their own consent or that of a guardian (n = 22). A percutaneous endoscopic gastrostomy (PEG) tube was used in 20 patients, with 4 being informed patients. There was a need to isolate and physically restrain one patient, who gained only 1.11 kg in 178 days. No outcome data were reported, but the difficulties encountered when treating such patients were clearly evident. There was evidence of "massive resistance," with a patient proclaiming, "So far I have beaten everybody and have not put on weight. Here too, I will win." There were anecdotal reports of patients "manipulating" their PEG, with major countertransference issues developing between patients and staff. It sounded much more like a battleground than a cooperative treatment environment. The authors of the trial recommended that patients needed to be kept on guardianship legislation for at least 2 years to allow for swift intervention should a relapse become evident. The challenging treatment environment evident in this study (Laakman et al., 2006) was not evident in similarly compulsorily detained patients in London, who gained weight without forced or tube feeding (Ramsay, Ward, Treasure, & Russell (1999). Thiels (2008) argues that the highly skilled nursing staff used in the London study most likely contributed to the more favorable therapeutic environment. Furthermore, the patients in London were admitted at a higher BMI of 14.2 (*SD* 7.3) kg/m², whereas the German patients had a BMI of only 12.09 (*SD* 1.51) kg/m². Thiels (2008) was of the opinion that preventing weight loss to a patient with a BMI of 12 by an earlier involuntary admission may result in the avoidance of forced feeding altogether.

Thiels and Paul (2007) have published a series of recommendations to best assist clinicians who find themselves having to use an involuntary admission with a resistant or recalcitrant patient. These include the following:

1. Coercion is not an exercise to preclude psychotherapy, nor does coercion mean that psychotherapy should not be forthcoming.
2. Because there is a need for ongoing core, guardianship applications should be made for between 3 and 6 months.
3. It is argued that since the risk of dying increases below a BMI of 13 kg/m², this cutoff should become the criterion for involuntary treatment. Clearly, this figure is only one indicator, and others such as suicidality, electrolyte imbalance, and cardiac arrhythmia need to be taken into consideration as well.
4. Coercion should be the least restrictive possible and for the shortest possible time. Ultimately, it is going to be the therapeutic relationship and a supportive milieu that will produce the best outcome.
5. Every effort needs to be made from the outset to encourage the patient to eat independently.
6. Although every effort is made to achieve independent eating, this, along with weight gain, should not be the focus of attention.
7. Patients should be treated with dignity and respect, recognizing their fragile mental state, especially in terms of self-esteem.
8. Wherever possible, consider the involvement of the family.
9. The goal is not to read a particular weight but rather to ensure a cooperative therapeutic relationship without the need for coercive powers.

Conclusions

There can be no doubt that those patients with AN who receive treatment under some form of legal compulsion do believe that it does impact on their lives. Such patients often report anxiety, anger, resentment, and a sense of powerlessness. However, this negative effect needs to be balanced with the knowledge that many such patients believe that it was this experience (i.e., the legal process) that ultimately gave them the "necessary permission" to accept change and treatment. However, in our Australian study there was no evidence of any of the "retrospective thank you" reported elsewhere in the literature.

So, does the law have a role to play in the management of AN? Clearly more research is warranted to better answer this question, but in the absence of a definitive statement, we can say that it does seem to play a constructive role "in overseeing proposed forcible detention and treatment and providing or overriding consent, and can play a more general role in setting up frameworks for protecting rights (Carney et al., 2006, p. 162). Ultimately, the management of AN should be a collaborative exercise to ensure greater protection for personal directives, improving the therapeutic environment to ensure that patients are engaged more effectively in their own treatment and are able to make informed choices and be treated in the least restrictive environment. We agree that if the above set of principles can be endorsed and followed, then there is the distinct possibility that the need for coercive treatments may, in fact, decline. However, in the meantime, the goal of providing the opportunity for a patient with severe and enduring AN to recover should be placed beyond individual autonomy. Thiels (2008, p. 498) has encapsulated this point rather well:

> Thus, detention of patients with severe AN is ethically justified, may be necessary and should be covered by legislation. Once the patient has been admitted to an eating disorder unit it is desirable and will usually be possible for improvement to be achieved with skilled nursing without the need to have recourse to forced or tube feeding.

References

Andersen A. (1998). Treatment of eating disorders in the context of managed health care in the United States: A clinician's perspective. In W Vandereycken & P Beumont (Eds.), *Treating eating disorders: Ethical, legal and personal issues* (pp. 261–282). London: Athlone.

Appelbaum P, & Rumpf T. (1998a). Civil commitment of the anorexic patient. *General Hospital Psychiatry*, 20:225–230.

Bartholomew T, & Paxton S. (2003). General practitioners' perspectives regarding competence and confidentiality in an adolescent with suspected anorexia nervosa: Legal and ethical considerations. *Journal of Law and Medicine*, 10:308–324.

Beumont P, & Carney T. (2003). Conceptual issues in theorising anorexia nervosa: Mere matters of semantics? *International Journal of Law and Psychiatry*, 26:585–598.

Beumont P, & Carney T. (2004). Can psychiatric terminology be translated into legal regulation?: The anorexia example. *Australian and New Zealand Journal of Psychiatry*, 38:819–829.

Braverman L. (1996). The application of the Health Care Consent Act to the force feeding of anorexic patients. *Health Law Review*, 5:25–32.

Carney T. (2001). Globalisation and guardianship: Harmonisation or (postmodern) diversity? *International Journal of Law and Psychiatry*, 24:95–116.

Carney T. (2002). Regulation of treatment of severe anorexia nervosa: Assessing the options? *Australian Health Law Bulletin*, 11:25–32.

Carney T. (2008). The mental health service crisis of neoliberalism: An Antipodean perspective. *International Journal of Law and Psychiatry*, 31:101–115.

Carney T, Tait D, Richardson A, & Touyz S. (2008). Why (and when) clinicians compel treatment of anorexia nervosa patients. *European Eating Disorders Review*, 16:199–206.

Carney T, Tait D, Saunders D, Touyz S, & Beumont P. (2003). Institutional options in management of coercion in anorexia treatment: The antipodean experiment. *International Journal Law and Psychiatry*, 26:647–675.

Carney T, Tait D, & Touyz S. (2007). Coercion is coercion?: Reflections on clinical trends in use of compulsion in treatment of anorexia nervosa patients. *Australasian Psychiatry*, 15:390–395.

Carney T, Tait D, Touyz S, Ingvarson M, Saunders D, & Wakefield A. (2006). *Managing anorexia nervosa: Clinical, legal and social perspectives on involuntary treatment.* New York: Nova Science.

Carney T, Tait D, Wakefield A, Ingvarson M, & Touyz S. (2005). Coercion in the treatment of anorexia nervosa: Clinical, demographic and legal implications. *Medicine and Law,* 24:21–40.

de Cruz P. (1999). Adolescent autonomy, detention for medical treatment and Re C. *Modern Law Review,* 62:595–604.

Devereux J, Jones D, & Dickenson D. (1993). Can children withhold consent to treatment? *British Medical Journal,* 306:1459–1461.

Dolan B. (1998). Food refusal, forced feeding and the law of England and Wales. In W Vandereycken & P Beumont (Eds.), *Treating eating disorders: Ethical, legal and personal issues* (pp. 151–178). London: Athlone.

Draper H. (2000). Anorexia nervosa and respecting a refusal of life-prolonging therapy: A limited justification. *Bioethics,* 14:120–133.

Dresser R. (1984). Feeding the hunger artists: Legal issues in treating anorexia nervosa. *Wisconsin Law Review,* pp. 297–374.

Fost N. (1984). Food for thought: Dresser on anorexia. *Wisconsin Law Review,* pp. 375–384.

Freckelton I. (2003). Involuntary detention decision-making criteria and hearing procedures: An opportunity for therapeutic jurisprudence in action. In K Diesfeld & I Freckelton (Eds.), *Involuntary detention and therapeutic jurisprudence* (pp. 293–337). Aldershot, UK: Ashgate.

Geist R, Katzman D, & Colangelo J. (1996). The consent to treatment act and an adolescent with anorexia nervosa. *Health Law in Canada,* 16:110–114.

Giordano S. (2005). *Understanding eating disorders: Conceptual and ethical issues in the treatment of anorexia and bulimia nervosa.* Oxford, UK: Oxford University Press.

Goldner E. (1989). Treatment of refusal in anorexia nervosa. *International Journal of Eating Disorders,* 8:297–306.

Griffiths R. (1996). Compulsory treatment and anorexia nervosa. *Australian Journal of Forensic Sciences,* 28:35–38.

Griffiths R, Beumont P, Russell J, Touyz S, & Moore G. (1997). The use of guardianship legislation for anorexia nervosa: A report of 15 cases. *Australian and New Zealand Journal of Psychiatry,* 31:525–531.

Griffiths R, & Russell J. (1998). Compulsory treatment of anorexia nervosa patients. In W Vandereycken & P Beumont (Eds.), *Treating eating disorders: Ethical, legal and personal issues* (pp. 127–150). London: Athlone.

Hartman R. (2000). Adolescent autonomy: Clarifying an ageless conundrum. *Hastings Law Journal,* 51:1265–1362.

Körner U, Bondolfi A, Bühler E, MacFie J, Meguid M, Messing B, et al. (2006). Ethical and legal aspects of enteral nutrition. *Clinical Nutrition,* 25:196–202.

Laakman G, Ortner M, Kamleiter M, Ufer S, Frodl T, Goldstein-Muller B, et al. (2006). Treatment of vitally endangered anorexia nervosa patients based on guardianship laws. *Nevenarzt,* 77:35–49.

Lee SC. (Ed.). (2007). *The family, medical decision-making and biotechnology: Critical reflections on Asian moral perspectives.* New York: Springer.

Meisel A. (1995). Decision making for children and newborns: Common-law approach. Mature minors: Rebuttability of presumption of incompetence. In A Meisel (Ed.), *The right to die* (2nd ed., pp. 276–281). New York: Wiley

Melamed Y, Mester R, Margolin J, & Kalian M. (2003). Involuntary treatment of anorexia nervosa. *International Journal of Law and Psychiatry,* 26:617–626.

Ramsay R, Ward A, Treasure J, & Russell GF. (1999). Compulsory treatment in anorexia nervosa: Short-term benefits and long-term mortality. *British Journal of Psychiatry,* 175:147–153.

Rothstein B. (1998). *Just institutions matter: The moral and political logic of the universal welfare state.* Cambridge, UK: Cambridge University Press.

Rumpf T, Gans M, & Bemporad B. (1998, June). *Life threatening issues and clinical decisionmaking in anorexia nervosa*. Paper presented at the 23rd Congress of the Academy of Law and Mental Health, Paris.

Schmidt W. (1985). Considerations of social science in a reconsideration of *Parham v. J.R.* and the commitment of children to public mental institutions. *Journal of Psychiatry and Law*, 13:339–359.

Serfaty M, & McCluskey S. (1998). Compulsory treatment of anorexia nervosa and the moribund patient. *European Eating Disorders Review*, 6:27–37.

Sigman G, & O'Connor C. (1991). Exploration for physicians of the mature minor doctrine. *Journal of Pediatrics*, 119:520–525.

Sjöstrand M, & Helgesson G. (2008). Coercive treatment and autonomy in psychiatry. *Bioethics*, 22:113–120.

Thiels A, & Paul T. (2007). Compulsory treatment in anorexia nervosa. *Psychotherapy and Psychosomatic Medical Psychology*, 57:128–135.

Thiels C. (2008). Forced treatment of patients with anorexia. *Current Opinion in Psychiatry*, 21:495–498.

Tiller J, Schmidt U, & Treasure J. (1993). Compulsory treatment for anorexia nervosa: Compassion or coercion? *British Journal of Psychiatry*, 162:679–680.

Torrey F, & Kress K. (2004). *The new neurobiology of severe psychiatric disorders and its implications for laws governing involuntary commitment and treatment*. Unpublished manuscript, University of Iowa, Iowa City.

Touyz SW, Polivy J, & Hay P. (2008). *Eating disorders*. Cambridge, MA: Hogrefe & Huber.

Traugott I, & Alpers A. (1997). In their own hands: Adolescents' refusals of medical treatment. *Archives of Paediatric Adolescent Medicine*, 151:922–927.

Vine R. (2003). Decision-making by psychiatrists about involuntary detention. In K Diesfeld & I Freckelton (Eds.), *Involuntary detention and therapeutic jurisprudence* (pp. 113–132). Aldershot, UK: Ashgate.

Werth J, Wright K, Archambault R, & Bardash R. (2003). When does the "duty to protect" apply with a client who has anorexia nervosa? *Counseling Psychologist*, 31:427–450.

CHAPTER 13

The Chronically Ill Patient
with Anorexia Nervosa

Development, Phenomenology,
and Therapeutic Considerations

Michael Strober

There are two uncontested points of unity among the many accounts of anorexia nervosa (AN) published following the seminal reports of Gull and Lasegue well over a century ago. The first is that there is no single, established way to approach its treatment. Clinicians easily agree that treatment is essential for an illness with such dire consequences, but there is no infallible source of knowledge as to how one should proceed. However strong a practitioner's belief as to what works and what doesn't, it is a personal belief—and neither predictably correct nor clinically illuminating as a general model of therapy. The second point is that no experienced clinician would expect a person with AN to welcome treatment unhesitatingly. We discover quickly that persons with AN do not form beliefs in the normal way. The risk, even the certainty, that disability or death will come if starvation persists can be entertained only when there is capacity for reason. However, introspection is not an important source of knowledge or justification for a person severely ill with AN. Thus, what is common sense to others—if one suffers from ill health, one should seek help—is vigorously disputed by those with AN, who casually dismiss the assertions of doctors and the impassioned pleas of family and friends about the possibility of death as blatant inconsistencies.

Thus, we readily accept that AN is a uniquely challenging illness not only because we lack a full understanding of its etiology, but because of how its seemingly willful character distinguishes it from other forms of human suffering. There are many areas of mental health in which the effects of treatment fall short. AN is not the only psychiatric disorder to bear tragic witness to debilitating and demoralizing consequences of odd, apparently volitional acts whose resistance to change frustrates even the most dedicated clinicians. But in conditions such as schizophrenia and bipolar disorder, headstrong acts emerge from a more pervasive decline of mental operations. The mechanisms involved in AN are understood differently. Outside of decisions relating to feeding and the appearance of their body, even very wasted patients remain capable of routine mental acts, their general reality sense is intact, and everyday attitudes are as reasonable as anyone else's. Instead, what specifically confounds these sensible applications of a reasoned mind is the isolated, delusive fear that they will suffer catastrophically lest acts of dieting and exercising are not followed exactly. All forms of psychopathology have their puzzling elements, but there is arguably no illness in which links between disturbances of biology, the consciousness of altered emotional states, and willfulness of behavior in the justification of senseless, injurious acts are as seamless.

Resolving the puzzle of AN remains a distant hope. However, new paradigms for approaching lingering questions are timely (Strober, 2004b; Strober, Freeman, Lampert, & Diamond, 2007), given accelerated progress in modern psychology, psychiatry, and neuroscience. Moreover, recent progress in neuroscience research has provided insights into how molecular, neural, and gene–environment mechanisms enable not only elementary programs of normal and maladaptive learning but complex systems of emotional memory, self-knowledge, and consciousness in normal and abnormal conditions (Charney & Nestler, 2009) and for AN (Kaye, Strober, & Jimerson, 2009). We know that genetic factors influence susceptibility to AN, and it is evident that AN is an illness triggered and sustained by powerful self-rewarding psychological drives. The knowledge that innate influences likely explain why some persons with AN suffer a chronic and refractory course throughout adult life is crucial for clinicians working with this population.

The Challenge of AN

If there is one uncontroversial fact about AN, it is that only rarely does it resolve quickly. Thus it is surprising that the modern literature has not investigated, in any comprehensive fashion, the metapsychology of those patients who will remain ill throughout their adult life, or considered how to best approach their care. Yet, even brief exposure to this population reveals how difficult a clinical challenge it is and why the therapist's task is hard to sustain. Unlike psychotherapy and family management with much younger, less morbidly ill patients with AN whose prospect for a satisfactory outcome is reasonably good (National Institute for Health and Clinical Excellence [NICE], 2004; Wilson, Grilo, & Vitousek, 2007), there is no consensus regarding therapeutic approaches for patients whose illness has advanced despite repeated treatments. Nevertheless, decisions a therapist is called upon to render soon after the first encounter with such patients are exceptionally complex, yet even the slightest misstep can provoke angry tirades, deepening resistance, or abrupt termination of a treatment scarcely begun. Facing such imperatives without any empirical foundation for direction, it is no surprise that a common response of many clinicians is to avoid the challenge entirely. What is bewildering and tragic about chronic AN, why the medical–legal predicaments family and friends often confront defy easy solution (Vandereycken & Beumont, 1998), is that no matter how crippling the illness is, there is no strain more terrible for the sufferer than being without it.

The symptoms manifest with startling suddenness, with a force that grows oddly stronger as the illness progresses. Many things about the apparent willfulness to starve are difficult to grasp, but what seems especially hard for family and friends is the unyielding intensity of it; that as weight decreases, avoidance of eating becomes even more determined and the claim of being too fat more irrefutable. Bewildering as these assertions are, for the patient they have a profound logical coherence that will withstand the eloquence of any challenge to the contrary.

Given that persons with AN express extreme sensitivity to arousal by emotions associated with threat or aversive outcomes, it is important to appreciate the meaningfulness of the developmental context in which the illness is embedded. As we know, most cases of AN unfold during transition to the teenage years—the stage of life whose hallmark is the strengthening of inward observation. This is a time for stepping out, for shedding any hints of culpability, so that emotion, thought, and impulse can lay siege to the heart and positive anticipation of future potentials can nourish self-development. Even so, the suddenness of this transition and its concomitant changes, signaling imminent new challenges with which to reckon, also set off pangs of doubt and angst. Neither is this response uncommon nor a reliable indication of future maladjustment. But for the person with AN, from a young age uncompromisingly rigid and compulsive, inhibited in expression, and prone to incessant worry over inconsequential mistakes and future uncertainties, the onset of puberty is a foreboding biological signal. This time period brings distressingly rapid changes in physicality and the rules of social and cognitive discourse—which arouse intense feelings of threat and the anticipation of future challenges perceived as insurmountable. Thus, arriving at this crucial point in development, when innate and social processes normally activate a wide range of appetitive drives, the adolescent experience is anticipated with dread, success in getting through it unscathed too wildly implausible to concede. For the girl vulnerable to AN, far more anxious and constrained than her peers and preferring a life rigidly structured to avoid need, novelty, and impulse, rather than a starry period of personal illumination, adolescence, and all that is innately and conditionally associated with it, is a painful, unforgiving visitation that heaps upon her all manner of personal offense. Instead of stumbling experimentation, building temptations, and moments of audacity, there is such suffocating unease with the trappings of change she is beset so far back that only the familiar traits of avoidance, compulsiveness of habit, and concealment of affections can offer welcome relief.

What then follows is utterly surreal. No matter how piercing their gasps of alarm and fury, loved ones soon discover that the compulsive nature of this illness yields nothing. They will plead many times for reason and sanity, but the protests go unheeded, silenced by a starvation so resolute it seems to be the only motivation about which their loved one is wholly serious.

Sadly, it is only a matter of time before even the strongest bond to the person chronically ill with AN withers, frayed by years of fury, despair, and resignation, unable to hold firm against the unrelenting defense of ideas for which there is no single shred of truth or evidence. It will come when the family has endured what they consider to be the final, painful offense, when the seductive strand of hope is declared lost to madness forever. It will start as before, how she is now ready to consider her poor health with a more reasoned mind, and that she truly wishes an end to the misery brought on by her illness. It is not that the wish for change at this particular moment is contrived, or that the dialogue in which sorrow for the agony she has caused is not reflected honestly. But when AN advances to this chronic state, the possibility that one day these splits in consciousness will cohere has passed. And so, too, will the moment of hope slip away yet again, flattened by the same well-worn litany of worries about becoming fat, of there being too much oil on her food. But no longer will anyone truly care.

A Neurodevelopmental Perspective

The question now arises: How does this come about? What transformations or what life circumstances could explain such seismic shifts in the psychological status among persons with AN? As noted, though time from onset of weight concerns to compulsive dieting is usually brief, a number of seemingly related characteristics are actually seen much earlier in life, suggesting a strong developmental continuity with the illness itself. These include tendencies toward worry and fearfulness, discomfort and stress aroused by change, regimentation of behavior and high levels of persistence in spite of non-reward, poor self-esteem, inhibition of expression, extreme perfectionism, and unease with self-soothing or pleasurable reinforcers, if not frank aversion to them (e.g., Anderluth, Tchanturia, Rabe-Hesketh, & Treasure, 2003; Karwautz, Rabe-Hesketh, Collier, & Treasure, 2002; Strober, 1991). From a developmental standpoint, then, there is strong support for the idea that early indicators of reduced emotional resiliency and heightened stress reactivity along with compulsive habit tendencies represent a pathway of vulnerability to AN, and that the mechanisms underlying these premorbid traits may possibly contribute directly to eating disorder (ED) symptoms as well (Steinglass & Walsh, 2006; Strober et al., 2007). Thus, potential causal mechanisms in AN are broad in scope and dynamic in the way they unfold, extending beyond consummatory aspects of feeding to motivational propensities that involve a range of appetitive and avoidance habit motives. The reader is referred to Kaye and colleagues (2009) for an overview of the neurobiology of EDs, which provides a foundation for these putative temperamental phenotypes in AN.

Implications for Clinical Understanding of Adaptive Crises

How the psyche evolves, how it forms intent around emotions of desire and fear, and why, for some, the prospect of change and new growth incites trepidation are matters of profound importance about which persons with chronic AN have little insight, and ones rich in meaning and implication for the therapist as well. Should the patient's motivation be challenged? Do I push hard with confrontational probing? Do I analyze resistances and point out the many instances of distractions, deflections, and manipulations? And how do I answer the questions: "Can I recover? Is there hope? Why do I act this way?"

In this regard, a reasonable argument can be made that innateness of anxiety, strong propensities to avoid appetitive experiences, and habit motives too inflexible for adaptive fitness are key elements that predispose some patients with AN to chronicity and constrain the effects of any treatment that is given regardless of experience or skill of the therapist. Reticence to treatment is common in AN generally, but it stands to reason it will be even more so among the most vulnerable of patients. And while we can assume their resistance to care is rooted in a deeply entrenched, fundamental dread of change, inflexibilities, and convictions of personal inadequacies, it will ultimately harden into seething mistrust of care providers if the treatment attempted is ill conceived, poorly executed, or coercive in approach. This will then be rationalized long after by an unshakable belief that further treatment will bring only more "callousness, mocking, and cruelty" (the reason given by a 69-pound, 26-year-old with a 13-year history of AN, in rejecting my recommendation of inpatient care).

What is evident is that if we are to understand the problem of AN across time and development in ways that parsimoniously explain its chronic course, the framework needed is one that is conceptual, and though inferential, sheds light on what limits our patients' capacities for getting through the disruptions of life that shake their preferred state of being. The adaptive crisis that sets AN in motion unfolds as the novelty and emotion-bearing events that signal puberty's approach bring unease. It is not an exaggeration to say that the suddenness with which these imperatives of development arrive makes for the unkindest of insults: a social world advancing too rapidly toward greater, more bewildering complexity; a life too unruly for her sensibilities, making demands for flexibility and tolerance that are beyond her reach; and a body sensing strange and compelling new energies, changing in shape unexpectedly.

But she soon learns, though not in ways immediately understood, that the unparalleled force of her temperament brings not only fear of change but order, routine, and blunting of need and arousal through avoidance habits well honed and disciplined by her proclivity toward repetitive behavior. To the observer, AN is an oddity—a perverse, uncontrollable madness that can thrive only in a person not in proper control of her mental faculties. But those who suffer with it support a very different view. Although they grudgingly concede that the insistence on losing even more weight lacks common sense, that a "weird" affliction has seized the mind, it is nonetheless a desperately needed solution to existential threat and seemingly well sustained by these very same traits. In addressing this point, L, a 31-year-old woman weighing 79 pounds at 5 feet, 8 inches, who has spent roughly 80% of her last 19 years in hospitals around the country, said:

> "It isn't that I want this illness, I just don't know any other way; it's evil, but I feel it makes me whole. I can remember even as a child hating any kind of change, and I felt disgusted whenever I wanted anything; it's weird, since I can't tell you why. I know I also liked being disciplined. My boyfriend said I was the most disciplined person he ever met, which surprised me, because this is what I thought about him."

The unfolding of AN is not any more intentional or purposive than melancholia, bipolar disorder, obsessive–compulsive disorder, or any other psychological illness, for that matter, but it is not without a volitional element. What is insidious about this psychopathology is that it is sustained, at least partly, by the irresistibly powerful allure of the safety it creates—the mock sanity of its welcoming discipline and the "distinct" sense of self that patients believe it affords. But what ultimately comes from diverting attention away from the natural pleasures of living and the possibility of new learning is impoverishment, invalidism, and despair. Eventually, the contents of her mind draw down, her interests narrow, and her soul withers, leaving only delusive ideas to fill the void that is left: "My illness is my friend." Reflecting these points, the therapist's reply to L's remarks was:

"Anorexia nervosa does not come to people at random. It requires a certain nature for its development, a certain temperament, one in which worry and discomfort with change is prominent, and discomfort is dealt with by avoiding change whenever possible. It is also almost always true that from early childhood people with anorexia nervosa have been plagued by terrible self-doubt and a near paralyzing fear of committing mistakes in what they set out to do, as if this would be an unacceptable blemish on their character that would bring shame or humiliation. But given that people who have this illness also tend to have enormous energy and discipline, which is certainly true of you, and they try to maintain as much routine in their life as possible, since what is new or unpredictable is generally uncomfortable, they create a day-to-day existence that lacks spontaneity, joy, or pleasure. Not only does this type of existence weaken the spirit, it deepens feelings of worthlessness to the point that they attribute whatever good comes from their actions not to true interest or ability but rather to hard work. Because little is taken in, because what is new is shunned for what is more familiar, few experiences are digested, and you suffer because of it. Consider the metaphor and symbolism here, for this is what you struggle with, not your weight."

Work with the chronically ill must rest on (1) a shared understanding of how development, biology, experience, and phenomenology intersect in what becomes a quest for psychic stability and compensatory adaptation, and then (2) a willingness to redress this in carefully measured ways. If there is no perception of shared knowledge, then meaningful dialogue within the intimate setting of psychological work is not possible. Working many years with patients young and old, I have found this framework to resonate strongly, to serve as the common language and the medium for this clinical work. Indeed, while much has been written about the limits of insight among patients with AN, I have not found this to be entirely accurate. Even when vehemently denying that they are too thin, chronically ill patients intuitively grasp the constraints of nature with which they are wrestling and the relevance to their illness: They have long sensed the impulse to avoid change, to narrow attention when confronted with whatever seems to be too complex and abstract, to suppress appetites and emotions that feel disruptive, and to seek affirmation of safety and worth through repetitious, excessively disciplined behaviors.

Midway into L's consultation, her parents railed at what they considered to be her many years of hardheadedness and, according to her father, "plain angry stubbornness," to which the therapist countered:

"By no means are you alone in this bitterness; other families struggling to make sense of this illness experience much the same. Yes, there is a certain kind of willfulness in anorexia nervosa, but it is driven more by fear and desperation and a rigidity of personality that show up in many other areas. Recall what both of you said about L: that from early on she was more nervous than your other children, resisted change, and worried constantly about all sorts of things in spite of all that you did to reassure her. What science has shown us in recent years is that people vary significantly in their sensitivity to change, in how quickly they experience worry and fear, and in their resilience in the face of stress. Certain genes can sensitize the brain to signs of change and thereby make some people prone to extreme levels of anxiety. And as it turns out, people who grow up worry prone tend to retain stronger memories of stressful experiences, compared to people who are less worry prone during childhood. In this same way, there are other genes that seem to reduce our sensitivity to desire and pleasure, and then again, numerous genes that influence the nature of our personality. Also, how we actually cope with the stress of change and other new challenges that arise throughout life very much depends on the unique qualities of our personality. What you describe as her headstrong nature is indeed one of these traits, and there is no question but that as her dieting strengthened, she exploited her disciplined nature to lose even more weight, but only because she was retreating from challenges she believed she could not tolerate because of this anxiety problem. After some time, people with this illness sometimes mistake the discipline of weight control for competence, but again, only because they need something of an antidote for the misery and embarrassment of carrying so much fear, anxiety, and rigidity all these years. But hardheaded for the sake of being hardheaded is not what lies beneath anorexia nervosa."

The circumstances of L's life experiences were of equal importance. Her father, a successful businessman involved in international commerce, traveled extensively, and her mother, a prominent trial attorney, was preoccupied with work throughout L's development. Discussing this family context, the therapist explained:

"Let's put L's timidity, self-discipline, and exaggerated feeling for security in the context of your family life. And I do not say this in accusation but rather to inform. Children have an inherent need for reassurance, whether they communicate this need or not. With few exceptions, neither of you was a very predictable presence in her life, given how often work kept you away from the family. And having heard admiring comments repeated throughout her childhood about her maturity, her poise, and her ability to look out for her self, L innocently took this to mean that to need, or to ask for, something or someone was impertinent, as if it were a sign of her failure at self-direction. So, when we map out the influences that bring someone to this terrible and confusing illness, we often see that there is a tie between biology and experience. For many parents, and for many patients, too, learning of this tie brings much pain and sorrow, so having a place to express those feelings will be important. But I hope it will also allow things to calm down by giving you a new way of looking at all of this."

And this is precisely what followed the consultation. The acrimony, accusations, and avoidance that had stained their relationships over several years lessened, and time spent together was better tolerated. It was, I would suggest, the level of detail given in the explanatory model of their suffering, and how it fit well with their own sense of what had transpired from early on, that allowed them to move forward.

Of course, in other cases, the life experiences that play a role in chronicity, trauma, and severe neglect are more problematic, and the resolutions not so straightforward. In such cases, it is often imperative for patient and family to keep healthy distances for extended periods of time.

The Desire for Marginal Comforts

For a woman with chronic AN, to "be in life" means to bear witness to experiences unwanted and disdained by her temperament. If she seems focused and dedicated, it is more likely than not that her affairs are driven less by zeal for new learning than her temperament's innate search for what is most predictable, tame, and familiar. Even though AN is sustained by malnutrition and predisposing biological traits, its psychopathology can be likened to an existential cocoon of marginal comforts: reassuring, esteem-enhancing successes that allow avoidance of psychosexual growth through a daily regimen of starvation dieting, exercise, and food- and/or weight-dependent rituals. And so it goes, day after day, quelling fear through unremittingly monotonous routines that nonetheless make life existentially bearable and knowable. Disrupt the routine, and the patient's sense of safety feels shattered. And it is for this reason that the clinical care required here is vastly different, and why anticipating the possibility of treatment failure is a justified premise. To approach the chronically ill patient assuming that anyone can be helped is a radically misconceived idea that can bring great harm. The notion may seem at odds with the ethical imperative to treat, but as Vandereycken and Meerman (1984) astutely point out, there is need for realism when confronting unbreakable resistances to change, and pressing the point will sometimes bring little more than angrier resistance, symptom exacerbation, family antagonism, or abrupt termination of a treatment scarcely begun.

The Illusion of Therapeutic Contracts and Dangers of Therapist Zeal

Caring for patients who seem so decidedly opposed to change is a paradox. The issue is made even more confusing by the fact that there is no singular definition of chronicity in AN, nor is there agreement among practitioners about how longstanding AN should be treated. Similarly, there is a wealth of follow-up data on AN from which conclusions have been drawn about variables predicting different outcome categories (Berkman, Lohr, & Bulik, 2007), but it is not clear that one can draw much meaning from the variables identified, given the many confounds inherent in follow-up research. But one unsettling truth is that the effects of psychological therapies in altering the short-term course of adults who have been ill with AN for many years are not impressive (Bulik, Berkman, Brownley, Sedway, & Lohr, 2007; NICE, 2004; see Wilson et al., 2007, for a review). So, as the duration of AN lengthens, the prospect of achieving complete recovery from the illness simultaneously lessens (Strober, Freeman, & Morrell, 1997).

It is evident, then, why our relationship with the chronic patient cannot be the usual one upon which traditional psychotherapy rests. Not welcoming treatment as a force of change, and too inflexible to tolerate the tedious process that psychotherapy is, the arrangement between therapist and patient requires a fundamentally different paradigm, one in which the therapist must expect little, seek nothing, and define the objectives carefully. Given that the forces maintaining chronic AN also sustain feelings of safety for these patients, any effort to peel back patients' dieting rituals, no matter how thoughtful and empathic the approach may be, is to ask patients to blindly accept a perilous journey into desire, appetites, and passions. The urge to move quickly with these frighteningly ill patients is understandable, but the likelihood of success is slim while the potential risks of intervening aggressively are high—and they are risks that medically and psychologically fragile patients can ill afford. I have consulted on many cases where efforts to restore weight rapidly with chronically ill patients were traumatizing, leaving patients embittered and resistant to any further treatment contact; in two cases described elsewhere (Strober, 2004a), the repercussions were more tragic.

The wish to help, to do well by people who suffer, is in the blood of every therapist, but the dangers involved cannot be ignored. Patients who are chronically ill and who thus rely on their disease for marginal comforts are easily unsettled, so what is deemed ethical, moral, and clinically sensible can nonetheless leave the patient feeling unstrung; and when this occurs, the only safety she seeks is that which is enabled by deprivation and further restraint.

A Different Paradigm of Management

When fragility and rigidity do not allow for contemplation of change, the goals are more simply framed: to create a palliative, holding management of carefully measured intensity. In this modified approach of support and comfort, the steps taken to cushion the effects of illness are necessarily small, but by no means is the work trivial or simple minded. The elements of the approach include the following:

1. A sufficiently long period of consultation before undertaking any intervention, in which the developmental model of chronicity is fully explained. The objective here is to reassure the patient that the care to be offered is predicated on deep understanding of the enduring strain she has suffered from an early age in attempting to manage intense fears of change with an unbearably rigid temperament, and of other life circumstances revealed in her history. In doing so, the therapist offers understanding that AN is as protective as it is debilitating and for this reason the goals of the care she is to receive will be worked out in very small steps.

2. Unambiguous reassurance that significant weight gain will not be a principal objective, unless the patients feels otherwise; that refeeding will be negotiated carefully, and collaboratively, so as to avoid panic and regression.

3. Establishing routines of social activity, however minimal, to prevent further invalidism and isolation. These may include contact with understanding and supportive family and friends, attendance at religious services and support groups, visits to a favorite coffee shop, and so forth. It is important that matters of timing and frequency of these contacts be considered carefully, particularly the ability of the people involved to tolerate time spent with the patient.

4. Encouraging involvement in hobbies, intellectual pursuits, and any activity that allows for feelings of pleasure or mastery, and which can also stimulate the patient cognitively.

5. Regular physical examinations with a psychologically informed collaborating physician so that patient and therapist are kept fully abreast of the patient's medical status and can thus make informed decisions about supportive steps to undertake.

6. Encouraging increases in nutrition that do not risk significant change in weight. Here, the point is made that the vast majority of chronically ill patients can increase

calories, easily reaching 1,200 kilocalories (kcal) per day, without weight gain because of elevations in energy metabolism. Naturally, if there is any one suggestion that will be viewed with suspicion it is this, and it should come only in time, and after the relationship is well secured. Input from other patients, if feasible, can be helpful here, though by no means does one patient necessarily take what another says at face value. At the same time, many chronically ill patients can, and do, improve their nutrition and increase weight. Not infrequently, agreement to do so comes after a medical crisis that spikes fear of deterioration or death. In most instances, however, it is simply with time and trust that the patient agrees to minimize the burden of disease by improving nutrition. However, the delicacy of the issue cannot be overstated. The therapist must shun any displays of relief or excitement and must similarly counsel family members to do the same. Instead, it must be stated in earnest to the patient that attempting any change in weight is recognized to be a complicated matter, that her fear in doing so is deeply understood, and that there will be no reproach if she backs off, as the challenge can be revisited another time.

7. Meeting adjunctively with family members and relevant others to educate them about the psychopathology of AN, to provide solace and support, and to discourage in the strongest possible way disparagement of the patient or overt displays of irritation or anger. Likewise, these sessions are used to assist the patient in accepting that there may be times when it is simply too painful for loved ones to be in her presence, and giving permission to family members to take time away from the patient when emotions are too raw for contact.

What is vital in this approach is succeeding in reassuring the patient that the compensatory aspects of AN are understood and that any changes in eating and weight gain will be measured against the patient's tolerance of the anxieties that are triggered so that risk of terminating treatment is minimized.

Returning to the case of L, she agreed to another course of hospital care, which, over 5 months of deliberately slow change, increased her weight to 104 pounds, at which point she felt she had reached her limit of tolerance. Her functioning is significantly improved, but her struggles remain.

Some Caveats

Although hospitalization is, in my experience, the ideal setting for implementing this approach with very malnourished patients, inpatient programs with the requisite experience are few in number and the realities of present-day managed care, at least in the United States, rarely permit the slow pace of treatment and long lengths of stay this type of care requires. General inpatient psychiatric hospitals are ill suited for this type of patient and should be avoided, as in many cases the treatment attempted is iatrogenic. Much the same can be said of refeeding in general medical services, except when the care is overseen by highly experienced and psychologically informed specialists. Similarly, when the care is being delivered in a routine outpatient setting in collaboration with a dietician and physician, the importance of having *all* nonmedical decisions negotiated and executed by the therapist, especially those involving nutrition and allowed types of activity, cannot be overstated, given the sensitive nature of the points elaborated above. Simply put, if the separate elements of care within this overarching paradigm do not cohere, the potential for disruption is great.

Countertransference with the Chronic Patient

Because management of the chronic patient is drastically different from conventional psychotherapy, rarely is the work as inherently rewarding. The self-ordered routine of the chronic patient offers preciously little hope that with analysis, probing, or confronting, new possibilities will emerge. Instead, the therapist will sit idly for long periods with a life that is, in all practical ways, sadly extinct, whose physical presence is but a lamentable footnote in a history that now seems too difficult to retrieve.

Transference and countertransference enter into any therapeutic experience, but it is different here. As the sessions come and go, the patient's presence seems but a perfunctory and formal appearance and the dialogue is tedious and draining, so much so that to manage more than several chronically ill patients at any one time is not advisable. In this same regard, undertaking this work without colleagues to confer with, or a supervision group to meet with, is not wise. With patients so ill, the work can seem grinding and boring, petty discomforts feeling like mountains of burden, and the wish to be free of the patient rippling scarcely beneath the skin. Therapists are not immune to self-deception and hiding inward discomforts may be a common vice, but trying to sanitize the countertransference with these patients, pushing it too far back to be acknowledged, will only deprive them of the respect they deserve. And this will surely be felt.

So, it isn't only the patient's temperament that needs understanding, as there is no illusion here about the qualities of therapist temperament essential for taking up work with chronically ill patients: an inexhaustible capacity for enduring monotony; deep compassion for human suffering, but one cushioned by an even-tempered manner; the ability to confront crises without feeling beleaguered or anxious; maintaining attentiveness in the presence of a life that flirts with death; and a capacity for deep and honest reflective talk about life's basic truths, and for exploring the sadness of a life not fully lived. Engaging the patient in painful reflections is a clinically delicate matter, so it must be undertaken with great caution, and only at a time that intuitively seems right, as it can sometimes bring things of importance into sharper relief. But what this section hopes to make unmistakably clear is that facing up to the "heaviness" of managing this type of patient is a formidable element of the therapist's task. Knowing in advance what emotions he/she will face allows the therapist to consider whether or not the undertaking can be tolerated, or if it is wanted at all.

Concluding Remarks

Work with the chronically ill patient with AN occupies a unique place in the larger arena of treating patients with EDs. The work is both challenging and difficult, for much is required of those who will undertake it: tolerance of sameness, a professional identity that does not require successes measured by patient progress, respect for solitude, the ability to face frailty and profound sickness with relative ease, the ability and willingness to explore the wounds and deprivations of a life passed by, and the ability to face frailty and profound sickness with ease. The goals of this management are circumscribed, reflecting the nature of the psychopathology of chronic AN, the patient's exquisite sensitivities, and the risks of treading too heavily on their efforts at salvaging "marginal comforts."

Acknowledgments

Preparation of this chapter was supported in part by the Franklin Mint Endowed Chair in Eating Disorders. I also thank Cynthia Pikus, PhD, for editorial assistance.

References

Anderluth MD, Tchanturia K, Rabe-Hesketh S, & Treasure J. (2003). Childhood obsessive–compulsive personality traits in adults in adult women with eating disorders. *American Journal of Psychiatry*, 160:242–247.

Berkman ND, Lohr KN, & Bulik CM. (2007). Outcomes of eating disorders: A systematic review of the literature. *International Journal of Eating Disorders*, 40:292–309.

Bulik CM, Berkman ND, Brownley KA, Sedway JA, & Lohr KN. (2007). Anorexia nervosa treatment: A systematic review of randomized controlled trials. *International Journal of Eating Disorders*, 40:310–320.

Bulik CM, Sullivan PF, Fear R, & Joyce PR. (1997). Eating disorders and antecedent anxiety disorders: A controlled study. *Acta Psychiatrica Scandanavica*, 96:101–107.

Charney DS, & Nestler EJ. (Eds.). *Neurobiology of mental illness* (3rd ed.). New York: Oxford University Press.

Karwautz A, Rabe-Hesketh S, Collier DA, & Treasure J. (2002). Premorbid psychiatric morbidity, comorbidity, and personality in patients with anorexia nervosa compared to their healthy sisters. *European Eating Disorders Review*, 10:255–270.

Kaye W, Strober M, & Jimerson D. (2009). The neurobiology of eating disorders. In DS Charney & EJ Nestler (Eds.), *Neurobiology of mental illness* (3rd ed., pp. 1349–1369). New York: Oxford University Press.

National Institute for Health and Clinical Excellence. (2004). *Eating disorders: Core interventions in the treatment and management of anorexia nervosa, bulimia nervosa and related eating disorders* (NICE Clinical Guideline No. 9). London: Author. Available online at *www.nice.org.uk*.

Steinglass J, & Walsh BT. (2006). Habit learning in anorexia nervosa: A cognitive neuroscience hypothesis. *International Journal of Eating Disorders*, 39:267–275.

Strober M. (1991). Disorders of the self in anorexia nervosa: An organismic developmental paradigm. In CL Johnson (Ed.), *Psychodynamic treatment for anorexia nervosa and bulimia* (pp. 354–373). New York: Guilford Press.

Strober M. (2004a). Managing the chronic, treatment resistant patient with anorexia nervosa. *International Journal of Eating Disorders*, 36:245–255.

Strober M. (2004b). Pathological fear conditioning and anorexia nervosa: On the search for new paradigms. *International Journal of Eating Disorders*, 35:504–508.

Strober M, Freeman R, Lampert C, & Diamond J. (2007). The association of anxiety disorders and obsessive compulsive personality disorder with anorexia nervosa: Evidence from a family study with discussion of nosological and neurodevelopmental implications. *International Journal of Eating Disorders*, 40:46–51.

Strober M, Freeman R, & Morrell W. (1997). The long-term course of severe anorexia nervosa in adolescents: Survival analysis of recovery, relapse, and outcome predictors over 10–15 years in a prospective study. *International Journal of Eating Disorders,* 22:339–360.

Vandereycken W, & Beumont PJV. (Eds.). (1998). *Treating eating disorders: Ethical, legal, and personal issues.* New York: New York University Press.

Vandereycken W, & Meermann R. (1984). *Anorexia nervosa: A clinician's guide to treatment.* Berlin: de Gruyter.

Wilson GT, Grilo CM, & Vitousek KM. (2007). Psychological treatment of eating disorders. *American Psychologist,* 62:199–216.

PART III

Treatment of Bulimia Nervosa and Binge-Eating Disorder

This section of the book details what is known concerning the available treatments for patients with bulimia nervosa (BN) and binge-eating disorder (BED). In contrast to the treatment of anorexia nervosa (AN), as reviewed in Part II, treatment research for BN and BED has shown much progress during the past two decades. The United Kingdom's National Institute for Health and Clinical Excellence (NICE) issued a detailed list of treatment guidelines for eating disorders (EDs) in 2004; these guidelines, based on available data, were assigned "grades" ranging from "A" (denoting strong empirical support from rigorous controlled trials) to "C" (denoting expert opinion without strong empirical data). NICE offered roughly 100 treatment recommendations across EDs, with most graded as "C," reflecting the need for continued treatment research. However, several treatment approaches received strong endorsements for BN and BED. Perhaps most noteworthy was the recommendation that a specific form of cognitive-behavioral therapy (CBT) be considered the "treatment of choice" for BN and BED, and this recommendation was given the "A" grade. This represents the first NICE recommendation of a psychological therapy as the initial treatment of choice for any psychiatric disorder. Other noteworthy recommendations for BN and BED, assigned "B" grades, included certain forms of pharmacotherapy, interpersonal psychotherapy, dialectical behavior therapy, and certain self-help approaches. Thus, clinicians have a number of evidence-supported treatments to consider. However, many patients with BN fail to benefit or improve sufficiently from these and other treatments. This section includes nine chapters describing a range of available treatments. Six of the treatment chapters include "mini-manuals" to provide the reader with guidance about how to deliver the treatments, as well as descriptions and examples about the specific techniques involved. The remaining chapters cover additional treatment methods, including self-help approaches and pharmacotherapy for BN and BED.

239

Chapter 14, by Zafra Cooper and Christopher G. Fairburn, describes an "enhanced version" of their evidence-based CBT (i.e., CBT-E). This second-generation CBT-E has two versions ("focused" and "broad") that were developed for the treatment of the full range of EDs. The CBT-E focused form is designed to target ED psychopathology, and the CBT-E broad form is a more complex approach that can be tailored to specific individual needs, based on the presence of additional psychopathology thought to either maintain or complicate the ED.

Chapter 15, by Marian Tanofsky-Kraff and Denise E. Wilfley, describes interpersonal psychotherapy (IPT) for BN and BED. This specialist psychotherapy, adapted from initial versions developed specifically for the treatment of depression, has received empirical support in both individual and group approaches for BN and BED. The authors also provide a description of initial adaptation of IPT to younger age groups.

Chapter 16, by Eunice Y. Chen and Debra L. Safer, describes dialectical behavior therapy (DBT) for BED and BN. This specialist therapy was initially developed for patient groups with severe emotional dysregulation problems, including self-destructive or parasuicidal patients and those with borderline personality disorder. DBT has received increasing empirical support with diverse patients groups, including Chen and Safer's recent applications to patients with BN and BED.

Chapter 17, by Stephen A. Wonderlich and his colleagues, describes integrative cognitive–affective therapy (ICAT) for BN. ICAT is a specialist therapy based on a programmatic line of empirical research that has suggested a number of putative maintaining mechanisms for BN. Conceptually, ICAT holds promise for intervening with patients with BN who have complex co-occurring problems.

Chapter 18, by Kathryn J. Zerbe, describes psychodynamic therapy for EDs. This chapter includes a cogent overview of the major psychodynamic aspects of EDs. This approach to treatment is widely applied yet there exist few descriptions of theory and methods. Zerbe provides details about the structure of treatment and rich clinical examples that bring specific techniques to life.

Chapter 19, by Varinia C. Sánchez-Ortiz and Ulrike Schmidt, describes self-help approaches for BN and BED. Emerging evidence supports the efficacy of certain approaches using guided self-help or even pure self-help, making use of specific forms of evidence-based CBT materials adapted for self-care. This is an exciting and important line of work in light of many barriers to treatment access and the shortage of specialist-clinicians in the ED field.

Chapter 20, by Daniel le Grange and James Lock, describes a family-based treatment for adolescents with BN. This chapter, which includes a detailed mini-manual, addresses a major clinical and research need. Remarkably little is known about how best to treat adolescents with BN. This chapter, which provides important clinical guidance for working with adolescent patients with BN and their families, should stimulate further research on this topic.

Part III closes with two chapters describing the status of pharmacotherapy for treating BN and BED. Allegra Broft, Laura A. Berner, and B. Timothy Walsh provide an overview of the pharmacotherapy for BN. Lindsay P. Bodell and Michael J. Devlin provide an overview of the pharmacotherapy literature for

BED. Both chapters present what is known regarding pharmacotherapy alone and in combination with psychological treatments for BN and BED. Unlike the case for AN, pharmacotherapy has demonstrated efficacy for both BN and BED, although both chapters highlight the pressing need for studies to include follow-up assessments, since almost nothing is known regarding maintenance following pharmacotherapy. The reader should benefit from close inspection of both chapters, which provide information about specific dosing methods for the available medications.

CHAPTER 14

Cognitive Behavior Therapy for Bulimia Nervosa

Zafra Cooper and Christopher G. Fairburn

The cognitive-behavioral treatment described in this chapter is not merely a treatment for bulimia nervosa (BN); rather, it is a treatment for all forms of eating disorder (ED) psychopathology, including that seen in anorexia nervosa (AN) and eating disorder not otherwise specified (EDNOS). However, this chapter focuses on its use with patients who have BN or BN-like states.

The treatment, CBT-E, is an "enhanced" version of the leading evidence-based treatment for BN, a specific form of cognitive behavior therapy (CBT-BN; Fairburn, Marcus, & Wilson, 1993). It is described as "enhanced" for three main reasons: (1) The strategies and procedures used to address the ED psychopathology have been refined and extended; (2) in certain subgroups of patients common additional maintaining mechanisms may be tackled, namely mood intolerance, clinical perfectionism, core low self-esteem, or major interpersonal difficulties; and (3), as noted above, the treatment has been adapted to make it suitable for all forms of ED rather than just BN. The rationale underpinning these changes is described in Fairburn, Cooper, and Shafran (2003) and Fairburn (2008a). The full transdiagnostic treatment is described in Fairburn, Cooper, and Shafran (2008) and Fairburn, Cooper, Shafran, Bohn, Hawker, and colleagues (2008b).

The Cognitive-Behavioral Theory of the Maintenance of BN

In common with most evidence-based cognitive-behavioral treatments, the theory that underpins CBT-E is primarily concerned with the processes that maintain psychopathology rather than those responsible for its development. According to the theory, central to the maintenance of BN is these patients' dysfunctional scheme for self-evaluation. Whereas most people evaluate themselves on the basis of their perceived performance in a variety of domains of life, people with EDs judge themselves largely, or even exclusively, in terms of their shape and weight and their ability to control them. As a result, their lives become focused on their shape, weight, and eating, with dietary control, thinness, and weight loss being actively pursued, while overeating, "fatness," and weight gain are avoided. Most of the other features of BN can be understood as stemming directly from this "core psychopathology," including the dietary restraint, the other forms of weight control behavior, the various forms of body checking and avoidance, and the preoccupation with thoughts about shape, weight, and eating. Figure 14.1 provides a schematic representation of the main processes involved in the persistence of ED psychopathology. Those specifically involved in the maintenance of the psychopathology seen in BN are highlighted in bold typeface.

The only feature of BN that is not obviously a direct expression of the core psychopathology is these patients' binge eating. The cognitive-behavioral theory proposes that binge eating is largely a product of these patients' distinctive form of dietary restraint (attempts to restrict their eating), which may or may not be accompanied by actual dietary restriction (true undereating in a physiological sense; Fairburn, 2008b). Rather than adopting general guidelines about how they should eat, these patients try to adhere to multiple, specific, and very demanding dietary rules. The accompanying tendency to react in an extreme and negative fashion to the (almost inevitable) breaking of these rules results in even minor dietary slips being viewed as evidence of lack of self-control. Patients respond to such rule-breaking by temporarily abandoning their attempts to restrict their eating, and, as a result, they succumb to the urge to eat that arises from their dietary restraint (and any accompanying dietary restriction). The result is an episode of binge eating (i.e., uncontrolled overeating), which is followed after a variable length of time by renewed attempts to restrict their eating (i.e., dietary restraint and restriction). These processes produce the distinctive pattern of eating that characterizes BN, in which attempts to restrict eating are interrupted by repeated

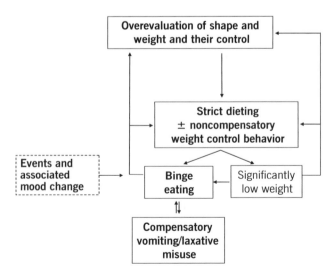

FIGURE 14.1. The composite transdiagnostic formulation of ED psychopathology with the features seen in BN highlighted in bold typeface. From Fairburn (2008b). Copyright 2008 by The Guilford Press. Reprinted by permission.

episodes of binge eating. The binge eating, in turn, maintains the core psychopathology by intensifying patients' concerns about their ability to control their eating, shape, and weight. As noted, it also encourages yet greater dietary restraint, thereby increasing the risk of further binge eating.

It is also important to note the influence of another set of mechanisms. These patients' dietary slips and binges are particularly prone to occur in response to adverse day-to-day events and negative moods. This arises, in part, because it is difficult to maintain dietary restraint under such circumstances and, in part, because binge eating both temporarily ameliorates negative mood states and distracts patients from aversive thoughts.

A further process maintains binge eating among those who practice compensatory purging (i.e., those who induce vomiting or take laxatives in response to specific episodes of binge eating). Patients' belief in the ability of purging to minimize weight gain results in a major deterrent against binge eating being undermined (i.e., the prospect of weight gain). They do not realize that vomiting only retrieves part of what has been eaten, and that laxative misuse has little or no effect on energy absorption (Fairburn, 1995).

As mentioned earlier, in addition to these core ED maintaining mechanisms, the theory underpinning CBT-E proposes that in certain patients there are additional mechanisms that also maintain the ED psychopathology and are therefore further obstacles to change. The role of each of these additional mechanisms (mood intolerance, clinical perfectionism, core low self-esteem, and major interpersonal difficulties) in the maintenance of BN and other forms of ED is discussed in detail in the complete treatment guide (Fairburn, Cooper, & Shafran, 2008; Fairburn, Cooper, Shafran, Bohn, & Hawker, 2008a).

This cognitive-behavioral theory of the maintenance of BN has clear implications for treatment. It suggests that if treatment is to have a lasting impact on these patients' binge eating and purging, the aspect of their disorder that they most want to change, it also needs to address their dieting, their overevaluation of shape and weight, their sensitivity to external events and negative moods, and any of the four additional maintaining mechanisms that may also be operating.

Research on the Treatment

Consistent with the current way of classifying EDs, the research on their treatment has focused on the particular disorders in isolation. This research has been reviewed by Wilson, Grilo, and Vitousek (2007). In addition, several "systematic reviews" and meta-analyses have been conducted (e.g., National Collaborating Centre for Mental Health, 2004; Shapiro et al., 2007). The general conclusion is that there is a clear leading treatment, namely, CBT-BN. However, the research findings also indicate that this treatment is far from being a panacea, since less than half the patients who start treatment make a full and lasting recovery.

To date, there has been just one trial of CBT-E, although others are in progress. This trial recruited adult patients with any form of ED, provided they had a body mass index (BMI) over 17.5 (Fairburn et al., 2009). Following DSM-IV diagnostic conventions, these patients met diagnostic criteria for either BN or for EDNOS. The mean duration of their ED was over 8 years. Few exclusion criteria were applied (unusual for randomized controlled trials), since one goal was to recruit a sample representative of patients seen in routine clinical practice. The outcome of the two diagnostic groups was similar. At the end of 20 weeks of treatment over half the randomized patients (52.7% of those with BN and 53.3% of those with EDNOS, respectively) had a level of ED features less than one standard deviation above the community mean, and at 60-week follow-up the comparable figures were 61% and 46%, respectively. These outcomes for CBT-E appear more favorable than those previously reported for CBT-BN in a major multisite study (Agras, Walsh, Fairburn, Wilson, & Kraemer, 2000), although a direct comparison of CBT-BN and CBT-E would be needed to determine their relative efficacy.

Overview of CBT-E

There are various versions of CBT-E. This chapter is concerned primarily with the "focused" treatment, the version that focuses exclusively on the ED psychopathology. This is suitable for the majority of patients with BN and is the default version. The "broad" version is designed for patients with marked coexisting mood intolerance, clinical perfectionism, low self-esteem, or interpersonal difficulties (Fairburn, Cooper, Shafran, Bohn, & Hawker, 2008a). It will be only briefly mentioned, given limitations on space. The results of the CBT-E trial mentioned above suggest that the broad version should be used only with patients who have extreme forms of the additional psychopathology of the type mentioned above, the focused treatment being more effective for the remainder (Fairburn et al., 2009).

CBT-E is time-limited and is best delivered on a one-to-one basis, as it is designed to be individualized. For the majority of patients 20 sessions are sufficient (preceded by an initial assessment session). The main advantages of a fixed time frame are that it concentrates the mind of both the patient and the clinician and it makes it much more likely that treatment will have a formal ending. A formal ending encourages clinicians to allocate time in the final sessions to the coverage of important future-oriented topics (as are discussed later in the chapter). There are circumstances under which it is appropriate to adjust the length of treatment. It rarely needs to be shortened, although this may apply in certain cases. Somewhat more often there is a case for extending treatment. The indications for doing this are also described toward the end of the chapter.

Readers should note that CBT-E is intended to be a complete treatment in its own right. It is not designed to be combined with other forms of treatment, nor is it desirable for it to coexist with them. Both risk undermining the treatment and thereby rendering it less effective. Thus we recommend using the full treatment rather than using elements in isolation or in combination with other forms of treatment.

CBT-E has four stages. In Stage 1 the aims are to engage the patient in treatment and the process of change, to jointly create a formulation of the processes maintaining the ED, to provide education, and to introduce two important procedures, "weekly weighing" and "regular eating." Appointments are twice weekly for 4 weeks, preceded by an initial assessment session. Stage 2 is a transitional stage whose aims are to review progress, identify barriers to change, modify the formulation as needed, and plan Stage 3. This stage generally comprises two appointments, each a week apart. The aim of Stage 3, which is the main body of treatment, is to address the key mechanisms that are maintaining the patient's ED; there are eight weekly appointments. Stage 4, the final stage in treatment, has two aims: (1) to ensure that the changes made in treatment are maintained over the following months, and (2) to minimize the risk of relapse in the long term. There are three appointments, each 2 weeks apart. Following the end of treatment, there is a review appointment 20 weeks later.

Assessing and Preparing Patients for Treatment

The essential first step in managing any psychiatric problem is an evaluation interview or interviews. The goals are to engage the patient, establish the nature and severity of the problem, and decide how best to proceed. Engaging the patient and beginning to forge a positive therapeutic relationship is particularly important. Many patients referred with a possible ED are ambivalent about treatment because aspects of their psychopathology may be positively valued (especially dietary control); there may be shame about other features (e.g., binge eating); and the patient may have had adverse treatment experiences in the past.

Toward the end of the initial interview we weigh patients and measure their height. Weighing is an extremely sensitive matter for most patients, and some are resistant to it. It is nevertheless essential if the assessment is to be complete. It is not appropriate to rely upon patients' self-reported weight, as this is sometimes inaccurate. The importance of being weighed is explained to patients by telling them that we *have* to check their weight in order to conduct a complete assessment and give them good advice. In our experience patients do not refuse. At this point we do not insist upon patients knowing their weight, if they do not wish to.

We are not in favor of lengthy assessment appointments because they are exhausting for the patient and, in our view, unnecessary; 90 minutes is our maximum. However, we routinely see patients twice as part of the assessment process, as we often find that a second appointment, a week or two later, adds new information of value. On this second occasion patients are more relaxed, they may disclose information previously withheld, and we have an opportunity to pursue matters that require particularly careful exploration (e.g., the nature and extent of coexisting depressive features; Fairburn, Cooper, & Waller, 2008a). The second appointment is also a good time to discuss the various treatment options in more detail.

We routinely ask patients to complete certain questionnaires prior to the initial assessment appointment. This is useful because it gives us standardized information on the nature and severity of the patient's ED. The two questionnaires we favor are the Eating Disorder Examination Questionnaire (EDE-Q; Fairburn & Beglin, 2008) and the Clinical Impairment Assessment (CIA; Bohn & Fairburn, 2008; Bohn et al., 2008), both of which can be downloaded from this website: *www.psychiatry.ox.ac.uk/credo*. The EDE-Q provides a measure of current ED features, and the CIA assesses the impact of this psychopathology on psychosocial functioning. Both questionnaires are short and easy to complete and both focus on the previous 28 days. In addition, we include one of the well-established measures of general psychiatric features.

By the end of the second appointment it should be possible to decide on the best treatment options. Outpatient-based CBT-E is appropriate for the vast majority of cases. When presenting treatment options, we inform patients about their prognosis, both with and without treatment. It is important that patients know that an established ED is unlikely to resolve in the absence of treatment.

There are certain contraindications to embarking upon CBT-E straightaway:

- *Compromised physical health.* Patients should be assessed by a physician before starting CBT-E if their physical state is of concern (see Fairburn, Cooper, & Waller, 2008b, for a list of indications).
- *Suicide risk.* This risk is largely, but not exclusively, confined to patients who have a coexisting clinical depression, although heightened suicide risk is also present in patients who feel hopeless about the prospect of recovery. All ED clinicians should be competent at assessing suicide risk.
- *Clinical depression.* It is our view that there is a sizeable subgroup of people who have both an ED and a clinical depression embedded within the population of patients with EDs. These people are easy to miss, yet to do so is regrettable, since they respond well to antidepressant medication (at high doses) and, as a result, are better able to make good use of psychological treatment directed at their ED. We are aware that there is no formal empirical work that supports this view: For example, the pretreatment level of clinical depression does not predict treatment response in BN, nor is there convincing evidence that combining psychological treatment with antidepressant medication enhances the effectiveness of the psychological treatment. Neither observation surprises us for the following two reasons: (1) the level of depressive features is no greater among those with a clinical depression than among those without—it is the pattern of depressive features that differs; and (2), the response to antidepressant medication typically only occurs at higher-than-usual dosages and so would not have been observed in the medication trials conducted to date. The identification and management of clinical depressions in patients with EDs is discussed in detail in Fairburn, Cooper, and Waller (2008a).
- *Persistent substance misuse.* Intoxication in treatment sessions renders the sessions virtually worthless, and persistent intoxication outside sessions undermines the patient's ability to utilize treatment. Both need to be addressed prior to embarking upon CBT-E.
- *Major life events or crises.* These are distracting and so interfere with treatment; it is often best to delay treatment until the crisis has passed.
- *Inability to attend treatment.* A central feature of CBT-E is establishing and maintaining therapeutic momentum. Achieving momentum requires that appointments be frequent (especially in the early stages) and regular. In our view it is essential that patients attend in this way, especially during the first 6 weeks. We ask patients to guarantee that there will be no breaks in their attendance during these 6 weeks and no breaks of longer than 2 consecutive weeks throughout the rest of treatment. If this is impossible, for example, because of a prebooked vacation, then we prefer to defer treatment. Patients generally understand and respect the rationale behind this firm stance.

Some patients realize that their day-to-day commitments or lifestyle are such that they are likely to interfere with treatment. In such cases we explore with them the possibility that they might take 6 months or a year off from their current work or other commitments so that they can fully devote themselves to overcoming their eating problem. Doing this is a major decision but is one that few patients come to regret.

The Treatment Protocol

Stage 1

This is the initial, intensive stage of treatment. The main elements are described below. Readers wishing to implement the treatment are advised to read the full treatment guide (Fairburn, Cooper, Shafran, Bohn, & Hawker, 2008a; Fairburn, Cooper, Shafran, Bohn, Hawker, et al., 2008b). The materials needed to implement the treatment (e.g., patient handouts, monitoring records) can be downloaded free of charge from this website: *www.psychiatry.ox.ac.uk/credo*.

Engaging the Patient in Treatment and the Prospect of Change

A particular challenge when working with patients with EDs is engaging them in treatment. As mentioned, there may be aspects of their disorder that they would like to change (e.g., binge eating), but generally there are other features that they value and with which they may even identify (e.g., maintaining strict control over their eating). It is essential that the clinician understands this and is sensitive at all times to the patient's likely ambivalence. The initial treatment session is especially important in this regard. Much has been written about engaging these patients in treatment; we particularly recommend the article by Vitousek, Watson, and Wilson (1998). Clinicians can enhance engagement as follows: by conveying that they understand eating problems and have expertise in their assessment and treatment; by actively involving the patient in the assessment process and in the creation of the formulation; and by instilling hope that the patient will be able to overcome the disorder. Also important is explaining what treatment involves.

Assessing the Eating Problem and Creating the Formulation

On the first occasion that the clinician and patient meet, the clinician will need to assess the nature and severity of the eating problem (unless he/she was involved in the initial evaluation interviews—see above). This assessment leads naturally to the creation of the formulation. The "formulation"—that is, a personalized visual representation (i.e., a diagram) of the processes that appear to be maintaining the patient's ED—is created in the initial session unless the form of the ED is particularly difficult to understand (in which case it is best delayed until the next session). Creating the formulation has a number of purposes:

1. It helps to engage patients in treatment, at least in part by indicating that the clinician understands the nature of the problem.
2. It conveys the notion that eating problems are understandable and are maintained by a number of interacting self-perpetuating mechanisms. Hence it explains why the patient has found it difficult to change.
3. It begins to distance patients from their problems by helping them step back and think about their difficulties and how they operate. The adoption of this "decentered" stance helps patients change.
4. Lastly, it provides a guide as to what needs to be targeted in treatment. Figure 14.2 provides an example of a personalized formulation (using the patient's own

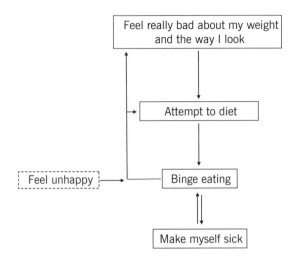

FIGURE 14.2. A formulation of a case of BN (using the patient's own words).

words) based on the relevant sections of the transdiagnostic template shown in Figure 14.1.

In creating the formulation two points need to be kept in mind. First, it should focus on the main mechanisms that appear to be maintaining the patient's eating problem. It does not need to include every clinical feature (as there is a risk that it might be overdetailed and confusing), nor is it concerned with the origins of the problem. Second, it is best to start drawing the formulation by focusing on something that the patient wants to change (e.g., binge eating). The clinician should take the lead in drawing out the formulation, but the patient should be actively involved and his/her own terms should be used wherever possible. Since the formulation is based on information only just obtained, it should be made clear that it is provisional and will be modified, as needed, during treatment.

Once the formulation has been created, the clinician should discuss its implications for treatment. The points to be made include the following: To overcome the eating problem the patient will need to address not only the features that he/she would like to change (e.g., loss of control over eating) but also the mechanisms responsible for maintaining them. Thus, for example, with patients who have BN, treatment commonly needs to focus on more than simply stopping binge eating; it also needs to address the patient's dieting, the patient's ability to deal with adverse events and moods without binge-eating, and the patient's overconcern with shape and weight. Failing to address the main maintaining processes markedly increases the likelihood of relapse.

Establishing Real-Time Self-Monitoring

Real-time self-monitoring involves the ongoing "in-the-moment" recording of relevant behavior, thoughts, feelings, and events (Figure 14.3 for an example monitoring record). Self-monitoring is initiated in the initial session, is fine-tuned in the subsequent session, and continues throughout treatment. We use monitoring records that are simple to complete. Exactly what is recorded evolves during treatment.

V = vomiting; L = laxative misuse; * = eating regarded as excessive.

Day ......Thursday...........   Date .....March 19th...........

Time	Food and drink consumed	Place	*	v/l	Context and comments
7:30	Glass water	Kitchen			Thirsty after yesterday
8:10	Half banana } Black coffee }	Cafe			Must be good and not binge today!
11:45	Smoked turkey on wheat bread } Light mayo Diet coke }	Cafe			Usual lunch
6:40–7:30	Piece of apple pie	Kitchen	*		Help—I can't stop eating. I'm completely out of control. I hate myself.
	1/2 gallon ice cream		*		
	4 slices of toast with peanut butter		*	V	
	Diet coke				
	Raisin bagel		*		
	2 slices of toast with peanut butter		*		
	Diet coke				
	Peanut butter from jar		*		
	Raisin bagel		*	V	
	Snickers bar		*		I am disgusting. Why do I do this? I started as soon as I got in. I've ruined another day.
	Diet coke—large				
9:30	Rice cake with fat-free cheese	Kitchen			Really lonely. Feel fat and ugly. Feel like giving up.
	Diet coke				

FIGURE 14.3. A completed monitoring record. From Fairburn (2008a). Copyright 2008 by The Guilford Press. Reprinted by permission.

Self-monitoring serves two purposes: It assists in the identification of the patient's problems and progress and, much more importantly, it facilitates change by helping patients examine and address problems as they occur. Fundamental to establishing accurate recording is going over the patient's records in detail, especially in the subsequent session when the patient brings them back for the first time. Reviewing the records should be a joint process, with the patient taking the clinician through each day's record in turn. Apart from the first time when the records are meticulously examined, this review should be brief.

Weekly Weighing

"Weekly weighing" is a new feature of treatment that is usually introduced in the second session. It is designed to address the unusual weighing practices seen among patients with EDs. These typically involve either very frequent weight checking, which leads to concern with trivial fluctuations in weight and thereby further dieting, or the avoidance of weighing, which allows patients' worst fears to persist unchallenged and leads them to continue to diet. Weekly weighing involves the checking of the patient's weight at the beginning of each session (twice weekly), followed by the joint plotting of the latest data point on an individualized weight graph. The clinician helps the patient interpret the emerging pattern by placing particular emphasis not on the latest reading but on trends over the previous 4 weeks. Patients are asked not to weigh themselves outside of these times and are given help doing so.

Patients are also educated about weight and weight changes. They are told their BMI and its significance from a health point of view. It is explained that body weight fluctuates (according to the level of one's hydration, the state of one's bowels and bladder, and in women the point in the menstrual cycle) and that, contrary to patients' beliefs, day-to-day weight fluctuations are not indicative of changes in fatness. Patients are advised against having an exact desired weight and are instead advised to accept a weight range of approximately 6 pounds (or 3 kg) in magnitude (see below).

Almost all patients are anxious about the effect that treatment will have on their weight. In practice patients with BN generally do not change much in weight. They should be told that it is the aim of treatment to give them control over their eating and thus they will have as much control over their weight as is generally possible. It is best that patients postpone deciding upon a specific goal weight range until near the end of treatment, when their eating habits have stabilized and they will be less acutely sensitive about their weight and shape. Once they reach this point they are advised against maintaining a weight that necessitates anything more than slight dietary restraint, since otherwise the risk of binge eating will be high, and they will continue to be preoccupied with food and eating.

Educating the Patient about Eating Problems

Many patients with eating problems have misconceptions about eating and weight that contribute to the persistence of their problems. We provide education using a procedure termed "guided reading." This involves patients being given one of the lay books on EDs, which we ask them to annotate to identify areas for discussion. We routinely use *Overcoming Binge Eating* (Fairburn, 1995), as it provides all the information needed and because it includes a CBT-E-compatible cognitive-behavioral perspective.[1]

Regular Eating

Establishing a pattern of regular eating is fundamental to regaining control over eating. It reliably results in a rapid and substantial decrease in the frequency of binge eating.

"Regular eating" is generally introduced shortly after the guided education, and it is the first time that patients are asked to change the way that they eat. There are two aspects to the intervention:

1. Patients are asked to eat three planned meals each day plus two planned snacks. Generally this involves eating breakfast, lunch, a midafternoon snack, an evening meal, and an evening snack.
2. Patients are asked to restrict their eating to these meals and snacks.

---

[1] Christopher G. Fairburn acknowledges the obvious conflict of interest.

A number of points about the intervention need to be stressed. (Further information is provided in the full treatment guide.)

- The new eating pattern should be given priority and be adhered to (in line with day-to-day commitments) whatever the patient's circumstances or appetite.
- Patients should plan ahead. They should always know when they are going to have their next meal or snack, and there should rarely be more than a 4-hour interval between the meals and snacks. If the day is going to be unpredictable, they should plan ahead as far as possible and identify a time when they can take stock and plan the rest of the day.
- Patients should choose what they eat in their planned meals and snacks. The only condition is that the meals and snacks must not be followed by vomiting, laxative misuse, or any other compensatory behavior. It is not helpful to suggest that patients change what they eat at this point in treatment, as this tends to result in their being unable to adopt the pattern of regular eating.
- Patients whose eating habits are chaotic and those whose eating is highly restrictive often need to introduce this pattern in stages. At first they should be advised to focus on the part of the day when their eating is least problematic (generally, the mornings) and then gradually extend the eating pattern until it encompasses the entire day.
- If patients seek advice about the quantity they should eat, and in particular whether they should eat until they feel full, they should be told that their sensations of appetite, hunger, and fullness are all likely to be disturbed at present and should not be used as a guide as to what to eat. Rather, they should adhere to the agreed pattern of eating and consume about average-sized portions of food.

Three difficulties commonly arise:

1. It is not uncommon for patients to say that they have never eaten in this way, nor do their family or friends. While this may be the case, adopting this pattern of eating will help them overcome their eating problem, and it will be the foundation upon which other changes will be built. Once they have overcome their eating problem, it will be up to them to decide exactly how they eat.

2. Some patients are reluctant to eat meals and snacks because they think that doing so will result in weight gain. They can be reassured that weight gain rarely occurs, since they have not been asked to change the amount that they eat or what they eat. Also, since regular eating results in a decrease in the frequency of binge eating and thereby a significant reduction in their overall energy intake (even if they vomit, they absorb a significant amount of energy each time that they binge), weight gain is most unlikely. Despite such assurances, it is common for patients to select meals and snacks that are low in energy. There should be no objections to this since at this point in treatment the focus is on their temporal pattern of eating.

3. Some patients are liable to feel full after eating relatively little, and this feeling produces a desire to vomit or take laxatives. Feelings of fullness are especially likely to occur after eating foods perceived as fattening. This reaction is usually largely cognitive in nature and involves, in part, paying undue attention to abdominal sensations that would normally pass unnoticed. They should be reassured that these feelings generally

subside within an hour and that their propensity to feel full will gradually decline with the adoption of this pattern of eating. Patients troubled by feelings of fullness often benefit from not wearing tight clothes at mealtimes and from engaging in distracting activities afterward.

Two rather different strategies may be used to help patients resist eating between the planned meals and snacks. The first is to help them identify and employ activities that are incompatible with eating or make it less likely (e.g., taking a shower, telephoning a friend). The other strategy involves asking patients to focus on the urge to eat and recognize that it is a temporary phenomenon and one on which they do not need to act. This latter strategy is a difficult one for most patients, especially in the early stages of treatment.

Involving Significant Others

CBT-E was developed as an individual treatment for adults and hence it does not actively involve others. Despite this, it is our practice to see "significant others" if this is likely to facilitate treatment and the patient is willing for this to happen. We do this with the aim of creating the optimum environment for the patient to change. There are two specific indications for involving others: (1) if they could be of help to the patient in making changes, and (2) if others are making it difficult for the patient to change (e.g., by commenting adversely on his/her appearance or eating).

Typically the sessions with others last about 45 minutes and take place immediately after a routine one. Generally the meeting involves the following, as agreed with the patient beforehand: (1) an introduction by the clinician and a statement about the aims of the meeting; (2) an explanation by the patient of the treatment rationale and what he/she is currently trying to do; (3) listening to the point of view of the significant other(s) and answering his/her questions; and (4) discussing how the significant other(s) could be of practical help to the patient (e.g., by responding to requests for help when the patient is having difficulty coping with urges to eat between planned meals and snacks). We hold up to three such sessions with about three-quarters of our patients and significant other(s).

Stage 2

Stage 2 is a transitional stage in treatment that has three aims: to conduct a joint review of progress; to revise the formulation, if needed; and to design Stage 3. At the same time the clinician continues to implement the procedures introduced in Stage 1. Sessions are now once weekly.

There is strong evidence across a variety of psychiatric disorders, including BN (Agras, Crow, et al., 2000a; Fairburn, Agras, Walsh, Wilson, & Stice, 2004), that the amount that the patient changes during the first few weeks of treatment is a potent predictor of outcome. Thus if the patient makes limited progress in Stage 1, this needs to be recognized early on and its explanation sought so that treatment can be adjusted to overcome the identified obstacle(s). The review of progress is best done systematically, with the patient once again completing the EDE-Q. In addition, the patient and clinician should consider the degree to which the patient has been complying with the various elements of treatment.

One important possible reason for progress not being as great as might be expected is the presence of a clinical depression. As noted earlier, ideally such depressions should be detected and treated before treatment is started, but inevitably some are missed and others develop afresh. If there appears to be a clinical depression it is our practice to treat it with antidepressant medication and consider suspending CBT until the patient has responded (Fairburn, Cooper, & Waller, 2008a).

It is also important to review the formulation in light of what has been learned during Stage 1. For example, it may have emerged that mood intolerance is a major factor contributing to the patient's binge eating. It is at this point that the decision about whether to use the broad form of CBT-E is made, based on the apparent contribution of the four additional maintaining mechanisms (i.e., mood intolerance, clinical perfectionism, core low self-esteem, and major interpersonal difficulties).

Lastly, it is at this stage that the clinician designs Stage 3 by deciding which strategies and procedures will be most relevant to the patient and in what order they should be implemented. Guidance for doing so is provided in the full treatment guide.

Stage 3

This is the main part of treatment, and its exact form differs substantially from patient to patient. The focus is on the mechanisms that are maintaining the particular patient's eating disorder. In the majority of cases these can be conceptualized under five broad headings:

1. The overevaluation of shape and weight and its various expressions
2. Dietary restraint
3. Event- or mood-related changes in eating (including mood intolerance)
4. Undereating and being underweight
5. Clinical perfectionism, core low self-esteem, and major interpersonal difficulties

The first three are considered in turn; the fourth is beyond the scope of this chapter, as the emphasis is on typical cases of BN (it is described in the complete treatment guide; Fairburn, Cooper, Shafran, Bohn, Hawker, et al., 2008b). Limitations of space also prevent discussion of the fifth group of mechanisms. For details, see Fairburn, Cooper, Shafran, Bohn, and Hawker (2008a).

The order in which the various mechanisms are addressed depends in part upon their relative importance in maintaining the patient's psychopathology and in part on the length of time it typically takes to implement the interventions. It is often best to begin by addressing the overconcern with shape and weight, as this psychopathology is complex and time consuming to tackle, and then add further strategies and procedures as needed. While doing this the clinician continues to implement the procedures introduced in Stage 1 and reinforces them, as needed.

Addressing the Overevaluation of Shape and Weight

At the heart of most EDs is the distinctive "core psychopathology": the overevaluation of shape and weight, that is, the judging of self-worth largely, or even exclusively, in terms of shape and weight and the ability to control them. As described earlier, most other features of these disorders appear to be secondary to this psychopathology and its consequences. Clinical experience and research evidence suggest that unless this psychopathology is successfully addressed, patients are at substantial risk of relapse. It is therefore a major target of treatment for all patients with an ED. Clinicians sometimes assume that it is understandable for overweight patients to dislike their appearance and that therefore weight and shape concerns do not need to be addressed. This is not the case. The strategies and procedures for tackling the overevaluation of shape and weight described below are also relevant to patients who are overweight (Fairburn, Cooper, Shafran, Bohn, Hawker, et al., 2008b; for further information on addressing shape concerns in people with obesity, see Cooper, Fairburn, & Hawker, 2003). The five main elements in tackling overevaluation of weight and shape are:

1. Identifying the overevaluation and its consequences
2. Developing marginalized self-evaluative domains
3. Addressing body checking and avoidance
4. Addressing "feeling fat"
5. Exploring the origins of the overevaluation
6. Learning to control the ED mindset

Other than the initial element, they are not necessarily introduced in this order.

Identifying the Overevaluation and Its Consequences

The starting point is educating patients about the notion of self-evaluation and helping them to identify their scheme for self-evaluation. The implications of this scheme are discussed, and a plan for addressing the expressions of the overevaluation is devised.

As clinicians are often unsure how to broach the subject of self-evaluation, an illustrative dialogue is provided below (Fairburn, Cooper, Shafran, Bohn, Hawker, et al., 2008b):

CLINICIAN: We've decided that today we are going to focus primarily on your shape concerns. I'd like to go back to why we are doing this. If we look back at our diagram showing the things that are keeping your eating problem going (*referring to the patient's formulation*), you can see that at the top are your concerns about your shape and weight. Clearly we need to focus on them, since they seem important in keeping the problem going and since they really worry you.

PATIENT: Yes, my shape really bothers me—the fact that I can't get it off my mind—and the fact that it is so awful ...

CLINICIAN: Well, to start with, we need to talk about the way we all evaluate or judge ourselves, something most of us don't even think about. We all have a way of judging ourselves and, if we are meeting our personal standards in this respect, we feel reasonably good about ourselves, whereas if we are not, we feel bad. So if we take a typical person, there will be various things that he or she will judge himself or herself by. For example, relationships with others are often important—say, one's relationships with one's parents (and children, if one has some) and one's relationships with friends. Other things may be how one is getting on at work and at important pastimes—say, sports or singing, music, cooking, or other things. And appearance may be important also. If things are going well in these areas of life, one feels fine about oneself, but if they are not, one feels bad. If one feels really bad when an aspect of life is not going well, this strongly suggests that this aspect is important to one's self-evaluation. Does that make sense?

PATIENT: Yes, I think so. The way I look, for example, it makes me feel really bad. I won't go out some days.

CLINICIAN: Exactly. So this indicates that your appearance is very important in how you see, or judge, yourself. A good way of representing all this is to draw a pie chart, with the various slices representing the various aspects of life that are important in the way you judge yourself, and the bigger the slice the more important that aspect is. Let me show you. (*Sketches out a "balanced" pie chart showing a number of "slices" of varying sizes, including areas such as work, family, friends, sports, and shape and weight [Figure 14.4].*)

CLINICIAN: Now what I would like us to do together is to try to draw your pie chart. What we first need to do is list the things that are important in the way you judge, or evaluate, yourself. What might they be?

The clinician and patient then generate a list of areas of life that are important and rank their relative importance. Using these rankings, a preliminary pie chart is drawn with the size of each slice representing the importance of that area in the patient's scheme for self-evaluation. A typical "unbalanced" pie chart is shown in Figure 14.5, illustrating that the pie charts of patients with EDs are typically dominated by their overevaluation of shape and appearance.

As homework, patients are asked to review their pie chart on several occasions over the next week or so in order that it can be discussed further and adjusted as needed. Generally, any revision involves expanding the size of the slice representing the contribution of shape and weight.

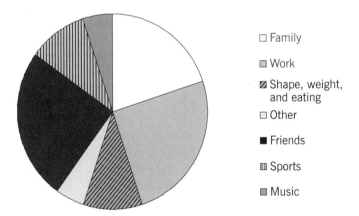

FIGURE 14.4. A pie chart of a young woman without an eating problem. From Fairburn, Cooper, Shafran, Bohn, Hawker, et al. (2008b). Copyright 2008 by The Guilford Press. Reprinted by permission.

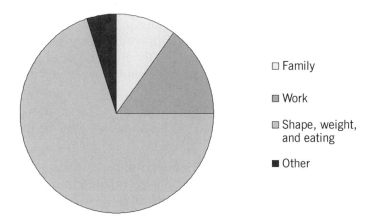

□ Family

▨ Work

▨ Shape, weight, and eating

■ Other

FIGURE 14.5. A pie chart representing a patient's overevaluation of control over shape, weight, and eating. From Fairburn, Cooper, Shafran, Bohn, Hawker, et al. (2008b). Copyright 2008 by The Guilford Press. Reprinted by permission.

The next step involves a discussion of the problems inherent in the patient's scheme for self-evaluation. There are three main problems:

1. Having a pie chart with a dominant slice is risky because self-evaluation is largely dependent upon one just aspect of life. Therefore, if difficulties are present or arise in this domain, self-esteem is likely to be substantially undermined.
2. Judging oneself largely on the basis of appearance is also problematic. Success in this area of life is elusive, and apparent failure is ever present due both to the effects of body checking and "feeling fat" (discussed below) and because shape and weight are only controllable to a limited extent.
3. Judging oneself in this way may lead to behavior that is unhelpful or even harmful, for example, repeated self-induced vomiting.

This discussion leads naturally to the creation of a new "extended" formulation that includes the consequences of the overevaluation (Figure 14.6). The clinician elicits this by asking patients what they do, or experience, as a result of the importance they place on shape and appearance and adds the upward feedback arrows explaining their role in maintaining the overevaluation (described below).

In collaboration with the patient, the clinician then devises a plan for addressing the overconcern about shape and weight. There are two overarching strategies:

1. Developing other domains for self-evaluation
2. Reducing the importance attached to shape and weight

Both are important and complement each another.

Developing Marginalized Domains for Self-Evaluation

Tackling the expressions of the overevaluation of shape and weight will gradually reduce the extent of the overevaluation, and the shape- and weight-related slice of the

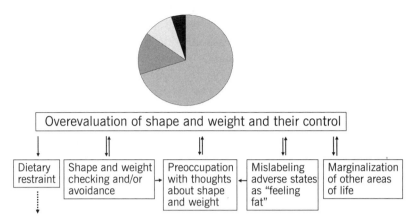

FIGURE 14.6. The overevaluation of control over shape and weight: An "extended formulation." From Fairburn, Cooper, Shafran, Bohn, Hawker, et al. (2008b).

pie chart will begin to shrink. At the same time, it is important to do the corollary: Increase the number and importance of other domains for self-evaluation to further diminish the relative importance placed on shape and weight. The goal is for patients to begin to get actively engaged in other aspects of life. This is done by explaining the rationale to patients, encouraging them to identify and engage in new activities (preferably social in nature), and subsequently to persist in their involvement with them. An active problem-solving approach is used (see below).

Simultaneously, the clinician directly targets the patient's overevaluation of shape and weight, often starting with body checking because this tends to be of central importance in maintaining the patient's concerns.

Addressing Body Checking

The importance of body checking and avoidance has only recently been appreciated. The reason is quite simple: Few clinicians were aware of it because patients do not disclose the behavior unless asked, and many patients are not fully aware of it.

The first step in addressing this is to provide information about body checking and avoidance and their consequences, stressing the following two points:

1. Most people check their body, to some extent, but many people with eating problems repeatedly check their bodies and may do so in unusual ways. Patients may not be immediately aware of such checking, but nevertheless it can serve to maintain dissatisfaction with shape and weight.
2. Some people with eating problems avoid seeing their bodies and also dislike other people seeing them. Body avoidance is also problematic because it allows concerns and fears about shape and appearance to persist in the absence of any information about actual appearance.

Using an adaptation of the usual monitoring record with an extra "body checking" column, patients are asked to record body checking for two 24-hour periods, one being a working day and one being a nonworking day. Because this form of recording may be distressing for patients, they are only asked to do it on two occasions, and they are forewarned that they may find it upsetting.

The various forms of body checking that are identified are divided into two groups: forms of behavior that are best stopped, and behavior that needs to be adjusted (principally, mirror use). In addition, the clinician discusses comparison making.

Behavior That Is Best Stopped. Most forms of body checking are best stopped altogether. Patients can usually stop such behavior, or phase it out, if the rationale is explained and they are provided with support. The points to emphasize are as follows:

- Rarely does one feel better after body checking, since one is focusing on aspects of one's appearance that one dislikes. Body checking also maintains preoccupation with shape and weight.
- Stopping body checking is generally experienced (after a week or so) as a relief.

Mirror Use. A different strategy needs to be adopted with mirror use. Here the problem is the way that the checking is done, patients' interpretation of what they find, and the frequency of the checking. The clinician needs to help patients consider the following questions each time that they are about to check themselves:

- What am I trying to find out?
- Do I need to find this out now?
- Can I find it out in this way?
- Might there be adverse effects from checking in this way?
- Is there a better alternative?

Mirror use deserves particular attention because mirrors have the potential to provide misleading, but highly credible, information, and it is likely that they play an important role in the maintenance of many patients' body dissatisfaction. The main point to stress is that, as with other forms of body checking, what one finds depends, to an extent, on how one checks (or looks in the mirror). Detailed scrutiny, especially of perceived defects, is prone to magnify these apparent flaws. Patients therefore need to question their use of mirrors. Mirrors are useful for applying makeup, arranging hair, and, for men, shaving, and full-length mirrors provide information about whether clothes go well together, but it could be argued that there are few reasons to scrutinize oneself (check one's body) in a full-length mirror, particularly when naked. This is not to recommend that patients engage in total avoidance; rather, the advice is (at least for the meantime) to restrict the use of mirrors to the purposes listed above.

Comparison Making. Another form of body checking that actively maintains dissatisfaction with shape involves making comparisons with other people. The nature of these comparisons generally results in patients' concluding that their bodies are large and unattractive. As noted above, patients' appraisal of their own shape often involves scrutiny and selective attention to supposed flaws. In contrast, patients' assessment of others is very different, as they tend to make more superficial and less critical judgments. Furthermore, when making comparisons they tend to compare themselves with people who are particularly thin or attractive. The steps involved in addressing comparison making are as follows:

1. The clinician helps the patient identify when and how such comparisons are made.
2. The clinician and patient explore whether these comparisons are inherently biased in terms of both the chosen subject of the comparison (e.g., an attractive, thin person) and how the comparison was made (typically, a superficial uncritical appraisal).
3. The clinician sets relevant homework tasks; for example, patients may be asked:
   • To experiment with being less biased when choosing someone with whom to compare themselves.
   • To scrutinize other people's bodies (e.g., in changing rooms), with the goal of recognizing the point that "What you see depends (to an extent) on how you look."
4. The clinician helps the patient explore the implications of the bias inherent in his/her comparison making in terms of the validity of the patient's views about his/her appearance. The goal is that patients become aware that their comparison making has yielded misleading information about other peoples' bodies in relation to their own and that they stop making these kinds of comparisons.

Addressing Body Avoidance

Some patients avoid seeing all or parts of their bodies. Clinicians need to help these patients get used to the sight and feel of their bodies, to be less sensitive to being seen by others, and to learn to make evenhanded comparisons with others. Dressing and undressing in the dark will need to be phased out, and patients should stop wearing baggy, shape-disguising clothes. Participation in activities that involve a degree of body exposure can be helpful, for example, swimming. Clinicians should be aware that there is a risk that patients will switch over to repeated body checking.

Addressing "Feeling Fat"

"Feeling fat" is an experience widely reported by women, but the intensity and frequency of this feeling appears to be greater among people with EDs. Since feeling fat tends to be equated with *being* fat, it is an important target for treatment. It tends to fluctuate markedly from day to day, and even within the day, and should be distinguished from the relatively more stable body dissatisfaction (to which it contributes) experienced by almost all those with an ED. It is our impression that feeling fat is a result of mislabeling certain emotions and bodily experiences. It is important to note that "feeling fat" and "being fat" are quite different, even though they can co-occur.

In general, it is best to address feeling fat once the patient has begun to make progress with body checking and avoidance, unless it is a particularly prominent feature—in which case the order may be reversed. The steps in addressing feeling fat are as follows:

1. The clinician explains that this phenomenon may mask other feelings or sensations that are occurring at the same time and stresses that it is important not to equate feeling fat with being fat. The clinician points out that while feelings of fatness fluctuate, body shape barely changes within such a short time frame. This suggests that something else must be responsible for the fluctuations in the feelings of fatness.

2. Patients are asked to monitor particularly intense feelings of fatness together with what else they are feeling at the time.

3. Each recorded occurrence of feeling fat is reviewed in terms of the context in which it occurred and the presence of any potentially masked feelings or sensations.

4. Over a few sessions the patient should become better at identifying the accompanying feelings and experiences and their triggers, and it should become clear that the patient's experience of feeling fat tends to be triggered either by the occurrence of certain negative mood states or by physical sensations that heighten body awareness. Examples of these two types of stimulus include:

- Feeling bored, depressed, lonely, or tired
- Feeling full, bloated, sweaty; feeling one's body wobble or thighs rub together; clothing feeling tight

5. Eventually patients should attempt to identify these triggers in real time and promptly address them (e.g., feeling bored) using the problem-solving approach (see below).

Addressing feeling fat typically takes many weeks. Generally, its frequency and intensity decline and patients' "relationship" to the experience alters such that it is no longer equated with being fat. This metacognitive change is important, since once it is achieved, the experience of feeling fat ceases to maintain body dissatisfaction.

Exploring the Origins of the Overevaluation of Shape and Weight

Toward the end of Stage 3 it is helpful to explore the origins of the patient's sensitivity to shape, weight, and eating. This exploration can help make sense of how the problem developed and evolved, and it can highlight how it might have served a useful function in its early stages—for example, exerting strict dietary control gives some people a sense of self-control in circumstances where they feel powerless. Occasionally specific events are identified that appear to have played a critical role in the development of the eating problem, such as the patient having been humiliated about his/her appearance. In such instances the clinician needs to help the patient reappraise the critical event from the vantage point of the present.

Learning to Control the ED Mindset

The core psychopathology of EDs may be viewed as a "mindset" or a frame of mind that has multiple effects. For example:

- It leads patients to filter external and internal stimuli in a distinctive way (e.g., preferentially noticing thin people of the same gender; interpreting clothing being tight as evidence of fatness).
- It results in the characteristic forms of behavior seen in people with EDs (e.g.,

rigid and extreme dieting, self-induced vomiting, laxative misuse, driven exercising).
- It results in the mislabeling of various physical and emotional experiences as
"feeling fat."

These consequences of the ED mindset tend to reinforce it through the mechanisms
described in the formulation and its expanded form (see above). As a result the mindset becomes "locked in place." The cognitive-behavioral strategies used in CBT-E are
designed to address the key features of the ED and the processes that are maintaining them. Thus as treatment progresses the mechanisms that have been holding the
ED mindset in place are gradually eroded and healthier and situationally appropriate
mindsets replace it. At first this happens only transitorily, but in patients who are making good progress, these periods free from the ED mindset become more frequent and
prolonged. The first signs are often reported spontaneously: For example, patients may
describe (sometimes with surprise) that they were able to eat out with no difficulty or
that they could watch a film without worrying about what they had eaten.

Once there are signs that the mindset is being displaced, patients should learn
about this phenomenon because they can be taught to influence it. When introducing
the topic, an analogy that we find useful is to compare the mind to a DVD player, suggesting that people with eating problems have an "ED DVD" that tends to get locked
into place so that it plays, whatever the circumstances. Most patients relate to this type
of explanation, especially in the later stages of treatment when their ED mindset is
liable to be displaced at times. Another way to raise the topic is to capitalize on a recent
setback (if there has been one), as this will typically have been preceded by the mindset
(ED DVD) coming back into place.

Having introduced the topic, the clinician should explain that now their ED mindset (DVD) is no longer permanently locked in place by the ED-maintaining mechanisms, they are in a position to influence whether or not they play it. More specifically,
they can learn to:

1. Identify potential stimuli that are likely to put the ED mindset back in place.
2. Recognize the first signs (the first track on the DVD) that their ED mindset is in
   place.
3. Displace the mindset (i.e., press the "eject" button).

It is not possible for patients to do these things earlier in treatment when their ED
mindset is firmly in place, as they have no other state with which to contrast it. Details
of the procedure are provided in the full treatment guide.

Addressing Dietary Restraint

A major goal of treatment is to reduce, if not eliminate altogether, the strong tendency
of these patients to diet. As noted earlier, this dieting has two aspects: attempts to limit
eating ("dietary restraint") and actual undereating in physiological terms ("dietary
restriction"). The latter always coexists with the former, whereas the opposite is not the
case. Dietary restriction may occur only during parts of the day—typically the first half,
as a result of delaying eating until late in the day—or there may be sustained undereat-

ing with the result that the patient loses weight. The "regular eating" intervention of Stage 1 addresses the former ("delayed eating"). Addressing sustained dietary restriction (which is not generally a major issue in the treatment of BN) is described in the full treatment guide.

The dietary restraint of patients with BN is usually manifested as multiple demanding rules concerning when to eat, how much to eat, and what to eat. The result is that patients' eating is inflexible and restricted in nature. Nevertheless, patients value dietary restraint and tend to be oblivious to its adverse effects. The main adverse effects that need to be brought to their attention are:

- It is a major cause of preoccupation with thoughts about food and eating.
- It restricts the ways in which patients can eat, often preventing them from eating with others and eating outside the home.
- It is a major contributory factor to binge eating.
- It may result in dietary restriction, which in turn may lead to weight loss or the maintenance of an unduly low weight.

Once it has been agreed that dietary restraint needs to be tackled, the clinician and patient identify the various dietary rules to which the patient is adhering. In each case the clinician needs to identify the exact nature of the rule and the concerns that are driving it. The patient should then be helped to practice breaking the rule, possibly in the form of behavioral experiments designed to test the concern in question. For example, many patients believe that eating certain foods will inevitably lead them to binge-eat. This belief can be disconfirmed by asking patients to introduce these foods into their planned meals or snacks on days when they are feeling in control over their eating and are capable of resisting binge eating. (They do not need to eat much of the avoided food, as eating even a small quantity will break the dietary rule.) By doing this repeatedly, patients learn that the feared consequence is not an inevitable result of breaking the rule. This has the effect of undermining and eroding the rule, thereby allowing the patient's eating to become more flexible.

For patients with BN it is important to pay particular attention to "food avoidance." Patients should be asked to identify the foods that they are avoiding and to then progressively introduce them into their diet, starting with the easiest and moving on to the most difficult. A good way of gaining a comprehensive list of patients' avoided foods is to ask them to visit a local supermarket and note down all foods that they would be reluctant to eat because of feared effects on their shape or weight or because they think that the food might trigger a binge.

A small number of patients may find it impossible to break their dietary rules without binge eating or purging afterward. With such patients some form of clinician-assisted exposure may be helpful.

Addressing Event- and Mood-Related Changes in Eating

Among patients with EDs eating habits may change in response to outside events and changes in mood. The change may involve eating less, stopping eating altogether, overeating, or frank binge eating (subjective or objective). A variety of different mechanisms may be involved, including the following:

- Patients may eat less or stop eating to gain a sense of personal control when external events feel outside their control; this is seen most often in underweight patients.
- Patients may eat less to influence others; for example, it may be a way of exhibiting feelings of distress or anger, or it may be an act of defiance.
- Overeating may be used by patients as a way of giving themselves a "treat" when they feel that they deserve one; this tends to be most characteristic of overweight patients.
- Binge eating may occur in response to adverse events and associated changes in mood. Binge eating has two properties that help people cope with negative events: (1) the act of binge eating is distracting, and (2) it has a direct mood-modulatory effect in that it dampens strong mood states, possibly because it is somewhat sedating. Often both mechanisms operate in tandem.

If event- or mood-related changes in eating persist into Stage 3, they should be directly addressed. Such changes should be identified through the use of real-time recording, with the clinician helping the patient understand the processes involved. Depending upon what appear to be the main mechanisms operating, the clinician will generally focus on one or more of the following:

- Enhancing patients' ability to deal with, and ideally forestall, day-to-day problems by training them in proactive problem solving.
- Helping patients accept the triggering moods states by introducing the notion that they do not necessarily have to be neutralized.
- Identifying ways in which patients can modulate their mood that do not do them harm (unlike binge eating, substance misuse, or self-harm).

Problem Solving

The patient should be taught how to use proactive problem solving to avoid event-triggered changes in eating. We do this with reference to the relevant section from *Overcoming Binge Eating*. The clinician explains that while many problems may seem overwhelming at first, if they are approached systematically, they usually turn out to be manageable or even preventable. By becoming effective problem solvers most patients can successfully tackle day-to-day events of the type that that have disrupted their eating in the past. Effective problem solving involves the following commonsense steps:

- *Step 1: Identifying the problem as early as possible.* Spotting problems early is of great importance. Almost invariably problems are easier to address if they are caught early on.
- *Step 2: Specifying the problem accurately.* Working out the true nature of the problem is essential if the best solution is to be found. Doing so may lead to the realization that there are two or more coexisting problems, in which case each should be addressed individually. Rephrasing the problem is often helpful.
- *Step 3: Considering as many solutions as possible.* All ways of dealing with the problem should be considered. The patient should generate as many potential solutions as possible. Some solutions may seem nonsensical or impractical. Nevertheless,

they should be included in the list of possible alternatives. The more solutions that are generated, the more likely a good one will emerge.

- *Step 4: Thinking through the implications of each solution.* The likely effectiveness and feasibility of each solution should be considered.
- *Step 5: Choosing the best solution or combination of solutions.* Interestingly, if Step 4 has been thorough, choosing the best solution (or combination of solutions) is usually a straightforward matter.
- *Step 6: Acting on the solution.*

The clinician and patient should go through a recent problem using the six problem-solving steps. This should be a collaborative endeavor, with patients being encouraged to take the lead whenever possible. As homework, patients should be asked to practice their problem-solving skills. More specifically, over the following week patients should identify events of the type that would be liable to trigger changes in their eating (especially binge eating) and address them using the problem-solving procedure. In each case they should review their attempt at problem solving the following day. The aim of this review is for patients to focus not on whether the problem was successfully solved but rather on enhancing their problem-solving skills. By becoming effective problem solvers, most patients can successfully tackle events of the type that have disrupted their eating in the past.

Binge Analysis

This procedure is used to address any residual binges. It involves identifying, in real time, the mechanisms contributing to each remaining binge. To start, the clinician explains that binges do not occur spontaneously; rather they are the product of four well-defined processes:

1. Breaking a dietary rule and reacting by temporarily abandoning dietary restraint.
2. Being disinhibited by alcohol or other psychoactive substance and therefore being unable to maintain dietary restraint.
3. Undereating and being under physiological and psychological pressure to eat.
4. Reacting to an adverse event or mood.

Once these mechanisms have been discussed, patients should be asked to conduct a "binge analysis" immediately after any binge, the goal being for them to consider which of these four mechanisms contributed to the binge and what can be learned as a result. This strategy reinforces those treatment procedures that are of most relevance to the elimination of the remaining binges, and it results in patients gaining from each of their binges rather than being simply demoralized by them.

Addressing Mood Intolerance

There is a subgroup of patients whose eating is markedly influenced by their mood. These patients are either extremely sensitive to certain mood states and have difficulty tolerating them, or they experience unusually intense moods, or both. This is termed "mood intolerance." Generally the moods in question are adverse moods, but this is not invariably the case. Patients may be sensitive to any intense mood, including, for example, excitement. This sensitivity leads them to engage in forms of behavior ("mood modulatory behavior") that help them cope either by reducing their awareness of the moods or by neutralizing them. Self-harm in the form of cutting is a common example, but binge eating, vomiting, and overexercising are others. In these patients aspects of the ED are therefore maintained by mechanisms "external" to the core ED, and treatment may therefore have to directly address these additional maintaining mechanisms.

The patients for whom these strategies and procedures are most relevant are best identified in Stage 2 when reviewing progress. By then it is generally clear that some of their ED behavior is being maintained by mood sensitivity. A clue is a history of dysfunctional mood modulatory behavior, such as self-injury or self-medication with psychoactive substances.

This aspect of treatment was originally one element of the broad form of CBT-E, but subsequent experience has shown that it can be readily and appropriately incorporated within the main focused version of the treatment. The approach overlaps with elements of dialectical behavior therapy (Linehan, 1993) and is described in detail in the full treatment guide.

Stage 4

This is the final stage in treatment, comprising three sessions over 5 weeks (i.e., the sessions are 2 weeks apart). It has two broad aims:

1. To ensure that the changes made in treatment are maintained
2. To minimize the risk of relapse in the future

At the same time patients discontinue self-monitoring and transfer from in-session weighing to weighing themselves at home.

Ensuring That the Changes are Maintained

The first step is to review in detail the patient's progress and identify problems that remain. This can be done in much the same way as in Stage 2, using the EDE-Q and CIA as a guide. On the basis of this review the clinician and patient jointly devise a specific plan for the patient to follow over the following 5 months (i.e., until the post-treatment review appointment, discussed below). Typically this includes further work on body checking, food avoidance, and perhaps further practice at problem solving. In addition, patients should be encouraged to continue developing new interests and activities.

Minimizing the Risk of Relapse in the Future

Our emerging experience with CBT-E (with over 300 patients) suggests that full-scale relapse is uncommon but that setbacks do occur, and it is important that they are dealt with effectively.

Relapse is not an all-or-nothing phenomenon. It occurs in degrees, often starting as a "lapse" that then escalates. Commonly the lapse involves the resumption of some form of dietary restraint, possibly triggered by an adverse shape-related event (e.g., a critical comment, clothes feeling tighter than usual). This return of dietary restraint may then lead to an episode of binge eating, which in turn will encourage further dietary restraint, thereby increasing the risk of further episodes of binge eating. The patient's response to this sequence of events is crucial because what started as a lapse can develop rapidly into a full-scale relapse.

To minimize the risk of relapse the clinician needs to do the following:

1. Educate the patient about the risk of relapse, highlighting common triggers and the likely sequence of events in the patient's case. The prior work with mindsets (DVDs) is crucial in this regard.
2. Stress the importance of detecting problems early, before they become entrenched. The clinician and patient should identify likely early warning signs of an impending relapse.
3. Construct with the patient a plan of action (a written personalized "maintenance plan") for use in the future should a problem arise. This plan should have two elements to it: it should focus (1) on the emerging eating problem and how to correct it, and (2) on how to address the trigger of the setback.
4. Discuss with the patient when it is appropriate to seek further help. We generally recommend that if the problem has not substantially resolved within 3 weeks, patients seek outside help.

Ending Treatment

It is unusual not to end CBT-E as planned. As long as patients have gotten to the point where the main maintaining mechanisms have been disrupted, then treatment can and should finish. Otherwise, patients (and clinicians) are at risk of ascribing continuing improvement to the ongoing therapy rather than the resolution of the disorder. In practice this means that it is acceptable to end treatment with patients still dieting to an extent, perhaps binge eating and vomiting on occasions, and having residual concerns about shape and weight.

At times there are grounds for extending treatment. In our view the main indication for doing this is the presence of ED features that are continuing to interfere significantly with the patient's functioning and are unlikely to resolve of their own accord. Another reason to extend treatment is to compensate for the deleterious impact of disruptions to treatment, generally due to the emergence of a clinical depression or the occurrence of a life crisis. The occasional patient benefits little from CBT-E. It is our practice to refer such patients for day or inpatient treatment.

The Posttreatment Review Appointment

We routinely hold a posttreatment review appointment about 20 weeks after the completion of treatment. During the intervening period patients do not receive any further therapeutic input. Instead, the intention is that they implement the agreed-upon short-term plan to maintain and consolidate the changes made in treatment and that they use strategies identified in their maintenance plan to address any setbacks.

In most cases we find that patients are managing well, that the changes made in treatment have been maintained, and that patients report having had only minor setbacks.

Concluding Remarks

A major challenge in developing evidence-based treatments is to balance the clinically appealing flexibility achieved with treatments based on an analysis of the individual patient's difficulties with the more structured and specified style of manual-based treatments. CBT-E attempts to strike this balance. While utilizing a range of well-specified treatment strategies and procedures, its exact form differs from patient to patient because it depends on a highly personalized case formulation. CBT-E is a treatment that is designed to fit the individual patient's psychopathology; it is not a treatment for a DSM diagnosis. And, as was noted at the outset of this chapter, CBT-E is a treatment for *all* forms of ED psychopathology, not just that seen in BN.

As for future developments, at least three important challenges remain. Two of these concern the treatment itself. First, the treatment needs to be made more effective. Despite its successes, CBT-E does not help everyone. There is a need to understand why certain patients do not benefit in order to improve the treatment further. The second related challenge is to better understand how the treatment works. Knowledge of its active ingredients would provide the basis for further enhancing these elements while omitting redundant ones. It might also suggest ways to simplify the treatment, more generally, or in certain cases. The third challenge concerns the dissemination of the treatment. There is a pressing need to determine how this might best be achieved.

Acknowledgments

A substantial proportion of this chapter has been reproduced from sections of the complete description of CBT-E (Fairburn, 2008a). Copyright 2008 by The Guilford Press. Adapted by permission. We are grateful to the Wellcome Trust for its support: Christopher G. Fairburn is supported by a Principal Research Fellowship (No. 046386), and Zafra Cooper is supported by a program grant (No. 046386).

References

Agras WS, Crow SJ, Halmi KA, Mitchell JE, Wilson GT, & Kraemer HC. (2000). Outcome predictors for the cognitive behavior treatment of bulimia nervosa: Data from a multisite study. *American Journal of Psychiatry,* 157:1302–1308.

Agras WS, Walsh BT, Fairburn CG, Wilson GT, & Kraemer HC. (2000). A multicenter comparison of cognitive-behavioral therapy and interpersonal psychotherapy for bulimia nervosa. *Archives of General Psychiatry,* 5:459–466.

Bohn K, Doll HA, Cooper Z, O'Connor M, Palmer RL, & Fairburn CG. (2008). The measurement of impairment due to eating disorder psychopathology. *Behavior Research and Therapy,* 46:1105–1110.

Bohn K, & Fairburn CG. (2008). Clinical Impairment Assessment questionnaire. In CG Fairburn (Ed.), *Cognitive behavior therapy and eating disorders* (pp. 315–318). New York: Guilford Press.

Cooper Z, Fairburn CG, & Hawker DM. (2003). *Cognitive-behavioral treatment of obesity: A clinician's guide.* New York: Guilford Press.

Fairburn CG. (1995). *Overcoming binge eating.* New York: Guilford Press.

Fairburn CG. (2008a). *Cognitive behavior therapy and eating disorders.* New York: Guilford Press.

Fairburn CG. (2008b). Eating disorders: The transdiagnostic view and the cognitive behavioral theory. In CG Fairburn (Ed.), *Cognitive behavior therapy and eating disorders* (pp. 7–22). New York: Guilford Press.

Fairburn CG, Agras WS, Walsh BT, Wilson GT, & Stice E. (2004). Prediction of outcome in bulimia nervosa by early change in treatment. *American Journal of Psychiatry*, 16:2322–2324.

Fairburn CG, & Beglin, S. (2008). Eating Disorder Examination Questionnaire. In CG Fairburn (Ed.), *Cognitive behavior therapy and eating disorders* (pp. 309–314). New York: Guilford Press.

Fairburn CG, Cooper Z, Doll HA, O'Connor ME, Bohn K, Hawker DM, et al. (2009). Transdiagnostic cognitive behavior therapy for patients with eating disorders: A two-site trial with 60-week follow-up. *American Journal of Psychiatry*, 166:311–319.

Fairburn CG, Cooper Z, & Shafran R. (2003). Cognitive behaviour therapy for eating disorders: A "transdiagnostic" theory and treatment. *Behavior Research and Therapy*, 4:509–528.

Fairburn CG, Cooper Z, & Shafran R. (2008). Enhanced cognitive behavior therapy for eating disorders: An overview. In CG Fairburn (Ed.), *Cognitive behavior therapy and eating disorders* (pp. 23–34). New York: Guilford Press.

Fairburn CG, Cooper Z, Shafran R, Bohn K, & Hawker D. (2008a). Clinical perfectionism, core low self-esteem, and interpersonal problems. In CG Fairburn (Ed.), *Cognitive behavior therapy and eating disorders* (pp. 197–220). New York: Guilford Press.

Fairburn CG, Cooper Z, Shafran R, Bohn K, Hawker DM, Murphy R, et al. (2008b). Enhanced cognitive behavior therapy for eating disorders: The core protocol. In CG Fairburn (Ed.), *Cognitive behavior therapy and eating disorders* (pp. 47–193). New York: Guilford Press.

Fairburn CG, Cooper Z, & Waller D. (2008a). "Complex cases" and comorbidity. In CG Fairburn (Ed.), *Cognitive behavior therapy and eating disorders* (pp. 245–258). New York: Guilford Press.

Fairburn CG, Cooper Z, & Waller D. (2008b). The patients: Their assessment, preparation for treatment and medical management. In CG Fairburn (Ed.), *Cognitive behavior therapy and eating disorders* (pp. 35–44). New York: Guilford Press.

Fairburn CG, Marcus MD, & Wilson GT. (1993). Cognitive behavior therapy for binge eating and bulimia nervosa: A comprehensive treatment manual. In CG Fairburn & GT Wilson (Eds.), *Binge eating: Nature, assessment and treatment.* New York: Guilford Press.

Linehan MM. (1993). *Cognitive-behavioral treatment of borderline personality disorder.* New York: Guilford Press.

National Collaborating Centre for Mental Health. (2004). *Eating disorders: Core interventions in the treatment and management of anorexia nervosa, bulimia nervosa and related eating disorders.* London: British Psychological Society and Royal College of Psychiatrists.

Shapiro J, Berkman ND, Brownley KA, Sedway JA, Lohr KN, & Bulik CM. (2007). Bulimia nervosa treatment: A systematic review of randomised controlled trials. *International Journal of Eating Disorders*, 40:321–336.

Vitousek KM, Watson S, & Wilson GT. (1998). Enhancing motivation for change in treatment-resistant eating disorders. *Clinical Psychology Review*, 1:391–420.

Wilson GT, Grilo CM, & Vitousek KM. (2007). Psychological treatment of eating disorders. *American Psychologist*, 62:199–216.

CHAPTER 15

Interpersonal Psychotherapy for Bulimia Nervosa and Binge-Eating Disorder

Marian Tanofsky-Kraff and Denise E. Wilfley

Interpersonal psychotherapy (IPT) was originally developed in the late 1960s by Gerald Klerman and colleagues (Klerman, Weissman, Rounsaville, & Chevron, 1984) for the treatment of unipolar depression. IPT is a brief, time-limited therapy that focuses on improving interpersonal functioning and, in turn, psychiatric symptoms, by relating symptoms to interpersonal problem areas and developing strategies for dealing with these problems (Freeman & Gil, 2004; Klerman et al., 1984). In the late 1980s, IPT was successfully modified for patients with BN (Fairburn et al., 1991; Fairburn, Peveler, Jones, Hope, & Doll, 1993) and shortly thereafter adapted into a group format for individuals with BED (Wilfley, Frank, Welch, Spurrell, & Rounsaville, 1998; Wilfley, MacKenzie, Welch, Ayres, & Weissman, 2000; Wilfley et al., 1993, 2002). IPT has been found to be an effective treatment for bulimia nervosa (BN) and binge-eating disorder (BED).

The present chapter reviews interpersonal theory and how it provides the foundation for IPT. The central role that interpersonal functioning plays in the development and manifestation of eating disorders (EDs) is discussed. Empirical evidence supporting the efficaciousness of IPT for the treatment of EDs is reviewed. The delivery of IPT for BN and BED are also explained, along with a description of the major tenets of the treatment and a novel adaptation of IPT for the prevention of obesity. Finally, we discuss how the delivery of IPT has been improved, and future directions are proposed.

Interpersonal Theory

IPT is grounded in theories developed independently by Meyer (1957), Sullivan (1953), and Bowlby (1982), which hypothesize that interpersonal function is a critical component of psychological adjustment and well-being. Meyer postulated that psychopathology was rooted in maladjustment to one's social environment (Frank & Spanier, 1995;

Klerman et al., 1984; Meyer, 1957). Sullivan theorized that a patient's interpersonal relationships, rather than intrapsychic processes alone, established the relevant focus of therapeutic attention (Sullivan, 1953). He believed that individuals could not be understood in isolation from their interpersonal relationships and posited that enduring patterns in these relationships could either encourage self-esteem or result in anxiety, hopelessness, and psychopathology. IPT is also associated with the work of Bowlby (1982), the originator of attachment theory. Bowlby emphasized the importance of early attachment in the later development of interpersonal relationships and emotional well-being, hypothesizing that failures in attachment resulted in later psychopathology.

The interpersonal roles of major interest to IPT occur within the nuclear family, the extended family, the friendship group, the work situation, and the neighborhood or community. IPT acknowledges a two-way relationship between social functioning and psychopathology: Disturbances in social roles can serve as antecedents for psychopathology, and mental illness can produce impairments in one's capacity to perform social roles (Bowlby, 1982). IPT is, therefore, derived from a theory in which interpersonal functioning is recognized as a critical component of psychological adjustment and well-being. It should be noted that IPT makes no assumptions about the causes of psychiatric illness; however, IPT does assume that the development and maintenance of some psychiatric illnesses occur in a social and interpersonal context and that the onset, response to treatment, and outcomes are influenced by the interpersonal relations between the patient and significant others. The major tenets of IPT for BN and BED are described in this chapter. The extensive empirical background and theoretical foundation, as well as the strategies and techniques of IPT, are fully described in a comprehensive book by Weissman, Markowitz, and Klerman (2000).

Interpersonal Functioning and EDs

A wealth of research has linked poor interpersonal functioning to EDs (Wilfley, Stein, & Welch, 2005). Individuals with BN and BED typically report past difficult social experiences, problematic family histories, and specific interpersonal stressors more often than non-eating-disordered individuals (Fairburn et al., 1997, 1998). Individuals with BN and BED also tend to experience a wide range of social problems, such as loneliness, lack of perceived social support, poor self-esteem and social adjustment, and difficulty with social problem-solving skills (Crow et al., 2002; Ghaderi & Scott, 1999; Grissett & Norvell, 1992; Gual et al., 2002; Johnson et al., 2001; O'Mahony & Hollwey, 1995; Rorty et al., 1999; Steiger et al., 1999; Troop et al., 1994; Wilfley et al., 2003). Heightened sensitivity to interpersonal interactions appears to be a common characteristic among individuals with bulimic tendencies (Evans & Wertheim, 1998; Humphrey, 1989; Steiger et al., 1999; Tasca et al., 2004; Troisi et al., 2005). Indeed, interactive paradigms suggest that interpersonal distress may trigger overeating (Steiger et al., 1999; Tanofsky-Kraff, Wilfley, & Spurrell, 2000) and potentially perpetuate binge eating. Furthermore, interpersonal difficulties, low self-esteem, and negative affect may be interconnected in a reciprocal fashion (Fairburn et al., 1997, 1998; Gual et al., 2002) and serve to perpetuate a cycle, each exacerbating the other and combining to precipitate and/or maintain dysfunctional bulimic or binge-eating patterns (Herzog, Keller, Lavori, & Ott, 1987). Therefore, the use of an interpersonally focused intervention appears to be especially suitable for the treatment of BN and BED and those with similar manifestations of these disorders. IPT is designed to improve interpersonal functioning and self-esteem, reduce negative affect, and, in turn, decrease ED symptoms.

Review of Outcome Studies
and Relevant Empirical Literature

IPT for BN

IPT has been shown to be effective for the treatment of BN. To date, cognitive-behavioral therapy (CBT) is currently the most researched, best established treatment for BN (Wilson, Grilo, & Vitousek, 2007). Nevertheless, IPT is the only psychological treatment for BN that has demonstrated long-term outcomes that are comparable to those of CBT (Wilson & Shafran, 2005). Currently, all *controlled* studies of IPT for BN have been comparison studies with CBT. Initially, similar short- and long-term outcomes for binge-eating remission between CBT and IPT were reported (Fairburn et al., 1993, 1995). In a subsequent multisite study (Agras, Walsh, Fairburn, Wilson, & Kraemer, 2000) comparing CBT and IPT as treatments for BN, in the short-term posttreatment, patients receiving CBT demonstrated higher rates of abstinence from binge eating and lower rates of purging. By 8- and 12-month follow-ups, however, patients receiving CBT tended to maintain their progress or slightly worsen, whereas patients receiving IPT experienced slight improvement such that the two treatments no longer differed significantly in their outcomes. The more impressive effect of CBT compared to IPT may be at least partially explained by a relative lack of focus on ED symptomatology in the research version of individual IPT for BN. Interestingly, IPT patients rated their treatment as more suitable and expected greater success than did CBT patients. Therefore, a potential advantage of IPT may be that many patients with BN perceive the interpersonal focus of IPT as particularly relevant to their ED and to their treatment needs, perhaps more so than a cognitive-behavioral focus on distortions related to weight and shape. Currently, IPT is considered an alternative to CBT for the treatment of BN (Wilson et al., 2007). Although, it has been recommended that clinicians inform patients of the slower response time for improvements compared to CBT (Wilson, 2005), our contention is that when IPT is delivered in a manner such that interpersonal problems are consistently linked to ED symptoms, response to treatment will likely occur more rapidly.

An emerging literature has provided some insight into predictors of success with IPT for the treatment of EDs. Chui, Safer, Bryson, Agras, and Wilson (2007) reported that although patients in the large multicenter trial responded with higher abstinence rates when randomized to CBT as opposed to IPT, African American participants showed greater reductions in binge-eating episode frequency when treated with IPT compared to CBT. This finding suggests that IPT may be particularly appropriate for African American women with BN, and speaks to the need for further study of IPT with different racial and ethnic groups. Since therapeutic alliance is associated with treatment outcome, researchers from this same study examined patient expectation of improvement (Constantino, Arnow, Blasey, & Agras, 2005). They found that expectation of improvement was positively associated with outcome for both CBT and IPT, emphasizing the important role of patient expectations in both treatments. Finally, in a study of postremission predictors of relapse, Keel and colleagues found that for women with BN, worse psychosocial functioning was associated with a greater risk for relapse, which, the authors posited, may partly help to explain the long-term effectiveness of IPT for BN (Keel, Dorer, Franko, Jackson, & Herzog, 2005).

IPT for BED

Based upon the initial success of IPT in BN (Fairburn et al., 1991), IPT for BED was developed. Wilfley and colleagues first adapted IPT to a group format for patients with BED (Wilfley et al., 1993, 2000). During their work, they found that a number of patients presented with chronically unfulfilling relationships that were well suited to be addressed in the group format. Therefore, new strategies were adapted to specifically address such interpersonal deficits. For example, in the current format of group IPT for BED, group members with interpersonal deficits are strongly encouraged to use the group as a "live" social network. This social milieu is designed to decrease social isolation, support the formation of new social relationships, and serve as a model for initiating and sustaining social relationships outside of the therapeutic context (Wilfley et al., 1998). Shame and self-stigmatization are common among patients with BED and may contribute to the maintenance of the disorder. By its very nature, group therapy offers a radically altered social environment for patients with BED, who typically keep shameful eating behaviors hidden from others.

IPT has demonstrated effectiveness in the treatment of BED. As in the case of CBT for BN, CBT for BED has been shown to have specific and robust treatment effects (Devlin et al., 2005; Grilo, Masheb, & Wilson, 2005; Kenardy, Mensch, Bowen, Green, & Walton, 2002; Nauta, Hospers, Kok, & Jansen, 2000; Ricca et al., 2001; Telch, Agras, Rossiter, Wilfley, & Kenardy, 1990; Wilfley et al., 1993). Two randomized trials have compared IPT with CBT and found that IPT has similar effects to CBT in the management of BED. The first study, comparing group CBT and IPT, revealed that both treatments were more effective than a wait-list control group at reducing binge eating and had similar significant reductions in binge eating in both the short and long term (Wilfley et al., 1993). In the second study, which included a substantially larger sample size, both CBT and IPT demonstrated equivalent short- and long-term efficacy in reducing binge eating and associated specific and general psychopathology, with approximately 60% of the patients remaining abstinent from binge eating at 1-year follow-up (Wilfley et al., 2002). In contrast to the literature on IPT for BN, the time course of almost all outcomes with IPT was identical to that of CBT.

In a follow-up analysis of treatment predictors of long-term outcome of the 2002 study, patients with a greater extent of interpersonal problems at both baseline and midtreatment showed poorer treatment response to both treatments (Hilbert et al., 2007). An important caveat of this finding, however, is that, not surprisingly, those individuals with greater interpersonal problems were also those who had more Axis I and Axis II psychiatric disorders and lower self-esteem than those with less severe interpersonal problems. Such individuals are likely in need of augmented or extended treatment. Supporting this assertion, in IPT adapted for individuals with borderline personality disorder, many of whom present with comorbid depression, Markowitz and colleagues suggest that extending IPT effectively improves the disorder (Markowitz, Skodol, & Bleiberg, 2006). A preliminary examination of patients in the larger BED cohort at least 5 years posttreatment indicated that those in IPT maintained reductions in binge eating and disordered eating cognitions (Bishop, Stein, Hilbert, Swenson, & Wilfley, 2007, October). These data may suggest evidence for good maintenance of change for patients with BED treated with IPT.

Results from a recently completed multisite trial that compared individual IPT to behavioral weight loss treatment or CBT guided self-help for the treatment of BED points to the importance of making a clear connection between interpersonal problems and binge-eating symptoms in the delivery of IPT. Similar to Wilfley and colleagues' 2002 trial, in this multisite study the clinicians linked interpersonal functioning to disordered-eating symptoms throughout the course of IPT. Findings from this study revealed that IPT was most acceptable to patients; the dropout rate was significantly lower in IPT compared to the other two interventions (Wilfley, Wilson, & Agras, 2008). IPT and CBT guided self-help were significantly more effective than behavioral weight loss in eliminating binge eating after 2 years. Furthermore, compared to the other two programs, IPT produced greater binge episode reductions for patients with low self-esteem and greater disordered-eating behaviors and cognitions, whereas CBT guided self-help was generally effective only for those with low ED psychopathology. It is notable that in this trial, compared to the 2002 study (Hilbert et al., 2007; Wilfley et al., 2002), individuals with more psychopathology showed greater improvements in IPT than with CBT guided self-help. This is in concert with Hilbert and colleagues' follow-up data suggesting that greater disordered eating serves as a moderator in predicting poorer outcome in CBT (Hilbert et al., 2007).

In general, compared to European American participants, individuals of other ethnic minorities demonstrated less retention in the multisite study (Wilfley et al., 2008). Although there was no treatment by ethnicity effects in this regard, there was very low attrition for minority participants in IPT and very high dropout rates by minorities in CBT guided self-help. The small sample size of minority participants across sites precludes definitive conclusions. Nevertheless, this pattern is in concert with the finding that IPT was particularly effective for African American participants in the previously described multisite study for individuals with BN (Chui et al., 2007). It is possible that the personalized nature of IPT (e.g., problem areas and goals are developed based upon each individual's social environment) is modifiable to, and thus particularly acceptable to, persons of various cultures and backgrounds.

A number of recommendations can be drawn from the recent multisite study. It is possible that CBT guided self-help could be considered the first-line treatment for the majority of individuals with BED, and that IPT is recommended for patients with low self-esteem and high eating-disorder psychopathology. Alternatively, IPT may be considered a first-line treatment for BED. This recommendation is based upon a number of factors: IPT has been shown to be effective across multiple research sites, is associated with high retention across different patient profiles (e.g., high negative affect, minority groups), and demonstrated superior outcomes to behavioral weight loss overall, and to CBT guided self-help among a subset of patients with high disordered-eating psychopathology and low-self-esteem. Clinicians and patients should consider these alternatives when deciding the best approach to treating their disorder. Finally, behavioral weight loss should not be considered as a first choice when treating individuals with BED.

In summary, the literature suggests that IPT represents an efficacious treatment alternative to CBT for BED. If delivering IPT for BED in a group format, as with all group therapies, developing member cohesion is paramount to the achievement of treatment success.

Additional Considerations When Choosing Treatment Modality

When determining the treatment approach for patients with EDs, the clinician and patient should together evaluate the advantages and disadvantages of utilizing IPT, CBT, or another therapeutic modality. Furthermore, as part of this determination, it is crucial for clinicians to also explore their own comfort level in terms of their expertise, theoretical knowledge, and propensity toward administering an interpersonally focused treatment. IPT, like CBT, is a specialty treatment and should be administered only by trained practitioners. It has been argued that experienced clinicians who have been trained in other treatment modalities tend to learn IPT quickly and are often able to implement IPT with a high degree of integrity despite minimal training (Birchall, 1999). Currently, there are more data in support of the efficacy of CBT. Based on the evolving literature, IPT may be well suited for patients presenting with or without exacerbated difficulties in social functioning. Although greater problems were associated with poorer outcomes for both CBT and IPT in the Hilbert and colleagues (2007) study, the moderator effect in the more recent multisite study—that patients presenting with greater psychopathology seem to respond well to IPT (Wilfley et al., 2008)—suggests that IPT (or another specialized treatment such as CBT) may be well suited for individuals with a broad range of disordered eating and general psychopathology. Moreover, IPT can be enhanced for individuals with exacerbated psychological problems (Markowitz et al., 2006). It is also possible that IPT may be especially fitting for some minority groups (e.g., African Americans) or specific age cohorts (e.g., adolescents, as described below). Lastly, some patients may express discomfort or difficulties with elements of CBT (e.g., self-monitoring), and IPT should be considered for these individuals.

IPT for Eating Disorders

Basic IPT Concepts

A number of basic concepts are common across all adaptations of IPT, including treatment for EDs. Specifically, adaptations for IPT all focus on interpersonal problem areas and maintain a similar treatment structure. Given the time-limited nature of IPT, treatment success hinges on the clinician's rapid discernment of patterns in interpersonal relationships and the linking of these patterns to eating-disordered symptoms that may have precipitated and maintain the disorder. Thus, early identification of the problem area(s) and treatment goals by the clinician and patient is crucial. Throughout every session, interpersonal functioning should be linked to the onset and maintenance of the eating disorder.

Interpersonal Problem Areas

A primary aim of IPT is to help patients identify and address *current* interpersonal problems. By focusing on current as opposed to past relationships, IPT makes no assumptions about the etiology of an ED. Treatment focuses on the resolution of problems within four social domains that are associated with the onset and/or maintenance of the ED: interpersonal deficits, interpersonal role disputes, role transitions, and grief. *Interpersonal deficits* apply to those patients who are either socially isolated or who are involved in chronically unfulfilling relationships. For clients with this problem area, unsatisfying relationships and/or inadequate social support are frequently the result of poor social skills. *Interpersonal role disputes* refer to conflicts with a significant other (e.g., a partner, other family member, coworker, or close friend) that emerge from differences in expectations about the relationship. *Role transitions* include difficulties associated with a change in life status (e.g., graduation, leaving a job, moving, marriage/divorce, retirement, changes in health). The problem area of *grief* is identified when the onset of the patient's symptoms is associated with either the recent or past loss of a person or a relationship. Making use of this framework for defining one or more interpersonal problem areas, IPT for EDs focuses on identifying and changing the maladaptive interpersonal context in which the eating problem has developed and been maintained. The four problem areas are discussed in detail in the section describing the "Intermediate Phase."

Treatment Structure

IPT for EDs is a time-delineated treatment that typically includes 15–20 sessions over 4–5 months. Regardless of the exact number of sessions, IPT is delivered in three phases. The *initial phase* is dedicated to identifying the problem area(s) that will be the target for treatment. The *intermediate phase* is devoted to working on the target problem area(s). The *termination phase* is devoted to consolidating gains made during treatment and preparing patients for future work on their own.

Implementing IPT for EDs

The Initial Phase

The first five sessions typically constitute the initial phase of IPT for EDs. The patient's current ED symptoms are assessed and a history of these symptoms is obtained. The clinician provides the patient with a formal diagnosis, which they then discuss, along with what can be expected from treatment. An assignment of the "sick role" (described in further detail below) during this phase serves several functions, including granting the patient the permission to recover, delineating recovery as a responsibility of the patient, and allowing the patient to be relieved of other responsibilities in order to recover. The clinician explains the rationale of IPT, emphasizing that therapy will focus on identifying and altering current dysfunctional interpersonal patterns related to ED features. In order to determine the precise focus of treatment, the clinician conducts an "interpersonal inventory" with the patient and, in doing so, develops an interpersonal formulation that specifically relates to the patient's ED. In the interpersonal formulation the clinician links the patient's ED to at least one of the four interpersonal problem areas. The patient's concurrence with the clinician's identification of the problem area and agreement to work on this area are essential before beginning the intermediate phase of treatment. Indeed, a collaborative effort is promoted throughout the interpersonal inventory and the ensuing therapy sessions.

Diagnosis and Assignment of the Sick Role

Following a psychiatric assessment, the patient is formally diagnosed with an ED and assigned what is termed the "sick role." The assignment of the sick role is theoretical and serves a practical purpose. Consistent with the medical model, receiving a formal diagnosis reinforces the understanding that the patient has a known condition that can be treated. Accurate diagnosis is essential to effective treatment. Providing a diagnosis also explicitly identifies the patient as in need of help. The sick role is assigned not to condescend to the patient but rather to temporarily exempt him/her from other responsibilities in order to devote full attention to recovery. This is particularly important for individuals with a tendency to set aside their own needs and desires in order to care for and please others. If appropriate, the IPT clinician might explicitly highlight the patient's excessive caretaking tendencies and encourage the patient to redirect this energy from others toward self-recovery.

The Interpersonal Inventory

An initial and critical component of IPT is the interpersonal inventory, which involves a thorough examination of the patient's interpersonal history. Although clinicians have historically taken up to three sessions to complete the interpersonal inventory, we have found that conducting a longer first session (approximately 2 hours) to complete the entire interpersonal inventory may increase the effectiveness of the treatment. This is likely because it allows patients to get "on board" early in terms of their understanding of IPT and how their ED fits into the IPT rationale (Wilfley et al., 2000). The interpersonal inventory is essential for adequate case formulation and the development of an optimal treatment plan. The clinical importance of investing the time to conduct a comprehensive interpersonal inventory cannot be overemphasized; accurate identification of the patient's primary problem area(s) is often complicated and is crucial to success in treatment.

The interpersonal inventory involves a review of the patient's current close relationships, social functioning, relationship patterns, and expectations of relationships. Interpersonal relationships—both patterns and changes—are explored and discussed with reference to the onset and maintenance of ED symptoms. For each significant relationship the following information is assessed: frequency of contact, activities shared, satisfactory and unsatisfactory aspects of the relationship, and ways in which the patient wishes to change the relationship. The clinician obtains a chronological history of significant life events, fluctuations in mood and self-esteem, interpersonal relationships, and ED symptoms. Throughout this process, the clinician works collaboratively with the patient to make connections between life experiences and ED development and symptoms. This exploration provides an opportunity for the patient to clearly understand the relationship between life events, social functioning, and the ED, and thereby clarifies the rationale behind IPT. Upon completion of the interpersonal inventory, the clinician and patient collaboratively identify a primary interpersonal problem area. In some cases, more than one problem area may be identified.

The Interpersonal Formulation

Following completion of the interpersonal inventory, the clinician develops an individualized interpersonal formulation that includes the identification of the patient's primary problem area. Although some patients may present for treatment with difficulties in several problem areas, the time-limited nature of the treatment necessitates a focused approach. Therefore, the clinician should focus treatment on the problem area(s) that appears to not only impact the patient's interpersonal functioning most, but also those most closely linked to the ED. The clinician, with the agreement of the patient, should assign one, or at most two, problem area(s) for which to develop a treatment plan. We recommend that clinicians write out the agreed-upon goals and present this write-up to patients. The presentation of documented goals can be a very effective technique that serves as a treatment "contract" of sorts. This document becomes a collaborative work agreement that can be revisited and revised throughout treatment to assess and plan future progress. The goals developed at this stage will be referenced at each future session and will guide the day-to-day work of the treatment. If more than one problem area is identified, the patient may choose to work simultaneously on both or may decide to first address the problem area that seems most likely to be responsive to treatment. For example, when a patient has role disputes and interpersonal deficits, clinical attention might first be focused on role disputes, since interpersonal deficits reflect long-term patterns that may require considerably more time and effort to change. Once the role dispute has been resolved, the clinician and patient would then decide how to best address the more entrenched interpersonal deficits. Once the primary problem area(s) has been identified and the treatment goals have been agreed upon, the initial phase of treatment is completed.

The Intermediate Phase

The intermediate phase typically contains a total of 8–10 sessions and constitutes the "work" stage of the therapy. As currently conceptualized, an essential task throughout the intermediate phase of IPT for EDs is to assist the patient in understanding the connection between difficulties in interpersonal functioning and the ED behaviors and symptoms. Therapeutic strategies and goals of this phase are shaped by the primary problem area targeted in the treatment. The following section describes the implementation of specific treatment strategies based upon the identified problem area.

Problem Areas

Grief. Grief is identified as the problem area when the onset of the patient's symptoms is associated with the death of a loved one, either recent or past. Grief is not seen as limited to the physical death of a loved one; it can also result from the loss of a significant relationship or the loss of an important aspect of one's identity. The goals for treating complicated bereavement include facilitating mourning and helping the patient find new activities and relationships to substitute for the loss. Reconstructing the relationship, both the positive and its negative aspects, is central to the assessment of not only what has been lost but also what is needed to counter the idealization that so commonly occurs. As patients become less focused on the past, they should be encouraged to consider new ways of becoming more involved with others and establishing new interests (Wilfley et al., 2005).

Role Transitions. Role transition includes any difficulties resulting from a change in life status. Common role transitions include a career change (promotion, firing, retirement, changing jobs), a family change (marriage, divorce, birth of a child, child moving out), the beginning or end of an important relationship, a move, graduation, or diagnosis of a medical illness. The goals of therapy include mourning and accepting loss of the old role, recognizing the positive and negative aspects of both the old and new roles, and restoring the patient's self-esteem by developing a sense of mastery in the new role. Key strategies in achieving these goals include a thorough exploration of the patient's feelings related to the role change as well as encouraging the patient to develop new skills and adequate social support for the new role (Wilfley et al., 2005b).

Interpersonal Role Disputes. Such disputes involve conflicts with a significant other (e.g., a partner, other family member, employer, coworker, teacher, close friend) that emerge from differences in expectations about the relationship. The goals of treatment include clearly identifying the nature of the dispute and exploring options to resolve it. It is important to determine the stage of the dispute; once the stage of the dispute becomes clear, it may be important to modify the patient's expectations and remedy faulty communication in order to bring about adequate resolution. It may be particularly helpful to explore how nonreciprocal role expectations relate to the dispute. If resolution is impossible, the clinician assists the patient in dissolving the relationship and in mourning its loss (Wilfley et al., 2005b).

Interpersonal Deficits. Interpersonal deficits are typically seen in patients who are socially isolated or who are in chronically unfulfilling relationships. The goal is to reduce the patient's social isolation by helping enhance the quality of existing relationships and encouraging the formation of new ones. To help these patients, it is necessary to determine why they have difficulty in forming or maintaining relationships. Carefully reviewing past significant relationships is particularly useful in making this assessment. During this review, attention should be given to both the positive and negative aspects of the relationships, as well as an investigation of potentially recurrent patterns in these relationships. It may also be appropriate to examine the nature of the patient–clinician relationship, since this may be the patient's only close relationship and it can be observed firsthand by the therapist (Wilfley et al., 2005b).

The Termination Phase

By the end of the intermediate phase, patients are often acutely aware that treatment will soon be ending. The clinician should begin to discuss termination explicitly and address any anxiety the patient may be experiencing. In doing so, the patient should be prepared for emotions that may arise with termination, including grief related to the ending of treatment. At times, patients deny any emotion with regard to the end of treatment and appear to have little reaction to termination. Nevertheless, the clinician should clearly address termination, as the patient may be unaware of, or avoiding, affects related to the end of treatment.

The termination phase typically lasts four or five sessions. During this phase, the patient should be encouraged to reflect on the progress that has been made during therapy—both within sessions and outside of the therapeutic milieu—and to outline goals for remaining work. IPT does not assume that the work toward changes in interpersonal functioning is complete after the last session of the therapy. Rather, patients and clinician collaboratively summarize the remaining work for the patient to continue outside of the therapeutic milieu. Patients are encouraged to identify early warning signs of relapse (e.g., binge eating, overeating or chaotic eating, excessive dietary restriction, negative mood) and to prepare plans of action. Patients are reminded that ED symptoms tend to arise in times of interpersonal stress and are encouraged to view such symptoms as important early warning signals. Identifying potential strategies to cope with such situations is designed to increase patients' sense of competence and security. Nevertheless, it is also essential to assist patients in identifying warning signs and symptoms that may indicate the need for professional intervention in the future.

Therapeutic Techniques

Therapeutic Stance

As with most therapies, IPT places importance on establishing a positive therapeutic alliance between clinician and patient. The IPT therapeutic stance is one of warmth, support, and empathy. Furthermore, throughout all phases of the treatment, the clinician is active and advocates for the patient rather than remaining neutral. Issues and discussions are framed positively so that the clinician can help the patient feel at ease throughout treatment. Such an approach promotes a safe and supportive working environment. Confrontations and clarifications are offered in a gentle and timely manner, and the clinician is careful to encourage the patient's positive expectations of the therapeutic relationship. Finally, the clinician conveys a hopeful and optimistic attitude about the patient's potential to recover.

Focusing on Goals

As a directed, goal-oriented therapy, IPT clinicians should maintain a focus each week on how the patient is working on his/her agreed-upon goals between sessions. Phrases such as "moving forward on your goals" and "making important changes" are used to encourage patients to be responsible for their treatment while also reminding them that altering interpersonal patterns requires attention and persistence. Sometimes during the course of therapy, unfocused discussions arise. The clinician should sensitively, but firmly, redirect the discussion to the key interpersonal issues. By explicitly addressing goals each week, the patient can work toward necessary changes. This goal-oriented focus has been supported by research on IPT maintenance treatment for recurrent depression, which has demonstrated that the clinician's ability to maintain focus on interpersonal themes is associated with better outcomes (Frank, Kupfer, Wagner, McEachran, & Cornes, 1991). In IPT for EDs, it is essential that the clinician facilitate and strengthen the recognition of connections between patients' problematic eating and difficulties in their interpersonal lives.

Making Connections

During the intermediate phase, it is crucial that the clinician assist patients in recognizing, and ultimately becoming more aware of, the connections between eating difficulties and interpersonal events during the week. As patients learn to make these connections, the clinician should guide them to develop strategies to alter the interpersonal context in which the disordered-eating symptoms occur. As a result, the cycle of the ED is interrupted. Patients are encouraged to make connections between interpersonal functioning and eating patterns that are positive as well. For example, an individual may recognize that communication improved with a significant other and, as a result, the patient did not engage in eating-disordered behaviors. To encourage positive and negative connections, clinicians should ask the patient about his/her eating patterns between sessions: if there were any changes and if the patient recognized any links between eating patterns and interpersonal functioning.

Redirecting Issues Related to ED Symptoms

During sessions, patients with EDs may raise issues relating to distressing eating behavior (e.g., binge episodes; overconcern about eating, shape, and weight) or want to engage in extended discussion related to these behaviors. These issues are relevant insofar as they reflect the clinical status of the patient's ED. The clinician must be cognizant of how these issues are being discussed during the sessions and vigilantly keep the session focused on the patient's treatment goals by gently, but firmly, redirecting discussion to work on the treatment goals. For example, a female patient who avoids intimacy with her husband may attribute her avoidance to body dissatisfaction related to her obesity. She may wish to discuss her body concerns at great length to circumvent actual difficulties in communication with her husband. Dialogue related to ED symptoms must be consistently and repeatedly linked to its functional role in the patient's interpersonal domain.

General Therapeutic Techniques

The IPT clinician differs from providers of other modalities in that throughout the course of treatment, a constant focus on the interpersonal context of the patient's life and its link to the ED symptoms is maintained. Although this approach is unique to IPT, a number of the therapeutic techniques utilized in IPT are similar to those used in other therapies. Such techniques include exploratory questions, encouragement of affect, clarification, communication analysis, and use of the therapeutic relationship.

Exploratory Questions. Use of general, open-ended questions or statements often facilitates the free discussion of material. This technique is especially useful during the beginning of a session. For example, the clinician might open a session with the statement "Tell me about your relationship with your husband." Progressively more specific questioning should follow, as the patient describes the relationship.

Encouraging Affect. IPT's focus throughout the therapeutic process involves affect evocation and exploration (Wilfley et al., 2000). This emphasis is particularly relevant for patients with EDs because problematic eating often serves to regulate negative affect. The IPT clinician should assist patients in (1) acknowledging and accepting painful emotions, (2) using affective experiences to facilitate desired interpersonal changes, and (3) experiencing suppressed affect (Wilfley, 2008; Wilfley et al., 2000).

1. *Encourage acceptance of painful affects.* Patients with BN and BED are often emotionally constricted in situations when others would typically experience strong emotions. These patients use food to cope with negative affect. Therapy provides an arena in which they can experience and express these feelings versus using food as an attempted coping mechanism. As the feelings are expressed, it is important for the IPT clinician to validate and help the patient accept them (Wilfley, 2008).

2. *Teach the patient how to use affect in interpersonal relationships.* Although the expression of strong feelings in the session is seen as an important starting point for much therapeutic work, the expression of feelings outside the session is not a goal in and of itself. The goal is to help the patient act more constructively (e.g., *not* binge eat or purge) in interpersonal relationships, and this may involve either expressing or suppressing affects, depending on the circumstances. A goal for the patient in IPT is to learn when his/her needs are met by expressing affect and when they are better met by suppressing affect. However, a primary goal is helping patients to identify, understand, and acknowledge their feelings whether or not they choose to verbalize them to others (Wilfley, 2008).

3. *Help the patient experience suppressed affects.* Many who struggle with BN or BED are emotionally constricted in situations where strong emotions are normally felt. An example might be the patient who is unassertive and does not feel anger when his/her rights are violated. On the other hand, the person may feel anger but may lack the courage to express it in an assertive manner. Sometimes patients deny being upset, when it is clear that an upsetting interaction has just occurred. The clinician might say, "Although you said you were not upset, it appears to me that you have shut down since you talked about the situation with your husband." In this way the clinician attempts to draw out affect when it is suppressed (Wilfley, 2008).

Clarification. Clarification is a useful technique that can serve to increase the patient's awareness about what he/she has actually communicated, and to draw awareness to contradictions that may have occurred in the patient's presentation of interactions or situations. An example might involve contradictions between the patient's affect and speech: "While you were telling me how upset you are about your father, you had a smile on your face. What do you think that's about?"

Communication Analysis. The technique of communication analysis is used to identify potential communication difficulties that the patient may be experiencing and to assist the patient in modifying these ineffective patterns. In using communication analysis, the clinician asks the patient to describe, in great detail, a recent interaction or argument with a significant other. The clinician and patient then work collaboratively to identify difficulties in the communication that may be impacting the process and outcome of the interaction and to find more effective strategies.

Use of the Therapeutic Relationship. The premise behind this technique is that all individuals have characteristic patterns of interacting with others. The technique is utilized by exploring the patient's thoughts, feelings, expectations, and behavior in the therapeutic relationship and relating these to the patient's characteristic way of behaving and/or feeling in other relationships. This technique is particularly relevant to, and useful for, patients with interpersonal deficits and interpersonal role disputes. Use of this technique offers the patient the opportunity to understand the nature of his/her difficulties in interacting with others and provides the patient with helpful feedback on his/her interactional style.

Use of a Group. The group setting frequently provides an optimal modality for conducting IPT (Wilfley et al., 2000). Following an individual session to conduct a thorough interpersonal inventory, the group is an ideal milieu in which to work on interpersonal skills with other patients struggling with similar eating problems. It also offers the clinician an opportunity to observe and identify characteristic interpersonal patterns with other individuals. Furthermore, when another group member recognizes and verbally identifies a dysfunctional pattern of communication in a fellow patient, it can be powerful for the patient as well as the other group members. The group setting allows patients to experiment with different ways of communicating within the safe confines of the group. Members can use the sessions to discuss problems they are having in their significant relationships and how these problems relate to their eating patterns. This format often allows patients to recognize that they are not alone in their difficulties, thereby helping to reduce feelings of isolation.

IPT for the Prevention of Excessive Weight Gain

A recent and novel adaptation of IPT has been developed, and is currently being tested, for the prevention of excessive weight gain in adolescents who report loss of control (LOC) eating patterns. LOC refers to the sense that one cannot control what or how much one is eating, regardless of the reported amount of food consumed (Tanofsky-Kraff, 2008). Common among youths, LOC eating is associated with distress and overweight (Tanofsky-Kraff, 2008) and predicts excessive weight gain over time (Tanofsky-Kraff et al., 2009). This adaptation makes use of IPT for the prevention of depression in adolescents (IPT Adolescent Skills Training, IPT-AST) (Young, Mufson, & Davies, 2006) and group IPT for BED (Wilfley et al., 2000), and evolved from the outcome data of psychotherapy trials for the treatment of BED. An unexpected finding of IPT and most psychological treatments for BED has been that individuals with BED who cease to binge-eat tend to maintain their body weight during and/or following treatment (Agras et al., 1995; Agras, Telch, Arnow, Eldredge, & Marnell, 1997; Devlin et al., 2005; Wilfley et al., 1993, 2002). Therefore, it has been hypothesized that treatment of binge eating in youths may reduce excessive weight gain and prevent full-syndrome EDs during development (Tanofsky-Kraff, Wilfley, et al., 2007).

A number of factors suggest that IPT is particularly appropriate for the prevention of obesity in high-risk adolescents with LOC eating patterns. Specifically, adolescents frequently use peer relationships as a crucial measure of self-evaluation (Mufson, Dorta, Moreau, & Weissman, 2004; Mufson, Moreau, Weissman, & Klerman, 1993). A recent study revealed the import of perceived social interactions and social standing on body weight gain over time (Lemeshow et al., 2008). In this prospective cohort study, adolescent girls who rated themselves lower on a subjective social standing scale were 69% more likely to gain more weight over time, compared to girls who rated themselves on the higher end of the scale (Lemeshow et al., 2008). Furthermore, overweight teens are more likely to experience negative feelings about themselves, particularly regarding their body shape and weight, compared to normal-weight adolescents (Fallon et al., 2005; Schwimmer, Burwinkle, & Varni, 2003; Striegel-Moore, Silberstein, & Rodin, 1986), perhaps because of their elevated rates of appearance-related teasing, rejection, and social isolation (Strauss & Pollack, 2003). The social isolation that overweight teens report can be directly targeted by IPT.

Several longitudinal studies have found depressive symptoms to predict weight gain and obesity onset in children and adolescents (Anderson, Cohen, Naumova, & Must, 2006; Goodman & Whitaker, 2002; Pine, Goldstein, Wolk, & Weissman, 2001; Stice, Presnell, Shaw, & Rohde, 2005). Thus, the proven efficacy of IPT in decreasing depressive symptoms in adolescents (Mufson, Dorta, Wickramaratne, et al., 2004) may serve to decrease an additional risk factor for inappropriate weight gain. In addition to ameliorating depressive symptomatology, IPT is posited to increase social support, which has been demonstrated to improve weight loss and weight maintenance in overweight adults (Wing & Jeffery, 1999) and children (Wilfley et al., 2007). Indeed, data suggest that low social problems predict better response to weight loss treatment in children (Wilfley et al., 2007).

IPT for the prevention of excessive weight gain (IPT-WG) in adolescents at high risk for adult obesity, delivered in a group format, maintains the key components of traditional IPT: (1) a focus on interpersonal problem areas that are related to the target behavior (LOC eating in the present adaptation); (2) the use of the interpersonal inventory at the outset of treatment to identify interpersonal problems that are contributing to the targeted behavior; and (3) the three- staged structure of the intervention (initial, middle, and termination). The primary activities of IPT-WG involve providing psychoeducation about risk factors for excessive weight gain and teaching general skill building to improve interpersonal problems. IPT-WG was founded on Young and Mufson's IPT-AST (Young & Mufson, 2003) and group IPT for the treatment of BED in adulthood (Wilfley et al., 2000). IPT-WG differs from other adaptations in that it was developed to specifically address the particular needs of adolescent girls at high risk for adult obesity due to their current body mass index (BMI) percentile and report of LOC eating behaviors.

Based on IPT-AST, IPT-WG is presented to teenagers as "Teen Talk" in order to be nonstigmatizing. As designed by Dr. Young, this preventive adaptation of IPT focuses on psychoeducation, communication analysis, and role playing (Young & Mufson, 2003). Specific interpersonal communications skills are taught, including "strike while the iron is cold," "use 'I' statements," "be specific" (when talking about a problem), and "put yourself in their shoes" (Young & Mufson, 2003). For IPT-WG, an additional skill, "what you don't say speaks volumes," has been added to teach adolescents how their body language has the ability to impact communication regardless of their words. During the interpersonal inventory, a "closeness circle" (Mufson, Dorta, Moreau, et al., 2004) is used to identify the close relationships of the participant. Sessions can be appropriately geared toward the adolescents' developmental level. For instance, younger adolescents, who may be uncomfortable talking about themselves, may respond better to hypothetical situations and games, whereas older teenagers may more readily discuss their own interpersonal issues from the outset.

Based on IPT for BED, IPT-WG focuses on linking negative affect to LOC eating, overeating, times when individuals eat in response to cues other than hunger, as well as overconcern about shape and weight. Furthermore, a timeline of personal eating and weight-related problems and life events is discussed individually with participants prior to the group program. Unlike IPT for BED, the problem area of grief is rarely relevant due to the young age of participants, but may be included on a case-by-case basis. Similar to both programs, IPT-WG is delivered in a group format. IPT-WG is 12 weeks in duration, longer than IPT-AST (8 sessions), but shorter than group IPT for BED (typically 20 sessions). Similar to IPT-AST, group size is smaller than in IPT-BED (five vs. nine members), enabling clinicians to keep adolescents engaged.

Progress in the Delivery of IPT for EDs

IPT interventions for major depression and associated disorders are uniform in that they include a consistent focus on the target symptoms of the respective disorders. By contrast, most research applications of IPT for EDs, especially BN, did not initially include a strong focus on ED symptoms. Initially, this lack of symptom focus was intentional in order to minimize procedural overlap with CBT and, in doing so, clearly distinguish IPT from CBT in comparative psychotherapy trials. Increasingly, however, in both clinical settings and research studies of IPT for BED and the prevention of adult obesity, consistent attention to the relationship between interpersonal functioning and disordered-eating symptoms is being utilized to achieve maximum therapeutic impact. Indeed, in each session of IPT for EDs, symptoms should be explicitly and repeatedly linked to problems in interpersonal functioning. In IPT-WG for adolescents at risk for adult obesity, linking LOC eating to interpersonal functioning is done consistently and frequently throughout the interpersonal inventory as well as the group sessions (Tanofsky-Kraff, Wilfley, et al., 2007). Indeed, preliminary findings suggest that IPT prevents excess weight gain among these high-risk adolescent girls (Tanofsky-Kraff, Wilfley, et al., 2008).

Future Directions for IPT in the Treatment of EDs

Several important areas require further study. An important next step is to determine whether IPT for EDs can be translated from specialty care centers to the primary care setting and other typically nonresearch clinical practice milieus where counselors are trained to deliver IPT. In an effort to continually improve IPT and broaden its utility, we propose other research directions in this section.

Enhancing IPT for BN and BED

As efforts to more frequently and consistently link ED symptoms to interpersonal functioning have evolved in the use of IPT for BED, clinical researchers involved in developing IPT for BN should also consider stressing this link during the delivery of IPT so that it offers the utmost potency. IPT, in its current form, already seamlessly incorporates aspects of other therapeutic modalities. For example, the collaborative, behavioral formulation during the interpersonal inventory is one of the ways in which IPT more closely resembles the behavior therapies than it does the supportive or psychodynamic therapies. Therefore, some aspects of CBT may support the efficacy of IPT. For example, IPT clinicians might wish to use self-monitoring as a method for patients to become more aware of their negative affect surrounding ED symptoms. Such an approach is already being tested in other treatment modalities. Indeed, Fairburn and colleagues have found the inclusion of an interpersonal module effective when administering a recently modified version of CBT for EDs (Enhanced CBT for Eating Disorders; Fairburn, 2008).

Adolescent– and Child–Parent Adaptations

Given the robust efficacy of IPT for adolescents with depressive disorders, and the initial promise of IPT-WG, future research should involve additional adolescent adaptations. Adolescence is a key developmental period for cultivating social and interpersonal patterns, which may explain why adolescents appear to relate well to IPT. From its inception, Mufson and colleagues made important adolescent-relevant adaptations to the treatment (Mufson, Dorta, Moreau, et al., 2004), for example, the inclusion of a parent component and the assignment of a "*limited* sick role," since adolescents are required to attend school and reducing their activities is likely to exacerbate their interpersonal difficulties. Given that this foundation has been established, the use of IPT for adolescents with BN and BED warrants investigation.

Utilizing IPT for younger children may also be effective. A pilot study of family-based IPT for the treatment of depressive symptoms in 9- to 12-year-old children was found to be feasible and acceptable to families (Dietz, Mufson, Irvine, & Brent, 2008). Currently, an effectiveness trial is underway. The moderating influence of social problems on weight loss outcome in a family-based program (Wilfley et al., 2007) suggests that targeting interpersonal functioning in the nuclear family milieu may serve as a point of intervention for the treatment of eating- and weight-related problems during middle childhood.

Developing IPT for the Prevention of Eating- and Weight-Related Problems

Given the increasingly high rates of obesity in the United States (Ogden et al., 2006), it may be reasonably posited that the increases in disordered eating will continue as well, considering that overweight is a significant risk factor for the development of eating pathology (Fairburn et al., 1997, 1998). Therefore, the use of IPT to prevent obesity and full-syndrome EDs should be explored by targeting other behaviors that promote both conditions. Since not all overweight individuals report LOC eating, reducing emotional eating and eating in the absence of hunger may also be suitable for IPT modalities. Recent studies suggest that LOC eating in youths is associated with eating in response to negative affect (Goossens, Braet, & Decaluwe, 2006), including anger, frustration, depression, and anxiety (Tanofsky-Kraff, Wilfley, et al., 2007). In studies of adolescents, emotional eating is significantly correlated with constructs of disturbed eating (van Strien, 1996; van Strien, Engels, Van Leeuwe, & Snoek, 2005) and symptoms of depression and anxiety (van Strien et al., 2005). Data also suggest that emotional eating may be associated with overweight in youths (Braet & van Strien, 1997) and predict overeating in cross-sectional structural models (van Strien et al., 2005). Considering that IPT for BED effectively reduces eating in response to negative affect in adults (Wilfley et al., 1993, 2002), preventive adaptations targeting emotional eating require investigation.

Eating in the absence of hunger has been associated with overweight (Moens & Braet, 2007) and excessive weight gain over time (Shunk & Birch, 2004). Reported eating in the absence of hunger has been shown to be associated with LOC eating, emotional eating, and elevations in general psychopathology (Tanofsky-Kraff, Ranzen-hofer, et al., 2008). Of concern are data indicating that eating in the absence of hunger is a stable trait throughout adolescence (Birch, Fisher, & Davison, 2003; Fisher & Birch, 2002). Promising findings indicate that young children can be trained to better regulate food intake (Johnson, 2000), and a number of intervention studies targeting eating in the absence of hunger are currently underway. IPT may serve as a natural extension on this work; in particular, negative affect associated with interpersonal problems might be linked to eating in the absence of hunger. Then, recognition of internal physiological hunger cues can be taught so that patients learn to differentiate true hunger from when they are already sated.

Finally, there has been a growing interest in, and awareness of, the role that social and interpersonal factors may play in behavioral health problems (Glass & McAtee, 2006). Particularly for obesity, moving away from focusing solely on individual behavioral changes (e.g., diet and exercise) and toward the greater social context has not been the norm. IPT may be particularly well suited for developing new approaches for the prevention of obesity and EDs on a broader social level.

Conclusion

IPT for BN and BED is a focused, time-limited treatment that targets interpersonal problems associated with the onset and/or maintenance of the ED. The interpersonal focus is highly relevant to individuals with EDs, many of whom experience difficulties in interpersonal functioning. Depending on the individual's primary problem area, specific treatment strategies and goals are incorporated into the treatment plan. The primary problem area is determined by conducting a thorough interpersonal inventory, a unique aspect of IPT, and by devising an individualized interpersonal formulation for each patient. IPT has demonstrated significant and well-maintained improvements for the treatment of BN and BED. Preliminary data support the utility of IPT for the prevention of excess weight gain in adolescent girls. Adaptations of IPT should be explored for adolescent populations and the treatment of other eating- and weight-related problems.

Acknowledgments

This work was supported by National Institute of Diabetes and Digestive and Kidney Diseases Grant No. 1R01DK080906-01A1 and Uniformed Services University of the Health Sciences Grant No. R072IC (to Marian Tanofsky-Kraff) and by National Institute of Mental Health Grant Nos. 5R01MH064153-06 and 1K24MH070446 (to Denise E. Wilfley). The opinions and assertions expressed herein are those of the authors and are not to be construed as reflecting the views of the Uniformed Services University of the Health Sciences or the U.S. Department of Defense.

References

Agras WS, Telch CF, Arnow B, Eldredge K, Detzer MJ, Henderson J, et al. (1995). Does interpersonal therapy help patients with binge eating disorder who fail to respond to cognitive-behavioral therapy? *Journal of Consulting and Clinical Psychology*, 63:356–360.

Agras WS, Telch CF, Arnow B, Eldredge K, & Marnell M. (1997). One-year follow-up of cognitive-behavioral therapy for obese individuals with binge eating disorder. *Journal of Consulting and Clinical Psychology*, 65:343–347.

Agras WS, Walsh BT, Fairburn CG, Wilson GT, & Kraemer HC. (2000). A multicenter comparison of cognitive-behavioral therapy and interpersonal psychotherapy for bulimia nervosa. *Archives of General Psychiatry*, 57:459–466.

Anderson SE, Cohen P, Naumova EN, & Must A. (2006). Association of depression and anxiety disorders with weight change in a prospective community-based study of children followed up into adulthood. *Archives of Pediatric Adolescent Medicine*, 160:285–291.

Birch LL, Fisher JO, & Davison KK. (2003). Learning to overeat: Maternal use of restrictive feeding practices promotes girls' eating in the absence of hunger. *American Journal of Clinical Nutrition*, 78:215–220.

Birchall H. (1999). Interpersonal psychotherapy in the treatment of eating disorder. *European Eating Disorders Review*, 7:315–320.

Bishop M, Stein R, Hilbert A, Swenson A, & Wilfley DE. (2007, October). *A five-year follow-up study of cognitive-behavioral therapy and interpersonal psychotherapy for the treatment of binge eating disorder*. Paper presented at the annual meeting of the Eating Disorders Research Society, Pittsburgh, PA.

Bowlby J. (1982). *Attachment and loss* (Vol. 1, 2nd ed.). New York: Basic Books.

Braet C, & Van Strien T. (1997). Assessment of emotional, externally induced and restrained eating behaviour in nine to twelve-year-old obese and non-obese children. *Behaviour Research and Therapy*, 35:863–873.

Chui W, Safer DL, Bryson SW, Agras WS, & Wilson GT. (2007). A comparison of ethnic groups in the treatment of bulimia nervosa. *Eating Behaviors*, 8:485–491.

Constantino MJ, Arnow BA, Blasey C, & Agras WS. (2005). The association between patient characteristics and the therapeutic alliance in cognitive-behavioral and interpersonal therapy for bulimia nervosa. *Journal of Consulting and Clinical Psychology*, 73:203–211.

Crow SJ, Agras WS, Halmi K, Mitchell JE, & Kraemer HC. (2002). Full syndromal versus subthreshold anorexia nervosa, bulimia nervosa, and binge eating disorder: A multicenter study. *International Journal of Eating Disorders*, 32:309–318.

Devlin MJ, Goldfein JA, Petkova E, Jiang H, Raizman PS, Wolk S, et al. (2005). Cognitive behavioral therapy and fluoxetine as adjuncts to group behavioral therapy for binge eating disorder. *Obesity Research*, 13:1077–1088.

Dietz LJ, Mufson L, Irvine H, & Brent DA. (2008). Family-based interpersonal psychotherapy (IPT) for depressed preadolescents: An open treatment trial. *Early Intervention Psychiatry*, 2:154–161.

Evans L, & Wertheim EH. (1998). Intimacy patterns and relationship satisfaction of women with eating problems and the mediating effects of depression, trait anxiety, and social anxiety. *Journal of Psychosomatic Research*, 44:355–365.

Fairburn CG. (2008). *Cognitive behavior therapy and eating disorders*. New York: Guilford Press.

Fairburn CG, Doll HA, Welch SL, Hay PJ, Davies BA, & O'Connor ME. (1998). Risk factors for binge eating disorder: A community-based, case-control study. *Archives of General Psychiatry*, 55:425–432.

Fairburn CG, Jones R, Peveler RC, Carr SJ, Solomon RA, O'Connor ME, et al. (1991). Three psychological treatments for bulimia nervosa. A comparative trial. *Archives of General Psychiatry*, 48:463–469.

Fairburn CG, Norman PA, Welch SL, O'Connor ME, Doll HA, & Peveler RC. (1995). A prospective study of outcome in bulimia nervosa and the long-term effects of three psychological treatments. *Archives of General Psychiatry*, 52:304–312.

Fairburn CG, Peveler RC, Jones R, Hope RA, & Doll HA. (1993). Predictors of 12-month outcome in bulimia nervosa and the influence of attitudes to shape and weight. *Journal of Consulting and Clinical Psychology*, 61:696–698.

Fairburn CG, Welch SL, Doll HA, Davies BA, & O'Connor ME. (1997). Risk factors for bulimia nervosa: A community-based case-control study. *Archives of General Psychiatry*, 54:509–517.

Fallon EM, Tanofsky-Kraff M, Norman AC, McDuffie JR, Taylor ED, Cohen ML, et al. (2005). Health-related quality of life in overweight and nonoverweight black and white adolescents. *Journal of Pediatrics*, 147:443–450.

Fisher JO, & Birch LL. (2002). Eating in the absence of hunger and overweight in girls from 5 to 7 y of age. *American Journal of Clinical Nutrition*, 76:226–231.

Frank E, Kupfer DJ, Wagner EF, McEachran AB, & Cornes C. (1991). Efficacy of interpersonal psychotherapy as a maintenance treatment of recurrent depression: Contributing factors. *Archives of General Psychiatry*, 48:1053–1059.

Frank E, & Spanier C. (1995). Interpersonal psychotherapy for depression: Overview, clinical efficacy, and future directions. *Clinical Psychology: Science and Practice*, 2:349–369.

Freeman LMY, & Gil KM. (2004). Daily stress, coping, and dietary restraint in binge eating. *International Journal of Eating Disorders*, 36:204–212.

Ghaderi A, & Scott B. (1999). Prevalence and psychological correlates of eating disorders among females aged 18–30 years in the general population. *Acta Psychiatrica Scandinavica*, 99:261–266.

Glass TA, & McAtee MJ. (2006). Behavioral science at the crossroads in public health: Extending horizons, envisioning the future. *Society of Science and Medicine*, 62:1650–1671.

Goodman E, & Whitaker RC. (2002). A prospective study of the role of depression in the development and persistence of adolescent obesity. *Pediatrics*, 110:497–504.

Goossens L, Braet C, & Decaluwe V. (2007). Loss of control over eating in obese youngsters. *Behaviour Research and Therapy*, 45(1):1–9.

Grilo CM, Masheb RM, & Wilson GT. (2005). Efficacy of cognitive behavioral therapy and fluoxetine for the treatment of binge eating disorder: A randomized double-blind placebo-controlled comparison. *Biological Psychiatry*, 57:301–309.

Grissett NI, & Norvell NK. (1992). Perceived social support, social skills, and quality of relationships in bulimic women. *Journal of Consulting and Clinical Psychology*, 60:293–299.

Gual P, Perez-Gaspar M, Martinez-Gonzalez MA, Lahortiga F, de Irala-Estevez J, & Cervera-Enguix S. (2002). Self-esteem, personality, and eating disorders: Baseline assessment of a prospective population-based cohort. *International Journal of Eating Disorders*, 31:261–273.

Herzog D, Keller M, Lavori P, & Ott I. (1987). Social impairment in bulimia. *International Journal of Eating Disorders*, 6:741–747.

Hilbert A, Saelens BE, Stein RI, Mockus DS, Welch RR, Matt GE, et al. (2007). Pretreatment and process predictors of outcome in interpersonal and cognitive behavioral psychotherapy for binge eating disorder. *Journal of Consulting and Clinical Psychology*, 75:645–651.

Humphrey LL. (1989). Observed family interactions among subtypes of eating disorders using structural analysis of social behavior. *Journal of Consulting and Clinical Psychology*, 57:206–214.

Johnson JG, Spitzer RL, & Williams JB. (2001). Health problems, impairment and illnesses associated with bulimia nervosa and binge eating disorder among primary care and obstetric gynaecology patients. *Psychological Medicine*, 31:1455–1466.

Johnson SL. (2000). Improving preschoolers' self-regulation of energy intake. *Pediatrics*, 106:1429–1435.

Keel PK, Dorer DJ, Franko DL, Jackson SC, & Herzog DB. (2005). Postremission predictors of relapse in women with eating disorders. *American Journal of Psychiatry*, 162:2263–2268.

Kenardy J, Mensch M, Bowen K, Green B, & Walton J. (2002). Group therapy for binge eating in Type 2 diabetes: A randomized trial. *Diabetes Medicine*, 19:234–239.

Klerman GL, Weissman MM, Rounsaville BJ, & Chevron ES. (1984). *Interpersonal psychotherapy of depression*. New York: Basic Books.

Lemeshow AR, Fisher L, Goodman E, Kawachi I, Berkey CS, & Colditz GA. (2008). Subjective social status in the school and change in adiposity in female adolescents: Findings from a prospective cohort study. *Archives of Pediatric and Adolescent Medicine*, 162:23–28.

Markowitz JC, Skodol AE, & Bleiberg K. (2006). Interpersonal psychotherapy for borderline personality disorder: Possible mechanisms of change. *Journal of Clinical Psychology*, 62:431–444.

Meyer A. (1957). *Psychobiology: A science of man*. Springfield, IL: Thomas.

Moens E, & Braet C. (2007). Predictors of disinhibited eating in children with and without overweight. *Behaviour Research and Therapy*, 45:1357–1368.

Mufson L, Dorta KP, Moreau D, & Weissman MM. (2004). *Interpersonal psychotherapy for depressed adolescents* (2nd ed.). New York: Guilford Press.

Mufson L, Dorta KP, Wickramaratne P, Nomura Y, Olfson M, & Weissman MM. (2004). A randomized effectiveness trial of interpersonal psychotherapy for depressed adolescents. *Archives of General Psychiatry*, 61:577–584.

Mufson L, Moreau D, Weissman MM, & Klerman GL. (1993). *Interpersonal psychotherapy for depressed adolescents*. New York: Guilford Press.

Nauta H, Hospers H, Kok G, & Jansen A. (2000). A comparison between a cognitive and a behavioral treatment for obese binge eaters and obese non-binge eaters. *Behavior Therapy*, 21:441–461.

Ogden CL, Carroll MD, Curtin LR, McDowell MA, Tabak CJ, & Flegal KM. (2006). Prevalence of overweight and obesity in the United States, 1999–2004. *Journal of the American Medical Association*, 295:1549–1555.

O'Mahony JF, & Hollwey S. (1995). The correlates of binge eating in two nonpatient samples. *Addictive Behaviors*, 20:471–480.

Pine DS, Goldstein RB, Wolk S, & Weissman MM. (2001). The association between childhood depression and adulthood body mass index. *Pediatrics*, 107:1049–1056.

Ricca V, Mannucci E, Mezzani B, Moretti S, Di Bernardo M, Bertelli M, et al. (2001). Fluoxetine and fluvoxamine combined with individual cognitive-behaviour therapy in binge eating disorder: A one-year follow-up study. *Psychotherapy and Psychosomatics*, 70:298–306.

Rorty M, Yager J, Buckwalter JG, & Rossotto E. (1999). Social support, social adjustment, and recovery status in bulimia nervosa. *International Journal of Eating Disorders*, 26:1–12.

Schwimmer JB, Burwinkle TM, & Varni JW. (2003). Health-related quality of life of severely obese children and adolescents. *Journal of the American Medical Association*, 289:1813–1819.

Shunk JA, & Birch LL. (2004). Girls at risk for overweight at age 5 are at risk for dietary restraint, disinhibited overeating, weight concerns, and greater weight gain from 5 to 9 years. *Journal of the American Dietetic Association*, 104:1120–1126.

Steiger H, Gauvin L, Jabalpurwala S, Seguin JR, & Stotland S. (1999). Hypersensitivity to social interactions in bulimic syndromes: Relationship to binge eating. *Journal of Consulting and Clinical Psychology*, 67:765–775.

Stice E, Presnell K, Shaw H, & Rohde P. (2005). Psychological and behavioral risk factors for obesity onset in adolescent girls: A prospective study. *Journal of Consulting and Clinical Psychology,* 73:195–202.

Strauss RS, & Pollack HA. (2003). Social marginalization of overweight children. *Archives of Pediatric and Adolescent Medicine,* 157:746–752.

Striegel-Moore RH, Silberstein LR, & Rodin J. (1986). Toward an understanding of risk factors for bulimia. *American Psychologist,* 41:246–263.

Sullivan H. (1953). *The interpersonal theory of psychiatry.* New York: Norton.

Tanofsky-Kraff M. (2008). Binge eating among children and adolescents. In E Jelalian & R Steele (Eds.), *Handbook of child and adolescent obesity* (pp. 41–57). New York: Springer.

Tanofsky-Kraff M, Ranzenhofer LM, Yanovski SZ, Schvey NA, Faith M, Gustafson J, et al. (2008). Psychometric properties of a new questionnaire to assess eating in the absence of hunger in children and adolescents. *Appetite,* 51:148–155.

Tanofsky-Kraff M, Theim KR, Yanovski SZ, Bassett AM, Burns NP, Ranzenhofer LM, et al. (2007). Validation of the Emotional Eating Scale adapted for use in children and adolescents (EES-C). *International Journal of Eating Disorders,* 40:232–240.

Tanofsky-Kraff M, Wilfley DE, & Spurrell EB. (2000). Impact of interpersonal and ego-related stress on restrained eaters. *International Journal of Eating Disorders,* 27:411–418.

Tanofsky-Kraff M, Wilfley DE, Young JF, Mufson L, Salaita CG, Glasofer DR, et al. (2008, September). *Interpersonal psychotherapy (IPT) for the prevention of excess weight gain in adolescents girls with and without loss of control eating: A pilot study.* Paper presented at the annual meeting of the Eating Disorders Research Society, Montreal.

Tanofsky-Kraff M, Wilfley DE, Young JF, Mufson L, Yanovski SZ, Glasofer DR, et al. (2007). Preventing excessive weight gain in adolescents: Interpersonal psychotherapy for binge eating. *Obesity,* 15:1345–1355.

Tanofsky-Kraff M, Yanovski SZ, Schvey NA, Olsen C, Gustafson J, & Yanovski JA. (2009). A prospective study of loss of control eating for body weight gain in children at high-risk for adult obesity. *International Journal of Eating Disorders,* 42:26–30.

Tasca GA, Taylor D, Ritchie K, & Balfour L. (2004). Attachment predicts treatment completion in an eating disorders partial hospital program among women with anorexia nervosa. *Journal of Personality Assessment,* 83:201–212.

Telch CF, Agras WS, Rossiter EM, Wilfley DE, & Kenardy J. (1990). Group cognitive-behavioral treatment for the nonpurging bulimic: An initial evaluation. *Journal of Consulting and Clinical Psychology,* 58:629–635.

Troisi A, Massaroni P, & Cuzzolaro M. (2005). Early separation anxiety and adult attachment style in women with eating disorders. *British Journal of Clinical Psychology,* 44:89–97.

Troop NA, Holbrey A, Trowler R, & Treasure JL. (1994). Ways of coping in women with eating disorders. *Journal of Nervous and Mental Disorders,* 182:535–540.

van Strien T. (1996). On the relationship between dieting and "obese" and bulimic eating patterns. *International Journal of Eating Disorders,* 19:83–92.

van Strien T, Engels RC, Van Leeuwe J, & Snoek HM. (2005). The Stice model of overeating: Tests in clinical and non-clinical samples. *Appetite,* 45:205–213.

Weissman MM, Markowitz J, & Klerman GL. (2000). *Comprehensive guide to interpersonal psychotherapy.* New York: Basic Books.

Wilfley DE. (2008). *Interpersonal psychotherapy for binge eating disorder (BED) therapist's manual.* Unpublished manuscript.

Wilfley DE, Agras WS, Telch CF, Rossiter EM, Schneider JA, Cole AG, et al. (1993). Group cognitive-behavioral therapy and group interpersonal psychotherapy for the nonpurging bulimic individual: A controlled comparison. *Journal of Consulting and Clinical Psychology,* 61:296–305.

Wilfley DE, Frank MA, Welch RR, Spurrell EB, & Rounsaville BJ. (1998). Adapting interpersonal psychotherapy to a group format (IPT-G) for binge eating disorder: Toward a model for adapting empirically supported treatments. *Psychotherapy Research*, 8:379–391.

Wilfley DE, MacKenzie KR, Welch RR, Ayres VE, & Weissman MM. (2000). *Interpersonal psychotherapy for group.* New York: Basic Books.

Wilfley DE, Stein RI, Saelens BE, Mockus DS, Matt GE, Hayden-Wade HA, et al. (2007). Efficacy of maintenance treatment approaches for childhood overweight: A randomized controlled trial. *Journal of the American Medical Association*, 298:1661–1673.

Wilfley DE, Stein RI, & Welch RR. (2005). Interpersonal psychotherapy. In J Treasure, U Schmidt, & E van Furth (Eds.), *The essential handbook of eating disorders* (pp. 137–154). West Sussex, UK: Wiley.

Wilfley DE, Welch RR, Stein RI, Spurrell EB, Cohen LR, Saelens BE, et al. (2002). A randomized comparison of group cognitive-behavioral therapy and group interpersonal psychotherapy for the treatment of overweight individuals with binge-eating disorder. *Archives of General Psychiatry*, 59:713–721.

Wilfley DE, Wilson GT, & Agras WS. (2003). The clinical significance of binge eating disorder. *International Journal of Eating Disorders*, 34:S96–S106.

Wilfley DE, Wilson GT, & Agras WS. (2008, September). *A multi-site randomized controlled trial of interpersonal psychotherapy, behavioral weight loss, and guided self-help in the treatment of overweight individuals with binge eating disorder.* Paper presented at the annual meeting of the Eating Disorders Research Society, Montreal.

Wilson GT. (2005). Psychological treatment of eating disorders. *Annual Review of Clinical Psychology*, 1:439–465.

Wilson GT, Grilo CM, & Vitousek KM. (2007). Psychological treatment of eating disorders. *American Psychologist*, 62:199–216.

Wilson GT, & Shafran R. (2005). Eating disorders guidelines from NICE. *Lancet*, 365:79–81.

Wing RR, & Jeffery RW. (1999). Benefits of recruiting participants with friends and increasing social support for weight loss and maintenance. *Journal of Consulting and Clinical Psychology*, 67:132–138.

Young JF, & Mufson L. (2003). *Manual for interpersonal psychotherapy—adolescent skills training (IPT-AST)*. New York: Columbia University.

Young JF, Mufson L, & Davies M. (2006). Efficacy of interpersonal psychotherapy—adolescent skills training: An indicated preventive intervention for depression. *Journal of Child Psychology and Psychiatry*, 47:1254–1262.

CHAPTER 16

Dialectical Behavior Therapy for Bulimia Nervosa and Binge-Eating Disorder

Eunice Y. Chen and Debra L. Safer

Standard dialectical behavior therapy (DBT) is an outpatient cognitive-behavioral therapy originally developed for women with extreme emotion dysregulation and recurrent suicidal behavior: that is, borderline personality disorder (BPD). This comprehensive skills-based treatment integrates behavioral principles with dialectical philosophy and acceptance-based strategies derived from Zen, such as mindfulness skills. For a more exhaustive description of this treatment, see Linehan's manuals (1993a, 1993b). Over time, standard DBT has been adapted to address a variety of problematic behaviors associated with emotion dysregulation, including eating disorders (EDs). This chapter focuses on adaptations of DBT for patients with bulimia nervosa (BN) or binge-eating disorder (BED) and coexisting BPD, and for patients with primary BN or BED. The former adaptation was researched at the University of Washington, Seattle, and the latter at Stanford University. DBT was adapted for these patients with EDs for several reasons. DBT offers an alternative for difficult-to-treat patients for whom existing treatments have failed. DBT is based on a broad affect regulation model of problems rather than a symptom-focused model, which may be particularly helpful for individuals with EDs and BPD, as this comorbidity is not uncommon among those with BN (Sansone, Levitt, & Sansone, 2005).

In addition to addressing a variety of problem behaviors associated with emotion dysregulation, DBT includes special protocols addressing life-threatening and therapy-interfering behavior (e.g., missing sessions), telephone coaching, and ancillary treatment; novel acceptance-based treatment strategies such as mindfulness; and comprehensive case-management strategies. In addition, DBT attends to the behaviors of both clinicians and patients.

Biosocial Theory

Emotion Dysregulation

The biosocial theory describes both etiological and maintaining factors associated with BPD, which is conceptualized as a disorder of extreme emotion dysregulation. "Emotion dysregulation" refers to the combination of emotional vulnerability and difficulties in modulating emotional reactions. "Emotional vulnerability" refers to a heightened sensitivity to emotional stimuli, intense emotional responses, and a slow return to emotional baseline. Difficulties in emotion modulation may include (1) trouble inhibiting mood-dependent behaviors such as self-injury; (2) difficulty organizing behavior to achieve goals, independent of current mood; (3) impaired up- or downregulation of physiological arousal; (4) trouble diverting attention from emotionally evocative stimuli; and/or (5) difficulty experiencing emotion without avoidance or an extreme secondary negative emotion. Emotion dysregulation results in a cycle of dysfunctional attempts to escape aversive emotions (e.g., using self-injurious behavior to escape anger). Secondary emotions are generated (e.g., shame) that lead in turn to more dysfunctional attempts to escape emotions, fueling the cycle.

The affect regulation model is utilized in adaptations of DBT for EDs. Intense affect is a frequent precursor to binge eating and other ED behaviors, which may provide a means, albeit maladaptive, of regulating emotions. ED behaviors in the absence of other adaptive emotion regulation skills may become negatively reinforced (i.e., as escape behaviors) or result in secondary emotions such as shame or guilt, which prompt further ED behaviors. Using this model, DBT is designed to teach adaptive affect regulation skills and to target behaviors resulting from emotion dysregulation.

Invalidating Environment

The biosocial theory asserts that BPD develops over time due to transactions between an invalidating environment and an emotionally vulnerable individual. The invalidating environment may negate, punish, and/or respond erratically and inappropriately to private experiences and self-generated behaviors, particularly emotional experiences, independent of the validity of the actual behavior. This pattern may lead to the punishment of emotional displays and thereby to an inadvertent intermittent reinforcement of emotional escalation over time. It may also lead to the oversimplification of goal-setting and problem-solving processes. This theory has been broadened to include individuals with EDs. The invalidating environment may include specific invalidation of ED behaviors (e.g., "Why can't you just stop eating?"), weight-related teasing, or overconcern with weight by peers and family.

Stages of Treatment and Targets

In standard DBT treatment is organized around the patient's level of disorder, as determined by the current severity, pervasiveness, complexity, disability, and imminent threat of the patient's problems. Each level of disorder is associated with a different treatment stage, with each stage associated with particular treatment goals. DBT stages involve

(1) *pretreatment*, in which patients are oriented to the treatment and to patient–clinician agreements and establish commitment to treatment goals (particularly to stopping suicidal and self-injurious behavior); (2) *Stage I*, stopping out-of-control behaviors; (3) *Stage II*, replacing "quiet desperation" with nontraumatic emotional experiencing; (4) *Stage III*, reducing ongoing disorders and problems in living; and (5) *Stage IV*, resolving a sense of incompleteness in order to achieve freedom. Each stage of treatment is associated with a target hierarchy. For example, Stage I target hierarchy is to (1) reduce life-threatening behaviors (e.g., suicide attempts, increase in suicide ideation, nonsuicidal self-injurious behaviors, homicidal threats and behaviors), (2) reduce therapy-interfering behaviors (e.g., missed sessions), and (3) reduce quality-of-life-interfering behaviors (e.g., substance abuse or other Axis I disorders, homelessness), and (4) increase behavioral skills.

Stage I individual DBT is organized around the highest-priority behaviors on the target hierarchy that are present at a session, as determined by a patient's current urges to commit suicide, to self-injure or to quit treatment and from the patient's diary card ratings (Wisniewski, Safer, & Chen, 2007) over the last week. Secondary targets are dialectical dilemmas characteristic of BPD patients that interfere with therapy. These include swinging between intense emotional vulnerability and self-invalidation of emotions, being engaged in passive problem-solving behavior yet being apparently competent, and shifting from the experience of unrelenting crises to inhibited grieving. Progression through targets is recursive rather than linear. The University of Washington model of DBT for BED or BN with BPD is an adaptation for Stage I patients, whereas the Stanford DBT model is an adaptation for Stage III patients.

Structure of Treatment

Stage I DBT functions to enhance patient and clinician behavioral capabilities and motivation. This goal is accomplished for patients by increasing skillful behavior, reducing reinforcement for dysfunctional or ineffective behavior (e.g., restructuring the environment), and generalizing behavior from the therapy setting to the natural environment. Modes of treatment include weekly individual psychotherapy, group skills training, a "therapist consultation team," and 24-hour telephone consultation. Each treatment mode involves a different hierarchy of targets. The individual clinician is responsible for assessment and problem solving of skills deficits and motivational problems, including organizing other treatment modes in service of these. Group skills training targets the acquisition of new behavioral skills in a structured psychoeducational format where four modules are taught: mindfulness, distress tolerance, emotion regulation, and interpersonal effectiveness skills. Telephone consultation provides emergency crisis intervention and disrupts potential reinforcement of suicidal behavior by having patients page clinicians before engaging in such behavior. This protocol utilizes a "24-hour rule," such that clinicians do not inadvertently reinforce suicidal behavior by responding to patients within the 24 hours after such an episode takes place. Telephone consultation also provides skills coaching to promote skill generalization and to repair patient–clinician relationships. DBT attends as much to clinician behavior as patient behavior. The therapist consultation team, which is regarded as therapy for the therapist, enhances clinicians' motivation, builds clinicians' skills, and manages problems arising in the delivery of DBT. DBT is seen as a treatment involving a community of clinicians treating a community of patients.

Treatment Strategies

The treatment strategies in DBT balance change and acceptance and include dialectical strategies, core strategies, stylistic strategies, case management strategies, and integrated strategies. The first four are outlined here.

1. *Dialectical strategies* highlight dichotomous thinking, behavior, and emotions to assist patients in finding balanced and synthesized responses to polarities. Patients learn, for instance, that polar viewpoints can coexist without the necessity of shifting between viewpoints. The fundamental dialectic underlying treatment is that of acceptance and change (e.g., acceptance of the patient's present ineffective behavior as well as the need for this behavior to change). Various dialectical strategies include the use of metaphors, stories, paradox, playing devil's advocate, fluctuating between ambiguity and certainty, using cognitive restructuring, highlighting continual change, and validating a patient's intuitive wisdom.

2. *Core strategies* that underlie DBT are based on facilitating acceptance and behavioral change. The latter strategies include the chain analysis: a meticulous analysis of the topography, intensity, frequency, duration, situation, antecedents, and consequences of a problem behavior. This strategy is typically conducted within individual psychotherapy. Repeated chain analyses of a problem behavior allow the clinician and patient to determine the cues, the maintaining factors, and the function of a behavior. In turn, this strategy enables the clinician to determine what prevented the patient from being effective in a prior situation and subsequently to teach new skills (e.g., using role play and rehearsal). These new skills might consist of emotion regulation skills, cognitive modification, or mindfulness to address faulty cognition. Environmental contingencies may also be clarified. Once having established a solution with the patient and a plan to prevent future problem behaviors, the clinician assesses the patient's commitment. A variety of commitment strategies are used, including evaluating pros and cons, playing devil's advocate, and using "foot in the door" (a therapist increases compliance by making an easier request first of the client followed by a more difficult request) and "door in the face" (a therapist requests the client of something much larger than the therapist expects and then asks for something easier) strategies. The clinician troubleshoots the plan, with the patient revising as necessary, and then ascertains the patient's commitment to the revised plan.

In every DBT encounter with a patient, change strategies are balanced with acceptance strategies. Validation, for example, is utilized to build and maintain a strong therapeutic relationship. Validation strategies include listening in an interested fashion, reflecting accurately, articulating unstated thoughts and emotions, communicating how behaviors make sense given the patient's learning history or present situation, and being radically genuine—that is, treating the patient as one would treat an equal.

3. *Stylistic strategies*, like the core strategies, are built upon a balance of acceptance and change-focused approaches. On the one hand, *reciprocal communication* involves interpersonal warmth, responsiveness to a patient's concerns, and strategic self-

disclosure (to provide a model of coping). On the other hand, *irreverent communication* involves an outrageous, humorous, or blunt style to be utilized when a clinician and patient become deadlocked and therapy becomes polarized.

4. *Case management strategies* include three specific tactics. First, the "consultation-to-the-patient strategy" teaches a patient how to interact with the environment rather than attempting to organize the environment to meet his/her needs. Second, "environmental interventions," in which the clinician acts directly on the patient's behalf, are utilized when a patient is in immediate danger or is powerless. Third, with the "consultation-to-the-clinician strategy" individual clinicians seek consultation in their team for support and assistance in delivering DBT effectively.

Treatment Literature

Standard DBT is currently the most empirically validated treatment for BPD, with seven randomized controlled trials providing evidence of its efficacy ([1] Linehan, Armstrong, Suarez, Allmon, & Heard [1991], with follow-up reported in Linehan, Tutek, Heard, & Armstrong [1994] and Linehan, Heard, & Armstrong [1993]; [2] Linehan et al. [1999]; [3] Linehan et al. [2002]; [4] Turner [2000]; [5] Koons et al. [2001]; [6] Verheul et al. [2003], with the study described in detail in van den Bosch, Verheul, Schippers, & van de Brink [2002]; and [7] Linehan et al. [2006]). Compared to treatment as usual or treatment by experts, 1 year of standard DBT was found to significantly reduce suicidal and nonsuicidal self-injurious behavior or other target behaviors (e.g., substance dependence) and to improve global and social adjustment as well as mood. Other randomized controlled trials of DBT have included medication (Simpson et al., 2004; Soler et al., 2005) as well as adaptations of standard DBT for older adults with depression (Lynch, Morse, Mendelson, & Robins, 2003) and individuals with treatment-resistant depression (Harley, Sprich, Safren, Jacobo, & Fava, 2008). A controlled trial was used to investigate DBT for suicidal adolescents with BPD symptoms (Rathus & Miller, 2002).

There are currently two published small open trials for individuals with both BPD and ED, each utilizing minimal adaptations of standard DBT (Chen, Matthews, Allen, Kuo, & Linehan, 2008; Palmer et al., 2003). The former study, conducted at the University of Washington, employed 6 months of a minimally adapted version of standard DBT with women with BED or BN and BPD ($N = 8$). Assessments were conducted pretreatment, posttreatment, and at 6-month follow-up. From pretreatment to 6-month follow-up, there were large reductions in suicidal behavior and nonsuicidal self-injury, binge eating, secondary ED concerns, the number of coexisting non-ED Axis I psychiatric disorders, and a large improvement in social functioning. The same large reductions were also found from pre- to posttreatment, with smaller reductions in the number of coexisting non-ED Axis I disorders and in suicidal behavior and self-injury. The latter study, which added five or six sessions of a psychoeducational skills module addressing ED behavior, found a substantial reduction in hospital days and self-injury ($N = 7$). Additionally, three of the seven patients remitted from their ED and four improved.

The only adaptation of DBT for EDs currently supported through randomized controlled trials is the Stanford model for BN and BED. Given this singularity, much of the chapter is devoted to describing this program. The Stanford DBT model for BN or BED differs from standard DBT program for BPD in a number of ways affecting treatment structure and content. These differences include the following: (1) only a single modality of treatment delivery is used (e.g., group DBT for BED and individual DBT for BN); (2) treatment involves 20 sessions; and (3) three DBT skills modules (mindfulness, emotion regulation, distress tolerance)—for reasons related to research design—are utilized instead of the four in standard DBT.

Following initial promising findings from a small (uncontrolled) case-series report of DBT for BED (Telch, Agras, & Linehan, 2000) and case reports of DBT for BED (Telch, 1997a) and for BN (Safer, Telch, & Agras, 2001a), three small randomized controlled trials have been performed to date (Safer, Robinson, & Jo, in press; Safer, Telch, & Agras, 2001b; Telch, Agras, & Linehan, 2001). Of the three randomized controlled trials testing the Stanford DBT Model for BED and BN, two involved BED (Safer et al., in press; Telch et al., 2001) and one BN (Safer et al., 2001b). In the first DBT for BED study, Telch and colleagues (2001) reported that 89% (16 of 18) women receiving DBT were abstinent from binge eating, compared to 12.5% (2 of 16) of the wait-list controls at the end of the 20-week treatment study. In addition, DBT showed significantly greater improvements than the wait-list control group on body image, eating concerns, and urges to eat when angry. At 3-month follow-up, 67% (12 of 18) of women receiving DBT were abstinent, and 56% (10 of 18) were abstinent at 6-month follow-up. Because of the wait-list design, those in the wait list were not followed up but were offered DBT. Of the 10 individuals in the wait-list group who later received DBT, 90% (9 of 10) were abstinent at posttreatment, 80% (8 of 10) at 3-month follow-up, and 67% (6 of 10) at 6-month follow-up.

Similar promising findings were found in a replication study of the Stanford DBT model for BED, in which the patient population was expanded to include both men and women and individuals on stable doses of psychotropic medication (Safer et al., in press). Participants in both the DBT and active supportive psychotherapy group improved substantially in achieving binge abstinence. Posttreatment abstinence rates were 64% for DBT and 36% for supportive psychotherapy, and at 12-month follow-up abstinence rates were 64% and 56% for DBT and supportive psychotherapy, respectively. DBT, however, had a significantly lower dropout rate (4%) compared to supportive psychotherapy (33.3%). Additionally, at 12-month follow-up, a significantly lower percentage of supportive psychotherapy participants completed assessments (76.5%) compared to those in the DBT group (98%). These differences suggest that although there were no significant differences in binge-eating abstinence between treatment groups at 12-month follow-up, DBT was superior to supportive psychotherapy in maintaining engagement in treatment—that is, in reducing therapy-interfering behavior.

In the randomized controlled trial of DBT for BN (Safer et al., 2001b), individually delivered DBT skills training for bulimic behaviors was compared to no training in the wait-list control group. Binge–purge abstinence rates at the end of 20 weeks of treatment were 28.6% (4 of 14) compared to 0% (0 of 15) for the wait-list control (Safer et al., 2001b), with both groups improving on secondary ED outcomes. The outcome of the wait-list group for this BN trial (Safer et al., 2001b) appeared to be lower than that for an earlier BED trial (Telch et al., 2001), which may be due to the greater severity of BN.

In conclusion, the study findings of DBT for EDs are promising, although more randomized controlled trials are needed to establish the efficacy and effectiveness of this treatment for this patient group. In particular, larger studies that utilize more active and specific control treatments are needed.

We first briefly describe the University of Washington model of DBT for individuals with BED or BN and BPD, because this model is closest to the original DBT treatment model for patients in Stage I. As noted, the remainder of the chapter focuses on the Stanford DBT model for BED or BN, an adaptation intended for Stage III patients whose BED or BN symptoms are the primary focus of treatment.

University of Washington
DBT Model for BPD with BED or BN

The model for Stage I BPD with BN or BED is briefly outlined below.

Target Hierarchy

The standard Stage I DBT targets outlined earlier (p. 296) are unchanged in this adaptation. In other words, ED behavior targets or weight loss are not specifically prioritized when addressing quality-of-life targets. In deciding which quality-of-life target to treat, the clinician prioritizes patient problems that are immediate, easily solved, functionally related to higher-priority targets such as life-threatening behavior, and that fit the patient's goals. For example, in one case, a patient with BED and BPD also complained of a hoarding problem. Her apartment was so full of belongings that it was difficult to move from room to room. For this patient, hoarding was functionally related to higher-order targets (i.e., the hoarding led to suicidal feelings), and this patient wanted to change her hoarding behavior but did not feel the same about her binge eating. Initially in treatment, when binge eating was prioritized over hoarding, this patient refused to continue therapy. However, when the second clinician on the consultation team reprioritized the hoarding ahead of the binge eating, the patient reengaged in therapy, and both behaviors improved.

Assessment prior to and frequently throughout the course of treatment is required for determining quality-of-life targets. Such assessment may involve examining the effect on life-threatening behaviors if various quality-of-life behaviors (including binge eating and hoarding) were to increase or decrease as well as the effect on life-threatening behaviors if binge eating or other quality-of-life behaviors were to stop. Overweight patients with BED are highly likely to list weight loss as a quality-of-life goal. For overweight patients, we recommend that clinicians establish realistic expectations about weight loss early in treatment to prevent later frustration with failures to lose unrealistic amounts of weight. Clinicians should be educated about the importance of focusing on specific achievable lifestyle changes (e.g., stopping binge eating, limiting eating out at restaurants) and the possible use of ancillary treatments such as walking groups.

Addressing multiple complex problems in one session is challenging but necessary. Tips for clinicians include finding common links between multiple behaviors (e.g., emotions or secondary targets) and coaching patients to skillfully address these; conducting a chain analysis on a day that the patient engaged in multiple target behaviors; and/or focusing on multiple brief chain analyses, asking, for example, "What would you have done differently to be more effective?"

Treatment Structure

The University of Washington DBT model for BPD with BED or BN utilizes the same treatment modalities as standard DBT (see pp. 294–300). For reasons related to the research design, the protocol is 6 months long. It is important to note that most Stage I DBT studies involve 12 months of treatment and that in some situations this greater duration may be preferable.

Individual DBT

In the pretreatment stage (see p. 304), patients are oriented to the structure of treatment, including the use of telephone consultation and the four-miss rule (patients in DBT who miss four consecutive scheduled group skills training sessions or four scheduled individual sessions are regarded as dropping out of treatment). Patients also are required to have their own physicians conduct an initial medical assessment as well as provide ongoing monitoring. In order to quickly stop problem behaviors such as binge eating, patients are taught crisis survival skills to identify cues to problem behaviors and to examine the pros and cons of these behaviors. A crisis plan to prevent life-threatening and other dysfunctional behaviors is formulated. Patients are asked to commit to ceasing life-threatening behaviors, maintain regular treatment attendance, and stop binge eating and drug use. At each individual DBT session the clinician greets the patient and asks him/her to rate urges (0–5) to commit suicide, quit therapy, and binge-eat or engage in any other target behavior. The diary card is then reviewed, skillful behavior reinforced, and problem behaviors noted. A chain analysis is carried out on any life-threatening behavior. Depending on the time remaining, chain analyses are also conducted on lower-ranking behaviors that occurred over the course of the week. If there are no such behaviors, chain analyses are conducted on urges connected with the highest-ranking behaviors in the hierarchy (if increased by at least 2 points from last week) or diary card.

DBT Skills Group

Participants with BPD and either BN or BED are placed in the same group. There is no module specifically addressing ED behaviors, and only minor adaptations are made to the skills program (i.e., modeling the use of skills to prevent binge-eating behaviors). For patients who also attempt to regulate their emotions through restriction or overexercise, more adaptive alternatives incompatible with binge eating are identified. Mindfulness exercises concerning eating and body awareness are utilized, including the "raisin exercise" adapted from Kabat-Zinn (1990), and observing and describing the taste and texture of a piece of melting chocolate. Patients are to note any judgmental thoughts that may arise (e.g., "Chocolate is bad"; "This is sinful").

Therapist Consultation Team

Members of the University of Washington DBT model for BPD with BED or BN team are trained in the identification and treatment of EDs (e.g., high-risk ED behaviors, consequences of ED behaviors, obesity) and information regarding activity, weight, and healthy eating. Training may take the form of lectures, journal clubs, engaging a consultant, and workshops.

24-Hour Phone Consultation

Whereas phone consultation rules are those of standard DBT, the time interval before the patient can call after engaging in binge eating (24-hour rule) is determined by examination of the patient's chain analysis, binge-eating frequency, the degree of reinforcement experienced by clinician contact, and patient and clinician agreements. During a typical 10-minute phone consultation the individual clinician, after assessing urges, may ask: "What skills have you tried to prevent binge eating? What help do you need to use skills?" After generating solutions and a plan, the clinician obtains the patient's commitment to this plan, troubleshoots the plan, and then asks the patient to page again if he/she runs into difficulty. Patients who avoid telephone consultation, despite its potential helpfulness, are given homework to make phone calls.

Ancillary Treatment

Patients are required to have a full medical workup and ongoing medical monitoring (e.g., regular assessment of electrolytes) by their own physicians. Attendance is monitored by the DBT individual clinician, and nonattendance is targeted as therapy-interfering behavior. Ancillary activities are also utilized for weight management or related medical issues (e.g., consultation with a dietician, personal trainer, gym, specialist in chronic pain or diabetes, attending Weight Watchers) or for other psychological treatment (e.g., Narcotics Anonymous, pharmacotherapy). Ancillary providers are often accustomed to speaking with the clinician rather than patient him/herself. The consultation-to-the-patient case consultation strategy in DBT encourages patients to skillfully interact directly with ancillary treatment providers after being coached by the clinician.

Dialectical Strategies

During pretreatment, patients are taught the concept of dialectical abstinence from objective binge eating (this concept is more fully described in the discussion of the Stanford DBT model, pp. 303–310). Secondary targets and dialectical dilemmas include "overcontrolled eating" versus "out-of-control objective binge eating," or the vacillation between extreme dieting and loss of control. The synthesis of this dialectical dilemma involves engaging in neither extreme but eating in moderation. Dialectical dilemmas to discuss with patients trying to lose weight include the dialectic of "no activity" versus "overexercise," with the synthesis being incorporating healthy activity into one's lifestyle.

Core Strategies

The standard DBT diary card was adapted to include assessment of ED behaviors. Chain analyses are conducted in individual DBT and often target binge eating or ED behaviors. Similar to standard DBT, the clinician validates the patient, as appropriate, during every interaction, paying particular attention to the shame many patients with ED feel regarding their eating behavior.

Stanford DBT Model for BED or BN

The Stanford model of DBT, initially developed by Telch (Safer, Telch, & Chen, 2009; Telch, 1997b), is an adaptation of standard DBT that targets patients whose BED or BN symptoms are the primary focus of treatment. Individuals with active suicidal or self-injurious behaviors should be offered a Stage I treatment, such as the University of Washington DBT model described above. This section describes the group DBT program adapted for BED, highlighting any exceptions for DBT for BN, which is delivered in an individual format.

Target Hierarchy

As per the standard DBT hierarchy, if suicidal or nonsuicidal self-injurious behaviors emerge during treatment, the focus of therapy shifts immediately to stopping life-threatening behaviors. For the majority of patients with primary BN or BED, however, the highest treatment target is reducing any behavior(s) that interferes with the successful delivery of treatment, followed by the targets in Figure 16.1.

"Mindless eating" refers to not attending to one's eating (e.g., eating popcorn while watching TV and finding that one has finished the bowl without being aware of this occurring). Unlike with binge eating, a loss of control is not experienced in mindless eating. "Food preoccupation" involves having one's thoughts or attention absorbed or focused on food to the point that functioning is adversely affected (e.g., inability to concentrate at work or school). "Capitulating" is giving up on one's goals to cope skillfully with emotions and stop binge eating and, instead, acting as if there were no other option than to cope by using food. Finally, "apparently irrelevant behaviors" are those that do not appear relevant to binge eating and purging or that a patient convinces him/herself do not matter but which, upon examination with the chain analysis, actually play an important role (e.g., buying extra dessert to have on hand "for company" may seem irrelevant but may lead to binge eating).

Treatment Structure

A distinctive feature of the Stanford model is that it combines individual and group functions of standard DBT into one 2-hour group session (for BED) or one 50-minute individual session (for BN). The Stanford model includes a pretreatment interview followed by 20 treatment sessions, as described below. The pretreatment interview as well as Sessions 1 and 2 comprise the pretreatment stage and include an orientation to the treatment model and targets, a review of group rules and agreements, attainment of a group commitment to stop binge eating, and explanation of the concept of dialecti-

1. Stop binge eating (and purging, for patients with BN).
2. Eliminate mindless eating.
3. Decrease cravings, urges, preoccupation with food.
4. Decrease capitulating.
5. Decrease apparently irrelevant behaviors.

FIGURE 16.1. Path to mindful eating.

cal abstinence. Sessions 3–5 cover the mindfulness module, Sessions 6–12 the emotion regulation module, and Sessions 14–18 the distress tolerance module. Sessions 19 and 20 are devoted to review and relapse prevention. As mentioned, the interpersonal effectiveness module is not included for reasons related to research design (i.e., time constraints, potential overlap with interpersonal psychotherapy). Clinicians not limited to 20 sessions or to a particular research protocol may wish to include this module.

Pretreatment Interview

Each patient meets individually with one of the clinicians (or, for BN, the individual clinician) for 30–45 minutes prior to beginning therapy. The major goals of this pretreatment visit involve (1) orienting patients to the DBT emotion regulation model of binge eating and the targets of treatment, (2) describing the expectations for group members (e.g., regular timely attendance, listening to tapes of any missed sessions, completing homework assignments), and (3) eliciting a commitment from the patient to stop binge eating and to address any treatment-interfering behaviors that may arise. Formal clinician and patient agreements are reviewed and signed during this visit.

Clinician Pointers for Pretreatment Interview

The clinician conducts this session and obtains a commitment using the same dialectical and irreverence strategies that would be used in standard DBT with an individual patient. For example, if a patient expresses hesitancy about his/her ability to attend all group sessions, the clinician might choose the stylistic strategy of irreverence to say, "Gosh, if you'd been able to stop binge eating on your own, you'd never have come in for treatment. I know that you don't want this program to be another that failed to help you stop binge eating. But the research on this treatment was based on those who came to sessions and completed treatment, not those that didn't come to sessions." Clinicians might also employ the metaphor of taking antibiotics, explaining that attending only some of the sessions is like being prescribed a course of antibiotics and stopping halfway or taking doses only intermittently. Such a situation can be less helpful than not having started any treatment at all.

Sessions 1–20: Format of Group Sessions—
Combining Elements of Individual and Skills Groups

The first half of a group or individual session (i.e., 1 hour for DBT for BED and 25 minutes for DBT for BN) is used to review homework. This review entails discussion of patient diary cards, chain analyses, and practice of the prior week's newly presented skills, including description of specific successes or difficulties in applying the skills to replace targeted problem eating behaviors. Groups consist of 8–10 patients and are run by two clinicians, who explain that each member will have about 5 minutes to report on his/her homework (see below for pointers). Group members are encouraged to help one another identify solutions to problems encountered in using the skills and to "cheerlead" each others' efforts. A 5- to 8-minute break separates the first half from the second of the DBT for BED sessions. This second half is devoted to skills instruction: teaching, practicing, and strengthening new and previously presented skills.

Therapeutic Pointers for Homework Review

Group members are assigned homework of filling out at least one chain analysis each week for at least the first 15 sessions. Even if they do not engage in binge eating, patients can use the chain to describe another targeted behavior or to identify a problem behavior unique to them that sets them up for binge eating. If patients have had absolutely no eating-related problem behaviors during a particular week, they could describe a past binge-eating episode or a non-eating-related problem behavior. By week 16, patients can begin to fill out chain analyses only as needed for any problematic eating-related episodes.

Because of the limited time available, clinicians should help patients stay focused. For example, group members are oriented to the importance of making maximal use of the allotted time by coming to sessions with their completed diary card, chain analysis, and specific skill homework sheets. This orientation is given briefly in Session 1 and in more detail in Session 2.

When discussing their chain analyses, group members are asked to focus on the highest-ranking problem behaviors on the treatment hierarchy (e.g., a binge-eating episode rather than a mindless eating episode). To maximize the use of group time, each group member is asked to be prepared to report on (1) the key dysfunctional link identified in the chain leading to the problem eating behavior, and (2) what skill or skills could have been used (and will be used next time) to replace that dysfunctional link. It is important to distinguish between "telling a story" and reporting from the chain. For group members who are having difficulty with their skills practice and application, clinicians should troubleshoot to determine whether the problem is a matter of not understanding the skill or needing additional practice using the skill in order to implement it effectively. Noncompletion of homework is identified and addressed as therapy-interfering behavior (i.e., an in-session chain analysis is then completed or assigned as homework).

In order to prevent a potential increase in urges or cravings by having group members discuss their problematic food behaviors (i.e., a potential contagion effect), members are asked to avoid mentioning specific food names during the first 10 or so sessions of the treatment (i.e., speak of "dessert" instead of "double chocolate fudge sundae"). After the 10th session, members are encouraged to use their skills to cope with any cravings or urges triggered by the mention of specific food names.

Session 1: Orientation to Treatment— Orientation to the Model and Targets, Review of Group Rules and Agreements, and Obtaining a Group Commitment to Stop Binge Eating

Clinicians begin by welcoming patients to the treatment program and expressing enthusiasm about embarking on this experience together. A major task of this first session is to obtain a group commitment to stop binge eating. After initial introductions by each group member and the clinicians, it is key that clinicians create a groundswell of motivation and commitment from group members by flexibly utilizing the commitment strategies of standard DBT. Clinicians might begin by using a devil's advocate strategy. In a somewhat puzzled and challenging manner, for example, they might say: "Okay, we're assuming that you are all here because you want to gain control over your eating behavior. Specifically, we're assuming that you want to stop binge eating, right? We're also assuming that you want to enjoy your life—that is, you want a quality of life in which you enjoy your relationships, feel a sense of mastery, and feel good about yourself most of the time. And as we understand it, binge eating is a problem because it interferes with feeling good about yourself and having the quality of life you desire. What isn't clear to us is this: Why can't you have a quality life and stay a binge eater? Why can't you do both? Explain that to us." (Safer et al., 2009; Telch, 1997a).

Playing devil's advocate encourages group members to argue that it is imperative for them to stop binge eating in order to lead a quality life. Clinicians must be sure to polarize the argument by describing the quality of life they believe group members can attain as one that is deeply rewarding, one in which group members are fully alive and feel very very good about themselves—a seeming impossibility to many patients with BED. In other words, clinicians must ensure that group members understand that references to "quality of life" involve more than simply existing, getting through, or minimizing pain.

Clinicians then use the group members' arguments as a starting point for eliciting the pros and cons of continuing life as a binge eater, listing these on the board. For example, they might say: "Okay, based on what we've just heard from you, there is absolutely no other choice than to stop binge eating. You've convinced us with your arguments. So let's face it and put this on the table before we get any farther. Binge eating is over. Whenever you last binged, that was the last one. You simply can't have the kind of life you want to lead and continue binge eating and problem eating. So we're all in agreement, right? We're all committed, right?" (Safer et al., 2009; Telch, 1997a). The goal is to obtain a verbal commitment from each group member. Some patients may fear making a commitment because of worries that they will fail. Clinicians might ask: "Are you worried about binge eating in this moment or are you worried about the future? We're not talking about the future but about this one moment. Can you make a commitment to try your absolute hardest to never ever binge again in this one moment, right now?" (this is an example of the DBT commitment strategy "foot in the door"; Safer et al., 2009; Telch, 1997a). If a patient insists "it's impossible" or that making a commitment would be a "setup," clinicians might query: "Would it literally be impossible? I mean, it would likely be very, very difficult and scary—but is it literally impossible, like pigs flying?" [irreverence]. If the patient concedes that it actually would be possible, clinicians can respond: "So, it sounds like you agree it might actually be possible to stop bingeing, but you are very certain that you would fail in the attempt. Therefore it feels easier to tell yourself that stopping binge eating is impossible than to try to stop. Because if you were to try your best but fail, you would have to feel awful about yourself not only for having binged but for failing in your attempt to stop. I can understand that kind of thinking [validation]. Yet we know from research on commitments that when people don't make a commitment or when they say they will accept less—this can become a self-fulfilling prophecy" (Safer et al., 2009; Telch, 1997a).

In addition to this group commitment, other tasks of Session 1 include orienting group members to (1) the emotion regulation model of binge eating, (2) the treatment targets and group agreements, (3) the biosocial model, and (4) the diary card and chain analysis.

Session 2: Explaining Dialectical Abstinence

In Session 2, after conducting homework review for the first half of the session (see above), clinicians introduce patients to the concept of dialectical abstinence, originally developed in DBT for substance use disorders (Linehan & Dimeff, 1997). Dialectical abstinence is a synthesis of a 100% commitment to abstinence and a 100% commitment to relapse prevention strategies. Before a patient engages in binge eating, there is an unrelenting insistence on total abstinence. After a patient has engaged in binge eating, however, the emphasis is on radical acceptance, nonjudgmental problem solving and effective relapse prevention, followed by a speedy return to an unrelenting insistence on abstinence.

Clinicians might introduce this concept with an explanation that a "dialectical view" recognizes that for every force or position there exists an opposing force or position: a thesis and antithesis; the yin and the yang. A dialectical view searches for a synthesis that is more than the sum of the opposite parts. For example, the yin and yang symbol is black and white, yet the synthesis of these is not merely the color gray. A synthesis transcends both.

This leads to discussion of a problem as well as its solution. On the one hand, group members have all made a 100% commitment to binge abstinence. Anything short would be failure. When faced with the urge to binge, one cannot have the idea that it is "okay" to binge-eat and fail and to "just try again." Such thinking is undermining and will make it more likely one will decide to binge-eat. On the other hand, it is clear that in not anticipating and preparing for a slip, patients will be less likely to handle such an event effectively, should it occur. This is the problem with which clinicians and group members are faced and which is presented for discussion: How can one deal with these two opposing forces of success and failure?

The Olympics metaphor described by Telch (Safer et al., 2009; Telch, 1997a) becomes quite useful here. The clinicians suggest that group members are like Olympic athletes and the clinicians, like coaches. Patients are participating in an incredibly important event, improving their lives by stopping binge eating. It takes tremendous effort. Absolutely nothing is discussed before a race in the Olympics except winning, or "going for the gold." An Olympian cannot think "maybe a bronze would be okay" or focus on what might happen if he/she falls down. Similarly, the only thing group members can possibly allow themselves to think about and discuss is absolute and total abstinence from binge eating. Yet, of course, athletes and group members must be prepared for the possibility of failure. The key is to be prepared to fail well. The dialectical dilemma is that both success and failure exist. The dialectical abstinence solution involves 100% certainty that binge eating is out of the question and 100% confidence that one will never binge again. Simultaneously, one keeps in mind ("way, way back in the very farthest part so that it never interferes with your resolve") that if one slips, one will deal with it effectively by accepting it nonjudgmentally and picking oneself back up, knowing one will never slip again.

Sessions 3–5: Mindfulness Skills

The mindfulness skills are introduced in these three sessions and reviewed in Session 12. These skills are the same as those taught in standard DBT (e.g., wise mind, the "what" skills, the "how" skills) except for an additional three described below: mindful eating, urge surfing, and alternate rebellion. The latter two skills have origins in earlier substance abuse work (Linehan & Dimeff, 1997; Marlatt & Gordon, 1985).

Mindful Eating. Mindful eating, as opposed to mindless eating, is the experience of full participation in eating: that is, observing and describing in one's mind the experience. It is eating with full awareness and attention ("one-mindfully"; only eating and not doing other things at the same time), but without self-consciousness or judgment.

Urge Surfing. Urge surfing involves mindful, nonattached observation of urges to binge-eat or eat mindlessly. Mindfulness skills teach one to accept the reality that there are cues in the world that trigger one's urges to binge-eat. Patients are taught how urges and cravings are classically conditioned responses that have been associated with a particular cue. Mindful urge surfing involves awareness without engaging in impulsive mood-dependent behavior. One simply notices and then describes the ebb and flow of the urge. This approach involves "letting go" or "detaching" from the object of the urge and "riding the wave" of the urge instead. Although similar to mindfulness of the current emotion, urge surfing is a mindfulness skill that involves nonjudgmental observation and description of urges, cravings, and food preoccupation.

Alternate Rebellion. The aim of this skill is to satisfy the wish to rebel without destroying one's overriding objective to stop binge eating. The purpose is not to suppress or judge the rebellion but to find creative ways to rebel so as not to "cut off your nose to spite your face." In other words, this skill makes use of the mindfulness skill of being *effective.* Many patients with BED describe a desire to "get back" at society, friends, and/or family members whom they perceive as judgmental about their weight. For these patients, "getting back" involves rebelling through consuming even more food. This behavior would not be viewed as an effective means to achieve one's goals. Clinicians encourage patients to observe the need to rebel, label this as such, and then, if patients decide to act on the wish, to do so effectively. Group members can be creative in thinking up alternate rebellion strategies. For example, a patient who feels judged by society for being obese might "rebel" by mindfully going to a restaurant and openly, unselfconsciously treating herself to a healthy and delicious bowl of soup.

Sessions 6–12: Emotion Regulation Skills

These sessions cover the emotion regulation skills taught in standard DBT, without any specific adaptations for BED. These skills involve observing and describing emotions, learning the function of emotions, decreasing vulnerability to "emotion mind," increasing positive events, and acting opposite to the current emotion.

Sessions 13–18: Distress Tolerance Skills

These sessions cover the distress tolerance skills of standard DBT. One skill, "burning bridges," has been added. Like many of the other skills adapted for BED, it was borrowed from DBT—substance use disorder (SUD; Linehan & Dimeff, 1997).

Burning Bridges. This radical acceptance skill involves accepting, at the deepest and most radical level, the idea that one is really not going to binge-eat or mindlessly eat or abuse oneself with food ever again—thus, burning the bridge to those behaviors. One accepts that one will no longer block, deny, or avoid reality with binge eating. Instead, one makes a covenant from deep within to accept reality and one's experiences.

Sessions 19–20: Relapse Prevention

Session 19 begins with a review of mindfulness, emotion regulation, and distress tolerance skills. In addition, patients are asked to fill out a "Planning for the Future" Worksheet for Session 20, which asks the following: "(1) Detail your specific plans for continuing to practice the skills taught. (2) Outline your specific plans for skillfully managing emotions in the future. Think of circumstances and emotions that previously set off binge eating. Outline your plans for dealing with the emotions that will prevent any problem eating behaviors. Write about at least 3 different emotions. (3) Write about what you need to do next in your life to continue to build a satisfying and rewarding quality of life for yourself."

In Session 20 each group member reviews his/her worksheet. Final goodbyes and perhaps a goodbye ritual (e.g., writing cards) are used to mark the end of treatment.

Therapist Consultation Team. Clinicians meet weekly with the treatment team to confer regarding the progress of treatment and adherence to DBT principles. Unlike standard DBT, only group or only individual session format is discussed, depending on the mode of delivery.

Telephone Consultation. Patients are encouraged to call clinicians if they have questions during the week (e.g., checking on what homework was assigned). However, 24-hour telephone consultation, as practiced by individual clinicians in standard DBT, is not used.

Ancillary Treatments. The research protocol proscribed patients from seeking concurrent outside treatment (e.g., psychotherapy, behavioral weight loss). Exceptions, such as visiting a medical doctor for physical complaints associated with obesity, would involve consultation to the patient as necessary. Given the research protocol's proscriptions, the utility of possibly combining DBT with other ancillary treatments is not known.

Dialectical Strategies. As described and highlighted earlier, dialectical strategies utilized in this treatment include the teaching of dialectical abstinence, metaphor, devil's advocate, and foot in the door/door in the face (used in eliciting commitment). It also includes the use of stylistic strategies such as irreverence, which is particularly useful in situations when patients and clinicians become polarized. Examples include the following:

PATIENT: My wise mind told me to binge.

CLINICIAN: (*laughing good-naturedly*) Come on! Your wise mind would never say that—was that the wise mind or the cookie monster?! [irreverent reframe, confronting]

PATIENT: Nothing has changed. This isn't working. [Patient has not been practicing skills.]

CLINICIAN: (*gently teasing tone*) What a mystery! I can't imagine why everything isn't totally different for you, since you're doing everything exactly the same! [irreverence]

PATIENT: I couldn't keep practicing the skills because they were taking too much time.

CLINICIAN: (*with a humorous tone*) Ah—I get it. Practicing the skills took up too much time ... but you *were* able to fit in time for a binge. [irreverent, confronting]

Or

If you had time to binge, you had time to practice the skills. (*speaking directly and to the point*)

PATIENT: The skills just aren't strong enough to help me stop binge eating!

CLINICIAN: Oh, I've certainly heard that one before. You're going to have to come up with something way more original and creative than that if you want to demoralize me! [irreverent reframe]

Core Strategies. Patients are given a diary card (see Figure 16.2) each week to chart targeted behaviors and use of skills, and they are advised to keep this with them during the day to facilitate accurate recording. Definitions for the treatment targets specific to DBT for BED are given above.

The chain analysis used in DBT for BED is the same as that used in standard DBT. Specific to DBT for BED or BN is how the problem behavior is defined (e.g., binge eating or one of the other targets listed in the treatment target hierarchy in Figure 16.1).

Available Resources

In order to be competent in the delivery of this adapted treatment, familiarity with behavioral principles and of the standard DBT program is essential. Readers are urged to read Linehan's two manuals: *Cognitive-Behavioral Treatment of BPD* (Linehan, 1993a) and the *Skills Training Manual for Treating BPD* (Linehan, 1993b). In addition, interested readers are referred to a descriptive chapter (Wisniewski, Safer, & Chen, 2007) as well as overviews of the Stanford model (Wiser & Telch, 1999) and the University of Washington model (Linehan & Chen, 2005). Descriptive case reports of the Stanford DBT manual (Safer et al., 2001a; Telch, 1997a) and *Dialectical Behavior Therapy for Binge Eating and Bulimia*, a manual by Safer, Telch, and Chen (2009), are also available. Finally, in order to receive more training in DBT, readers are referred to Behavioral Tech. LLC (*http://behavioraltech.org*), a company focused on the dissemination of DBT and other empirically validated treatments.

Instructions for Completing Your Diary Card

Urge to Binge: Refer to the legend and choose the number from the scale (0–6) that best represents your highest rating for the day. The key characteristics of the urge to consider when making your rating are intensity (how strongly you felt the urge) and duration (how long the urge lasted).

Binge Episodes: Write the number of objective binge episodes (OBEs) and subjective binge episodes (SBEs) you had each day. Both OBEs and SBEs involve eating episodes in which you felt a loss of control during the eating. An "OBE" involves eating a large amount of food that others would regard as large for the situation in a short period of time. A "SBE" involves eating an amount of food that others would regard as normal for the situation.

Mindless Eating: Write in the number of mindless eating episodes that you had each day. "Mindless eating" refers to not paying attention to what you are eating, although you do not feel the sense of loss of control that you do during binge episodes. A typical example of mindless eating would be sitting in front of the TV and eating a bag of microwave popcorn without any awareness of the eating (i.e., somehow, the popcorn was gone, and you were only vaguely aware of having eaten it). Again, however, you didn't feel a sense of being out of control during the eating.

Apparently Irrelevant Behaviors (AIBs): Circle either "yes" or "no" depending on whether you did or did not have any AIBs that day. If you did, briefly describe the AIB in the place provided or on another sheet of paper. An "AIB" refers to behaviors that, upon first glance, do not seem relevant to binge eating and purging but which actually are important in the behavior chain leading to these behaviors. You may convince yourself that the behavior doesn't matter or really won't affect your goal to stop bingeing and purging when, in fact, the behavior matters a great deal. A typical AIB might be buying several boxes of your favorite Girl Scout cookies because you wanted to help out a neighbor's daughter (of course, you could buy the cookies and donate them to the neighbor).

Capitulating: Refer to the legend and choose the number from the scale (0–6) that best represents your highest rating for the day. The key characteristics to consider when making your rating are intensity (strength of the capitulating) and duration (how long it lasted). "Capitulating" refers to giving up on your goals to stop binge eating and skillfully cope with emotions. Instead, you capitulate or surrender to bingeing, acting as if there were no other option or way to cope than with food.

Food Preoccupation: Refer to the legend and choose the number from the scale (0–6) that best represents your highest rating for the day. "Food preoccupation" refers to your thoughts or attention being absorbed by, or focused on, food. For example, your thoughts of a dinner party and the presence of your favorite foods may absorb your attention so much that you have trouble concentrating at work.

Emotion Columns: Refer to the legend and choose the number from the scale (0–6) that best represents your highest rating for the day. The key characteristics to consider when making your rating are intensity (strength of the emotion) and duration (how long it lasted).

(cont.)

FIGURE 16.2. Stanford DBT model diary card.

Used Skills: Refer to the legend and choose the number from the scale (0–6) that best represents your attempts to use the skills each day. When making your rating, consider whether or not you thought about using any of the skills that day, whether or not you actually used any of the skills, and whether or not the skills helped.

Weight: Weigh yourself once each week and record your weight in pounds in the space provided. Please write in the date you weighed. It is best if you choose the same day each week to weigh. Many women find that arriving a few minutes early to the session and weighing at the clinic is a good way to remember to weigh.

Urge to Quit Therapy: Indicate your urge to quit therapy before and after the session each week. Both of these ratings should be made for the same session as the one in which you received the diary card. It is best to make both of these ratings as soon as possible following that day's session. Use a 0–6 scale of intensity of the urge, with 0 indicating no urge to quit and a 6 indicating the strongest urge to quit.

Completing the Skills Side of the Diary Card

How Often Did You Fill Out This Side? Place a check mark to indicate how frequently you filled out the skills side of the diary card during the week.

Skills Practice: Go down the column for each day of the week and circle each skill that you practiced/used that day. If you did not practice or use any of the skills that particular day, then circle on the last line, which states, "Did not practice/use any skills."

(cont.)

FIGURE 16.2. *(cont.)*

Diary Card

Initials _____ ID # _____

How often did you fill out this side?
_____ Daily _____ 4–6x _____ 2–3x _____ Once

Day and Date	Urge to Binge[1] (0–6)	Binge Episodes # OBE lg	Binge Episodes # SBE sm	Mindless Eating # episodes	AIBs[2] Circle one	Capitulating[1] (0–6)	Food[1] Craving (0–6)	Food[1] Preoccupation (0–6)	Anger[1] (0–6)	Sadness[1] (0–6)	Fear[1] (0–6)	Shame[1] (0–6)	Pride[1] (0–6)	Happiness[1] (0–6)	Used[3] Skills (0–7)
Mon					yes/no										
Tues					yes/no										
Wed					yes/no										
Thurs					yes/no										
Fri					yes/no										
Sat					yes/no										
Sun					yes/no										

[1]Use the following scale to indicate the highest rating for the day:

0 = urge/thought/feeling not experienced
1 = urge/thought/feeling experienced slightly and briefly
2 = urge/thought/feeling experienced moderately and briefly
3 = urge/thought/feeling experienced intensely and briefly
4 = urge/thought/feeling experienced slightly and endured
5 = urge/thought/feeling experienced moderately and endured
6 = urge/thought/feeling experienced intensely and endured

[2]Describe apparently irrelevant behaviors (AIBs): _____

[3]USED SKILLS:

0 = Not thought about or used
1 = Thought about, not used, didn't want to
2 = Thought about, not used, wanted to
3 = Tried but couldn't use them
4 = Tried, could do them, but they didn't help
5 = Tried, could use them, helped
6 = Didn't try, used them, didn't help
7 = Didn't try, used them, helped

Weight _____ Date Weighed _____

Urge to quit therapy (0–5): _____ Before therapy session: _____ After therapy session: _____

NIMH 1997–2000

Note. OBE, objective binge episode; SBE, subjective binge episode.

SKILLS DIARY CARD	Instructions: Circle the days you worked on each skill.			How often did you fill out this side? ____ Daily ____ 4–6x ____ 2–3x ____ Once			
1. Diaphragmatic breathing	Mon	Tues	Wed	Thurs	Fri	Sat	Sun
2. Wise mind	Mon	Tues	Wed	Thurs	Fri	Sat	Sun
3. Observe: just notice	Mon	Tues	Wed	Thurs	Fri	Sat	Sun
4. Describe: put words on	Mon	Tues	Wed	Thurs	Fri	Sat	Sun
5. Participate: enter into the experience	Mon	Tues	Wed	Thurs	Fri	Sat	Sun
6. Mindful eating	Mon	Tues	Wed	Thurs	Fri	Sat	Sun
7. Nonjudgemental stance	Mon	Tues	Wed	Thurs	Fri	Sat	Sun
8. One-mindfully: in-the-moment	Mon	Tues	Wed	Thurs	Fri	Sat	Sun
9. Effectiveness: focus on what works	Mon	Tues	Wed	Thurs	Fri	Sat	Sun
10. Urge surfing	Mon	Tues	Wed	Thurs	Fri	Sat	Sun
11. Alternate rebellion	Mon	Tues	Wed	Thurs	Fri	Sat	Sun
12. Mindful of current emotion	Mon	Tues	Wed	Thurs	Fri	Sat	Sun
13. Loving your emotions	Mon	Tues	Wed	Thurs	Fri	Sat	Sun
14. Reduce vulnerability: PLEASE (Physical illness, Eating, Avoid drugs, Sleep, Exercise)	Mon	Tues	Wed	Thurs	Fri	Sat	Sun
15. Build MASTERy (doing one new thing a day to build confidence)	Mon	Tues	Wed	Thurs	Fri	Sat	Sun
16. Build positive experiences	Mon	Tues	Wed	Thurs	Fri	Sat	Sun
17. Mindful of positive experiences	Mon	Tues	Wed	Thurs	Fri	Sat	Sun
18. Opposite-to-emotion action	Mon	Tues	Wed	Thurs	Fri	Sat	Sun
19. Observing your breath	Mon	Tues	Wed	Thurs	Fri	Sat	Sun
20. Half-smiling	Mon	Tues	Wed	Thurs	Fri	Sat	Sun
21. Awareness exercises	Mon	Tues	Wed	Thurs	Fri	Sat	Sun
22. Radical acceptance	Mon	Tues	Wed	Thurs	Fri	Sat	Sun
23. Turning the mind	Mon	Tues	Wed	Thurs	Fri	Sat	Sun
24. Willingness	Mon	Tues	Wed	Thurs	Fri		
25. Burning your bridges	Mon	Tues	Wed	Thurs	Fri	Sat	Sun
26. Distract	Mon	Tues	Wed	Thurs	Fri	Sat	Sun
27. Self-soothe	Mon	Tues	Wed	Thurs	Fri	Sat	Sun
28. Improve the moment	Mon	Tues	Wed	Thurs	Fri	Sat	Sun
29. Pros and cons	Mon	Tues	Wed	Thurs	Fri	Sat	Sun
30. Commitment	Mon	Tues	Wed	Thurs	Fri	Sat	Sun
30. Did not practice any skills	Mon	Tues	Wed	Thurs	Fri	Sat	Sun

References

Chen EY, Matthews L, Allen C, Kuo J, & Linehan MM. (2008). Dialectical behavior therapy for clients with binge-eating disorder or bulimia nervosa and borderline personality disorder. *International Journal of Eating Disorders*, 41:505–512.

Harley R, Sprich S, Safren S, Jacobo M, & Fava M. (2008). Adaptation of dialectical behavior therapy skills training group for treatment-resistant depression. *Journal of Nervous and Mental Disease*, 196:136–143.

Kabat-Zinn J. (1990). *Full-catastrophe living*. New York: Delta.

Koons CR, Robins CJ, Tweed JL, Lynch TR, Gonzalez AM, Morse JQ, et al. (2001). Efficacy of dialectical behavior therapy in women veterans with borderline personality disorder. *Behavior Therapy*, 32:371–390.

Linehan MM. (1993a). *Cognitive-behavioral treatment of borderline personality disorder*. New York: Guilford Press.

Linehan MM. (1993b). *Skills training manual for treating borderline personality disorder*. New York: Guilford Press.

Linehan MM, Armstrong HE, Suarez A, Allmon D, & Heard HL. (1991). Cognitive-behavioral treatment of chronically parasuicidal borderline patients. *Archives of General Psychiatry*, 48:1060–1064.

Linehan MM, & Chen EY. (2005). Dialectical behavior therapy for eating disorders. In S Felgoise, AM Nezu, CM Nezu, MA Reinecke, & A Freeman (Eds.), *The encyclopedia for cognitive-behavioral therapy*. New York: Springer.

Linehan MM, Comtois KA, Murray AM, Brown MZ, Gallop RJ, Heard HL, et al. (2006). Two-year randomized controlled trial and follow-up of dialectical behavior therapy vs. therapy by experts for suicidal behaviors and borderline personality disorder. *Archives of General Psychiatry*, 63:757–766.

Linehan MM, & Dimeff LA. (1997). *Dialectical behavior therapy manual of treatment interventions for drug abusers with borderline personality disorder*. Unpublished manuscript, University of Washington, Seattle.

Linehan MM, Dimeff LA, Reynolds SK, Comtois KA, Welch SS, Heagerty P, et al. (2002). Dialectical behavior therapy versus comprehensive validation therapy plus 12-step for the treatment of opioid dependent women meeting criteria for borderline personality disorder. *Drug and Alcohol Dependence*, 67:13–26.

Linehan MM, Heard HL, & Armstrong HE. (1993). Naturalistic follow-up of a behavioral treatment for chronically parasuicidal borderline patients. *Archives of General Psychiatry*, 50:971–974.

Linehan MM, Schmidt H, III, Dimeff LA, Craft JC, Kanter J, & Comtois KA. (1999). Dialectical behavior therapy for patients with borderline personality disorder and drug dependence. *American Journal of Addiction*, 8:279–292.

Linehan MM, Tutek DA, Heard HL, & Armstrong HE. (1994). Interpersonal outcome of cognitive behavioral treatment for chronically suicidal borderline patients. *American Journal of Psychiatry*, 151:1771–1776.

Lynch TR, Morse JQ, Mendelson T, & Robins CJ. (2003). Dialectical behavior therapy for depressed older adults: A randomized pilot study. *American Journal of Geriatric Psychiatry*, 11:33–45.

Marlatt G, & Gordon JR. (1985). *Relapse prevention and maintenance strategies in the treatment of addictive behaviors*. New York: Guilford Press.

Palmer RL, Birchall H, Damani S, Gatward N, McGrain L, & Parker L. (2003). A dialectical behavior therapy program for people with an eating disorder and borderline personality disorder—description and outcome. *International Journal of Eating Disorders*, 33:281–286.

Rathus JH, & Miller AL. (2002). Dialectical behavior therapy adapted for suicidal adolescents. *Suicide and Life Threatening Behavior*, 32:146–157.

Safer DL, Robinson AH, & Jo B. (in press). Outcome from a randomized controlled trial of group therapy for binge eating disorder: Comparing dialectical behavior therapy adapted for binge eating to an active comparison group therapy. *Behavior Therapy*.

Safer DL, Telch CF, & Agras W. (2001a). Dialectical behavior therapy adapted for bulimia: A case report. *International Journal of Eating Disorders*, 30:101–106.

Safer DL, Telch CF, & Agras WS. (2001b). Dialectical behavior therapy for bulimia nervosa. *American Journal of Psychiatry*, 158:632–634.

Safer DL, Telch CF, & Chen EY. (2009). *Dialectical behavior therapy for binge eating and bulimia*. New York: Guilford Press.

Sansone RA, Levitt JL, & Sansone LA. (2005). The prevalence of personality disorders among those with eating disorders. *Eating Disorders: The Journal of Treatment and Prevention*, 13:7–21.

Simpson EB, Yen S, Costello E, Rosen K, Begin A, Pistorello J, et al. (2004). Combined dialectical behavior therapy and fluoxetine in the treatment of borderline personality disorder. *Journal of Clinical Psychiatry*, 65:379–385.

Soler J, Pascual JC, Campins J, Barrachina J, Puigdemont D, Alvarez E, et al. (2005). Double-blind, placebo-controlled study of dialectical behavior therapy plus olanzapine for borderline personality disorder. *American Journal of Psychiatry*, 162:1221–1224.

Telch CF. (1997a). *Emotion regulation skills training treatment for binge eating disorder: Therapist manual*. Unpublished manuscript, Stanford University.

Telch CF. (1997b). Skills training treatment for adaptive affect regulation in a woman with binge-eating disorder. *International Journal of Eating Disorders*, 22:77–81.

Telch CF, Agras WS, & Linehan MM. (2000). Group dialectical behavior therapy for binge-eating disorder: A preliminary, uncontrolled trial. *Behavior Therapy*, 31:569–582.

Telch CF, Agras WS, & Linehan MM. (2001). Dialectical behavior therapy for binge eating disorder. *Journal of Consulting and Clinical Psychology*, 69:1061–1065.

Turner RM. (2000). Naturalistic evaluation of dialectical behavior therapy-oriented treatment for borderline-personality disorder. *Cognitive and Behavioral Practice*, 7:413–419.

van den Bosch LM, Verheul R, Schippers GM, & van den Brink W. (2002). Dialectical behavior therapy of borderline patients with and without substance use problems. Implementation and long-term effects. *Addictive Behaviors*, 27:911–923.

Verheul R, van den Bosch LM, Koeter MW, De Ridder MA, Stijnen T, & Van Den Brink W. (2003). Dialectical behaviour therapy for women with borderline personality disorder: 12-month, randomised clinical trial in The Netherlands. *British Journal of Psychiatry*, 182:135–140.

Wiser S, & Telch CF. (1999). Dialectical behavior therapy for binge-eating disorder. *Journal of Clinical Psychology*, 55:755–768.

Wisniewski L, Safer D, & Chen E. (2007). Dialectical behavior therapy and eating disorders. In LA Dimeff & K Koerner (Eds.), *Dialectical behavior therapy in clinical practice: Applications across disorders and settings* (pp. 174–221). New York: Guilford Press.

CHAPTER 17

Integrative Cognitive–Affective Therapy for Bulimia Nervosa

Stephen A. Wonderlich, Carol B. Peterson, Tracey L. Smith,
Marj Klein, James E. Mitchell, Scott J. Crow, and Scott G. Engel

Cognitive-behavioral therapy (CBT) received an "A" grade in the National Institute for Health and Clinical Excellence Guidelines (NICE, 2004) and is generally regarded as the most empirically supported psychotherapy for the treatment of bulimia nervosa (BN) (Wilson, Grilo, & Vitouske, 2007). CBT, however, does not sufficiently help many patients with BN, and the limitations of CBT have been described (e.g., Mitchell, Hoberman, Peterson, Mussell, & Pyle, 1996). Similar criticisms of existing CBT approaches have also emerged in the broader psychotherapy research community (e.g., Safran & Segal, 1996; Westen, 2000; Zinbarg, 2000). Clark (1995) summarized the criticisms of CBT into four categories. These include (1) a limited view of emotional responding, (2) inadequate consideration of interpersonal factors, (3) insufficient attention to the clinician–client relationship, and (4) an overemphasis on consciously controlled cognitive processing. Samoilov and Goldfried (2000) also suggested that by eliciting rather than suppressing emotion in CBT, the long-term effectiveness of CBT interventions can be further enhanced. Zinbarg (2000) went on to suggest that CBT might also be criticized for failing to address issues of resistance, or ambivalence, which may influence compliance with CBT techniques and consequent magnitude of change, although CBT practitioners have discussed issues of resistance for some time (e.g., Wachtel, 1982).

In response to these criticisms of CBT, efforts have been made to extend or modify traditional cognitive theory and therapy. For example, it has been argued that CBT might be improved further in a number of ways, including maintaining a stronger focus on interpersonal and affective issues (Safran & Segal, 1996; Samoilov & Goldfried, 2000); borrowing and integrating concepts from constructivist theories to enhance treatment technique (Neimeyer, 1993); including narrative and metaphorical strategies (Meichenbaum, 1993); utilizing the therapeutic relationship more thoroughly as a clinical technique (Safran & Segal, 1996; Westen, 2000; Zinbarg, 2000); and placing greater emphasis on developmental and systemic issues (Guidano, 1986).

Clinical research in eating disorders (EDs) has also supported expanding or extending the range of interventions in CBT for BN. Recently, the most empirically supported CBT model of BN (i.e., Fairburn, Marcus, & Wilson, 1993) was tested and found to have more power in predicting bulimic symptoms when factors such as impulsivity and thin-ideal internalization were included (Von Ranson & Schnitzler, 2007). Such findings suggest the importance of developing a broader conceptual model. Additionally, Fairburn (2008) adapted his original CBT for BN to create a new treatment (i.e., Cognitive Behavior Therapy—Enhanced, or CBT-E), which includes interventions that target perfectionism, low self-esteem, interpersonal factors, and emotional factors. Such adaptations were included because these factors were thought to play significant roles in maintaining the disorder but did not receive sufficient attention in the original CBT for BN. Also, recent developments in the application of dialectical behavior therapy (DBT) to BN (e.g., Safer, Telch, & Agras, 2001; Chen & Safer, Chapter 16, this volume) reflect another attempt to modify and apply a specific form of CBT for the treatment of BN. Although modified from its original form, current DBT treatment for BN retains an emphasis on emotion regulation, distress tolerance, and interpersonal factors and has been shown to be at least somewhat effective in a randomized control trial with CBT as the comparison condition (Safer et al., 2001).

Paralleling developments in cognitive therapy, emotion-focused models of psychopathology and associated treatments have rapidly emerged in the broader behavioral therapy literature (e.g., *Clinical Psychology: Science and Practice*, 2007, Vol. 14, No. 4). For example, Allen, McHugh, and Barlow (2008) outlined a unified protocol for emotional disorders that highlights identification of typically avoided emotional responses and exposure to such disavowed emotions as a core of treatment. Similarly, Hayes and colleagues (Hayes, Strosahl, & Wilson, 2002) argued that behavioral analysts should carefully consider the functional relationships between emotional states and efforts to manage or cope with such states in treatment. Hayes and colleagues' (2002) acceptance and commitment therapy (ACT) emphasizes minimizing the avoidance of negative emotions and experience as a core intervention. Greenberg's (2002) emotion-focused therapy (EFT) also emphasizes identification, experience, expression, and modification of emotional states for various forms of psychopathology, including depression and marital dysfunction. All of these approaches reflect an increased emphasis on emotional experience, which in turn is posited to reduce psychopathology.

Integrative cognitive–affective therapy (ICAT) resembles many of these emotion-focused interventions but also retains some elements of previous CBT-based treatment approaches for BN that have been found to be efficacious. Several recent psychotherapy approaches have emphasized the importance of emotion and interpersonal behavior, and these serve as cornerstones of ICAT. In these respects, ICAT is, as it is named, integrative. ICAT incorporates interventions to enhance motivation for treatment; an explicit behaviorally oriented meal planning system; careful attention to emotional responding and exposure to emotions (including emotions regarding food, shape, and weight); and strategies to identify patterns of interpersonal and self-directed behavior, which may promote the avoidance of underlying negative feelings. These extensions and modifications reflect a growing perspective that a broader model with associated interventions for previously untargeted maintenance factors could provide incremental treatment efficacy for BN. ICAT has evolved in the context of developing treatment based on empirically supported models of psychopathology (Strauman & Merrill, 2004) and deriving treatments that target specific features of these models.

ICAT Model of BN

The model of BN maintenance that underlies this approach to treatment is multifactorial and attempts to integrate a broad array of emotional, interpersonal, cognitive, and biological factors thought to increase the risk of developing and maintaining the behaviors associated with BN. It differs from other cognitive or interpersonal models of BN (e.g., Fairburn et al., 1993; Fairburn, Welch, & Doll, 1997) in that there is a greater emphasis on self-discrepancy, interpersonal patterns, self-directed styles of behavior, and emotional experience. Similar to other recently developed BN treatments (e.g., CBT-E, DBT) these constructs are targeted because of their potential maintenance role in BN.

In its simplest form, the model (see Figure 17.1) posits that life experiences (e.g., criticism, social comparison, rejection, loss) interact with temperamental predispositions (e.g., harm avoidance) to produce mental representations of the self and others that are strongly associated with emotional states that organize and guide future interpersonal perceptions and behavior. Representations of the self in the individual with BN are often characterized as deficient or inadequate, which can be specifically operationalized as a *discrepancy* between the individuals' perception of their *actual self* and their standards for evaluating that self (Higgins, 1987). These standards are referred to as the *desired self.* This perceived self-discrepancy is thought to have motivational significance in the ICAT model because high levels of self-discrepancy are thought to elicit associated negative emotions, which individuals with BN will attempt to avoid or reduce. Individuals with BN are posited to engage in a variety of interpersonal and self-directed behaviors that represent efforts to avoid negative emotions and reduce self-discrepancy. That is, many of the bulimic behaviors (e.g., dieting, purging, exercise) may be efforts

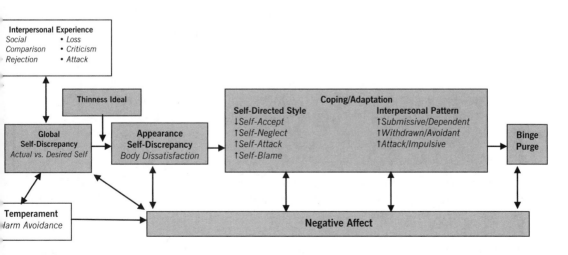

FIGURE 17.1. ICAT model of BN.

to reduce the discrepancy between the actual and desired self, while other aspects of BN (e.g., binge eating) may be viewed as an effort to avoid negative emotions, some of which may be associated with self-discrepancy.

Temperament

The model posits that individuals with BN display a temperament that is characterized by a propensity to avoid change and generally avoid situations that are perceived as threatening or harmful to their self-esteem. The model relies on the theoretical work of Cloninger, Svrakic, and Przybeck (1993), which has been previously applied to EDs (e.g., Brewerton, Lydiard, Laraia, Shook, & Ballenger, 1992; Bulik, Sullivan, Joyce, & Carter, 1995). Empirical reports using Cloninger's measure have consistently revealed that individuals with BN show elevated harm avoidance scores in comparison to normal controls (e.g., Brewerton et al., 1992). Novelty seeking has also frequently, though not consistently, been shown to be associated with BN (e.g., Bulik et al., 1995). Although a propensity to pursue novel and exciting stimuli may be present in some individuals with BN, it is also possible that this trait is primarily present in only one subgroup of individuals with BN (Lilenfield et al., 1997).

Interpersonal Experiences

The model posits that individuals with BN are likely to experience a broad array of events or circumstances in their life that threaten or interfere with attachment processes (i.e., increase risk of harm). For example, individuals with BN have been shown to be more likely than normal controls to have been adopted (Holden, 1991), to have experienced childhood physical or sexual abuse (Wonderlich, Brewerton, Jocic, Dansky, & Abbott, 1997), and to have parental histories of psychopathology, including depression and substance abuse (Fairburn et al., 1997), although these are not considered specific risk factors. Furthermore, there is considerable research indicating that adolescents and adults with BN perceive their relationships with their parents and their overall family environments as conflicted, disengaged, and non-nurturant (Kendler, Maclean, & Neale, 1991). Supporting these descriptions, observational studies of the families of individuals with BN in the laboratory suggest that their relationships are best described as disengaged, conflicted, and lacking in effective communication (Humphrey, 1989). The present model implies that such experiences, along with any other experience that threatens their feelings of interpersonal security and self-esteem (e.g., criticism, teasing, social comparison) will be emotionally significant for individuals with BN, especially given their temperamental sensitivity to harm.

Self-Discrepancy

Consistent with recent risk-factor studies (e.g., Fairburn et al., 1997; Jacobi, Hayward, de Zwaan, Kraemer, & Agras, 2004), the model posits that negative self-evaluation is associated with BN and is the consequence of the previously described interpersonal experiences and temperament/personality traits. However, the model predicts that it is not simply negative self-evaluation that is most important etiologically; according to the model, individuals with BN perceive a deficit in themselves that reflects a discrepancy between their perceived actual self and a comparative ideal standard, which they apply to themselves or believe others apply to them. These hypotheses are derived from self-discrepancy theory (Higgins, 1987) and its application to depression (Strauman, 1989) as well as to ED behaviors (Strauman, Vookles, Berenstein, Chaiken, & Higgins, 1991). Specifically, self-discrepancy theory postulates various domains of the self, including the *actual* self (i.e., a mental representation of the attributes or features the individual believes he/she actually possesses), the *ideal* self (i.e., a representation of the attributes that the individual or significant other would ideally like him/her to possess), and the *ought* self (a representation of the attributes that the individual or a significant other believes it is his/her obligation or duty to possess; Strauman et al., 1991).

Central to the theory that forms the basis of ICAT are Strauman's findings (Strauman et al., 1991), suggesting that discrepancies between actual and ideal selves are related to negative mood and, importantly, body dissatisfaction, body size overestimation, and BN symptoms. It is further hypothesized that such body dissatisfaction, as a specific facet of self-concept, may exacerbate negative affective states (Altabe & Thompson, 1996). Together, these findings suggest that discrepancies between the actual and ideal selves elicit negative affect, body dissatisfaction, and body size overestimation, which in turn exacerbate one another.

Several recent investigations have tested the self-discrepancy component of the ICAT model of BN (Wonderlich et al., 2008). In two independent studies, individuals with BN have been shown to have significantly higher levels of both actual–ideal and actual–ought discrepancies than control subjects. Furthermore, self-discrepancies were shown to be predictive of higher levels of negative mood in both in BN and control participants. In addition, the relationship between self-discrepancy and BN was mediated by significant elevations in negative mood states, thus empirically supporting the hypothesis that self-discrepancy is related to negative emotion in BN.

In the ICAT model, self-discrepancies are significant not only as cognitive phenomena relating to one's own standards but also as interpersonal phenomena. That is, failure to meet desired standards is considered significant to the individual because of the implications it poses for the individual's level of interpersonal security. The evaluative standards (e.g., ideal and ought selves) that the person holds represent the internalization of external behavioral standards modeled or reinforced by others (e.g., family, friends, culture). The perceived failure to meet these standards is associated with a negative reaction from others (e.g., rejection). Thus, the presence of self-discrepancy and associated affective states is expected to be a motivational stimulus for interpersonal and intrapsychic behavior in the individual.

Negative Emotion

There is considerable evidence to suggest that individuals with BN experience exaggerated states of aversive self-awareness and a propensity for negative affectivity (e.g., Smyth et al., 2007). In fact, there continues to be evidence that a subset of individuals with BN have significant emotional disturbance, which is correlated with worse overall psychopathology and a more negative outcome than patients with less emotional disturbance (e.g., Stice, Bohon, Marti, & Fischer, 2008). The present model posits that such negative emotions are often precipitated by the previously described self-discrepancy or difficult interpersonal situations. Consistent with escape theory (Heatherton & Baumeister,

1991), it is predicted that individuals with BN experience prolonged states of aversive, self-oriented cognitive preoccupation focused on their perceived self-deficits and the implication of such deficits for their interpersonal security. Prolonged states of such negative affect may be associated with the high levels of mood and anxiety problems that individuals with BN report (Wonderlich & Mitchell, 1997), particularly worrying, rumination, and guilt (Cooper & Fairburn, 1986). The ICAT hypothesis that for individuals with BN, the correlation of such negative affectivity and self-oriented discrepancies will be particularly significant was supported in a recent empirical investigation (Wonderlich et al., 2008).

There is some evidence in the cognitive psychology literature that individuals reporting high levels of BN attitudes may attend more to emotionally threatening stimuli (Waller, Quinton, & Watson, 1995). Research has also found that the induction of negative mood appears to increase the likelihood of binge eating in some individuals (Agras & Telch, 1998). Thus, individuals with BN may experience more negative emotion and may have difficulty regulating behavior in the face of such negative emotion.

Recent investigations have used ecological momentary assessment (EMA), a naturalistic technology-based method that reduces cognitive biases in self-reported recall data, to examine the link between emotion and BN symptoms. Smyth and colleagues (2007) found a significant increase in negative emotions in the 4–6 hours preceding BN behavior and a complementary decrease in negative emotions in the several hours following BN behavior. The findings support the premise that increased states of negative mood may serve as a significant antecedent for BN behavior and that BN behavior may have negative reinforcing properties, which could help to explain part of the maintenance of this behavioral constellation in the context of negative emotion.

Avoidance of Emotions Related to Food, Shape, and Weight

Although ICAT emphasizes the importance of all emotion, emotions related specifically to eating, shape, and weight issues are especially important. ICAT posits that these emotions are particularly distressing and therefore frequently avoided by individuals with BN. In addition, ICAT posits that many BN behaviors function to facilitate such avoidance. Specifically, it is thought that individuals engage in a variety of emotional avoidance behaviors, including skipping meals, exercising, purging, restricting food intake, and following rigid eating rules to help them minimize intense anxiety about weight, food, and body shape.

Thinness Ideal and Appearance Self-Discrepancy

The impact of sociocultural variables is important in the development of BN symptoms (Striegel-Moore, Silberstein, & Rodin, 1986), particularly the internalization of the thinness ideal of Western society, which appears to be a specific risk factor for eating pathology (Stice, 2002). Internalization of the thinness ideal has been found to correlate with eating problems and body image disturbance (Stice, Schupak-Neuberg, Shaw, & Stein, 1994), and to predict the development of body dissatisfaction (Stice, 2001) and BN symptoms (Stice & Agras, 1998) among adolescent females. According to the ICAT model, internalization of the thinness ideal, in conjunction with high levels of self-discrepancy, will result in appearance self-discrepancy. This internalization occurs, in part, as a result of repeated exposure to media images. Indeed, it is the internalization of the appearance ideal that is predictive of body dissatisfaction rather than media exposure itself (Cusumano & Thompson, 1997). In addition to the media, peers and family members facilitate the internalization of the thin ideal by providing social reinforcement: Weight loss and thinness are praised; weight gain and obesity are criticized (Thompson & Stice, 2001). In the ICAT model, the internalization of the thinness ideal and global self-discrepancy interact to influence appearance self-discrepancy in the form of body dissatisfaction. Because the ideal of thinness is unattainable for most females, the inevitable result is that the individual's desired appearance is much thinner than the perceived actual size and shape. This discrepancy results in emotional distress as well as an attempt to cope with this distress with maladaptive self-directed styles, interpersonal patterns, and BN symptoms that act as emotion avoidance strategies.

Interpersonal Patterns and Self-Directed Styles

In addition to the influence of early attachment relationships, the ICAT model emphasizes the role of current interpersonal patterns and self-directed style as maintenance factors of BN symptoms. Specifically, the model posits that individuals with BN will enact specific repetitive interpersonal patterns across a wide variety of relationships as a means of regulating underlying emotions. Based on Benjamin's (2003) model of social behavior, the present model implies that these interpersonal patterns are oriented toward avoiding interpersonal rejection or abandonment. Two of the primary patterns posited to be associated with BN in the model are a *submission* pattern and a *withdrawal/wall-off* pattern. In the submission pattern the individual with BN is likely to appease and satisfy key attachment figures in an effort to avoid rejection and associated negative emotional experience. For similar reasons, the withdrawal pattern may develop when relationships are perceived as threatening to attachment status and associated self-esteem, and the individual sees no way to reduce the relational problem through engagement. An additional interpersonal pattern, *blame*, is also hypothesized to be present in some individuals with BN. This pattern is predicted to be most common in the highly impulsive borderline-type individual with BN and is seen primarily when these individuals perceive attachment figures as withdrawing or being unavailable to them. The pattern is based on the fundamental interpersonal idea that such relationship-sensitive individuals will engage in hostile control behaviors in an effort to prevent the withdrawal of significant others (Benjamin, 2003).

In addition to interpersonal patterns, the ICAT model emphasizes four types of self-directed styles: *self-control, self-blame, self-attack,* and *self-neglect*. Some individuals with BN may engage in extreme efforts to control the self and attain perfection in order to reduce their self-discrepancy and associated negative emotions. Others may rely on a more hostile pattern of self-control in which they blame and criticize themselves in an effort to reduce their self-discrepancy. Others may attempt to avoid the discrepancy through self-neglect and engage in more reckless, unpredictable behaviors. It is important to note that such self-directed styles are used by the individual with BN in an effort to manage the underlying negative emotion that is ultimately linked to a fundamental self-discrepancy.

Summary of the ICAT Model

In summary, the theoretical model underlying ICAT emphasizes the importance of cognitive, interpersonal, and affective factors in the maintenance of BN symptoms. Preliminary investigations have provided initial empirical support of the ICAT model. ICAT has been developed as an intervention that specifically targets these core aspects that underlie and maintain BN and emphasizes changes in behavior, self-discrepancy, self-directed styles, interpersonal patterns, and emotions.

Treatment Outcome Research

Given ICAT's recent development, empirical testing of this treatment is in its early stages. Two uncontrolled multisite pilot studies have been conducted and a randomized control trial is currently underway. Although the data from the pilot studies are preliminary, they provide initial support for the efficacy of ICAT in reducing bulimic and associated symptoms.

Pilot Testing

To test ICAT, two waves of adult, female participants ($n = 10$ and $n = 11$; average age = 27.5, $SD = 8.8$) meeting DSM-IV diagnostic criteria for BN or subthreshold BN were enrolled in a 20-session trial. Seventy-one percent ($n = 15$) met diagnostic criteria for BN. Twenty-nine percent ($n = 6$) were classified as subthreshold BN because they reported binge-eating episodes that were not objectively large but were accompanied by a subjective experience of loss of control and followed by purging, or engaged in objectively large binge-eating episodes and purging at a frequency of less than twice per week. Potential participants with low body weight (i.e., less than 85% of ideal), psychotic symptoms, bipolar disorder, history of gastric bypass surgery, or current ED treatment were excluded. The psychotherapy in both treatment waves was provided by doctoral-level psychologists. All clinicians delivering ICAT received an initial didactic workshop on the model and treatment techniques, along with weekly teleconference supervision. Psychotherapy sessions were audiotaped and reviewed by the primary investigators for quality and adherence.

Of the 10 participants enrolled in the first wave, 1 (10%) dropped out of treatment before the final session. Three of 11 participants (27.3%) in the second wave dropped out of treatment before completion. Thus, a total of 17 of 21(80.9%) participants enrolled in ICAT were considered treatment completers. In the first wave, the average number of self-reported binge-eating episodes at baseline was 4.3 per week, and the average number of purging episodes was 6.7 per week. At the final session, the average number of binge-eating episodes was 0.6 per week, and the average number of purging episodes was 0.3 per week. The second wave of pilot cases revealed a similar reduction in symptoms, with the average number of binge-eating episodes dropping from 10.6 episodes per week to 0.2 episodes per week, and vomiting dropping from 14.1 episodes per week to 1.1 episodes per week on the Eating Disorder Examination (EDE). Furthermore, at the end of the 20-session treatment, 70% of the combined sample of 17 treatment-completing participants was abstinent from binge eating and 65% of the participants were abstinent from vomiting for the final 2 weeks of treatment. In addition, acceptability ratings of the ICAT components by the second-wave participants were high, indicating that they found all aspects of the treatment helpful. Variables hypothesized to be central to ICAT were also examined and improvements were found in both self-discrepancy and positive directed style. However, changes in negative self-directed style were minimal.

In summary, initial pilot data from two treatment waves provide preliminary support for the efficacy of ICAT with notable reductions in bulimic symptoms and abstinence from binge eating and purging among the majority of treatment completers. In addition, attrition was minimal, and acceptability ratings were high. Improvements were also observed in self-discrepancy and self-directed style, two key components of the ICAT model of bulimic symptoms. Clearly, a larger randomized controlled trial, currently underway, is essential to test the efficacy and acceptability of ICAT.

ICAT Mini-Manual

ICAT is a structured short-term psychotherapeutic treatment for BN behavior that includes four phases that are described in detail in the following sections. Phase I (approximately 1–2 sessions) introduces ICAT and emphasizes motivational enhancement and the importance of emotional responding. The main focus of Phase II (approximately 3–8 sessions) is nutritional rehabilitation, facilitated by structured meal planning and coping skills. Phase III (approximately 9–18 sessions) focuses on the relationship of emotional states, interpersonal behavior, and self-directed behavior, referred to as "self-directed style." Phase IV (approximately 19–20 sessions) emphasizes relapse prevention and healthy lifestyle planning, along with termination.

The various treatment strategies and interventions of ICAT for BN are outlined in Table 17.1. The therapy starts by attempting to engage patients in a collaborative therapeutic relationship that addresses an emotionally meaningful discrepancy between their current life and the way in which they would like to live. The treatment then begins to emphasize a normalization of the eating process. It is assumed that this will be somewhat difficult for patients to do, and the treatment actively attempts to support patients' efforts to normalize their eating by introducing numerous coping skills, some of which are included in a personal digital assistant (PDA) handheld computer. An emphasis on eating patterns is maintained throughout the remainder of treatment; however, there is a decided shift in emphasis to interpersonal factors just before the midpoint of treatment, at the beginning of Phase III. At that time the patient and clinician collaboratively set goals for the balance of therapy regarding interpersonal patterns and self-directed style. Ultimately, the treatment concludes by helping the patient prepare for the risk of symptomatic lapse and relapse as well as establishing a healthy lifestyle. The identification and expression of emotion is emphasized in each phase of ICAT.

Core Skills

As shown in Table 17.2, ICAT introduces five core behavioral skills. These skills are discussed in psychotherapy sessions, outlined in the Patient Workbook, and presented

TABLE 17.1. Summary of ICAT Phases

Phase of ICAT	Treatment strategies	Specific interventions
Phase I: Introduction and Motivation	1. Conduct motivational enhancement 2. Present psychoeducational material 3. Engage in emotion identification	1. Discuss current behavior vs. broader goals and emotional significance 2. Self-monitor food intake and context 3. Introduce FEEL skill
Phase II: Nutritional Rehabilitation	1. Begin meal planning 2. Continue food logs 3. Identify emotions associated with eating	1. Encourage meal plan and regular consumption of meals/snacks (CARE skill) 2. Actively teach coping skills for purpose of assisting meal planning (PDA) 3. Monitor context of symptoms 4. Monitor and elicit affect regarding meal plan, especially monitoring emotional avoidance
Phase III: Interpersonal Patterns and Self-Directed Styles	1. Conduct interpersonal pattern and self-directed style analysis 2. Conduct historical analysis of patterns (optional) 3. Focus on changing interpersonal patterns and self-directed styles 4. Focus on reducing self-discrepancy 5. Continue food logs	1. Identify interpersonal patterns of patient and specific others as well as self-directed style 2. Attempt to identify historical factors associated with underlying beliefs and interpersonal rules that inform and direct the interpersonal pattern (optional) 3. Carefully elicit and clarify affect in interpersonal situations 4. Focus on assertiveness training and increasing self-accepting self-regulatory style (SAID, SPA, WAIT skills) 5. Address and modify maladaptive evaluative standards; heavy emphasis on workbook 6. Elicit and monitor affect
Phase IV: Relapse Prevention	1. Discuss components of a healthy lifestyle 2. Develop written relapse prevention plan 3. Address feelings related to termination	1. Review progress in treatment 2. Formalize relapse prevention plan 3. Elicit and monitor affect

Note. CARE, calmly arrange regular eating; FEEL, focus, experience, examine, and label; PDA, personal digital assistance; SAID, sensitively assert ideas and desires; SPA, self-protect and accept; WAIT, watch all impulses today.

TABLE 17.2. Core Skills in ICAT

Coping skill	Phase	Acronym for skill	Elements in acronym
Emotion identification	I	FEEL	Focus, experience, examine, and label
Meal planning	II	CARE	Calmly arrange regular eating
Assertiveness	III	SAID	Sensitively assert ideas and desires
Self-regulation	III	SPA	Self-protect and accept
Impulse control	III	WAIT	Watch all impulses today

in the PDA modules. Patients are encouraged to access and review these skills on the handheld computer at least twice a day and focus on the skills being emphasized in that particular phase of treatment. Clinicians emphasize these skills, using their acronyms, throughout treatment, encouraging their use.

ICAT Treatment Materials

In order to generalize therapeutic work and behavior change outside of therapy sessions, patients are provided with a Patient Workbook and their PDA. At the present time, the technology employed is a palm-based PDA, but other technological media are being considered as technological advancements continue. The PDA and Patient Workbook have been developed to be used adjunctively, to individual therapy sessions. Although patients are instructed to use the Patient Workbook and PDA on their own, the clinician should plan to "check in" about usage at each session. For example, the clinician can ask the patient to turn on the handheld computer in session to review aspects that have been helpful and clarify any questions. Similarly, the clinician should provide information to the patient about when particular sections of the Patient Workbook are most relevant; however, the patient should also be encouraged to read and review the materials independently, and therapy sessions should not be focused on reiterating materials that are provided in the Patient Workbook. The clinician's primary goals with the workbook and computer are to (1) encourage the frequent use of the Patient Workbook and the PDA between sessions and praise the patient for using them; (2) emphasize the most important material; (3) explore any emotions that the workbook or computer elicit from the patient; and (4) answer any questions that are raised by the workbook or PDA.

Detailed Description of ICAT

In the sections that follow, each phase of ICAT is described in detail, including goals, background information, and specific therapeutic techniques.

Phase I: Motivation Enhancement and Introducing Emotions

Goals of Phase I (Sessions 1–2)

1. Establish a treatment relationship that clearly includes the patient as a significant collaborator in the process.
2. Enhance motivation by noting discrepancies between the effects of the ED symptoms and broader life goals.
3. "Side with the disorder" in terms of acknowledging possible benefits of the symptoms.
4. Remain sensitive to patients' emotional state and make efforts to identify emotional reactions (this goal serves as a basic strategy that is employed throughout the therapy).
5. Introduce FEEL skill.
6. Begin self-monitoring of food intake.

Therapeutic Techniques

The first few sessions of ICAT focus on clarifying and enhancing the patient's motivation for treatment. The fundamental techniques of motivational interviewing, originally developed by Miller and Rollnick (2002), are utilized to facilitate these goals. Clinicians focus on two main tasks in motivational interviewing. First, they attempt to assist patients in articulating the discrepancy that exists between how they would like to be functioning and how they are actually functioning in their lives, particularly in terms of how the ED behavior may contribute to this discrepancy. Second, clinicians align themselves with the potentially positive aspects of the disorder in an effort to provide a balanced perspective on the costs and benefits of the BN. For example, in spite of numerous medical, psychological, or financial costs of the bulimic behavior, clinicians may explore with patients the possible benefits in the form of emotion regulation or perceived weight management. Clinicians examine the possibility that patients are indeed ambivalent about making changes because of fears about losing the positive aspects of the symptoms, were recovery achieved. The interviewing process is a highly empathic one in which clinicians make every effort to avoid any confrontational strategies to pressure patients into treatment. Many of these techniques can be seen in the dialogue below, which illustrates motivational interviewing in the early phases of ICAT.

> CLINICIAN: In what ways have your bulimic symptoms been helpful to you?
>
> PATIENT: No one has ever asked me that before. Everyone just talks about how dangerous it is.
>
> CLINICIAN: Actually, we do think it's very important to understand what might actually be positive for you about having bulimia, especially at this point when you are just starting treatment.
>
> PATIENT: Well, I do get to eat whatever I want and know that I can get rid of it without gaining weight. And if I have had a bad day, bingeing makes me forget about whatever is upsetting me.
>
> CLINICIAN: So having bulimia helps you feel less scared about weight gain and makes you feel more freedom to eat what you want?
>
> PATIENT: Yes, exactly. But there are problems, too, which is why I decided to get help.
>
> CLINICIAN: Tell me about those.
>
> PATIENT: Well, it's like I have this secret life. I eat in secret, I purge in secret. None of my family or friends knows, and I feel like I am living a lie, which is awful.
>
> CLINICIAN: So the dishonesty feels bad to you.
>
> PATIENT: Yes. And I feel really sick after I binge and purge. I feel weak and dizzy. Also, I am obsessed with food. All I ever think about is what I've eaten, what I shouldn't eat, and what I'm going to eat. It's hard to concentrate on anything else.
>
> CLINICIAN: What other things do you wish you could concentrate on instead of thinking about food?

PATIENT: Well, like when my friends are talking. And also my music. Being a musician is really important to me and sometimes it's hard to focus on it because I'm bingeing or obsessing about food.

CLINICIAN: So when you think of your life 5 years from now, what do you hope it will be like?

PATIENT: I think about having a successful music career, close friends, travel, stuff like that.

CLINICIAN: Where does the bulimia fit in?

PATIENT: It doesn't.

CLINICIAN: So, if I am understanding you correctly, I hear that there is a real split for you in this area. On one hand, the binge eating helps soothe you when you are upset, and the purging helps you worry less about gaining weight and gives you more freedom to eat. But the bulimia makes it hard to concentrate on things you care about; it takes a lot of time away from other things you value, it makes you feel sick, and it causes you to feel badly about yourself for being dishonest. And, I'm struck by the fact that when you think about the future and the life you want to be leading, there is really no room for the bulimia, and you really don't want to be dealing with it.

PATIENT: Yes, that's right.

Occasionally a patient's ambivalence about moving ahead at the end of Phase I is pronounced, and the clinician may be unsure whether the transition into Phase II is appropriate. In this case the clinician should acknowledge that the patient's uncertainty about wanting to change is extreme, but given the person's incipient interest in coming to the session, Phase II would be offered in order to help him/her explore whether or not ICAT might be appropriate.

The other primary task in Phase I is to introduce the FEEL skill—focus, experience, examine, and label—which is designed to help patients gain a greater understanding of underlying emotions. Patients are provided basic education about emotional functioning. For example, in ICAT emotion is assumed to be a normal process that indicates that something of significance to the patient is occurring. Also, there is an emphasis placed on the somatic experience of emotions and attempting to use bodily cues to detect emotional experiences. Finally, an emphasis is placed on "action dispositions," which are the types of behavioral choices typically made in response to negative emotions. All of these elements are emphasized throughout the treatment, and patients are encouraged to practice the FEEL skill twice a day during Phases I and II. A clinician's introduction of the FEEL skill can be seen in the transcript below.

CLINICIAN: In this treatment we believe that emotions are linked to bulimic behavior and that often people with eating disorders are not aware of their emotions. Because emotions are such a normal part of life, we think it is important to attend to them, understand them, and frequently express them, particularly in therapy. If you are willing, I would be very interested in knowing about your emotional experience. We even have a specific skill in this treatment designed to help with that.

PATIENT: Yeah, I am pretty good at knowing what I am feeling.

CLINICIAN: Great. This might be really easy for you then. We call it the FEEL skill, which stands for *focus, experience, examine,* and *label,* and we have even put it on the PDA and in your workbook as one of the core parts of the treatment. We find that it works best if people practice this skill a couple of times a day.

PATIENT: If I know what I'm feeling, do I really have to do it?

CLINICIAN: Well, that's a good question. Maybe we will find that your skills are so good that practicing with our FEEL skill doesn't help you much, but it still might be worth trying. Would you be willing to hear a little more about it and what we think is most helpful?

PATIENT: Yeah, I suppose, I am willing to try things.

CLINICIAN: Great.

Phase II: Meal Planning and Identification of Feelings

Goals of Phase II (Sessions 3–8)

1. Continue self-monitoring food intake.
2. Implement formal meal planning with an emphasis on nutritionally adequate meals and snacks.
3. Introduce CARE skill while continuing to practice FEEL skill within and outside of session.
4. Remain sensitive to patients' emotional states and make efforts to identify emotional reactions.

Therapeutic Techniques

The primary task of Phase II is introducing the CARE plan (*calmly arrange regular eating*) through self-monitoring of eating behavior and meal planning. Simultaneously, the clinician continues to emphasize the FEEL skill in an effort to enhance patients' awareness of underlying emotional experiences as they are making changes in their eating behavior.

As can be seen in Figure 17.2, the typical food record is utilized to record foods consumed, location of eating, and feeling states. Early in Phase II, patients are provided with their CARE plan, which is a relatively detailed meal planning system that includes meal planning forms and sample menus. The clinician and patient collaboratively identify the starting calorie level for the patient, which can range from 1,600 to 2,200 calories per day. The following points are emphasized to patients when they are developing their CARE plans:

1. All eating should be planned.
2. Patients should spend time each day devising their CARE plan for the next day.
3. Patients should plan to have no more than 2–3 hours elapse between a meal or snack.

SAMPLE DAILY FOOD RECORD

Date _Tuesday_

TIME	TYPE* (B, L, D, S, O, V, L, D, R, Exercise)	FOOD/ BEVERAGE	ON-CARE PLAN	NOTES (Location, Feelings)
7:00	B, R	½ Bagel, plain Water (1 bottle)	Yes	Breakfast at home Feeling fat, trying to cut back
10:00		Coffee (1 cup)		Work, stressed about meeting
12:00	L, R	Salad (2 cups) Water (1 bottle)	Yes	At work, preparing for meeting Feeling worried about meeting Trying not to eat much, skipped salad dressing
2:30	S, R	Nonfat yogurt (½ cup)	Yes	Worried about meeting Saw cookies in the break room Had yogurt instead of cookies
3:00	S	2 cookies (chocolate chip)	No	Ate during meeting Unhappy about meeting Mad at myself for not doing a better presentation
3:30	O	5 cookies (chocolate chip)	No	Can't stop eating; mad, sad

TYPE: B = breakfast; L = lunch; D = dinner; S = snack; O = overeating/binge/more than planned/loss of control; V = vomiting; L = laxative; D = diuretic; R = restricting; E = exercise (specify type and how long).

FIGURE 17.2. Abbreviated sample food record.

4. Bulimic episodes are likely to continue as the CARE plan is evolving and should be recorded so that the clinician and patient can identify antecedents for these behaviors.
5. In the early stages, the variety of food is less important than the frequency and overall amount eaten.

It is important for the clinician and patient to review meal plans and food logs at the beginning of each session. The early Phase II session should focus almost exclusively on reviewing the CARE plans and food records, with considerable attention paid to the precipitants of problematic eating or episodes of restriction.

PDA-Based Coping Modules. During Phase II, patients receive a series of modules on the PDA that helps them deal with particular high-risk situations as they are modifying their eating pattern and planning their meals. For example, there are modules focusing on the five core skills (i.e., FEEL, CARE, WAIT, SAID, SPA) on the PDA and can be accessed by the patient at will. It is possible to determine how much time patients spend in given modules or core skills on the PDA by synchronizing the PDA at each clinic visit. Clinicians are encouraged to discuss the utilization of the PDA so that the patients optimize its portability and immediacy in terms of providing support during high-risk times.

Phase III: Interpersonal Patterns, Self-Directed Styles, and Cognitive Processes

Goals of Phase III (Sessions 9–18)

1. Identify and modify maladaptive self-directed styles.
2. Identify and modify maladaptive interpersonal patterns.
3. Identify the connection between emotion, interpersonal patterns, and self-directed styles and how these relate to bulimic symptoms.
4. Continue to modify extreme discrepancies between actual self and evaluative standards for the patient.
5. Implement SPA, SAID, and WAIT core skills.

Overview of Phase III

This phase shifts the therapeutic focus from nutritional rehabilitation to interpersonal patterns and self-directed styles. Of particular importance is how these behaviors may be related to negative emotions, potentially related to self-discrepancy, and may ultimately lead to emotion-driven BN behaviors. After carefully listening to patients' descriptions of their interpersonal transactions and self-directed behavior, the clinician hypothesizes about the repetitive pattern of typical behaviors with others and the self (Benjamin, 2003) so that patients gain an understanding of their interpersonal and self-directed behavior in "if–then" terms (i.e., "if others do x, then I do y"). For example, a patient may have an interpersonal pattern that implicitly incorporates the if–then statement "If I submit to others, then others will be nice to me." Alternatively, a patient may have developed a self-directed style that relies on the if–then statement "If I can control myself perfectly, I will be okay."

Identifying Repetitive Interpersonal Patterns and Self-Directed Styles. Self-monitoring in Phase III focuses on social situations that are either closely linked in time to BN behavior or to significant emotional distress, as noted in patients' food logging sheets; an explicit interpersonal transaction log can also be used. Patients are encouraged to monitor and record interpersonal transactions on a regular basis, and this information will provide a focus for the third phase of treatment. Patients are encouraged, of course, to continue using their CARE plan, which is also monitored by the clinician. When a patient provides a particular social transaction for review, the clinician carefully assesses the transaction in terms of who was involved, what was said or done, what was the patient's emotional experience, and if there was any ED behavior that may be linked in some way to the transaction. Benjamin's (2003) structural analysis of social behavior is used to facilitate identification of repetitive patterns or "self-directed styles," a term that refers to patterns of behavior directed toward the self, so these patterns become a primary target in the modification of social behavior in BN patients. Self-directed styles include attributes such as self-control, self-acceptance, self-protection, self-blame, and self-attack, which are described in the workbook. The clinician attempts to understand the transaction from the perspective of the patient, including the perception of the other person (e.g., attacking, blaming, controlling, protecting, affirming, ignoring) and the perception of the patient (e.g., defending, walling off, submitting, expressing). The Patient Workbook describes ample examples of interpersonal patterns, and the patient and clinician work together to identify typical patterns experienced by the patient. Interventions are then developed to help the patient engage in new patterns. For example, assertiveness or expression of feelings is frequently introduced as a possible alternative behavior to various problematic response styles, such as excessive submission or angry withdrawal. Also, patients who tend to be embroiled in hostile, controlling transactions can be helped to develop greater degrees of interpersonal separation from these relationships. Alternatively, individuals who are highly withdrawn and disengaged can be helped to engage in more trusting and disclosing patterns of behavior.

A typical pattern analysis from ICAT can be seen in the following excerpt. In the first section of the example, the clinician is trying to gather the general facts and details surrounding the social transaction. Then the clinician attempts to clarify the interpersonal pattern, beginning with the patient's perception of her boyfriend's behavior.

CLINICIAN: Okay, so something happened last night when you were talking to your boyfriend on the phone.

PATIENT: Yeah.

CLINICIAN: Can you tell me about what took place last night, all of what happened with him?

PATIENT: Well, it was a bad night. I got home from work and called him, and I just got the feeling he was preoccupied. Some of the guys from his softball team wanted him to go out later and I had thought we were going to do something. [She sees him as SEPARATE.]

Next, the clinician begins to clarify the patient's emotional reaction to her perception of the boyfriend's interpersonal pattern. This emotion exploration should be quite detailed. Then the clinician attempts to assess the patient's interpersonal behavior, which appears to consist of an initial effort to BLAME the boyfriend for being SEPARATE, but then in the face of the boyfriend's intensified WALLING OFF, she becomes SUBMISSIVE and also unaware of her feeling state.

CLINICIAN: Can you say what it was like, that is, what you were feeling, when he was talking about going out with his friends on the phone?

PATIENT: I was mad! He always does this. He has got softball games all summer, and every time he has a softball game, he has to be with his friends. But then when he has got time free, he expects me to drop everything and be available. ["Mad" is obviously an emotion word and explored further below.]

CLINICIAN: So you saw him as sort of doing his own thing and not being very available to you, and you noticed that you were angry? Can you describe more completely what that was like for you when you were angry? [Further effort to clarify feelings]

PATIENT: I don't know, I just get mad.

CLINICIAN: Yes, I understand that, but what happens when you get mad? What does it feel like internally and what do you do? [Continued emotion exploration]

PATIENT: I just get crazy. I feel like I want to cry and scream. I pace and I don't seem to be able to sit still. That's when I do my [bulimic] behaviors. [Beginning to see the action tendency]

CLINICIAN: Did you in this case?

PATIENT: Yeah.

CLINICIAN: Did those behaviors help you?

PATIENT: For a little while, but I was still freaking out.

CLINICIAN: Can you tell me what you wound up doing, then, after your behaviors, when you were feeling so upset and your boyfriend was not going to be available to you?

PATIENT: Well, I talked to him later and screamed at him and told him what a jerk I thought he was. I told him that he was insensitive and spoiled and that I was sick of being treated like dirt. [Clinician is beginning to identify a possible ATTACK pattern.]

CLINICIAN: So you really sort of let him have it?

PATIENT: Yeah, I did, and he really deserved it.

CLINICIAN: And what happened then? [Looking for consequences of behavior]

PATIENT: Well, then he got really quiet. He wouldn't talk to me, and I got sort of nervous. I kept asking him to talk to me, and he told me that he thought that maybe we needed a break from each other and that he was sick of dealing with my tantrums. [Boyfriend appears to be WALLING-OFF.]

CLINICIAN: So he sort of pulled back. Sounds like he was threatening to leave.

PATIENT: Yeah, that freaked me out. ["Freaked-out" is an emotion word.]

CLINICIAN: Freaked you out? What did you do? [Directly explores action tendency]

PATIENT: Well, I did what I always do. I told him I was sorry, and I would never do it again. That I was out of line. That I was acting like a bitch and I would try and do better next time. [Possible evidence of SUBMISSION and self-directed behavior of SELF-BLAME]

CLINICIAN: Do you remember what you what you were feeling once you started to take the blame?

PATIENT: I'm not sure. I know I get really nervous when he threatens to leave me. I think that I just keep telling him I'll be better and kind of begging him to stay. I don't know what I feel. Probably something like scared.

Interventions in Phase III

Early in Phase III patients are given feedback about what appears to be their typical interpersonal and self-directed style patterns. An agreement is sought to target a particular interpersonal or self-directed style that seems relevant to the BN behavior. The

Patient Workbook and PDA modules include strategies for modifying interpersonal behavior. Also, clinician modeling of patterns and role plays in session are often useful in terms of modifying interpersonal patterns. Changing self-directed styles typically necessitates a focus on the patient's self-discrepancy between perceived actual self and desired self, including extreme and unattainable personal standards. Interventions can focus on reducing perfectionist standards and acknowledgment of disavowed, but potentially valuable, aspects of the actual self. As discrepancy is clarified, ICAT promotes a greater level of self-acceptance and pursuit of more reasonable standards.

It is important to emphasize that although Phase III places a strong emphasis on interpersonal patterns, there is also a continuing focus on emotional responding and eating behavior, carried over from Phases I and II. Thus, patients may work on modifying interpersonal behavior in the hope that it will provide an increase in positive, and decrease in negative, emotions, which in turn may reduce the likelihood of BN behaviors. However, it is important that patients understand that they need to keep working on directly modifying eating behavior and gaining a greater understanding of their emotional behavior while they are trying to modify typical interpersonal patterns. Simply changing interpersonal patterns is unlikely to modify BN behavior unless those remain a direct focus of the treatment.

Core Skills in Phase III

Early in Phase III patients are introduced to the WAIT skill—watch all impulses today—as an effort to foster the ability to delay gratification and reduce impulsive action. Patients are encouraged to monitor feeling states and consider action alternatives. Additionally, as ICAT focuses on interpersonal patterns and self-directed styles, the SAID (sensitively assert ideas and desires) and SPA (self-protect and accept) skills are increasingly emphasized as mnemonic strategies for encouraging assertiveness, self-acceptance, and self-protection. Again, all core skills are emphasized in the Patient Workbook as well as the PDA modules.

Phase IV: Relapse Prevention and Treatment Termination

Goals of Phase IV (Sessions 19–20)

1. Review progress in treatment and identify skills that have been particularly helpful.
2. Construct healthy lifestyle plan.
3. Educate about relapse.
4. Address emotions related to termination.

Therapeutic Techniques

The final phase of ICAT consolidates gains and promotes a healthy lifestyle for the patient. Typical relapse prevention strategies are included; many of the skills emphasized in ICAT, particularly the five core skills, are embedded in all relapse prevention procedures. Patients are educated about the difference between a "lapse" and a "relapse" and given an explicit coping strategy intervention to use in the face of a lapse situation in order to prevent a full return of bulimia behavior (i.e., relapse). Further-more, they are encouraged to write out the fundamental components of their lapse prevention plan and to construct a healthy lifestyle plan that encompasses a broader array of goals than those explicitly targeted in ICAT. Again, the Patient Workbook pro-vides considerable instruction and education about these interventions and becomes a particular focus in Phase IV.

Summary

ICAT is a new promising psychosocial treatment for BN that presently has minimal empirical support. Initial studies of the underlying conceptual model have generally supported the ICAT theory, but continued psychopathology-oriented research is clearly needed. The developers of ICAT have secured a grant from the National Institute of Mental Health, which will allow treatment refinement and development, with an ulti-mate comparison to the narrow form of CBT-E (Fairburn, 2008). This study began in March 2009 and should take approximately 2 years to complete. It will provide prelimi-nary data regarding the relative efficacy of ICAT.

In terms of clinical technique, ICAT represents a relatively unique approach to BN treatment. Although certain elements of traditional behavioral therapies (e.g., self-monitoring) are emphasized, other interventions focusing on emotion regulation and interpersonal behavior are quite different. Furthermore, utilization of the Patient Workbook and PDA modules is unique. Nonetheless, in spite of these interesting theo-retical and clinical features, it remains to be seen if ICAT will generate evidence to support its ultimate utilization by clinicians.

References

Agras WS, & Telch CF. (1998). The effects of caloric deprivation and negative affect on binge eating in obese binge-eating disordered women. *Behavior Therapy*, 29:491–503.

Allen LB, McHugh RK, & Barlow DH. (2008). Emotional disorders: A unified protocol. In DH Barlow (Ed.), *Clinical handbook of psychological disorders: A step-by-step treatment manual* (4th ed., pp. 216–249). New York: Guilford Press.

Altabe M, & Thompson KJ. (1996). Body image: A cognitive self-schema construct. *Cognitive Therapy and Research*, 20:171–193.

Benjamin LS. (2003). *Interpersonal reconstructive therapy: An integrative, personality-based treatment for complex cases.* New York: Guilford Press.

Brewerton TD, Lydiard RB, Laraia MT, Shook JE, & Ballenger JC. (1992). CSF beta-endorphin and dynorphin in bulimia nervosa. *American Journal of Psychiatry*, 149:1086–1090.

Bulik CM, Sullivan PF, Joyce PR, & Carter FA. (1995). Temperament, character, and personality disorder in bulimia nervosa. *Journal of Nervous and Mental Disease*, 183:593–598.

Clark DA. (1995). Perceived limitations of standard cognitive therapy: A consideration of efforts to revise Beck's theory and therapy. *Journal of Cognitive Psychotherapy: An International Quarterly*, 9:153–172.

Cloninger CR, Svrakic D, & Przybeck T. (1993). A psychobiological model of temperament and character. *Archives of General Psychiatry*, 50:975–990.

Cooper PJ, & Fairburn CG. (1986). The depressive symptoms of bulimia nervosa. *British Journal of Psychiatry*, 148:268–274.

Cusumano DL, & Thompson JK. (1997). Body image and body shape ideals in magazines: Exposure, awareness, and internalization. *Sex Roles*, 37:701–721.

Fairburn CG. (2008). *Cognitive behavior therapy and eating disorders.* New York: Guilford Press.

Fairburn CG, Marcus MD, & Wilson GT. (1993). Cognitive-behavioral therapy for binge eating and bulimia nervosa: A comprehensive treatment manual. In CG Fairburn & GT Wilson (Eds.), *Binge eating: Nature, assessment and treatment* (pp. 361–404). New York: Guilford Press.

Fairburn CG, Welch SL, & Doll HA. (1997). Risk factors for bulimia nervosa: A community-based case-control study. *Archives of General Psychiatry*, 54:509–517.

Greenberg LS. (2002). *Emotion-focused therapy: Coaching clients to work through their feelings.* Washington, DC: American Psychological Association.

Guidano VF. (1986). The self as mediator of cognitive change in psychotherapy. In LM Hartman & KR Blankstein (Eds.), *Perception of self in emotional disorder and psychotherapy* (pp. 305–330). New York: Plenum Press.

Hayes SC, Strosahl KD, & Wilson KG. (2002). Acceptance and commitment therapy: An experiential approach to behavior change. *Cognitive and Behavioral Practice*, 9:164–166.

Heatherton TF, & Baumeister RF. (1991). Binge eating as escape from self awareness. *Psychological Bulletin*, 110:86–108.

Higgins ET. (1987). Self-discrepancy: A theory relating self and affect. *Psychological Review*, 94:319–340.

Holden NL. (1991). Adoption and eating disorders: A high-risk group? *British Journal of Psychiatry*, 158:829–833.

Humphrey LL. (1989). Observed family interactions among subtypes of eating disorders using structural analysis of social behavior. *Journal of Consulting and Clinical Psychology*, 57:206–214.

Jacobi C, Hayward C, de Zwaan M, Kraemer H, & Agras WS. (2004a). Coming to terms with risk factors for eating disorders: Application of risk terminology and suggestions for a general taxonomy. *Psychological Bulletin*, 130:19–65.

Kendler KS, Maclean C, & Neale M. (1991). The genetic epidemiology of bulimia nervosa. *American Journal of Psychiatry*, 148:1627–1637.

Lilenfeld LR, Kaye WH, Greeno CG, Merikangas KR, Plotnicov K, Pollice C, et al. (1997). Psychiatric disorders in women with bulimia nervosa and their first-degree relatives: Effects of comorbid substance dependence. *International Journal of Eating Disorders*, 22:253–264.

Meichenbaum D. (1993). Changing conceptions of cognitive behavior modification: Retrospect and prospect. *Journal of Consulting and Clinical Psychology*, 61:202–204.

Miller WR, & Rollnick S. (2002). *Motivational interviewing: Preparing people for change* (2nd ed.). New York: Guilford Press.

Mitchell JE, Hoberman HN, Peterson CB, Mussell M, & Pyle RL. (1996). Research on psychotherapy of bulimia nervosa: Half empty or half full? *International Journal of Eating Disorders*, 20:219–229.

Neimeyer RA. (1993). An appraisal of constructivist psychotherapies. *Journal of Consulting and Clinical Psychology*, 61:221–234.

Safer DL, Telch CF, & Agras WS. (2001). Dialectical behavior therapy for bulimia nervosa. *American Journal of Psychiatry*, 158:632–634.

Safran JD, & Segal ZV. (1996). *Interpersonal process in cognitive therapy.* Northvale, NJ: Aronson.

Samoilov A, & Goldfried MR. (2000). Role of emotion in cognitive-behavior therapy. *Clinical Psychology: Science and Practice*, 7:373–385.

Smyth J, Wonderlich SA, Heron K, Sliwinski M, Crosby RD, Mitchell JE, et al. (2007). Daily and momentary mood and stress predict binge eating and vomiting in bulimia nervosa patients in the natural environment. *Journal of Consulting and Clinical Psychology*, 75:629–638.

Stice E. (2002). Risk and maintenance factors for eating pathology: A meta-analytic review. *Psychological Bulletin*, 128:825–848.

Stice E, Bohon C, Marti CN, & Fischer K. (2008). Subtyping women with bulimia nervosa along dietary and negative affect dimensions: Further evidence of reliability and validity. *Journal of Consulting and Clinical Psychology*, 76:1022–1033.

Stice E, Schupak-Neuberg E, Shaw HE, & Stein RI. (1994). Relation of media exposure to eating disorder symptomatology: An examination of mediating mechanisms. *Journal of Abnormal Psychology*, 103:836–840.

Strauman TJ, & Merrill KM. (2004). The basic science/clinical science interface and treatment development. *Clinical Psychology: Science and Practice*, 11:263–266.

Strauman TJ, Vookles J, Berenstein V, Chaiken S, & Higgins ET. (1991). Self-discrepancies and vulnerability to body dissatisfaction and disordered eating. *Journal of Personality and Social Psychology*, 61:946–956.

Striegel-Moore RH, Silbertstein LR, & Rodin J. (1986). Toward an understanding of risk factors for bulimia. *American Psychologist*, 41:246–263.

Thompson JK, & Stice E. (2001). Thin-ideal internalization: Mounting evidence for a new risk factor for body-image disturbance and eating pathology. *Current Directions in Psychological Science*, 10:181–184.

Von Ranson K, & Schnitzler C. (2007, October). *Adding impulsivity and thin-ideal internalization to the cognitive-behavioral model of bulimic symptoms.* Paper presented at the annual meeting of the Eating Disorder Research Society, Pittsburgh, PA.

Wachtel PL. (1982). *Resistance: Psychodynamic and behavioral approaches.* New York: Plenum Press.

Waller G, Quinton S, & Watson D. (1995). Processing of threat-related information by women with bulimic eating attitudes. *International Journal of Eating Disorders*, 18:189–193.

Westen D. (2000). Commentary: Implicit and emotional processes in cognitive-behavioral therapy. *Clinical Psychology: Science and Practice*, 7:386–390.

Wilson GT, Grilo CM, & Vitousek K. (2007). Psychological treatments for eating disorders. *American Psychologist*, 62:199–216.

Wonderlich SA, Brewerton T, Jocic Z, Dansky B, & Abbott DW. (1997). The relationship between childhood sexual abuse and eating disorders. *Journal of the American Academy of Child and Adolescent Psychiatry*, 36:1107–1115.

Wonderlich SA, Engel SG, Peterson CB, Robinson MD, Crosby RD, Mitchell JE, et al. (2008). Examining the conceptual model for integrative cognitive–affective therapy for BN: Two assessment studies. *International Journal of Eating Disorders*, 41:748–754.

Wonderlich SA, & Mitchell JE. (1997). Eating disorders and comorbidity: Empirical, conceptual, and clinical implications. *Psychopharmacology Bulletin*, 33:3981–3901.

Zinbarg RE. (2000). Comment on "role of emotion in cognitive behavior therapy": Some quibbles, a call for greater attention to patient motivation for change, and implications of adopting a hierarchical model of emotion. *Clinical Psychology: Science and Practice*, 7:394–399.

CHAPTER 18

Psychodynamic Therapy for Eating Disorders

Kathryn J. Zerbe

Psychodynamic psychotherapy is a uniquely useful modality in the treatment of patients with eating disorders (EDs) because it emphasizes personal narrative and subjective experience. Clinical experience demonstrates that many patients with EDs do not improve with short-term, behaviorally oriented therapies or medication alone; this group of patients may place a particularly high demand on their therapists, and individual treatment plans must be adapted to meet specific interpersonal issues and areas of functioning and deficit that imperil the patients' capacity to develop themselves over the life cycle.

Psychodynamic psychotherapy aims to explore and rectify those interpersonal and intrapsychic issues of the patient in the relationship with the therapist toward attenuation of the patient's self-destructive symptom patterns and to significantly improve quality of life. By the conclusion of a successful psychodynamic course of therapy, patients should also have newfound ego strength with which they can face what were once overpowering but often unconscious fears, set better interpersonal boundaries in their daily lives, and respond to their impulses and affects constructively.

Clinicians working with psychodynamic principles will expand upon their initial formulation of the patient's difficulties by attending to details of the patient's individual life history as it enfolds in the therapeutic setting. The psychodynamic approach is usually a longer-term endeavor (at least 1 year, frequently 2–4 or more) because the crucial data needed to understand the specific individual and family dynamics that undergird a long-standing ED take time to uncover and work through. Just as no two case histories are alike, every psychodynamic psychotherapeutic process must be adapted to the pertinent, vexing concerns, and healthy strengths, that the patient brings to the treatment process.

Contemporary psychodynamic practitioners rely upon an ever-expanding theoretical repertoire and research base to do their work. The majority of therapists who incorporate psychodynamic methods into clinical work with patients with EDs borrow, blend, and amalgamate their technical interventions from a variety of approaches or "schools" that have challenged and shaped the discipline over the past 110 years. In the next section of this chapter, the evolution of psychodynamic theory, as applied to eating problems since the time of Freud, is reviewed, including the particular methods derived from classical and contemporary Freudian viewpoints, ego psychology, object relations, self psychology, and attachment theories. Despite many differences, this noninclusive list of psychodynamic theories has in common the exploration of feelings, perceptions, memories, fantasies, wishes, conflicts, and defenses, as well as the relationship patients have within themselves and with others, to assist them in facing their pathological relationship to food, to their body, and to themselves as individuals. The long-standing aim of psychoanalysts, dating back to the first quarter century of the field, of "making the unconscious conscious" is still applied in order for patients to explore and eventually gain greater mastery over those long buried but toxic factors that may play a role in the maintenance of any manifest symptoms.

Through the examination of the most pertinent transference and countertransference paradigms that arise within a given patient's therapy, both participants in the therapeutic dyad gain a clear view of subjective experience, negotiation within interpersonal interactions, and potential stalemates that can and often do derail the patient's life. To enhance the patient's well-being and to counter the therapist burnout that arises when one works with patients who present extraordinary challenges, it is necessary to deconstruct the transference–countertransference matrix—a potent force for understanding the individual and what may be getting in the way of partial or full recovery. Because EDs are among the most life-threatening of psychiatric illnesses, they elicit powerful affects in members of the clinical team. These affects must be understood and worked through to assist the patient in countering self-destructive behaviors.

Psychodynamic psychotherapeutic principles and methods could be summed up as the method of investigating the unique power and pitfalls that accompany any "therapeutic couple." With respect to treating EDs, in particular, working with the transference–countertransference relationship is a powerful means of assisting the patient in dealing with self-representations, long-held character traits, body image, comorbid symptoms, family stories, and individual metaphors surrounding food, eating, and mealtime rituals. The therapeutic dyad is also the milieu in which to explore multifaceted aspects of abuse, deficits in early caregiving, and psychological and psychophysiological regulation. Table 18.1 contains a glossary of selected psychoanalytic terms that are used throughout the chapter.

Theoretical Models

Disturbances related to eating too much or too little, the impact of one's body image on one's sense of self, the role that early feeding patterns with primary caretakers may play in personal development, and the psychological meaning of eating and food have been of great interest in psychoanalysis since its inception. Many of Sigmund Freud's early, detailed case studies contained an element related to choice of food or eating (e.g., the Rat Man; the Wolf Man). According to analytic theory in the first half of the 20th century, problems negotiating the oral phase of development were seen as leading

TABLE 18.1. Glossary of Selected Psychoanalytic Terms

Transference and countertransference paradigms. Repetitive patterns that are enacted in the therapeutic relationship.

Drive discharge. The biological and psychological processes by which an individual achieves homeostasis by reducing or sublimating innate libido and aggression.

Object relations, object constancy, rapprochement. As the primary caretaker (e.g., object) is internalized during infancy, the toddler attains a sense of him/herself that allows him/her to feel safe in leaving the mother and returning to her (rapprochement) without experiencing trauma or significant loss. This psychological process heralds a developmental achievement that permits the child to experience others, especially the primary caretaker, as a constant object even when the child is away from them (object constancy).

Process of separation–individuation. The psychological process whereby the child gradually steps away from his/her primary caretakers and establishes a sense of self as a separate person.

Internal working model. A transgenerational cognitive model proposed by attachment theorist John Bowlby that predicts how a child's expectations of relationships derive from his/her caretaker's earliest responses to him/her. Our behaviors and views of ourselves are shaped by the model of relationships we experienced in our earliest years.

Internal objects, good object, depressive position. Originally conceptualized by psychoanalyst Melanie Klein, the process by which an individual comes to believe in his/her capacity to repair relationships and that his/her love survives destructiveness.

Mirroring. The process by which one feels seen and recognized by the primary caretaker and therefore more real. If this process is disrupted in early life, the therapist is co-opted by the patient to provide a developmental experience of having his/her emotions and desires adequately mirrored.

Projection of a critical superego. The tendency to find fault or see "the speck in the other person's eye" rather than owning up to the "log" in oneself. In other words, ridding oneself of critical feelings so as to feel better about oneself.

Observational ego. The capacity to step back and observe oneself. Observation, taking stock of one's feelings and thoughts, and reflection are strengths of a healthy ego that should develop during a successful treatment, allowing the person to observe destructive tendencies and act to correct them.

to a broad array of difficulties, including anorexia, compulsive overeating, addictions, gambling, and depression. In essence, eating disturbances were first understood as disturbances in drive discharge and maintaining a sense of control. Impaired regulation of one's capacity to love and to hate in a developmentally appropriate manner resulted in the ego's incapacity to perform its necessary functions and to the significant pathology in self-representation observed in persons with eating difficulties.

Denial, repression, reaction formation, and over- and undercontrol of impulses were primary defensive patterns observed among patients with anorexia nervosa (AN) or obesity. AN was described as a monosymptomatic hypochondriacal delusion due to the extreme denial that accompanied extraordinary control of normal oral impulses and an excessively harsh superego. Early formulations also centered on psychogenic vomiting and other hysterical symptoms related to eating as the individual's unconscious oedipal wish to become pregnant through oral means. Again, distortions in the oral developmental phase and unresolved sexual conflicts were viewed by the early psychoanalysts as the primary cause that underlay the majority of eating problems (Bruch, 1973; Wilson, Hogan, & Mintz, 1985).

During the second half of the 20th century, observational studies of infants and toddlers and a shift in psychoanalytic theory that emphasized internal object relations and the development of a sense of self augmented what had heretofore been understood about AN, bulimia nervosa (BN), and compulsive overeating. When the normal process of separation–individuation was thwarted by pathology in the primary caretaker, the child sustains intrapsychic injury resulting in impaired object constancy, intense anxiety, and desperate efforts to cling to the primary object or to find other means of self-soothing (Mahler, Pine, & Bergman, 1975). Because the rapprochement stage of development (usually occurring at 16–22 months) is not negotiated in a phase-appropriate and sustaining manner (e.g., the primary caretaker turning away from the child as he/she seeks nourishment; the primary caretaker conveys anger, anxiety, or other averse emotions in response to the child's striving toward independence), other modes of self-soothing and solace are sought. Food in such situations can be viewed as a transitional object that can help the person withstand separation because of its ready availability; it "replaces" the disappointing object who is not there to assist or mirror the individual's independent strivings. Using the theory base derived from the studies of Mahler and colleagues (1975), EDs can be formulated as attempts to aid individuals in their struggle for independence, autonomy, and age-appropriate dependence on other people.

The seminal work of Hilda Bruch (1973, 1974, 1985) also highlighted the conflict between separation and individuation in patients with AN. Her extensive clinical work with adolescents and young adults led her to theorize that the patient's striving for thinness was an interpersonal event aimed at helping her separate from an intrusive parent, usually the mother. The patient was forced into a stance from childhood onward where she could never say no or complain to her mother. Difficulties identifying affect and articulating basic needs are anathema for such patients, whose mother directly or indirectly forbade them to develop ideas, thoughts, or a personality of their own. Bruch advised therapists to resist making interpretations to these patients but instead to use questions and to reframe what patients had just said as a way of abetting a necessary process of separation–individuation and cultivating their sense of self. Because BN can be understood in some cases as failed AN, Bruch's methods, which emphasize the urge to separate and to have a sense of oneself, were adapted for the treatment of patients with BN or obesity as well.

As object relations, self psychology, and attachment theory sequentially influenced psychoanalysis as a whole, a number of papers emerged that applied these concepts to the treatment of patients with EDs, in particular. Through the 1940s, 50s, 60s, and 70s, psychodynamic psychotherapists who studied the work of Melanie Klein, W. R. D. Fairbairn, and D. W. Winnicott began to envision the internal world of the patient as a failed attachment to, and a struggle to disengage from, "bad" internal objects (Greenberg & Mitchell, 1983; Hughes, 1989). Patients with EDs, particularly those with BN, were understood as holding onto self-destructive behaviors such as overexercise or purging because of a need to be punished based on a rejecting internal object (such as a sexually and/or physically abusive or abandoning caretaker in the past). These patients have significant difficulty attaining internal self-esteem and maintaining bodily self-regulation because they cannot evoke in themselves "good enough" others to help them in times of duress. The ED becomes a rigidified source of comfort and solace despite its consciously recognized propensity to medically and psychologically wreak havoc on the individual. Moreover, as in other psychosomatic illnesses, patients with EDs are known to have difficulty putting their feelings into words. The pervasive problem of having the body express what cannot be symbolically expressed in words derives from deficits in the external environment, such as the deficits of a caretaker who is emotionally or physically unavailable to comfort the child.

Self psychological perspectives have expanded upon the initial work of Heinz Kohut in the 1970s to the present in order to address specific diagnoses and problems of living. In normal development, the needs of the infant are transformed by the parents' ministrations and optimally result in the capacity to regulate the self. Contemporary infant research demonstrates how verbal and nonverbal communication that occur bidirectionally between infant and primary caretaker guide affect regulation and influence both participants in the dyad over time (Beebe & Lachman, 2002). Feeding is a paramount experience that spontaneously lends itself to the development of self-regulatory capacities that can perilously go awry if the primary caretaker (usually the mother) has difficulty in recognizing, empathically responding to, and providing for the infant's needs. One might say that the first experience humans have of love in the extra-uterine environment is being cuddled, fed, and attended to by our mother, and in the process, under usual circumstances, this leads to interactive regulation, including the opportunity to feed ourselves and to eat with others at mealtime.

As in the case of patients with other addictions, patients with EDs can make use of their affliction as a "psychic organizer" that provides a sense of self cohesion (de Groot & Rodin, 1998). Therapists view patients with EDs as exquisitely sensitive to feeling deflated and narcissistically wounded and frame interpretations from an "experience-near" perspective. Empathizing with and helping the patient become more curious about and conscious of her own self-experience alleviates the need to turn toward the ED because she now feels heard and understood. Rather than tout an interpretation or point of view derived from the therapist's perception, the dyad works to understand the ED in terms of the patient's singular experience and create a "joint construction of meaning within the therapeutic situation" (de Groot & Rodin, 1998, p. 361). In this way, therapists help to transform the patient's capacity to self-regulate and to honor his/her need to be mirrored, tend to his/her physiological needs, and be psychologically nourished by others.

Since the seminal work of psychoanalyst and researcher John Bowlby began in the 1970s, attachment theory has increasingly been applied to our understanding and treatment of patients with severe mental disorders such as borderline and narcissistic personality disorders, posttraumatic stress disorder, substance-related disorders, and EDs. According to Bowlby and the researchers/clinicians who continue to elaborate his work (Bowlby, 1988; Fonagy, Gergely, Jurist, & Target, 2002; Goldberg, Muir, & Kerr, 1995; Stein, Fonagy, Ferguson, & Wisman, 2000), human beings (and animals) are born with a biological need to make safe connections with others and maintain affirming affiliations. These early bonds help establish those "working models" in the mind from which the infant optimally develops a sense of reliable, secure attachments and a "secure base" from which he/she will later launch into the world. In a sense, Bowlby's and Mahler's work demonstrated similar concepts but used different methodologies and language. In order for individuals to grow up and face the world relatively free of psychopathology, they have to establish within themselves a "sense of object constancy"

(Mahler) or an "internal working model" (Bowlby) based on responsive, loving caretakers who are available when their children need to return in times of need.

There are many circumstances that can disrupt early attachment that profoundly impact the psychological growth of the child, adolescent, and adult. An insecurely attached infant or a person who endures significant loss at any developmental stage may not have available the "feedback loop" that Bowlby found essential for processing feelings of anger, rage, and abandonment; emotional growth and development will be restricted because a secure base may never have formed at the beginning of life or because the attachment system fails when it is most needed (Holmes, 1993). These individuals will experience a variety of psychopathological difficulties, including "hypervigilance, angry threats, compulsively congenial behaviors" (Armstrong & Roth, 1989, p. 143) and other self-regulatory problems, such as AN, BN, or compulsive overeating. Bowlby, and the attachment researchers who followed him, underscored that separation anxiety is a normal experience for all people, but it is those significant impairments, mismatches, and disruptions with reliable providers of care that result in anxious, ambivalent, dysregulated attachment patterns that eventuate in emotional illness, including (but not limited to) pathological bereavement, the anxiety disorders, and eating problems.

In contrast to persons who are more securely attached and can reach out over their entire lifespan to others when in need of comfort, some patients with EDs are, indeed, fearful, lack self-reliance, are subject to feelings of abandonment, and even lack curiosity and an interest in learning (Armstrong & Roth, 1989). Utilizing attachment theory in case formulation can alert the psychodynamic psychotherapist to consider that a particular patient with an ED may attempt "to avoid the experience and hurt of separation [but] are not successful in muting separation pain [and are therefore subject to] overreaction to minor separations and considerable self-blame, anger, and rejection as well as denial of these painful experiences" (Armstrong & Roth, 1989, p. 151).

Disturbances in early attachment are likely one root of the difficulties eating disorder patients with EDs have in sustaining a working alliance in therapy and maintaining intimate relationships in adulthood. Some clinicians now suspect that as babies, these individuals lacked responsiveness and a containing envelope from their primary caretakers, perhaps especially during the feeding situation (Winters, 2002), and the restrictive dieting may paradoxically provide a sense of security that abnegates need for another human being. Binge eating or overeating may provide a sense of nurturance or self-soothing "for individuals who cannot trust that an intimate relationship with significant others can meet these same needs" (Armstrong & Roth, 1989, p. 153). Finally, unresolved loss, excessive mourning, and pathological bereavement are implicated in the etiology of some EDs (Zerbe, 1993a, 1996, 2008). If attachment figures are unable, unwilling, or simply unavailable, withstanding and processing the inevitable myriad of affects that accompany loss is impossible. Restrictive eating, overexercise, or identification with a lost object who was thin at the time of death due to illness, may be the only ways the individual has to "withstand and process hostility" (Holmes, 1993, p. 94) or covertly give expression to "knowing what you are not supposed to know and feeling what you are not supposed to feel" (Bowlby, 1979, p. 403; see also Zerbe, 1996, 2001, 2008). Each of these formulations is a way to posit how the eating problem *may* have developed, based on application of Bowlby's attachment theory.

Controlled Trials

To date there are few controlled trials of the psychodynamic treatment of EDs. A notable exception is the work of Christopher Dare and colleagues at the Maudsley Hospital in London (Dare, 1993, 1997; Dare & Crowther, 1995; Dare, Eisler, Russell, Treasure, & Dodge, 2001). These reports yield a number of important findings, including confirmation of how a strong alliance between therapist and patient is an essential ingredient in overcoming a treatment stalemate. In once weekly, time-limited (1 year) psychodynamic psychotherapy for adults suffering from AN, patients were significantly helped when the therapist was viewed as "on the patient's side" (Dare & Crowther, p. 295) and pushed the patient to see hidden meaning, feelings, wishes, and fears that lie behind the ED. A focal hypothesis that examines losses, oedipal conflicts, and enactments, and also aims less for symptomatic cure than for patients "to discover and explore additional pathways for the expression of their psychological organization, in the expectation that people have more ways of being themselves than they usually display" (Dare, 1993, p. 18) result in an experience of healthy aggression and assertion. A truer sense of self evolves to challenge the central "paradox of starving to death" (Dare, p. 19) to save the self.

In a randomized study of 84 patients, even patients with a poor prognosis who were considered "chronic" by any standard made significant strides in the psychoanalytic psychotherapy and family therapy cohorts compared to those who received low-intensity, education-based, "routine" treatment. This research group goes further to confirm the long-held, clinically championed axioms that dynamic therapies assist patients by (1) demonstrating how symptoms are used to ward off painful affects and unconsciously serve as self-protective defenses against danger situations; (2) exploring how the disorder is experienced as self-imposed punishment; (3) making use of countertransference responses as information gleaned about the patient's inner experience (i.e., via projection, displacement, or projective identification of affects); and (4) facilitating the normative developmental tasks of separation, individuation, and the attainment of mature dependence.

In Germany, a specific psychodynamic method for treating severely disturbed patients (i.e., those with borderline personality disorder, perversion, addictions, and EDs), called "psychoanalytic–interactional psychotherapy" (PIP) (Streeck, 2006) ,emphasizes interpersonal processes and the subjective experience of the here and now with the therapist. Therapists verbalize the affect and experiences they observe in their patients and encourage patients' reflections and feelings about those perceptions, thereby enhancing the experience of interpersonal boundaries and subjectivity. Therapists actively respond to dysfunctional behavior patterns with the explicit goal of fostering differentiation of self from other and the development of reflective function (i.e., the ability to think about and understand one's and others' psychological and emotional processes). Interpersonal problems and comorbid difficulties such as EDs, suicide attempts, substance abuse, and self-mutilation decreased in severity in groups of very ill patients, suggesting that this modality holds promise for patients with EDs who do not share the same Cluster B personality profiles (Roth & Fonagy, 2005; Shadish, Matt, Navarro, & Phillips, 2000; Streeck, 2006). Although follow-up studies are required to examine the stability of treatment effects for ED symptoms, PIP researchers maintain that both naturalistic and randomized controlled trials (RCTs) are important and necessary because they complement each other. An effectiveness (naturalistic) study is carried out under the conditions of clinical practice but may not necessarily overestimate treatment effects compared to an RCT, which examines if treatment works under controlled, experimental conditions.

In a naturalistic study of 145 patients with bulimic symptoms (Thompson-Brenner & Westen, 2005), clinicians were found to tailor their practice techniques to the patient's specific problems. Psychodynamic psychotherapists incorporated more CBT interventions (e.g., practicing new coping strategies, suggesting tasks such as writing in a journal, encouraging patients to be less self-critical, challenging irrational thoughts), and cognitive-behavioral therapists implicitly increased their use of psychodynamic interventions, such as addressing traumatic experience, asking about shifts in topic or mood, addressing interpersonal difficulties, confronting perfectionism, and targeting affect regulation. This research demonstrates that interventions that are practiced in a community have "little relationship to RCTs," which are usually short term and "have been too brief to expect the distinctive goal of psychodynamic therapies ... namely characterological change or treatment of personality diatheses" (Thompson-Brenner & Westen, 2005, p. 593).

Because clinicians in the "real world" of everyday practice integrate symptom-focused and personality-focused interventions that may take longer to administer but are actually found to improve outcome, Thompson-Brenner and Westen (2005) argue for more naturalistic studies to be conducted. Their findings also suggest that some patients will benefit from a limited intervention, but the majority of their sample needed those additional interventions that psychodynamic therapies specifically address. In particular, recovering from bulimic symptoms necessitates "addressing enduring personality disposition toward emotional dysregulation and constriction which appear to influence outcome above and beyond Axis I symptoms" (p. 593). Including techniques that take into account issues that usually fall under the "psychodynamic domain," such as "exploring the patient's feelings, conflicts, impulses, significant relationships, defenses, and so forth" (p. 592), resulted in better global outcome in patients with bulimic symptoms.

Lastly, another promising area of research lies in mentalization-based therapy for EDs. Studies in the past decade indicate that insecure attachment (Ward, Ramsay, & Treasure, 2000) and dismissive attachment styles (Ward, Ramsay, Turnbull, Steele, Steele & Treasure, 2001) are linked with the development of EDs, especially AN. Evidence points to the fact that some mothers may transmit faulty attachment patterns to their daughters, resulting in an inability to emotionally process feelings, particularly loss. Manuals are being developed and tested that help individuals with EDs rehabilitate the mentalizing function. Data from this important work are forthcoming and will likely enhance the therapist's armamentarium "to investigate concretely the experiences with body and food, and connect them with emotional, cognitive and relational experiences" (Skarderud, 2007, p. 333). A derivative of psychodynamic principles, attachment theory, and contemporary cognitive and neuroscience research, mentalization-based therapy for EDs addresses a repertoire of patient difficulties in a refined manualized approach that aids in teaching students and in conducting RCTs in diverse populations of patients (Bateman & Fonagy, 2006; Skarderud, 2007).

Mini-Manual and Clinical Dialogues

Working Through Projection and Projective Identification

Projection and projective identification are frequently used defense mechanisms encountered in treating individuals with EDs and other severe mental illnesses, which are "used as a form of defense against internal and external realities" (Rozen, 1993, p. 262). Painful aspects of the self are psychologically evacuated in order to spoil a relationship, control another person, or rid oneself of a powerful affect that cannot yet be processed. Bion (1967) first observed that projective identification can also serve as a form of communication from a patient who has difficulty feeling and working on his/her emotions directly or needs to disclaim or eliminate an aspect of the self. Therapists also play a role in this regard. It is not merely the patient's splitting off and projection of feelings; through transference–countertransference the therapist may experience the way the patient feels unconsciously. For example, if a patient feels ineffectual but this is too painful, he/she may act in such a manner that under certain circumstances the therapist may feel that it is he/she who is powerless to help the patient make important changes.

Although eventually the patient must integrate these intolerable aspects into "a more thinkable form" (Rozen, 1993, p. 263) in order for the self to be experienced as whole and integrated, initially this is not possible. Like the mother of an infant, the therapist must provide a silent, containing function for the individual's split-off, dissociated, or repressed affects or self experience (Zerbe, 1993b, 2001, 2008).

In the following example of Ms. A, a 42-year-old patient with BN who survived a gang rape at age 18 and subsequently developed severe difficulties in self-regulation, two steps of working with the defense of projective identification, depending on the phase of treatment, are described. In the first sample dialogue, Ms. A's therapist works to help her contain her strong feelings as the therapeutic alliance gets established and solidifies. As the treatment moves along, Ms. A is able to have greater success maintaining steady employment and has developed a long-term relationship; her self-regulatory difficulties (e.g., binge eating, vomiting, using laxatives) go into significant remission. The therapist now feels ready to decisively intervene by interpreting projected elements based on countertransference feelings. Ms. A nondefensively accepts her therapist's confrontation and interpretation. She goes on to modify her actions based on the intervention and thereby demonstrates a stronger sense of herself. Extensive clinical experience with patients who have EDs reveals how often these patients use food, their eating behaviors, memories of family mealtime or lack thereof, and fantasies about eating, exercise, and food as elements of their lives to be "rid of quickly" via the projective mechanisms.

Phase I (11 Months into Therapy)

MS. A: You're going to be really mad at me today because I binged and purged all weekend long.

THERAPIST: Any guess as to why you did this?

MS. A: None whatsoever.

THERAPIST: (*sensing the patient's demoralization and anger that has been projected by the patient*) You seem to think I'll be as upset with you as you are with yourself, but that mode keeps us from understanding what might have triggered your bingeing and purging this weekend.

MS. A: I bet it's the old "abandonment" stuff you and I have talked about.

THERAPIST: Could be, but we can't know for sure until you can say what was going on in your mind.

Here the therapist contains the patient's feelings and gently probes to get more historical details or fantasies of what might have provoked the weekend regression. Rather than suggest that Ms. A was angry and demoralized, the therapist notes the feelings within herself and attempts to help soothe the patient by opening up the session for more dialogue and understanding. The motif of a mother silently tuning in to her infant's need for more comfort by singing a lullaby or attending to basic needs balances the more active, playful, overtly growth-promoting ministrations. Containment in the therapeutic situation is a similar notion.

Phase II (12 Months Later)

MS. A: I couldn't believe what happened last night. I've been doing better lately. But I binged and purged 10 times. Maybe it's because Joe forgot my birthday last week. He got defensive when I confronted him and walked out. He called and we got back together but I still went out, bought three quarts of ice cream, two dozen doughnuts, and down the hatch they went. Then you know where else they went!

THERAPIST: So you get upset with Joe for missing your special day and you had to put your anger into gobbling up the food and discharging it into the john?

MS. A: No. I wasn't angry. It was the abandonment thing again.

THERAPIST: "Abandonment" is only a jargon word until you can describe what you were actually feeling and thinking that made you feel so empty and alone.

MS. A: I really have no idea.

THERAPIST: (*confronting*) I bet you do. Give it another try. Why might you get so provoked with Joe forgetting your birthday and not let it go, even when you talked the situation over? Your relationship had been going pretty well for a few months before this wound.

MS. A: I hate myself for needing him, missing him, and loving him at the same time. When he messed up, I felt like he'd forgotten me. I didn't want to keep fighting and punishing him because he forgot, but I had to get those icky feelings out of my system some way.

THERAPIST: (*interpreting Ms. A's projection of her anger and abandonment onto the food*) Now we're getting somewhere. You have *mixed feelings* about Joe. It's understandable that you were hurt when he failed you by missing your birthday. But rather than keep talking, thinking, and even writing in your journal about the tender and angry sides, you soothed yourself temporarily with the soft ice cream and doughnuts and them spit them out as if to say, "Joe, you're in the toilet with me still. I'm not over being hurt by what you did."

MS. A: Maybe this has something to with why the bulimia started after the rape. I was ashamed and enraged but didn't have anywhere to turn, or so it seemed.

THERAPIST: Makes sense to me. When violence happens, it has to go somewhere. You coped as best you could when there didn't seem to be a safe, secure spot, inside or outside of yourself.

MS. A: (*winsomely*) I'm glad Joe gets back today. I want to do something nice for him, like cook dinner or take him on a hike at his favorite place. I think I'll wait to tell him what we talked about in here. I will be open with him about my relapse. I have the sense that he'll understand.

With the therapist's help over time, Ms. A is able to see that her binge–purge episodes have powerful historical antecedents. In each segment of these two dialogues, the patient deals with her inability to control another person by turning to food and purging, each time with somewhat greater insight and command of her symptoms. Although she projects her anger, anxiety, and abandonment–depression onto others (her therapist and boyfriend), in the first dialogue the therapist primarily contains the affects that are both intellectually understandable but also interpersonally felt. When symptoms are used unconsciously to rid the self of an unwanted experience and the therapist picks up on it by emotional resonance, successful projective identification has already occurred—which could potentially drive a nurturing other away if not understood as a form of emotional communication.

In the patients' lives outside the office, note how often this dynamic occurs in vignettes about how often others misunderstand, give up on, or get angry with them. These patients make others feel how they themselves feel but cannot experience—that is projective identification. In Ms. A's case, her gradual capacity to acknowledge and express realistic, mixed feelings signal that she has less need to split off feelings and potentially alienate others, in this case her boyfriend. Despite the regression into a bulimic pattern, she can own her behavior and look at what may have been behind it. She stops before she "evacuates" the feelings that led to the behavior prior to her boyfriend's return and instead is determined not to spoil his return.

Note also the patient's acknowledgment of a need for succor and safety as she recalls her history of trauma. Her choice of a creamy, easily consumed food may have several psychological meanings; here Ms. A appears to let her therapist in on the fact that she yearns for connection and closeness. Guilty and ashamed of her powerful need to consume as a way of warding off the experience of the abuse, she attacks herself and her internal objects by the evacuations. The symptomatic regression in the second dialogue does not deter the therapist's probing of Ms. A about what lay beneath her current need to binge and purge. By the end of that segment of the dialogue, Ms. A signals that she is now internalizing the therapist's interpretation and takes back her projection by demonstrating her ability to link her history to her symptomatic expression. She even intends to care for her "good object" (i.e., Joe, her boyfriend), which demonstrates functioning in the realm of the depressive position (Klein, 1975; Segal, 1980).

Confronting Narcissistic Self-Sufficiency

For patients who have experienced or believe that others are not reliable or dependable, disturbances in reaching out and receiving necessary support are ubiquitous and lead to character patterns that are counterproductive and often frankly destructive. Examining patients' defensive response, in the "real time" of therapy, to turn to their ED symptoms as a way to avoid making or using connections with other people encourages new modes of adaptation to life's vicissitudes. Over time patients learn that others can be trusted to meet needs for love and safety (i.e., using attachment and self psychology theories) and master a sense of powerlessness and humiliation when they would heretofore feel alone, damaged, and helpless (blending ego psychology, affect theory, and object relations approaches). Consider the following excerpt.

> MR. B: When I started treatment with you, I binged a lot more when you went on vacation. Last week Sally [his girlfriend of 2 years] went to visit her folks for 2 weeks in Maine. I was sad and upset because I couldn't go due to my work, but I didn't chow-down on everything in sight. I only did my routine workout, too, instead of running for 4 hours and then dashing to the gym. I was lonely, but it wasn't the same.
>
> THERAPIST: What do you think made the difference this time?
>
> MR. B: I knew Sally would call me because she said she would. In fact, she let me know when her plane landed and has rung me up every day since, even if it was just to leave a message. She knew I was a little irritable because she was going away, and we talked about it first. I also knew I would come in here and tell you that I was angry, even though I don't think it is fair of me to be upset with her. After all, I go away alone, too, sometimes.
>
> THERAPIST: It occurs to me that "traveling alone" inside of yourself disturbs you less than it did in the past. We've talked a good bit about your resolve to turn to people instead of food or exercise when you feel a need or have a strong feeling.
>
> MR. B: Sometimes I hate myself for being so needy. It makes me feel like a little boy.
>
> THERAPIST: It still seems hard for you to believe that even adults must rely on others. I bet it is hard to fully own the fact that Sally needs you, too, even though she shows that by calling you on her trip.

In this example, the therapist gently confronts the patient's ambivalence about making good use of a human attachment and clarifies that mature dependence helps him mollify his old symptoms. Including the girlfriend's name in the intervention and her own reaching out to Mr. B both personalizes and reifies the intervention. Helping patients recognize and own the counterdependent stance that once made them turn to food, overexercise, or even deny any need by aesthetically refusing to eat moves the treatment forward by recognizing positive attachments, demonstrating that overeating and overexercising are outmoded defensive styles, and mirroring how the new sense of trust in others to process positive and negative affects meets needs in a sustaining way that inanimate objects or activities never can.

Exploring the Psychological Meaning of Food and Eating

Although all persons have conscious and unconscious thoughts about food and eating, the symbolic, relational, and familial meanings embedded in this subject often go unaddressed, even in a psychodynamic treatment process. In part this occurs because most of us therapists have little training in discussing food and nutrition, prefer to leave this subject to those who have greater knowledge and experience (the nutritionist on the multidisciplinary team), and gravitated to a career in this field because of an interest in working with other people's life stories or an inherent ability in using a particular psychotherapeutic technique or application of a theory that "works" for us. Exploring how food is or was misused in the family of origin, the patient's thoughts and fantasies about particular food groups or eating in general, and clarifying distortions and perceptions about food brings into the open an area of psychological life that was previously unknown and unspoken. A psychodynamic approach to eating necessitates that the patient look at food as more than a biological necessity for the body but as a test for a psychological process with many potential and discoverable meanings.

> MS. C: Even though I trust Gretchen [her nutritionist] completely, I still believe that yogurt and cheese will make me fat. She keeps telling me about portion control and that no one food group can make a person fat. I know she is right because I read about this stuff all the time, but I can't seem to follow my meal plan on my own without getting mad at her and myself and feeling like a total failure.

> THERAPIST: Do you think that has anything to do with how your mother and father felt about food when you were a little girl?

> MS. C: Nope. I just don't want to get fat. I don't even like being this close to my "so-called target BMI" since I left the residential program. Cheese *will always* be on my forbidden food list.

> THERAPIST: I wonder why? Why cheese, specifically?

> MS. C: Don't play shrink with me by making this psychological. It is a *food* issue. I will take it up with Gretchen.

> THERAPIST: Sounds like you are trying to prove that it's not psychological to me. I wonder if a part of you knows that it is not rational, because you bring the issue here as well as to Gretchen.

> MS. C: (*angrily*) Just don't go there—OK? I don't want you tying this to my family or anything else like you *always* do.

> THERAPIST: (*undeterred but playfully*) Sounds like you want to try to forbid me from taking in or even thinking about what you think are my "cheesy" psychological theories! You're convinced I'll feed you something forbidden, like yogurt or cheese. In this case, it's a forbidden thought about your family issues!

> MS. C: (*reluctantly*) Maybe it's plausible, but I'm not about to swallow any of your psychological jibber jabber whole!

> THERAPIST: (*staying in the patient's metaphor*). As if I could make you do that. Who says you have to take it whole or swallow even a bit of it, really? We don't insist on a "clean plate club" in therapy.

Ms. C: Gretchen says pretty much the same thing. I get to pick what I want and to take small bites, as long as I can keep trying to raise my BMI to 18.5.

THERAPIST: Gretchen and I seem to be on the same page, and I wonder if that bugs you. I recall how you said in our first few sessions that your folks seemed, from your perspective, to debate what you should do and where you could go after school. Eating seems to have fit right in.

Ms. C: Food was never an issue. There was only so much to go around. Mom would sneak us kids out for a Tastycake or a pack of M&M's if we would go grocery shopping with her. Dad would say that we didn't have enough money for treats. He would insist that they would rot our teeth anyway.

THERAPIST: (*making an obvious interpretation of triangulation*) It must have felt sinful to have a sweet snack. And behind your father's back, no less. What a bind for the kids.

Ms. C: (*responding to the interpretation by providing some new data the therapist was not aware of previously*) I never got the "we have no money" part of this. They always got to do cool things. They belonged to a swim club, played bridge and golf. Sometimes they even drank like fish with their friends.

THERAPIST: You're telling me that there was a big double standard for the adults and the kids. You were in the middle of it all. Your eating disorder might have something to do with staying loyal to the "no money, no snack" mentality.

Ms. C: Do you think this has anything to do with why it feels awful to see Gretchen even though I really like her and get a lot out of our meetings? I like her as a person and she talks to me like an adult. Some days we don't even discuss my meal plan or food. She's cool. I always feel like I should not go back after I leave.

THERAPIST: (*understanding that the patient is unconsciously testing, in part, to see if both clinicians will not create a loyalty bind for the patient that repeats salient family issues*) Gretchen has become like a forbidden treat in some ways, and you want to know if that is okay with me because we both work with you individually and are part of "your team," so to speak. When you see Gretchen, I think it brings up a big conflict inside you because a part of you knows that seeing her won't make you fat or disloyal. It is one part of your treatment to help you get better.

Ms. C: That makes sense, but it makes me sad, too.

THERAPIST: Perhaps it makes you sad because when you were a child, you felt as though you were committing a big indiscretion when you ate a Tastycake or a pack of M&M's. Our work is about sorting this out, but I think that we can agree today that food issues are important in all kinds of ways, in part because they carry special meanings that aren't apparent on the surface.

Ms. C: When I see Gretchen next week, I'm going to tell her what we talked about! I might even try to add some milk products to my regimen. She will tell me that she is proud of my resolve.

THERAPIST: (*keeping within the metaphor of food and eating concerns, clarifying and inter-*

preting the unconscious test that both clinicians can and will work together without competing): It seems as though you and Gretchen are working well together, and she is helping you face down some core beliefs about foods that are "bad." Unlike your past, you are taking a step ahead by telling me about the importance of your work with her. You are checking out if you must keep your relationship with her and your discussions with her a secret or if you can have both of us working with you at the same time.

MS. C: The three of us—me, Gretchen, and you working together! That's like three different food groups.

THERAPIST: (*mirroring the newfound capacity to face down the loyalty bind*) Indeed, it is! What a concept that you can have us both and work with us both.

Here the therapist begins by skirting the patient's initial reluctance to address problems with food as a psychological issue that can be spoken about directly and understood historically and symbolically. The history about the use and misuse of food in the family nexus usually comes to the surface over time and can then be discussed naturally. Both therapist and nutritionist are calling attention to the patient's unrealistic assessment about certain foods and are working collaboratively to provide a new emotional experience within which the patient can learn and grow.

With time Ms. C not only comes to recognize and incorporate the notion that certain foods had special and significant meaning in her family of origin but the role they played in her development of an eating problem. She has identified with her father's projection of a critical superego onto the children in the family and has internalized her mother's experience that certain food-related activities must be hidden. In order for the patient to improve, she will need more opportunities to address her loyalty bind and weather the loss of these internalized images of each parent. Hence, in psychodynamic therapy, tincture of time must be an essential ingredient in the treatment plan. Sadness of this sort is "the vitamin of growth," according to the late Harvard psychoanalyst and educator Elvin Semrad (see Rako & Mazur, 1980, p. 45), because it necessitates coming to grips with the "necessary condition of human health to be able to bear what has to borne, to be able to think what has to be thought" (p. 47). Patients with EDs respond slowly but consistently to explorations of food-related symptoms and will accept clinician interventions without feeling that they are betraying themselves, their bodies, or significant people in their lives only after they can defy and work through a severe inner critic (e.g., internalized negative introject) by treating themselves benevolently (Schafer, 1960).

Facing Down Excessive Shame and Guilt

One area where psychodynamic theory and CBT converge is the use of the therapeutic relationship to attenuate excessive guilt and shame (Wurmser, 1994, 1995). Identifying and working through conflicts and concern with a severe inner critic reduce the punitive superego (psychodynamic conceptualization) and can diminish catastrophic thinking while countering negative attributes about oneself (cognitive-behavioral conceptualization). Extreme alterations between ego synchronicity and self-criticism may lead to symptomatic patterns that reflect an ideal self in conflict with a defective self. As a patient becomes aware of a flaw or imperfection, retreat may ensue via a pathway of extraordinary self-criticism and lack of worthiness for care.

In the case of Ms. D that follows, no historical antecedents are provided in the dialogue played out in this typical scene from her thrice weekly individual psychotherapy. Working within the here-and-now relationship with the therapist in the transference alone begins to mollify and modify the patient's experience of herself as seriously damaged. At the time of this vignette, Ms. D has been in treatment for BN for about 1 year and is making gains in symptom control and experiencing her life as fulfilling. A serendipitous encounter of seeing her therapist and his wife at a public event reactivates Ms. D's sense of defectiveness that is played out in a symptomatic regression and displacement onto her body. Her therapist chooses to address Ms. D's difficulties at this therapeutic moment by again pointing out hidden affects of shame and guilt.

Significant psychotherapeutic work has already paved the way for Ms. D to more readily take in her therapist's observations without "spitting them back." One might formulate what has happened as the cultivation of a more "loving and beloved" superego (Schafer, 1960). While adhering to customary and essential therapeutic boundaries, the therapist comments on how all human beings may at times feel weak, flawed, and vulnerable and then goes on to emphasize the steps the patient is making by risking talking about her recrudescence of symptoms, making observations about her own reactions, and trusting her therapist with those affects that can lead to otherwise "traumatic isolation and loss of control" (Wurmser, 1994, p. 55).

> MS. D: I saw you [her therapist] at the concert with your wife. I left at intermission because I could not stand it anymore. I went home and took laxatives again, but I didn't binge.
>
> THERAPIST: Might you have been angry with yourself for being curious about me being out with my spouse?
>
> MS. D: I'm bored today. My job is a wreck. I can't decide if I want to return to college next semester. I have no idea how I'd pay for it anyway.
>
> THERAPIST: I notice you quickly got off the subject of having feelings about seeing me at the concert. Might that incident have anything to do with your returning to using laxatives?
>
> MS. D: Do we always have to get back to bringing you into the picture? I hate it when you do that—even though I did mention it first this time.
>
> THERAPIST: (*moving right into the defense*) I think you hate bringing it up because it makes you feel embarrassed and "dirty" to have feelings about seeing me outside the office. It feels somehow elicit, even though it's actually pretty natural to have all kinds of feeling and thoughts about one's therapist and his family. I wonder what makes it difficult to talk about now.
>
> MS. D: I noticed a guy in the waiting room after my last session. I thought that maybe you like working with him more than you do me. I bet he's doing better, too. I've been working with you for months, and I still purge with laxatives sometimes despite all we have done. Sometimes I bet you must be really frustrated with me.

THERAPIST: You become quite self-critical about many things—having some feelings about seeing me at the concert with my wife, observing another person in the waiting room. I wonder if we could also think of it as progress that you can be more open about some of these things than when you began.

MS. D: I think it is ridiculous for a grown woman to get so caught up in this kind of crap.

THERAPIST: It feels better to try and cleanse the crap out with laxatives than to feel ridiculous and vulnerable.

MS. D: Maybe.

THERAPIST: I think that it also keeps you at a distance from me and our work—you put a "brake" on what we can talk about in here, and we both end up experiencing a brief stalemate that is uncomfortable. In this situation, I wonder if guilt and shame aren't holding you back.

MS. D: It helps me to know that you have feelings, too, sometimes.

THERAPIST: And that I can "call a spade a spade" and not be upset with either of us, because our task is to understand as best we can and to help you feel more human overall.

MS. D: Like jealousy and anger might be normal sometimes, even?

THERAPIST: They're part of the human condition and much better managed when they are out in the open.

When a punitive superego is addressed in treatment, the patient's observational ego grows and the therapeutic alliance strengthens. Ms. D "digests" her therapist's interventions, slowly regarding her competition and rivalry that led to her psychic retreat in this instance. Not surprisingly, Ms. D's history was laden with stories about her workaholic and self-involved father who delighted in devaluing and berating his progeny. Her youthful importuning for attention that was frequently derided and went often unheeded resulted in feeling exposed and belittled. She eschewed mature dependence in order to emulate what she falsely believed was her father's perfection. Unconsciously, her symptoms also spoke to the transformation of passive rage into an active psychophysiological symptom of BN, whereby she spuriously staved off unbearable affects and needs for connection to others.

Available Resources

Some residential and inpatient treatment programs do include individual and group approaches that incorporate psychodynamic perspectives, although the majority of these programs are relatively short term, focus on medical complications and symptom control, and stress educative and cognitive-behavioral methods to stabilize the patient and prevent relapse. This integrated, multidisciplinary approach is essential for all patients, and the majority of psychodynamic practitioners incorporate elements (e.g., medication, behavioral strategies, homework assignments) of evidence-based methods into a more insight-oriented, less-directive exploratory psychotherapy process.

Locating a psychodynamic practitioner is usually not difficult, even in smaller communities. The Academy for Eating Disorders and the International Association of Eating Disorder Professionals has members with specialized interest and training in this approach. Additionally, one may contact local professional societies (psychology, psychiatry, social work, etc.) or national organizations such as the American Psychoanalytic Association (*www.info.apsa.org*) or Division 39 of the American Psychological Association (*www.apa.org/about/division/div39.html*) for potential referrals.

To date there are no manual-based psychodynamic treatment books for EDs, as there are for other problem areas such as panic disorder (Milrod, Busch, Cooper, & Shapiro, 1997) or depression (Busch, Rudden, & Shapiro, 2004). Many clinicians graduating from residency, doctoral programs in psychology, and postmaster's programs in social work, nursing, etc., seek out additional training in psychodynamic psychotherapy by attending continuing education courses at national meetings or pursuing more formal training through a psychoanalytic institute.

Today most psychoanalytic institutes offer a 2-year certificate program in psychodynamic psychotherapy in addition to the traditional program of full analytic training that can take 4–7 years. Consultation and supervision are also readily available for clinicians through local psychodynamically trained practitioners. Individuals with an interest in learning more might begin by availing themselves of one or more of the excellent, contemporary texts (Gabbard, 2004, 2005; Hall, 1998; McWilliams, 1994, 1999, 2004) or explore a course of study such as Diana Fosha's (2000, 2007) accelerated experiential–dynamic psychotherapy.

References

Armstrong JG, & Roth DM. (1989). Attachment and separation difficulties in eating disorders: A preliminary investigation. *International Journal of Eating Disorders*, 8:141–155.

Bateman A, & Fonagy P. (2006). *Mentalization-based treatment for borderline personality disorder: A practical guide.* Oxford, UK: Oxford University Press.

Beebe B, & Lachman FM. (2002). *Infant research and adult treatment: Co-constructing interactions.* New York: Analytic Press.

Bion W. (1967). *Second thoughts: Selected papers on psychoanalysis.* London: Heinemann.

Bowlby J. (1979). On knowing what you are not supposed to know and feeling what you are not supposed to feel. *Canadian Journal of Psychiatry*, 241:403–408.

Bowlby J. (1988). *A secure base: Clinical applications of attachment theory.* London: Routledge.

Bruch H. (1973). *Eating disorders: Obesity, anorexia nervosa, and the person within.* New York: Basic Books.

Bruch H. (1974). *Eating disorders.* London: Routledge & Kegan Paul.

Bruch H. (1988). *Conversations with anorexics.* In D Czyzewski & M Suhr (Eds.), New York: Basic Books.

Busch FN, Rudden M, & Shapiro T. (2004). *Psychodynamic treatment of depression.* Washington, DC: American Psychiatric Association.

Dare C. (1993). The starving and the greedy. *Journal of Child Psychotherapy*, 19:3–20.

Dare C. (1997). Chronic eating disorders in therapy: Clinical stories using family systems and psychoanalytic approaches. *Journal of Family Therapy*, 19:319–351.

Dare C, & Crowther C. (1995). Living dangerously: Psychoanalytic psychotherapy for anorexia nervosa. In G Szmukler, C Dare, & J Treasure (Eds.), *Handbook of eating disorders* (pp. 293–308). London: Wiley.

Dare C, Eisler I, Russell G, Treasure J, & Dodge L. (2001). Psychological therapies for adults with anorexia nervosa: Randomised controlled trial of out-patient treatments. *British Journal of Psychiatry*, 178:216–221.

De Groot J, & Rodin G. (1998). Coming alive: The psychotherapeutic treatment of patients with eating disorders. *Canadian Journal of Psychiatry*, 43:359–366.

Fonagy P, Gergely G, Jurist E, & Target M (Eds.). (2002). *Affect regulation, mentalization, and the development of self.* New York: Other Press.

Fosha D. (2000). *The transforming power of affect: A model for accelerating change.* New York: Basic Books.

Fosha D. (2007). *Accelerated experiential dynamic psychotherapy* [DVD]. Washington, DC: American Psychological Association.

Gabbard GO. (2004). *Long-term psychodynamic psychotherapy: A basic text.* Washington, DC: American Psychiatric Association.

Gabbard GO. (2005). *Psychodynamic psychiatry in clinical practice* (4th ed.). Washington, DC: American Psychiatric Association.

Greenberg JR, & Mitchell SA. (1983). *Object relations in psychoanalytic theory.* Cambridge, MA: Harvard University Press.

Hall J. (1998). *Deepening the treatment.* Northvale, NJ: Jason Aronson.

Holmes J. (1993). *John Bowlby and attachment theory.* London: Routledge.

Hughes J. (1989). *Reshaping the psychoanalytic domain: The work of Melanie Klein, WRD Fairbairn, & DW Winnicott.* Los Angeles: University of California Press.

Klein, M. (1975). *Love, guilt, and reparation & other works 1925–1945.* London: Hogarth Press.

Mahler, M, Pine, F, & Bergman, A. (1975). *The psychological birth of the human infant.* New York: Basic Books.

McWilliams, N. (1994). *Psychoanalytic diagnosis: Understanding personality structure in the clinical process.* New York: Guilford Press.

McWilliams, N. (1999). *Psychoanalytic case formulation.* New York: Guilford Press.

McWilliams, N. (2004). *Psychoanalytic psychotherapy: A practitioner's guide.* New York: Guilford Press.

Milrod BL, Busch FN, Cooper AN, & Shapiro T (1997). *Manual of panic-focused psychodynamic psychotherapy.* Washington, DC: American Psychiatric Association.

Rako S, & Mazer H. (Eds.). (1980). *Semrad: The heart of a therapist.* New York: Jason Aronson.

Roth A, & Fonagy P. (2005). *What works for whom?: A critical review of psychotherapy research* (2nd ed.). New York: Guilford Press.

Rozen DL. (1993). Projective identification and bulimia. *Psychoanalytic Psychology*, 10:261–273.

Schafer R. (1960). The loving and beloved superego in Freud's structural theory. *Psychoanalytic Study of the Child*, 15:163–188.

Segal H. (1980). *Melanie Klein.* New York: Penguin Books.

Shadish W, Matt G, Navarro A, & Phillips G. (2000). The effects of psychological therapies under clinically representative conditions: A meta-analysis. *Journal of Consulting and Clinical Psychology*, 126:512–529.

Skarderud F. (2007). Eating one's words: Part III. Mentalization-based psychotherapy for anorexia nervosa—an outline for a treatment and training manual. *European Eating Disorders Review*, 15:323–339.

Stein H, Fonagy P, Ferguson KS, & Wisman M. (2000). Lives through time: An ideographic approach to the study of resilience. *Bulletin of the Menninger Clinic*, 64:281–305.

Streeck U. (2006). *Psychoanalytisch–interaktionelle therapie* [Psychoanalytic–interactional therapy]. In C Reimer & U Ruger (Eds.), *Psychodynamische psychotherapien* (pp. 108–135). Heidelberg: Springer.

Thompson-Brenner H, & Westen D. (2005). A naturalistic study of psychotherapy for bulimia nervosa: Part 2. *Journal of Nervous and Mental Diseases*, 193:585–595.

Ward A, Ramsay R, & Treasure J. (2000). Attachment research in eating disorders. *British Journal of Medical Psychology*, 73:35–51.

Wilson CP, Hogan CC, & Mintz IL. (1985). *Fear of being fat: The treatment of anorexia nervosa and bulimia*. Northvale, NJ: Aronson.

Winters NC. (2002). Feeding problems in infancy and early childhood. *Primary Psychiatry*, 10:30–34.

Wurmser L. (1994). *The mask of shame*. Northvale, NJ: Jason Aronson.

Wurmser L. (1995). *The hidden dimension*. Northvale, NJ: Jason Aronson.

Zerbe K. (1993a). *The body betrayed: Women, eating disorders, and treatment*. Washington, DC: American Psychiatric Association.

Zerbe K. (1993b). Selves that starve and suffocate: The continuum of eating disorders and dissociative phenomena. *Bulletin of the Menninger Clinic*, 57:319–327.

Zerbe K. (1996). Feminist psychodynamic psychotherapy of eating disorders: Theoretic integration informing clinical practice. *Psychiatric Clinics of North America*, 19:811–827.

Zerbe K. (2001). The crucial role of psychodynamic understanding in the treatment of eating disorders. *Psychiatric Clinics of North America*, 24:305–313.

Zerbe K. (2008). *Integrated treatment of eating disorders: Beyond the body betrayed*. New York: Norton.

CHAPTER 19

Self-Help Approaches for Bulimia Nervosa and Binge-Eating Disorder

Varinia C. Sánchez-Ortiz and Ulrike Schmidt

Most eating disorder (ED) experts endorse the notion that psychological interventions are the best available treatment for bulimia nervosa (BN) and binge-eating disorder (BED) (Wilson, Grilo, & Vitousek, 2007). Evidence-based clinical guidelines support this view, highlighting the efficacy of cognitive-behavioral therapy (CBT) for BN and BED (e.g., National Institute for Health and Clinical Excellence [NICE], 2004). In contrast, the public perception is that psychotherapy is of limited value for binge eating, whereas self-help treatments were thought to be very helpful (Mond & Hay, 2008). This perception fits in with surveys on common mental disorders, which suggest that self-help interventions are held in higher regard, compared to medication or treatments delivered by health professionals (Jorm et al., 1997). The service utilization of people with EDs reflects these views: In one large survey on this topic the majority of people with EDs had not received any professional treatment for their problem (60%), whereas all had tried self-help treatments (Mond, Hay, Rodgers, & Owen, 2007).

Definitions of self-help treatment have varied widely. Jorm, Christiansen, Griffiths, and Rodgers (2002) define this genre as any treatment that can be used by a person without necessarily consulting a health professional, including over-the-counter medicines, exercise, and bibliotherapy. We define self-help approaches more narrowly as those interventions that require limited or no involvement from a clinician, teach users relevant skills for dealing with their difficulties, and are based on a clear therapeutic model and a structure that centers on the problems of the patient (Lewis et al., 2003). This definition excludes self-help books that mainly give advice or information and self-help groups where people meet to provide each other with support.

The aims of this chapter are to review what is known about self-help approaches for BN and BED and to discuss the rationale for using self-help. A further aim is to review what is known about the perceptions that people hold regarding self-help approaches.

Treatment Models, Modes, and Delivery of Self-Help Interventions

Most self-help interventions for BN and BED are manual based, although some video, CD-ROM, and Web-based interventions are also available. Most self-help interventions for BN and BED have been based on a cognitive-behavioral or behavioral treatment model. The two most widely evaluated CBT manuals for these disorders are *Overcoming Binge Eating* (Fairburn, 1995) and *Getting Better Bite by Bite* (Schmidt & Treasure, 1993). Delivery of self-help interventions has been mainly on an individual basis, although group interventions have also been used. Self-help approaches have been delivered with or without therapist guidance, leading to a distinction between guided self help (GSH) and pure self-help (PSH). Intensity of guidance, training of self-help guides, and modality of guidance (face to face, telephone, e-mail) have also varied widely. Self-help interventions have been delivered in a range of settings, from primary care to highly specialist tertiary care settings.

Do Self-Help Interventions Work?

Manual-Based Self-Help Interventions

Two systematic and one narrative review have specifically addressed the topic of the efficacy and effectiveness of manual-based self-help interventions for EDs (Perkins, Murphy, Schmidt, & Williams, 2006) or BN, eating disorders not otherwise specified (EDNOS), and BED (Stefano, Bacaltchuk, Blay, & Hay, 2006; Sysko & Walsh, 2008). This section summarizes the key findings and conclusions from the two systematic reviews and any other relevant new study not included in the reviews.

A Cochrane review by Perkins and colleagues (2006) aimed to evaluate the evidence from controlled clinical trials (CCTs) and randomized controlled trials (RCTs) for the efficacy of PSH and GSH treatments in people with EDs with respect to ED symptoms, other psychiatric symptoms, interpersonal functioning, and cost. Self-help treatments were compared to waiting-list or placebo/attention control and other psychological or pharmacological treatments.

Thirteen RCTs and three CCTs were identified. All studies focused on adults with BN, BED, EDNOS, or combinations of these, and all used manual-based self-help in a variety of settings. Six studies included at least one arm with PSH, and the others evaluated GSH. The individuals giving guidance included laypersons, psychology students, general nurses, junior psychiatrists, doctoral-level psychologists, research clinicians, psychotherapists, specialist ED therapists, general practitioners, and people recovered from an ED. The amount of guidance provided varied from 90 minutes to 8 hours. Study settings included primary care, university and community settings, and secondary or tertiary ED services. Six studies were conducted in the United States or Canada, seven in European countries, and two in Australia. A number of comparisons and meta-analyses were conducted, which are summarized below:

1. Studies comparing PSH or GSH with a waiting-list control ($N = 4$ studies; Banasiak, Paxton, & Hay, 2005; Carter & Fairburn, 1998; Carter et al., 2003; Palmer, Birchall, McGrain, & Sullivan, 2002) did not find any difference in abstinence from binge

eating or purging at the end of treatment (average abstinence from bingeing after PSH or GSH was 35.2% and after waiting list was 11.2%; average abstinence from purging after PSH or GHS was 21.8% and 10.4% after waiting list). However, self-help treatments produced greater improvement than waiting list on ED symptoms, psychiatric symptomatology, and interpersonal functioning.

2. Only one study compared GSH to a placebo/attention control treatment in BED (Grilo & Masheb, 2005). GSH produced greater improvements in abstinence rates from binge eating (46 vs. 13.4% in the control group) and ED symptoms, but not on depression.

3. When compared to other psychological therapies, self-help treatments (with or without guidance) did not differ in terms of abstinence rates from binge eating and purging, improvement on ED symptomatology, interpersonal functioning, or depression at the end of treatment and at follow-up ($N = 4$ studies; Bailer et al., 2004; Durand & King, 2003; Thiels, Schmidt, Treasure, Garthe, & Troop, 1998; Treasure et al., 1996). In PSH or GSH, average abstinence rates from bingeing or purging at the end of treatment were 11 and 15.5%, respectively, and at follow-up were 35 and 42%. In other psychological treatments abstinence rates were 33% for bingeing and 31% for purging at the end of treatment, and 32 and 32% at follow-up, respectively.

4. Studies comparing PSH to GSH ($N = 5$ studies; Carter & Fairburn, 1998; Ghaderi & Scott, 2003; Huon, 1985; Loeb, Wilson, Gilbert, & Labouvie, 2000; Palmer et al., 2002) found no differences between groups on any of the outcome measures at end of treatment or at follow-up. Abstinence rates were as follows: *end of treatment*: bingeing— PSH (35.7%) versus GSH (42.9%); purging—PSH (53.4%) versus GSH (68%); *follow-up*: bingeing—PSH (40%) versus GSH (50%). One study reported adherence to self-help treatment at 6% in PSH and 50% in GSH (Carter & Fairburn, 1998).

5. Two studies comparing different types of self-help failed to find any differences on abstinence rates from binge eating and purging, depression scores, and body mass index (BMI), but found some differences on ED symptoms and in interpersonal functioning. Average abstinence from binge eating at the end of treatment was 29% in those using a CBT-based self-help treatment, compared with 17% in those using another type of self-help treatment (behavioral weight loss control treatment [Grilo & Masheb, 2005] or self-help for self-assertion [Carter et al., 2003]). In the latter study, abstinence from purging at the end of treatment was 7% for CBT self-help and 18% for the other form of self-help.

6. Three studies compared self-help with pharmacological interventions. One of these compared GSH plus orlistat to GSH plus placebo in BED, and found that participants with added orlistat achieved a larger posttreatment weight reduction and were more likely to maintain this loss at 3-month follow-up (Grilo, Masheb, & Salant, 2005). The addition of orlistat was also associated with a greater reduction of binge-eating episodes at posttreatment but not at follow-up. Two other studies compared fluoxetine only, placebo only, fluoxetine and PSH or GSH, and placebo and PSH or GSH in patients with BN (Mitchell et al., 2001; Walsh, Fairburn, Mickley, Sysko, & Parides, 2004). The Walsh and colleagues (2004) study had very high dropout rates, making it impossible to draw any conclusions. The Mitchell and colleagues (2001) study suggested that both fluoxetine and PSH were effective in reducing the frequency of self-induced vomiting episodes at the end of treatment, and both interventions acted additively on the outcome measures in this study.

The second systematic review of self-help treatments for binge eating in BN or BED was more limited in scope and included nine RCTs (Stefano et al., 2006). The main outcome was abstinence from binge eating at the end of treatment. Secondary outcomes were bulimic symptoms scores, weight, and treatment noncompletion rates. Purging and comorbidity were not included as outcomes. The authors carried out a number of meta-analyses, including comparisons of any kind of self-help (PSH or GSH) compared with waiting list, GSH versus PSH, and any form of self-help versus CBT. On abstinence from binge eating, only the meta-analysis of "any kind of self-help" versus waiting list (WL) found the self-help group to have significantly higher abstinence rates compared with those on the waiting list (26.5 vs. 6.5%). There were similar nonsignificant trends on the other comparisons (PSH vs. WL; GSH vs. WL); that is, participants who were offered a self-help intervention had higher rates of abstinence than waiting-list control groups, but the number of studies and participants included was probably too low to reach significance. There was no difference in treatment noncompletion between self-help approaches and control therapies or waiting-list control groups.

Two additional RCTs were reviewed by Sysko and Walsh (2008). Both studies focused on how to improve patients' motivation to take up and adhere to self-help treatments. In one of these studies (Dunn, Neighbors, & Larimer, 2006), the effect of adding one session of motivational enhancement therapy (MET) prior to self-help treatment was examined in people with BN or BED. Participants were randomly assigned either to have a 1-hour MET session prior to PSH with a manual or to PSH only. Participants in the MET group showed increased readiness to change binge eating compared to those in the PSH-only group. Few other differences were found between groups in terms of eating attitudes, frequency of binge eating and compensatory behaviors, and treatment adherence.

A second trial compared GSH with or without repeated personalized feedback (Schmidt et al., 2006) in adults with BN or EDNOS. The study found that added feedback did not have an effect on take-up or dropout rates from treatment. However, it did lead to greater improvements in self-induced vomiting and dietary restriction than GSH without feedback.

Finally, a recent RCT not included in the reviews previously mentioned, compared the efficacy and cost-effectiveness of family therapy to GSH in adolescents with BN or EDNOS (Schmidt et al., 2007). GSH produced a greater reduction of binge eating at 6 months than family therapy. However, there were no significant differences in ED outcomes at 1 year, suggesting that both treatments were equally effective in the longer term. Importantly, GSH was more acceptable to young people eligible for the study than family therapy. This preference was reflected in a significant proportion of adolescents (28%) citing not wanting their families involved as a reason for nonparticipation. In addition, direct treatment costs of GSH were lower than for family therapy, although other costs did not differ between groups.

In summary, the conclusions that can be drawn from the available evidence, and in particular the meta-analytic analyses, is limited by the low number, small size, and the heterogeneity of the trials included. For example, there were major differences in study populations, duration of interventions, and levels of training/expertise of the therapists. Overall, one can cautiously conclude that PSH/GSH has some utility as a first step in treatment of BN, EDNOS, and BED, and may have potential as an alternative to formal therapist-delivered psychological therapy. Where follow-up data are available, these suggest that gains are maintained or that there has been further improvement during the follow-up period. There is as yet insufficient evidence to support any single approach over any other, or PSH versus GSH. Very little is known about the cost-effectiveness of these kinds of interventions, as only one trial has formally studied this area.

Many important clinical questions can only be tentatively answered from the evidence. In terms of who is best positioned to support GSH, it is of note that a study that used general nurses to support a self-help intervention produced exceptionally high dropout rates (Walsh et al., 2004). This may suggest that specialists supporting these kinds of interventions may do so more effectively. Another important clinical question is who benefits most from self-help treatments. To date only two studies have examined pretreatment predictors of outcome. High levels of binge eating predicted poor outcome from self-help in patients with BN, whereas long duration of illness predicted good outcome (Turnbull et al., 1997), and personality disorders and negative affect predicted poor outcome from self-help in patients with BED (Masheb & Grilo, 2008). Two studies have examined adherence to self-help as a predictor and found high adherence to be associated with good clinical outcome (Thields, Schmidt, Troop, Treasure, & Garthe, 2000; Troop et al., 1996). Clearly, more research needs to be done to add to these findings.

Clinicians will also want to know about the relative merits of medication and self-help or whether to combine these approaches. The available evidence suggests that combining self-help with medication may improve outcomes. Likewise motivational enhancement appears to strengthen the efficacy of self-help approaches.

Computerized Self-Help Treatments

Computerized CBT interventions (delivered via CD-ROM or the Internet) are an alternative to manual-based self-help. Such interventions have advantages because they are more interactive and can be individually tailored. Such interventions have been successfully used with people with other mental disorders (e.g., obsessive–compulsive disorder, depression) (Kaltenthaler, Parry, Beverley, & Ferriter, 2008; Tumur, Kaltenthaler, Ferriter, Beverley, & Parry, 2007). Several CD-ROM and Internet-based treatments for BN, EDNOS, and BED have been developed and are being tested. As these were not included in the reviews described above, we discuss them here separately.

Overcoming Bulimia

A CBT multimedia self-help treatment for BN (*Overcoming Bulimia*; Williams, Aubin, Cottrell, & Harkin, 1998; Williams, Schmidt, & Aubin, 2005) was developed as a stand-alone CD-ROM and later adapted for use over the Internet. It consists of eight interactive modules combining cognitive-behavioral, motivational, and educational strategies. A key feature is the template for a personalized CBT formulation of the factors maintaining bulimic symptoms. Strategies for healthy regular eating and for eliminating bulimic behaviors are taught in early modules. Later modules focus on challenging extreme and unhelpful thinking, particularly in relation to weight, shape, and appearance. A range of basic CBT techniques address skills deficits commonly found in people with bulimia (e.g., poor problem solving, low assertiveness) to enable participants to lead fuller, more balanced lives. Each module takes between 30 and 45 minutes to complete at the computer. These have to be worked through in sequence. Each module finishes with a set of homework tasks. Patient workbooks that contain a condensed version of the module contents accompany each session. Self-assessment tools provide patients with feedback on their progress.

The CD-ROM program was tested in two pilot studies and one RCT. In the first pilot, patients with BN used the CD-ROM in the clinic without any therapist support. There were significant pre- to posttreatment reductions in bingeing and self-induced vomiting (Bara-Carril et al., 2004). The second pilot study compared data from the first cohort with data from a second cohort from the same center, in which patients were offered three brief support sessions with a trainee psychologist (Murray et al., 2007) to examine whether the addition of therapist support to the CD-ROM intervention would improve treatment uptake, adherence, or outcome. Patients in both cohorts improved significantly in their bulimic symptoms without any differences between the groups in treatment uptake, adherence, or outcome.

The RCT of the CD-ROM intervention tested its effectiveness in 97 patients with BN or EDNOS referred to a specialist ED service (Schmidt et al., 2008). There were two comparison groups. The first group accessed the CD-ROM intervention in the clinic over 3 months with no clinician guidance, followed by a flexible number of therapist sessions. The second group was on a waiting list for 3 months, followed by 15 sessions of face-to-face CBT. Treatment uptake in both groups was low, with only two-thirds of study patients starting treatment. While there were significant group-by-time interactions for binge eating and vomiting, favoring CD-ROM at 3 months and the other group at 7 months, post hoc group comparisons at 3 and 7 months found no significant differences on binge eating or vomiting frequency. This study was conducted in a routine clinical setting where patients had lengthy waiting periods prior to being assessed by the specialist service and prior to inclusion in the trial. The authors concluded that accessing the CD-ROM in clinic without support from a clinician may not be the best way of exploiting the benefits of this intervention.

More recently, two studies have used an Internet-based version of the same program—that is, *Overcoming Bulimia Online*. The first of these was conducted in 101 adolescents with BN or EDNOS. The intervention consisted of the interactive CBT Web program together with weekly e-mail support and a message board for participants and their parents (Pretorius et al., in press). There were significant pre- to postintervention improvements in binge-eating episodes, vomiting episodes, and in most ED symptoms. These changes were maintained at 6-month follow-up.

The second study was an RCT comparing *Overcoming Bulimia Online* with a delayed treatment control group of students with BN or EDNOS, recruited via the university networks, that had waited 3 months for treatment (Sánchez-Ortiz et al., 2008). At 3 months the group receiving immediate Internet-based CBT showed a greater reduction in binge-eating episodes, improvement in ED symptomatology, depression, anxiety, and quality of life, compared to participants in the delayed treatment group (who had not yet received any treatment). Improvements in the immediate treatment group were maintained at 6 months. At 6 months, waiting-list participants had not fully caught up with those who received immediate treatment.

Other Technology-Based Interventions

Three other RCTs investigated other technology-based interventions. The first of these compared face-to-face CBT groups to a CD-ROM-based CBT program and to a waiting-list control group in 66 overweight adults with BED, recruited via advertisements (Shapiro et al., 2007). Participants in the group CBT condition had a significantly higher dropout rate than those receiving CD-ROM or waiting-list controls. At the end of treatment, both the CD-ROM and the group CBT participants had a significantly greater reduction in the number of binge-eating days compared to the waiting-list group.

A European multicenter project developed an Internet-based CBT self-help guide for the treatment of BN. Treatment consisted of seven lessons and lasted for 4 months. Cohort studies evaluating the efficacy and acceptability of the intervention were conducted in Switzerland, Sweden, Germany, and Spain (Carrard et al., 2006; Fernández-Aranda et al., 2008; Liwowsky, Cebulla, & Fichter, 2006; Rouget, Carrard, & Archinard, 2005). Initial results from the Swiss and Spanish samples found a significant improvement in ED symptoms (Carrard et al., 2006; Fernández-Aranda et al., 2008). Results from the full study are not yet available.

A recent RCT including sufferers of BN or BED assessed the efficacy of a manual-based CBT self-help intervention combined with e-mail support and an online discussion forum for participants (Ljotsson et al., 2007). The treatment lasted for 12 weeks and was compared to waiting list. A significant improvement was found in the treatment group, compared to the waiting-list group, in the number of binge-eating episodes and in ED symptoms such as eating, shape, and weight concern and dietary restraint.

Taken together these studies suggest that CD-ROM and Web-based treatments hold considerable promise as first-step interventions in the treatment of people with BN, EDNOS, or BED. However, further studies are needed to compare technology-based treatments against manual-based self-care and face-to-face treatments in different populations and settings.

Service Users' Views
of Self-Help Interventions and Ability to Use Them

In general, most people appear to like the idea of self-help and many prefer this to therapist-aided treatments (e.g., Graham, Franses, Kenwright, & Marks, 2000). However, very little is known about what factors determine interest in, and benefits from, self-help treatments in EDs and what factors contribute to, or impede, treatment efficacy or effectiveness (Perkins et al., 2006; Schmidt & Sánchez-Ortiz, 2007). One qualitative study examined the views of 36 women on GSH for BN (Banasiak, Paxton, & Hay, 2007). Factors perceived to contribute to treatment effectiveness included accessibility of treatment, support from the general practitioner (GP) guiding the program, and the empathic and practical style of the manual, all of which were thought to lead to improved eating behaviors, body image, and well-being. Factors perceived as contributing to lack of treatment effectiveness included concerns about the adequacy and dose of the treatment and poor support from the GP who facilitated the program.

Murray and colleagues (2003) and Bara-Carril and colleagues (2004) assessed the characteristics of patients who were offered the CD-ROM package *Overcoming Buli-*

mia. Differences between those who did or did not take up the package were minimal, although Bara-Carril and colleagues found that those who did not take up the intervention had more severe bulimic symptoms.

The larger and more comprehensive study by Murray and colleagues (2003), which combined quantitative and qualitative elements, found no differences between those who did or did not take up the CD-ROM intervention in terms of previous experience of using self-help, participants' views on previous self-help, and views on the usefulness of self-help in general, computer literacy, or knowledge about BN. However, those who did take up the package were more positive about the usefulness of self-help for themselves. They were also more willing to try this treatment and understood that other treatments would be available to them if self-help did not lead to improvements. Those who did not take up the treatment felt that the CD-ROM was a "cheap and inferior" option compared to seeing a therapist.

Finally, a study using qualitative interviews explored the views and perceptions of people using the Internet-based version of *Overcoming Bulimia Online* (Sánchez-Ortiz, Munro, & Schmidt, 2007). Participants identified a number of reasons for choosing to participate, such as valuing the flexibility in terms of time and location of access that this approach offers. Some participants who had had previous treatment with a therapist commented that they preferred the Internet-based approach on the grounds that this did not make them feel judged. Moreover, they valued the content of the CBT sessions. Confidentiality seemed to be important, as most participants expressed concerns about other people finding out about their problem. E-mail support was seen as a factor that complemented the treatment package.

These studies suggest that participants' personal preferences may be key in their uptake and ability to benefit from self-help, but more research in this area is needed. Table 19.1 outlines points for how to introduce a self-help intervention to patients.

Public Health and Service Implications of Self-Help Interventions

BED and EDNOS are the most common EDs and have a significant burden for sufferers (Hay, Mond, Buttner, & Darby, 2008). Because the majority of people with BN do not seek treatment, being able to easily access evidence-based self-help interventions could make a real difference to the health and quality of life of this "silent majority." The marked increase in prevalence of BN and EDNOS is likely to lead to increased demands for treatment, putting additional pressure on resource-strapped mental health services and leading to long waiting lists. So how can precious resources be targeted on those with the greatest need? Lovell and Richards (2000) suggest that psychological treatment services need to get away from a one-size-fits-all approach of offering everyone once weekly sessions for a defined period of time. Instead, the treatment patients are offered should be tailored to the complexity of the problem they have. Specifically, there should be different levels of treatment intensity available in psychological services, and self-help interventions should be the most basic level of treatment offered.

An alternative approach is suggested by Haaga (2000), who proposes a stepped-care model starting with the least intensive intervention, and stepping up to more intensive ones. In this model self-help treatments with or without guidance could be the first step

TABLE 19.1. Points for Introducing an Evidence-Based Self-Help Intervention to Patients

What to say to the patient

- "As a first step in treatment we suggest that you work through a self-help book for people with BN or BED, which has been found to be effective in several clinical trials."

- "This book contains all the elements of cognitive-behavioral therapy, which is the treatment of choice for BN and BED. It is a structured program, and all the necessary steps to overcome your problem are presented in a user-friendly, easy-to-follow way."

- "Working through this book is useful as a preparation for further treatment with a therapist, should this be required."

- "One of the temptations with a book like this is to 'have a bit of a binge' and read most of it quickly in one go, or to dip in and out. This does not work well."

- "In order to make changes to your eating disorder, what works best is if people go through one chapter at a time. This can be done by making time at a particular point of the week."

- "It is very important to do the homework tasks. This helps you put into practice what you have read. Previous research has shown that people who do these tasks have a much better outcome than people who don't."

- "It can be helpful to review progress on a regular/weekly basis with a person you trust."

- "We know that people who do stick with the book and work through the material often make significant progress toward recovery, and a proportion totally overcome their problem."

- "The more you put in, the more you will get out of it."

- "You need to be clear that this is a first step in treatment only."

in the treatment of patients with BN, BED, or EDNOS presenting to services, and only if people do not respond adequately are they offered more intensive and more expensive treatments. This approach is supported by the findings from two RCTs in BED reporting that early rapid response to GSH predicts better outcomes (Grilo & Masheb, 2007; Masheb & Grilo, 2007). These findings are noteworthy because the pretreatment patient characteristics differed little between patients with or without a rapid response to GSH (i.e., it was not merely "easy" patients who got better quickly with GSH).

More research is needed on the optimal delivery and sequencing of self-help and other interventions for BN, BED, and EDNOS—an important task for the future.

Conclusion

Our knowledge in the field of self-help treatments continues to develop. The growth of self-help approaches to treatment has been motivated not only by health economic factors but, importantly, also by the fact that many people with mental health problems have become more active in their approach to their difficulties and search for help (Schmidt & Sánchez-Ortiz, 2007). We need to learn much more about these approaches and for whom they work best, in order to target them optimally at those who are willing and able to use them.

Acknowledgments

Varinia C. Sánchez-Ortiz was supported by a PhD scholarship from CONACyT (Consejo Nacional de Ciencia y Tecnología). This work was supported by a grant from the Biomedical Research

Centre of the National Institute for Health Research (NIHR) (Institute of Psychiatry, King's College London) and by a Department of Health (DH) NIHR Programme Grant for Applied Research (No. RP-PG-0606-1043) to U. Schmidt, J. Treasure, K. Tchanturia, H. Startup, S. Ringwood, S. Landau, M. Grover, I. Eisler, I. Campbell, J. Beecham, M. Allen, and G. Wolff. The views expressed herein are not necessarily those of DH/NIHR.

References

Bailer U, de Zwaan M, Leisch F, Strnad A, Lennkh-Wolfsberg C, El-Giamal N., et al. (2004). Guided self-help versus cognitive-behavioral group therapy in the treatment of bulimia nervosa. *International Journal of Eating Disorders*, 35:522–537.

Banasiak SJ, Paxton SJ, & Hay PJ. (2005). Guided self-help for bulimia nervosa in primary care: A randomized controlled trial. *Psychological Medicine*, 35:1283–1294.

Banasiak SJ, Paxton SJ, Hay PJ. (2007). Perceptions of cognitive behavioural guided self-help treatment for bulimia nervosa in primary care. *Eating Disorders* 15:23–40.

Bara-Carril N, Williams CJ, Pombo-Carril MG, Reid Y, Murray K, Aubin S. et al. (2004). A preliminary investigation into the feasibility and efficacy of a CD-ROM-based cognitive-behavioral self-help intervention for bulimia nervosa. *International Journal of Eating Disorders*, 35:538–548.

Carrard I, Rouget P, Fernández-Aranda F, Volkart AC, Damoiseau M, & Lam T. (2006). Evaluation and deployment of evidence based patient self-management support program for Bulimia Nervosa. *International Journal of Medical Informatics*, 75:101–109.

Carter JC, & Fairburn CG. (1998). Cognitive-behavioral self-help for binge eating disorder: A controlled effectiveness study. *Journal of Consulting and Clinical Psychology*, 66:616–623.

Carter JC, Olmsted MP, Kaplan AS, McCabe RE, Mills JS, & Aime A. (2003). Self-help for bulimia nervosa: A randomized controlled trial. *American Journal of Psychiatry*, 160:973–978.

Dunn EC, Neighbors C, & Larimer ME. (2006). Motivational enhancement therapy and self-help treatment for binge eaters. *Psychology of Addictive Behaviours*, 20:44–52.

Durand MA, & King M. (2003). Specialist treatment versus self-help for bulimia nervosa: A randomised controlled trial in general practice. *British Journal of General Practice*, 53:371–377.

Fairburn CG. (1995). *Overcoming binge eating.* New York: Guilford Press.

Fernández-Aranda F, Núñez A, Martínez C, Krug I, Cappozzo M, Carrard I, et al. (2008). Internet-based cognitive-behavioral therapy for bulimia nervosa: A controlled study. *CyberPsychology and Behaviour*, 12(1):37–41.

Ghaderi A, & Scott B. (2003). Pure and guided self-help for full and sub-threshold bulimia nervosa and binge eating disorder. *British Journal of Clinical Psychology*, 42:257–269.

Graham C, Franses A, Kenwright M, & Marks I. (2000). Psychotherapy by computer: A postal survey of responders to a teletext article. *Psychiatric Bulletin*, 24:331–332.

Grilo CM, & Masheb RM. (2005). A randomized controlled comparison of guided self-help cognitive behavioral therapy and behavioral weight loss for binge eating disorder. *Behaviour Research and Therapy*, 43:1509–1525.

Grilo CM, & Masheb RM. (2007). Rapid response predicts binge eating and weight loss in binge eating disorder: Findings from a controlled trial of orlistat with guided self-help cognitive behavioral therapy. *Behaviour Research and Therapy*, 45:2537–2550.

Grilo CM, Masheb RM, & Salant SL. (2005). Cognitive behavioral therapy guided self-help and orlistat for the treatment of binge eating disorder: A randomized, double-blind, placebo-controlled trial. *Biological Psychiatry*, 57:1193–1201.

Haaga DAF. (2000). Introduction to the special section on stepped care models in psychotherapy. *Journal of Consulting and Clinical Psychology*, 68:547–548.

Hay PJ, Mond J, Buttner P, & Darby A. (2008). Eating disorder behaviors are increasing: Findings from two sequential community surveys in South Australia. *PLoS ONE*, 3:e1541.

Huon GF. (1985). An initial validation of a self-help program for bulimia. *International Journal of Eating Disorder*, 4:573–578.

Jorm AF, Christensen H, Griffiths KM, & Rodgers B. (2002). Effectiveness of complementary and self-help treatments for depression. *Medical Journal of Australia*, 176:S84–S95.

Jorm AF, Korten AE, Jacomb PA, Rodgers B, Pollitt P, Christensen H, et al. (1997). Helpfulness of interventions for mental disorders: Beliefs of health professionals compared with the general public. *British Journal of Psychiatry*, 171:233–237.

Kaltenthaler E, Parry G, Beverley C, & Ferriter M. (2008). Computerised cognitive-behavioural therapy for depression: Systematic review. *British Journal of Psychiatry*, 193:181–184.

Lewis G, Anderson L, Araya R, Elgie R, Harrison G, Proudfoot J, et al. (2003). *Self-help interventions for mental health problems* (Expert briefing). Leeds, UK: National Institute for Mental Health.

Liwowsky I, Cebulla M, & Fichter M. (2006). New ways to combat eating disorders: Evaluation of an Internet-based self-help program in bulimia nervosa. *Münchener Medizinische Wochenschrift Fortschritte der Medizin*, 148:31–33.

Ljotsson B, Lundin C, Mitsell K, Carlbring P, Ramklint M, & Ghaderi A. (2007). Remote treatment of bulimia nervosa and binge eating disorder: A randomized trial of Internet-assisted cognitive behavioural therapy. *Behaviour Research and Therapy*, 45:649–661.

Loeb KL, Wilson GT, Gilbert JS, & Labouvie E. (2000). Guided and unguided self-help for binge eating. *Behaviour Research and Therapy*, 38:259–272.

Lovell K, & Richards D. (2000). Multiple access points and levels of entry (MAPLE): Ensuring choice, accessibility and equity for CBT services. *Behavioural and Cognitive Psychotherapy*, 28:379–391.

Masheb RM, & Grilo CM. (2007). Rapid response predicts treatment outcomes in binge eating disorder: Implications for stepped care. *Journal of Consulting and Clinical Psychology*, 75:639–644.

Masheb RM, & Grilo CM. (2008). Examination of predictors and moderators for self-help treatments of binge-eating disorder. *Journal of Consulting and Clinical Psychology*, 76:900–904.

Mitchell JE, Fletcher L, Hanson K, Mussell MP, Seim H, Crosby, R, et al. (2001). The relative efficacy of fluoxetine and manual-based self-help in the treatment of outpatients with bulimia nervosa. *Journal of Clinical Psychopharmacology*, 21:298–304.

Mond JM, & Hay PJ. (2008). Public perceptions of binge eating and its treatment. *International Journal of Eating Disorders*, 41:419–426.

Mond JM, Hay PJ, Rodgers B, & Owen C. (2007). Health service utilization for eating disorders: Findings from a community-based study. *International Journal of Eating Disorders*, 40:399–408.

Murray K, Pombo-Carril MG, Bara-Carril N, Grover M, Reid Y, Langham C, et al. (2003). Factors determining uptake of a CD-ROM-based CBT self-help treatment for bulimia: Patient characteristics and subjective appraisals of self-help treatment. *European Eating Disorders Review*, 11:243–260.

Murray K, Schmidt U, Pombo-Carril MG, Grover M, Alenya J, Treasure J, et al. (2007). Does therapist guidance improve uptake, adherence, and outcome from a CD-ROM based cognitive-behavioral intervention for the treatment of bulimia nervosa? *Computers in Human Behavior*, 23:850–859.

National Institute for Health and Clinical Excellence. (2004). *Eating disorders: Core interventions in the treatment and management of anorexia nervosa, bulimia nervosa, and related eating disorders. Clinical Guideline 9*. London: British Psychological Society.

Palmer RL, Birchall H, McGrain L, & Sullivan V. (2002). Self-help for bulimic disorders: A randomised controlled trial comparing minimal guidance with face-to-face or telephone guidance. *British Journal of Psychiatry*, 181:230–235.

Perkins SS, Murphy R, Schmidt U, & Williams C. (2006). Self-help and guided self-help for eating disorders. *Cochrane Database of Systematic Reviews*, Issue 3 (Article No. CD004191), DOI: 10.1002/14651858.CD004191.pub2.

Pretorius N, Arcelus J, Beecham J, Dawson H, Doherty F, Eisler I, et al. (in press). Cognitive-behavioural therapy for adolescents with bulimia nervosa: The acceptability and effectiveness of Internet-based delivery. *Behaviour Research and Therapy*.

Rouget P, Carrard I, & Archinard M. (2005). [Self-treatment for bulimia on the Internet: First results in Switzerland]. *Revue Medicale Suisse*, 1:359–361.

Sánchez-Ortiz VC, Munro C, & Schmidt U. (2007, May). *Views and perceptions of an Internet based CBT package*. Paper presented at the annual conference of the Academy of Eating Disorders, Baltimore, MD.

Sánchez-Ortiz VC, Munro C, Stahl D, House J, Startup H, Treasure J, et al. (2008). *A randomised controlled trial of Internet-based cognitive-behavioural therapy for bulimia nervosa in a student*. Manuscript submitted for publication.

Schmidt U, Andiappan M, Grover M, Robinson S, Perkins S, Dugmore O, et al. (2008). A randomised controlled trial of the effectiveness of a CD-ROM based cognitive behavioural self-care intervention for bulimia nervosa. *British Journal of Psychiatry*, 193:493–499.

Schmidt U, Landau S, Pombo-Carril MG, Bara-Carril N, Reid Y, Murray K, et al. (2006). Does personalized feedback improve the outcome of cognitive-behavioural guided self-care in bulimia nervosa?: A preliminary randomized controlled trial. *British Journal of Clinical Psychology*, 45:111–121.

Schmidt U, Lee S, Beecham J, Perkins S, Treasure J, Yi I, et al. (2007). A randomized controlled trial of family therapy and cognitive behavior therapy guided self-care for adolescents with bulimia nervosa and related disorders. *American Journal of Psychiatry*, 164:591–598.

Schmidt U, & Sánchez-Ortiz V. (2007). Self help and healing narratives. In M Nasser, K Baistow, & J Treasure (2007). *Minding the body* (pp. 214–227). London: Routledge.

Schmidt U, & Treasure J. (1993). *Getting better bit(e) by bit(e): Survival kit for sufferers of bulimia nervosa and binge eating disorders*. London: Psychology Press.

Shapiro JR, Reba-Harrelson L, Dymek-Valentine M, Woolson SL, Hamer RM, & Bulik CM. (2007). Feasibility and acceptability of CD-ROM-based cognitive-behavioural treatment for binge-eating disorder. *European Eating Disorders Review*, 15:175–184.

Stefano SC, Bacaltchuk J, Blay SL, & Hay P. (2006). Self-help treatments for disorders of recurrent binge eating: A systematic review. *Acta Psychiatrica Scandinavica*, 113:452–459.

Sysko R, & Walsh BT. (2008). A critical evaluation of the efficacy of self-help interventions for the treatment of bulimia nervosa and binge-eating disorder. *International Journal of Eating Disorders*, 41:97–112.

Thiels C, Schmidt U, Treasure J, Garthe R, & Troop N. (1998). Guided self-change for bulimia nervosa incorporating use of a self-care manual. *American Journal of Psychiatry*, 155:947–953.

Thiels C, Schmidt U, Troop N, Treasure J, & Garthe R. (2000). Binge frequency predicts outcome in guided self-care treatment of bulimia nervosa. *European Eating Disorders Review*, 8:272–278.

Treasure J, Schmidt U, Troop N, Tiller J, Todd G, & Turnbull S. (1996). Sequential treatment for bulimia nervosa incorporating a self-care manual. *British Journal of Psychiatry*, 168:94–98.

Troop N, Schmidt U, Tiller J, Todd G, Keilen M,, & Treasure J.(1996). Compliance with a self-care manual for bulimia nervosa: Predictors and outcome. *British Journal of Clinical Psychology*, 35(3):435–438.

Tumur I, Kaltenthaler E, Ferriter M, Beverley C, & Parry G. (2007). Computerised cognitive behaviour therapy for obsessive–compulsive disorder: A systematic review. *Psychotherapy and Psychosomatics*, 76:196–202.

Turnbull SJ, Schmidt U, Troop NA, Tiller J, Todd G, & Treasure J. (1997). Predictors of outcome for two treatments for bulimia nervosa: Short and long-term. *International Journal of Eating Disorders*, 21:17–22.

Walsh BT, Fairburn CG, Mickley D, Sysko R, & Parides MK. (2004). Treatment of bulimia nervosa in a primary care setting. *American Journal of Psychiatry*, 161:556–561.

Williams C, Schmidt U, & Aubin S. (2005). *Overcoming bulimia—Internet version*. Leeds, UK: Calipso Media Innovations.

Williams CJ, Aubin SD, Cottrell D, & Harkin PJR. (1998). *Overcoming bulimia: A self-help package*. Leeds, UK: University of Leeds Press.

Wilson GT, Grilo CM, & Vitousek KM. (2007). Psychological treatment of eating disorders. *American Psychologist*, 62:199–216.

CHAPTER 20

Family-Based Treatment for Adolescents with Bulimia Nervosa

Daniel le Grange and James Lock

As many as 2–3% of adolescents in the population binge-eat and purge, and 1–2% meet full criteria for bulimia nervosa (BN) (Herzog, Keller, Lavori, & Sacks, 1991; Lock, Reisel, & Steiner, 2001; Mussell et al., 1995; Stice & Agras, 1998). Until recently, however, most systematic research in the treatment of BN has focused on adults with the disorder. Significant progress has been made in understanding a range of efficacious treatments for this older patient population with BN (Wilson, Grilo, & Vitousek, 2007). Efficacious treatments include cognitive-behavioral therapy (CBT), interpersonal psychotherapy (IPT), and antidepressant medications, but the average age of participants in research studies of these treatment approaches is roughly 28 years (minimum age for entry is typically 18 years), and the duration of the disorder is approximately 10 years (Agras, Walsh, Fairburn, Wilson, & Kraemer, 2000).

In contrast to the sizeable empirical literature for adults with BN, very few studies have been performed with adolescents with BN and, to date, only two randomized controlled trials (RCTs) have been published (see Table 20.1). These two RCTs support the use of family-based therapy (FBT-BN) for this disorder (Le Grange, Crosby, Rathouz, & Leventhal, 2007; Schmidt et al., 2007). In this chapter we discuss FBT-BN to provide a description of the limited empirical support for this treatment, its theoretical rationale, and a summary description of the main elements of this therapy.

Theoretical Model for FBT-BN

FBT-BN (Le Grange & Lock, 2007) is adapted from FBT for anorexia nervosa (AN)—that is, FBT-AN (see Eisler, Lock, & Le Grange, Chapter 8, this volume). Like its precursor, this treatment is designed for adolescents. There are strong theoretical and clinical arguments that parents should be involved in the therapy of their children if ultimate success in treatment is to be accomplished. In FBT-AN, parents' love and understand-

TABLE 20.1. Psychosocial Studies for Adolescent BN

Study	Study Type	N	Age[1]	Type of treatment
Dodge et al. (1995)	Case series	8	16.5 (1.2)	FT
Le Grange et al. (2003)	Case study	1	17 yrs	FBT-BN
Lock et al. (2005)	Case series	34	15.8	CBT-A
Schapman et al. (2006)	Case series	7	16.3 (1.3)	CBT-A
Schmidt et al. (2007)	RCT	85	17.6 (0.3)	FT vs. CBT-GSC
Le Grange et al. (2007)	RCT	80	16.1 (1.6)	FBT-BN vs. SPT

Note. FT, family therapy; FBT-BN, family-based treatment for BN; CBT-A, cognitive-behavioral therapy for adolescents; CBT-GSC, cognitive-behavioral guided self-care; SPT, supportive psychotherapy; RCT, randomized controlled trial.
[1]Mean (*SD*), actual years, age range, or mean age with no *SD*.

ing of their child and family are mobilized to promote behavioral change around eating and weight. There is considerable research consensus that mobilizing parents to take charge of weight restoration in the treatment of teens with AN has been beneficial. Although modified from the approach employed with adolescent AN, this treatment shares many characteristics with FBT-AN.

Adolescents with BN tend to deny the alarming nature of their symptoms and are therefore mostly unable to appreciate the seriousness of BN. Then again, unlike the "typical" adolescent with AN, adolescents with BN tend to have heightened feelings of shame and guilt that isolate them from parental support and can reinforce the symptomatic behavior. As in FBT-AN, FBT-BN views the parents as a resource for resolving the eating disorder (ED) and attempts to assuage misperceptions of blame directed to either the parents or the adolescent. Insofar as the adolescent is suffering from BN and unable to recognize or effectively manage his/her dysfunctional eating pattern, parents are recruited to help their adolescent make necessary behavioral changes toward recovery. If the adolescent with BN is defined in the same way as Robin and colleagues (Robin et al., 1999) conceptualize the teenager with AN—that is, as "unable to take care of him- or herself," then the parents of the adolescent with BN should be coached to work as a team with their offspring to develop ways to restore healthy eating. FBT-BN seeks to show respect and regard for the adolescent's point of view and experience. Therefore, information about the ED is shared with the parents and the adolescent, and struggles around mealtimes and the impact of the ED on family relationships are addressed.

FBT-BN is primarily *symptom focused* and it does not delve into what caused BN. Instead, the treatment focuses on what can be done to resolve the disorder. FBT-BN assumes that the secrecy, shame, and dysfunctional eating patterns associated with BN have negatively affected adolescent development and have confused and disempowered parents and other family members. In addition, FBT-BN assumes that parents' guilt about having possibly caused the illness and anxiety about how best to proceed have further disabled them. Treatment aims at empowering parents and the adolescent to disrupt binge eating, purging, restrictive dieting, and any other pathological weight control behaviors in a *collaborative effort*. It also aims to *externalize* and separate the disordered behaviors from the affected adolescent to promote parents' action and decrease adolescent resistance to their assistance. Once successful in these tasks, the parents agree to return full control over eating to the adolescent and assist his/her in negotiating predictable adolescent development tasks. Siblings are protected from the job assigned to the parents and are encouraged to play a supportive role that does not involve mealtimes. Throughout treatment the therapist aims to take a nondirective stance and serves as an educator, consultant, and sounding board for the family, while leaving decision making up to the parents. This stance facilitates parental ownership of decisions made in treatment and thereby promotes an increased sense of empowerment.

Treatment Literature with Emphasis on RCTs

As noted, data supportive of treatments for adolescents with BN are sparse. Initial enthusiasm for FBT for BN developed because of the observation that the binge–purge subtype of AN responded to FBT-AN. In treatment studies for adolescents with AN, where binge–purge subtype typically comprises about 20% of cases, FBT has been found to be as effective for weight gain as it is for curtailing binge and purge episodes (Eisler et al., 2000; Lock, Agras, Bryson, & Kraemer, 2005). These data suggested that by following FBT-BN, parents would be able to effectively help their adolescent children decrease bulimic behaviors in addition to reversing severe dieting. Although AN and BN are distinct syndromes, there is considerable overlap in symptomatology. Consequently, it was reasonable to consider that FBT might also be effective for adolescents with BN.

FBT was first applied to adolescents with BN in a small case series by Dodge, Hodes, Eisler, and Dare (1995). This study demonstrated significant reductions in bulimic behaviors through educating the family about the ED and helping the parents disrupt binge-eating and purging episodes. This case series was followed by the detailed description of an adolescent progressing in FBT-BN (Le Grange, Lock, & Dymek, 2003). Both of these studies concluded that utilizing families in the recovery of adolescent BN was a promising treatment avenue for this younger population. These preliminary findings were recently supplemented with the publication of two RCTs for adolescents with BN utilizing forms of FBT (Le Grange et al., 2007; Schmidt et al., 2007).

Le Grange and colleagues (2007) assigned 80 patients with DSM-IV BN and partial BN, ages 12–19 years ($M = 16.1$ years, $SD = 1.6$), to FBT-BN ($n = 41$) or to individual supportive psychotherapy (SPT) ($n = 39$). Patients in both treatment conditions received 20 therapy sessions over a period of 6 months ($M = 17.5$, $SD = 4.6$), and assessments were conducted at baseline, midtreatment, end of treatment, and at 6-month follow-up. Adherence to treatment was satisfactory across modalities, with only 11% of patients dropping out of therapy prematurely. Moreover, the therapeutic alliance was acceptable and also did not differ between FBT-BN and SPT (Zaitsoff, Celio Doyle, Hoste, & Le Grange, 2008).

FBT-BN showed a clinical and statistical advantage over SPT at posttreatment and at 6-month follow-up. Significantly more patients in FBT-BN than in SPT were binge–purge abstinent at posttreatment (39 vs. 18%). Although abstinence rates at 6-month follow-up were reduced for both treatments, significantly more patients in FBT-BN were binge and purge free compared to those in SPT (29 vs. 10%). Secondary analyses of continuous outcome variables, using random regression models, revealed that the FBT-

BN had significantly greater improvements on measures of the behavioral and attitudinal features of ED psychopathology. In addition, FBT-BN appeared to show a more rapid rate of improvement in core bulimic symptoms, as shown in Figure 20.1. These results suggest that FBT-BN is superior to SPT on both the behavioral and attitudinal aspects of BN; they add additional support for further examination of FBT-BN for adolescent BN. Underscoring the generalizability of these findings, no differences were found in terms of treatment response for those with DSM-IV BN and partial BN at posttreatment or at follow-up.

In addition to comparing the effectiveness of FBT-BN and SPT, we have examined nonspecific predictors, moderators, and mediators of outcome (Le Grange, Crosby, & Lock, 2008; Lock, Le Grange, & Crosby, 2008) following Kraemer and colleagues' (Kraemer, Stice, Kasdin, Offord, & Kupfer, 2001) approach. The clearest predictor to emerge from our analyses was that patients with lower baseline eating concern scores

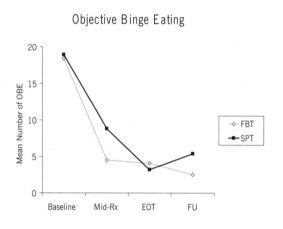

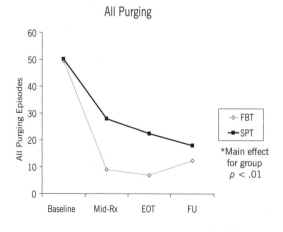

FIGURE 20.1. Objective binge eating and purging for FBT-BN and SPT. OBE, objective binge eating; Mid-Rx, midtreatment; EOT, end of treatment; FU, follow-up; FBT, family-based treatment; SPT, supportive psychotherapy.

(based on the Eating Disorder Examination [EDE]) were more likely to have remitted (binge and purge abstinent) at posttreatment and follow-up, regardless of the treatment received. Lower baseline depression scores predicted partial remission at posttreatment, and fewer binge–purge episodes at baseline predicted partial remission at follow-up. Thus, higher levels of both ED psychopathology and depressed mood predicted BN outcomes at posttreatment and follow-up. These findings are similar to those previously reported for FBT-AN (Lock, Couturier, Bryson, & Agras, 2006). In that study, Lock and colleagues (2006) found that comorbid symptoms of depression, anxiety, and obsessiveness predicted remission rates in a cohort of adolescent patients with AN receiving FBT.

Univariate analyses for predictors and moderators of outcome at 6-month follow-up revealed that higher baseline binge and purge frequency was related to reduced probability of meeting criteria for partial remission at end of treatment. In addition, the effects of treatment on partial remission were significantly moderated by four EDE variables (weight concerns, shape concerns, eating concerns, and global score). Partial remission rates were much higher for participants with low EDE scores receiving FBT-BN, whereas participants receiving SPT showed similar rates of partial remission regardless of EDE scores.

Multivariate analyses for partial remission revealed that binge and purge frequency at baseline remained a significant predictor of partial remission status. In addition, EDE Global score uniquely moderated the effects of treatment. That is, for those participants who received FBT-BN, 38.9% with high EDE Global scores (median split) and 56.5% of those with low EDE Global scores met criteria for partial remission. In contrast, 40.9% of SPT participants with high EDE Global scores met criteria for partial remission at follow-up, compared to 35.3% of those with low EDE Global scores (Le Grange et al., 2008). Taken together, these results support the use of FBT-BN as a particularly effective intervention with adolescents who are identified before their level of psychopathology reaches levels that might be less responsive to treatment.

In terms of exploring mediators, changes in the Restraint subscale on the EDE score measured at midtreatment suggest that changes in this score, consistent with findings in the literature on CBT, may mediate outcome for FBT-BN, but not for SPT (Lock et al., 2008). Furthermore, cognitive changes are not explained by changes in ED behaviors (i.e., greater reductions in binge eating and purging episodes), as these are not significantly associated with remission status. Thus, FBT-BN may exert its effects by changing disordered thinking. Since disordered thinking is not a direct therapeutic target of FBT-BN (as it is in CBT), a question about how thinking is changed in FBT-BN arises. Perhaps the FBT-BN therapist's externalization of BN symptoms increases challenges to BN thinking from this objective perspective. Another possibility is that the close attention to behavior through monitoring of binge and purge episodes by charting rates of these behaviors, provides an ongoing challenge to disordered thinking, not dissimilar to self-monitoring by means of food records in CBT (e.g., Wilson, Fairburn, Agras, & Kraemer, 2002). These exploratory findings await further testing in future controlled studies.

In the only other RCT to date, Schmidt and colleagues (2007) compared a form of FBT ($n = 41$) to cognitive-behavior therapy guided self-care ($n = 44$; CBT-GSC) for adolescents with DSM-IV BN and EDNOS, ages 12–20 years ($M = 17.6$ years, $SD = 0.3$). Significantly more patients in CBT-GSC, compared to those in family therapy, were abstinent from binge eating at posttreatment, although this difference disappeared at 6-month follow-up. There were no differences between the two groups in terms of vomiting at either time point. Looking at combined abstinence from binge eating and vomiting, findings from this study show that there were no significant differences between treatment groups at posttreatment (12.5% for family therapy vs. 19.4% for CBT-GSC) or 6-month follow-up (41.4% for family therapy vs. 36% for CBT-GSC). Direct cost of treatment was lower for CBT-GSC, but there were no differences in other cost categories. Schmidt and her colleagues acknowledge that their sample size was likely too small to detect differences between two active treatments for some outcomes. These authors also argue that the absence of a waiting-list or placebo-attention control group may have prevented them from ruling out that improvement was simply due to passage of time or nonspecific effects.

Family therapy, as described by these authors, resembles FBT-BN, although no published manual of their approach is available. One key difference between FBT-BN and the family therapy provided by Schmidt and colleagues (2007) is that in the latter, "family" is defined as any "close other" rather than specifically requiring that a parent or legal guardian be defined as "family." Participants who utilized a "close other" accounted for one-quarter of all cases. This definition of family was likely utilized because the mean age of participants in this study was 17.6 years ($SD = 0.3$), an age quite close to adulthood, especially in the United Kingdom where the age of consent is 16 years. While defining family as a "close other" may fit well with this older age group, such a definition of family might not be the most effective way to approach FBT-BN with younger adolescents who are still legally dependent on parents. Nonetheless, the abstinence rate of 41% that was achieved for family therapy in Schmidt and colleagues' study was comparable to those achieved using FBT-BN in the study by Le Grange and colleagues (2007).

From a practical and dissemination perspective for family-based treatment, some important questions need to be considered. A substantial number of eligible subjects in the Schmidt trial (28%) refused participation in the study because they did not want their families involved in treatment. The CBT-GSC approach appeared to present with fewer barriers, as it had less refusal to participate. Moreover, CBT-GSC performed at least at well as the family therapy in Schmidt's study or FBT-BN in Le Grange's study. The cost of providing CBT-GSC was also significantly less than the cost of delivering family therapy and underscores the fact that treatment studies for adolescents with BN are still in their infancy, and further evaluation of effective treatments is needed. To this point, a multisite comparison of FBT-BN and CBT for adolescent BN is currently in progress at the University of Chicago and Stanford University.

Mini-Manual with Clinical Illustrations and Dialogue

FBT for BN was developed as an adaptation from FBT for AN for the use in the aforementioned RCT (Le Grange et al., 2007). This manual was first piloted with a small number of cases before adjusted for implementation in the RCT. Upon completion of the study, this manual was further refined for publication as a detailed clinician's manual (Le Grange & Lock, 2007). FBT for BN, as outlined in this manual, proceeds through three phases with 20 sessions over a period of 6 months. Phase I lasts between

2 and 3 months, with sessions typically scheduled at weekly intervals. Toward Phase II, sessions are scheduled every second week, whereas sessions every third week or even monthly are advisable toward the conclusion of treatment (Phase III).

Phase I: Reestablishing Healthy Eating (Sessions 1–10)

Treatment in Phase I is almost entirely focused on helping parents devise effective strategies to confront the ED and its destructive impact on their adolescent child. From the outset, the therapist encourages united action from the parents to challenge and disrupt pathological eating and purging behaviors in a persistent and consistent fashion. Every treatment session starts with a brief meeting between the therapist and the patient lasting no more than 15 minutes before the rest of the family joins the meeting. The therapist emphasizes that it will be important to keep a close check on illness behaviors and will utilize this point in time to introduce a way in which the adolescent will be required to monitor and report her weekly binge and purge symptoms (i.e., the Patient Binge–Purge Log). It is explained to the patient and her family that this information will be shared with the parents, and that their task will be to reconcile their daughter's report with their own impressions of her symptomatic behaviors. This reconciled report will be logged in the therapist's Binge–Purge Chart (see Figures 20.2 and 20.3 as well as page 385 for a more detailed description of these charts).

In the meetings with the family, the therapist directs the discussion in such a way as to create and reinforce a strong parental alliance around their efforts at reinforcing healthy eating in their offspring. However, the therapist will also invite the adolescent to be a part of the decision-making process and make it clear that her collaboration is desired. This aspect of FBT-BN sets it apart from its AN counterpart, where the parents are guided to take charge of weight restoration without the adolescent's input.

This first phase of treatment is characterized by attempts to absolve the parents from the responsibility of having caused the illness and to diminish any blame or guilt that they may feel. This is achieved by complimenting them as much as possible on the positive aspects of their parenting as well as reminding them that research has not found parents to be at fault for their child's ED. The therapist can express this attitude best by saying something along these lines:

> "I am glad you brought your whole family along to this meeting today. This allows me to observe firsthand what a great job you've done as parents in raising your family. You have no doubt acquired many parenting skills along the way, especially ones that helped you achieve these earlier successes. It is these skills that you already have that you will also have to implement now as you figure out a way to help your daughter resolve the current eating problems."

This approach emphasizes the therapist's role as a caring and concerned expert rather than an authoritarian force.

Early in this phase the therapist reviews the medical and psychiatric consequences of BN with family members. This action is taken to increase their anxiety so that they can grasp the severity of the disorder and take action to help find a resolution rather than become critical and angry about the behaviors. To help parents achieve this goal, the therapist separates the disorder from the adolescent. This strategy permits the ther-

Binges

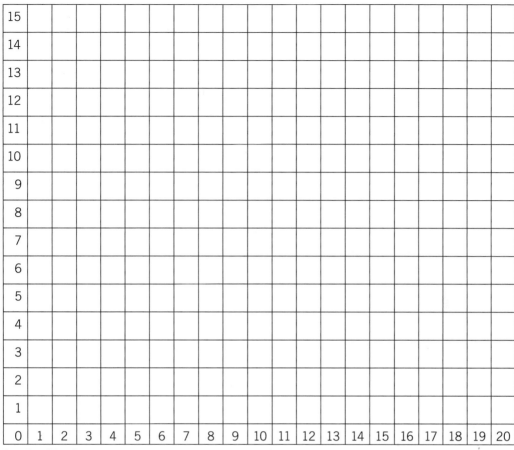

Session Number

(cont.)

FIGURE 20.2. Therapist Binge–Purge Chart. These two logs are completed by the therapist after he/she reconciles the patient's weekly report (from the Patient's Binge–Purge Log) with the parents' estimate of bulimic symptom frequency. Only once the patient and parents can agree upon the binge–purge frequency of the past week does the therapist note the numbers on the Therapist Binge–Purge Logs.

PURGES

Session Number

FIGURE 20.2. *(cont.)*

Day	Binge	Purge
1.		
2.		
3.		
4.		
5.		
6.		
7.		

FIGURE 20.3. Patient Binge–Purge Log. This log is completed by the patient. A separate log is utilized for each week of treatment and given to the therapist at the start of the session.

apist to disclaim the notion that the parents have caused the eating problem or that it is the adolescent's fault. Instead, the strategy aims to convey sympathy for the parents' plight as well as reduce shame in the adolescent. A metaphor that is often helpful in illustrating this point is to equate the ED with cancer. The therapist can explain this by saying:

> "The bulimia is like a malignant tumor; the tumor is not your daughter, it is something separate, and no one caused it. However, if it is left unchecked, it will continue to exert control over your daughter's thoughts and behaviors and physical health."

The primary goal with this intervention is to enable the parents to attribute symptomatic behaviors to "the illness" rather than blaming their offspring for willfully displaying such frustrating and disturbing behaviors.

With this background and new context in which the disorder is separated from the adolescent, intensive focus on confronting the BN behaviors follows. Families are encouraged to work out for themselves how best to stabilize their child's eating. This does not imply that the therapist withholds guidance or suggestions. However, empowerment of the family to address the ED symptoms will be easier to achieve when family members are allowed to figure out how they will supervise mealtimes and what appropriate steps they can take to ensure that purging is also addressed. The therapist does not allow family members to flounder—should they be unable to come up with reasonable and appropriate solutions, the therapist might say:

> "I realize that these are challenging steps to implement, and many families are at a loss for what to do. When confronted with a similar dilemma in deciding portion sizes or supervision post mealtimes, family X decided to do Y, and family A decided to do B. How might any of their solutions work for your family?"

In such a scenario family members are allowed to work out for themselves how they can assist their daughter in overcoming her symptoms rather than being told what they should do.

As is the case in FBT-AN, the therapist convenes a family meal early in treatment. This session usually serves to start the process of parental involvement and provides the therapist with an opportunity for direct observation of the familial interaction patterns around eating. The expectation for most cases is that the patient is at a healthy weight, and that reestablishing healthy eating habits (regular healthy meal consumption with no binge eating or purging) rather than weight is the priority.

The family is required to bring a regular meal plus an item that would constitute a "forbidden food" for the adolescent. The first goal would be for the adolescent to eat what is expected under the circumstances, and then for the parents to encourage their teenager to eat some of the forbidden food. The rationale for this maneuver is the benefit gained when parents are able to help their adolescent relax these unreasonable expectations around certain foods. The therapist also encourages the adolescent to let her parents know some of the internal turmoil that is usually associated with such transgressions—that is, to let them know how bad she might be feeling for being so "weak" as to eat the forbidden food item, how she should "just as well go ahead and eat the whole packet of cookies now," and that she would "in any case get rid of it afterward." This scenario might help the adolescent to take the first step toward being less secretive about her symptoms as well as help the parents understand just how much this disorder has come to occupy their daughter's mind and feelings. In addition, the family meal is an opportunity for parents to serve as a resource to their child as he/she struggles with the challenge of eating a forbidden or feared food.

The family meal session also allows the therapist to help the family work out some ground rules around eating times. For example, the adolescent is not to leave the therapist's room for at least 20 minutes after eating, thereby preventing purging. The therapist should encourage the adolescent to verbalize some of her thoughts and fears around eating forbidden foods and just how anxious she might get to rid herself of these foods, even after consuming only a small portion. This might be the parents' first opportunity to begin to appreciate their daughter's agonizing struggle around food, given the fact that the patient has probably been quite successful so far at keeping her parents uninformed about her dilemma. It will be the task of the parent to make sure that they can come to an agreement with their teen about how best to spend time after mealtimes in order to make their supervision feel more like spending quality time as a family—for example, watch a movie, play a card game, surf the Internet.

Parents are encouraged to seek the collaboration of their adolescent in their efforts to confront the BN. This collaborative stance is one of the differentiating aspects of FBT for BN compared to AN. In a general sense, though, the stance of the therapist is similar to that in AN. Specifically, he/she holds the family consistently and resolutely in positive regard, looking for opportunities to provide positive reinforcement and support by complimenting parents as much as possible on the positive aspects of their parenting. At the same time, it is important that the therapist show respect for the developmental status of the adolescent. This almost always means helping to ameliorate the shame associated with binge-eating and purging behaviors and sympathizing with the plight the disorder is creating for the patient. The therapist also acknowledges that allowing parents to be involved in normally autonomous eating and weight behaviors is out of sync with what parents of teenagers typically expect. However, it is made clear that this degree of involvement by parents is temporary and only needed to help change the course of BN at the outset of treatment.

Phase II: Helping the Adolescent Eat on Her Own (Sessions 11–16)

When eating patterns return to normal and binge eating and purging are largely eliminated, a change in the mood of the family is evident (i.e., relief after having taken charge of the ED). At this point, the therapist can move to the second phase of treatment. Disordered-eating symptoms remain central in the discussions, as the therapist monitors a return to regular meals that occur with minimum tension. Such monitoring occurs primarily through a detailed inquiry at each session: The therapist asks the parents and the adolescent to provide him/her with a detailed account of what a typical day looks like. This description should emphasize mealtimes. Using this account, the therapist makes a clinical judgment about whether these meals now occur without the tension and anxieties that characterized mealtimes when treatment started.

The aim of this phase is to return control of problematic eating behaviors that have been under the parents' watchful eye, back to the adolescent. The goal is for the adolescent to master these dilemmas with the support of her parents. In practice, this means that the parents might still monitor eating, but they allow the adolescent to make his/her own food choices and ensure that these choices are not influenced by the ED. This is possible during Phase 2 because the parents and adolescent, having worked together in Phase 1, have successfully broken the hold that excessive weight concern, inappropriate dieting strategies, and binge eating and purging have held on the teenager. In this context, family issues that relate to attitudes toward weight, dieting, and food can be brought forward in relation to BN and its emergence in the family. However, this discussion occurs only in relationship to the effect these issues have on the parents in their task of assuring regular eating in the absence of bulimic symptoms. In other words, while it is now appropriate for the parents to encourage the adolescent's integration with his/her peer group once more, such attempts are tempered by the parents' continuing vigilance over possible bulimic symptoms. What this means in practice is that parents would encourage their teen to join her friends at the mall for a movie, but that she should have a healthy meal with her parents either before or after such an outing.

Phase III: Adolescent Issues and Termination (Sessions 17–20)

The third phase is initiated when the patient maintains a stable weight and binge-eating and purging symptoms have mostly subsided. The central theme here is the establishment of a healthy relationship between the adolescent or young adult and his/her parents, in which the illness does not interfere or constitute the basis of their interaction. This entails, among other endeavors, working toward increased personal autonomy for the adolescent and more appropriate family boundaries. It also includes the need for the parents to reorganize their life together when the adolescent is nearing college age. Both patient and parents are usually focused on the adolescent's pending departure from her family, with the parents concerned about a possible relapse of the ED, whereas the adolescent/young adult is seemingly more focused on her pending freedom from parental oversight. Achieving some balance around both these important issues is a challenge for many families as they conclude treatment.

Taken together, the FBT-BN approach differs from that in adolescent AN in some significant ways. First, the emphasis is not on weight restoration but rather on regulating eating and curtailing purging. Second, whereas in FBT-AN the parents take charge of restoring the adolescent's weight, treatment in BN is more collaborative between the adolescent and his/her parents. Because adolescents with BN are typically about 2 years older than most adolescents with AN when they present for treatment, many are developmentally more autonomous, making it all the more important for therapists to encourage collaboration between the adolescent and his/her parents in treatment. Adolescents with BN are typically more interactive and talkative in treatment, even early on, than those with AN. This makes therapy seem more interactive and productive for the adolescent's development than sometimes appears to be the case with more silent and withdrawn adolescents with AN. Third, the secretive nature of BN, as well as the guilt and shame that are caused by these symptoms, make it more probable that the illness, and its severity, can be overlooked by the parents. These factors increase the discomfort of BN and contribute the largely ego-dystonic aspect of BN, compared to the usually ego-syntonic experience of AN. The emaciated state of a patient with AN is usually more obvious than any size/shape concerns attributable to BN and allows for the therapist to help the parents remain focused on the seriousness of his/her condition.

It should be noted that FBT-BN is often complicated by comorbid illnesses and other problems (Fischer & Le Grange, 2007). It is sometimes difficult to maintain treatment focus on BN when other important issues (drug use, sexual behavior, academic failure) come to the fore. FBT-BN is a focused treatment specifically tailored to BN and sometimes, because of comorbidity, developmental challenges, and other family dilemmas, other therapy to address these problems may need to follow the focused work of FBT-BN. Without the cognitively and emotionally disorganizing symptoms of BN as a constant concern, therapy to address these other psychological issues is more likely to be efficient and effective.

Forms and Worksheets

A *Binge–Purge Log* for the patient and *Binge–Purge Charts* for the therapist are utilized in FBT-BN (see Figures 20.2 and 20.3). At the time of the first meeting with the patient and his/her family the therapist explains that it is important to get an accurate account of binge-eating and purging behaviors. The therapist provides clear definitions of these behaviors and asks the adolescent to record these on a separate Binge–Purge Log for every week of treatment. The therapist also explains that he/she will collect this log from the adolescent at the start of every session when they (therapist and patient) meet for about 10 minutes before the rest of the family joins them. Once the parents have joined the session, the therapist attempts to reconcile the patient's report with his/her parents' impressions of binge–purge frequency. It is the agreed-upon binge–purge frequencies that are noted on the therapist's Binge–Purge Chart, and it is this chart that is utilized in treatment to reflect a change in symptomatic behaviors. The therapist explains to the adolescent and his/her parents that progress in symptomatic behaviors (or lack thereof) will set the tone of each session. If the log is not brought to a session, the therapist expresses concern but still asks the patient to try to recall any such episodes over the preceding 7 days. This recalled account is then reviewed with the parents once they join the session.

Additional Resources

Treatment

- See *www.maudsleyparents.org* and *www.feast-ed.org* for a list of providers.

Manual

- Le Grange D, & Lock J. (2007). *Treating bulimia in adolescents: A family-based approach.* New York: Guilford Press.

Training

- *Training Institute for Child and Adolescent Eating Disorders* (for details, visit *www. train2treat4ed.com*).

References

Agras WS, Rossiter EM, Arnow B, Schneider JA, Telch CF, Raeburn SD, et al. (1992). Pharmacologic and cognitive-behavioral treatment for bulimia nervosa: A controlled comparison. *American Journal of Psychiatry*, 149:82–87.

Agras WS, Walsh BT, Fairburn CG, Wilson GT, & Kraemer HC. (2000). A multicenter comparison of cognitive-behavioral therapy and interpersonal psychotherapy for bulimia nervosa. *Archives of General Psychiatry*, 57:459–466.

Dodge E, Hodes M, Eisler I, & Dare C. (1995). Family therapy for bulimia nervosa in adolescents: An exploratory study. *Journal of Family Therapy*, 17:59–77.

Eisler I, Dare C, Hodes M, Russell G, Dodge E, & Le Grange D. (2000). Family therapy for adolescent anorexia nervosa: The results of a controlled comparison of two family interventions. *Journal of Child Psychology and Psychiatry*, 41:727–736.

Fischer S, & Le Grange D. (2007). Co-morbidity and high-risk behaviors in treatment seeking adolescents with bulimia nervosa. *International Journal of Eating Disorders*, 40:751–753.

Herzog D, Keller M, Lavori P, & Sacks N. (1991). The course and outcome of bulimia nervosa. *Journal of Clinical Psychiatry*, 52(Suppl.), 4–8.

Hoek HW, & van Hoeken D. (2003). Review of the prevalence and incidence of eating disorders. *International Journal of Eating Disorders*, 34:383–396.

Kraemer H, Stice E, Kasdin A, Offord D, & Kupfer D. (2001). How do risk factors work together?: Mediators, moderators, and independent, overlapping, and proxy risk factors. *American Journal of Psychiatry*, 158:848–56.

Le Grange D, Crosby R, & Lock J. (2008). Predictors and moderators of outcome in family-based treatment for adolescent bulimia nervosa. *Journal of the American Academy of Child and Adolescent Psychiatry*, 47:464–470.

Le Grange D, Crosby R, Rathouz P, & Leventhal B. (2007). A controlled comparison of family-based treatment and supportive psychotherapy for adolescent bulimia nervosa. *Archives of General Psychiatry*, 64:1049–1056.

Le Grange D, & Lock J. (2007). *Treating bulimia in adolescents: A family-based approach*. New York: Guilford Press.

Le Grange D, Lock J, & Dymek M. (2003). Family-based therapy for adolescents with bulimia nervosa. *American Journal of Psychotherapy*, 67:237–251.

Lock J, Agras WS, Bryson S, & Kraemer H. (2005). A comparison of short- and long-term family therapy for adolescent anorexia nervosa. *Journal of the American Academy of Child and Adolescent Psychiatry*, 44:632–639.

Lock J, Couturier J, Bryson S, & Agras WS. (2006). Predictors of dropout and remission in family therapy for adolescent anorexia nervosa in a randomized clinical trial. *International Journal of Eating Disorders*, 39:639–647.

Lock J, Le Grange D, & Crosby R. (2008). Exploring possible mechanisms of change in family-based treatment for adolescent bulimia nervosa. *Journal of Family Therapy*, 30:260–271.

Lock J, Reisel B, & Steiner H. (2001). Associated health risks of adolescents with disordered eating: How different are they from their peers?: Results from a high school survey. *Child Psychiatry and Human Development*, 31:249–265.

Mussell MP, Mitchell JE, Weller CL, Raymond NC, Crow SJ, & Crosby RD. (1995). Onset of binge eating, dieting, obesity, and mood disorders among subjects seeking treatment for binge eating disorder. *International Journal of Eating Disorders*, 17:395–401.

Robin AL, Siegal PT, Moye A, Gilroy M, Dennis AB, & Sikand A. (1999). A controlled comparison of family versus individual therapy for adolescents with anorexia nervosa. *Journal of the American Academy for Child and Adolescent Psychiatry*, 38:1482–1489.

Schapman A, Lock J, & Conturier J. (2006). Cognitive-behavioral therapy for adolescents with binge eating syndromes: A case series. *International Journal of Eating Disorders*, 39:252–255.

Schmidt U, Lee S, Beecham J, Perkins S, Treasure J, Yi I, et al. (2007). A randomized controlled trial of family therapy and cognitive behavioral guided self-help for adolescents with bulimia nervosa and related conditions. *American Journal of Psychiatry*, 164:591–598.

Stice E, & Agras WS. (1998). Predicting onset and cessation of bulimic behaviors during adolescence. *Behavior Therapy*, 29:257–276.

Wilson GT, Fairburn CG, Agras WS, & Kraemer H. (2002). Cognitive-behavioral therapy for bulimia nervosa: Time course and mechanisms of change. *Journal of Consulting and Clinical Psychology*, 70:267–274.

Wilson GT, Grilo CM, & Vitousek K. (2007). Psychological treatments for eating disorders. *American Psychologist*, 62:199–216.

Zaitsoff S, Celio Doyle A, Hoste R, & Le Grange D. (2008). Therapeutic alliance and treatment acceptability with adolescents with bulimia nervosa: A comparison between individual and family based treatments. *International Journal of Eating Disorders*, 41:390–398.

CHAPTER 21

Pharmacotherapy for Bulimia Nervosa

Allegra Broft, Laura A. Berner, and B. Timothy Walsh

Theoretical Model(s)

Both an explanatory model for bulimia nervosa (BN) and an understanding of the neuroscience of BN remain limited. Consequently, the field has not yet developed a definitive rationale for psychopharmacological treatment strategies for this condition. Despite our limited understanding of the mechanisms underlying BN, some models that offer explanations for the initiation and maintenance of BN are relevant to the current main psychopharmacological strategies for the treatment of the disorder.

The cognitive-behavioral therapy (CBT) model of BN (Fairburn, 1997) is frequently utilized in clinical settings and provides one basis for the approach to the pharmacological treatment of the disorder. In this model, disruption of normal mechanisms for affective regulation, impairments in self-esteem, and other deficits in ego function may predispose some individuals to an overvaluation of shape and weight concerns, leading to increased preoccupation with dietary rules and an increase in dietary restrictions. This sequence, for some, may ultimately lead to binge eating and compensatory measures for binge-eating episodes. The emergence of the binge-eating and purging symptoms may, in turn, amplify the preexisting difficulties with affective regulation, self-esteem, and other deficits in ego function. The CBT model provides a rationale for the targeting of mood/affective symptoms in the treatment—pharmacological or psychotherapeutic—of BN. Additionally, the comorbidity of BN with depressive disorders (Hudson, Hiripi, Pope, & Kessler, 2007) and the clinically observed link between dysphoric mood states and binge-eating and purging episodes (Hsu, 1990) have led to controlled pharmacological trials in BN, focusing on the various classes of antidepressant medication.

A second model for the pharmacological treatment of BN has come from clinical studies of addiction and clinical research suggesting some overlap between eating disorders (EDs; particularly the binge type) and substance use disorders. The eating binges of individuals with BN are often described as a source of relief from depression or anxiety, just as drugs of abuse are sources of relief from these negative moods for those who abuse them (Gendall, Joyce, Sullivan, & Bulik, 1998; Gold, Frost-Pineda, & Jacobs, 2003). Furthermore, rates of BN are high among patients with substance use disorders, and the converse relationship has also been supported by several studies (Gold et al., 2003; Grilo, Sinha, & O'Malley, 2002; Holderness, Brooks-Gunn, & Warren, 1994). In animal models of BN, the neurochemical modifications, particularly in the ventral tegmental area (VTA) and the mesolimbic dopamine (DA) system, associated with a binge–fast schedule of palatable food intake (a schedule that resembles that of an individual with BN) result in neurological changes analogous to those of drug addictions (Colantuoni et al., 2002; Van Ree, 2000). Clinical trials research, driven in part by this model, has started to examine the efficacy of medications that target reward pathways involved in the development and maintenance of addictions.

Other pharmacological treatment models of BN have been directed by knowledge of neurocircuitry involved in feeding and natural rewards. Studies have indicated a role for the serotonergic system in feeding and promotion of the satiety response (Leibowitz & Alexander, 1998; Leibowitz, Weiss, & Suh, 1990) and a role for mesolimbic brain circuits (i.e., gamma-aminobutyric acid [GABA], glutamate, and DA-rich circuits involving the brainstem, VTA, and the basal ganglia–amygdala–anterior cingulate and associated areas) in the mediation of the acquisition of natural rewards such as food (Salamone, Correa, Farrar, & Mingote, 2007). For example, prior studies in rats have found that the intake of palatable foods on an intermittent schedule, as occurs during binge-eating episodes, results in a cyclic release of DA and upregulation of endogenous mu-opioid receptors, stimulating the neural reward system and consequently further stimulating palatable food intake (Colantuoni et al., 2001). Human neuroimaging studies have indicated involvement of these circuits in response to palatable food reward as well (Small, Jones-Gotman, & Dagher 2003; Volkow et al., 2002). Despite our limited knowledge regarding the neurobiology of BN, these models have provided some basis for current psychopharmacological treatment trials and strategies.

Treatment Literature

The pharmacological treatment of BN has been the focus of several review papers, including a recent excellent review by Shapiro and colleagues (2007) of randomized controlled trials up to 2005 of both medications alone and medications plus behavioral interventions. This systematic review, recommended for consultation for further details of trials discussed in this chapter, included double-blinded, single-blinded, and crossover designs that were initiated with 30 or more patients who were followed for a minimum of 3 months. The Cochrane Database of Systematic Reviews has compiled a comprehensive review of all randomized controlled trials of antidepressant medication in BN (Bacaltchuk & Hay, 2003), and is another excellent reference. The criteria for inclusion in this review are slightly more liberal, in that clinical trials as short as 4 weeks are included.

The synopsis of medication trials presented here has been organized in the following manner: Medication studies that meet criteria for inclusion by application of the Shapiro criteria are reviewed first, and these are the studies incorporated into the tables and figures in this chapter. Other remaining studies are more briefly reviewed next ("Medications with Less Empirical Support"). We note that some studies were close to meeting the Shapiro criteria and were ultimately included later in the chapter (e.g., Pope, Hudson, Jonas, & Yurgelun-Todd, 1983; Walsh et al., 1988). The review presented here is not meant to be exhaustive in referencing every existing pharmacological study, but rather to provide an overview of the current state of the field.

A search using criteria similar to Shapiro and colleagues, but including trials conducted up to 2008, produced 14 controlled medication trials for the treatment of BN, with individual studies including between 26 and 298 participants. The majority (11 of 14) of these studies were conducted with medications traditionally used as antidepressants—that is, selective serotonin reuptake inhibitors (SSRIs) and other serotonergic antidepressants, tricyclic antidepressants, and monoamine oxidase inhibitors. The majority of these studies (9 of 11) have investigated the serotonergic antidepressants. None of these studies was conducted in children or adolescents. Outcome measures have generally included a measure of frequency of binge eating and purging episodes. Various other secondary outcomes have been examined in these trials, including ratings of depression and anxiety, body image dissatisfaction, food preoccupation, shape and weight concern, "drive for thinness," and weight change. Other studies have examined the efficacy of combining medications and psychotherapy, but these are beyond the scope of this chapter.

Fluoxetine: The Gold Standard

Fluoxetine, approved by the Food and Drug Administration for, and currently considered the "gold standard" of, psychopharmacological treatment of BN, is an SSRI, with pharmacological action primarily at the serotonin reuptake transporter. The mechanism of action specific to its efficacy in BN is unknown. Six trials, one including concomitant inpatient treatment, one including concomitant nutritional counseling, and one aimed at preventing relapse, compared fluoxetine to placebo for the treatment of BN (Beumont et al., 1997; Fichter et al., 1991; Fluoxetine Bulimia Nervosa Collaborative Study Group, 1992; Goldstein et al., 1995; Kanerva, Rissanen, & Sarna, 1995; Romano, Halmi, Sarkar, Koke, & Lee, 2002). Five out of the six of these trials indicated significant efficacy of fluoxetine at a dose of 60 mg/day (Beumont et al., 1997; Fluoxetine Bulimia Nervosa Collaborative Study Group, 1992; Goldstein et al., 1995; Kanerva et al., 1995; Romano et al., 2002). More specifically, two of the three studies that examined the efficacy of fluoxetine versus placebo (PBO) for acute reduction of symptoms, and in the absence of supplemental behavioral treatments, found that fluoxetine significantly reduced binge eating and purging behaviors compared to PBO. Furthermore, all but one study (Fichter et al., 1991) found that fluoxetine was associated with significant improvement in other psychological symptoms, compared to PBO (see Tables 21.1 and 21.2). This number of controlled and successful clinical trials far exceeds the number of controlled trials conducted on any other medication in BN.

Fluoxetine has been specifically demonstrated to have increased efficacy for symptoms of BN at a higher (60 mg/day) dose compared to a lower dose (20 mg/day), and patients with BN can be started on this higher dose of 60 mg/day or titrated to it rapidly (Fluoxetine Bulimia Nervosa Collaborative Study Group, 1992). Of note, the one negative trial of fluoxetine was conducted in inpatients who were receiving concurrent

TABLE 21.1. Results of Double-Blind, Placebo-Controlled Psychopharmacological Interventions for BN

Source	N	Treatment	Medication superior to placebo		Comments
			For binge eating/ purging?	For other relevant measures?	
Fichter et al. (1991)	40	FLX vs. PBO, IP	No	No	No significant differences were found between FLX and PBO groups.
Fluoxetine BN Collaborative Study Group (1992)	387	FLX (20 mg) vs. FLX (60 mg) vs. PBO, OP	Yes	Yes	FLX, specifically at high dose (60 mg), was associated with the greatest reductions in binge eating and purging.
Goldstein et al. (1995)	398	FLX vs. PBO, OP	Yes	Yes	FLX group demonstrated a greater reduction in drive for thinness scores and greater median percentage reduction in purging and binge eating compared to PBO.
Kanerva et al. (1995)	50	FLX vs. PBO, OP	No	Yes	Binge reduction with FLX was not significantly different compared to PBO, but FLX was associated with a greater reduction in depressed and anxious mood, EAT, BITE, and EDI scores, and food preoccupation over 8 weeks.
Beumont et al. (1997)	67	Nutritional counseling + FLX vs. PBO, OP	No	Yes	FLX was associated with lower restraint, weight concern, and shape concern EDE subscale scores at week 8, but no difference in binge–purge reduction compared to PBO.
Walsh et al. (1991)	78	DES vs. PBO, OP	Yes	Yes	DES, compared to PBO, was associated with a significant reduction in binge and vomiting frequency, ED symptoms and body shape concerns, symptoms of depression, and ratings of obsessive–compulsiveness.
Kennedy et al. (1993)	36	BRF vs. PBO, OP	Yes*	No	BRF was associated with a greater reduction in vomiting episodes, but not with a reduction of binge-eating episodes* or improvements in self-report ratings of depression and anxiety.
Pope et al. (1989)	46	TRZ vs. PBO, OP	Yes	Yes	TRZ resulted in a greater percent decrease in binge eating and vomiting frequencies and greater subjective assessments of improvement compared to PBO.

(cont.)

TABLE 21.1. *(cont.)*

Source	N	Treatment	Medication superior to placebo		Comments
			For binge eating/ purging?	For other relevant measures?	
Hoopes et al. (2003); Hedges et al. (2003)	68	TPT vs. PBO, OP	Yes	Yes	TPT associated with greater percentage reduction in carbohydrate craving score and improved self-esteem, eating attitudes, body image, and anxiety; also resulted in greater reduction of binge–purge frequency.
Nickel et al. (2005)	30	TPT vs. PBO, OP	Yes	Yes	TPT resulted in significantly greater reductions in binge–purge frequency and significant improvements in health-related quality of life.
Faris et al. (2000)	26	ODT vs. PBO, OP	Yes	Yes	ODT associated with a greater reduction in binge–purge frequencies and in time spent engaging in BN behaviors and a greater increase in normal meals over 4 weeks.

Note. Studies presented include those initiated with 30 or more patients who were followed for a minimum of 3 months and met the criteria of Shapiro et al. (2007). *N*, sample size; FLX, fluoxetine; PBO, placebo; IP, inpatient; OP, outpatient; EAT, Eating Attitudes Test; BITE, Bulimic Investigatory Test, Edinburgh; EDI, Eating Disorder Inventory; EDE, Eating Disorder Examination; DES, desipramine; ED, eating disorder; BRF, brofaromine; TRZ, trazodone; TPT, topiramate; ODT, ondansetron.

TABLE 21.2. Results of Double-Blind, Placebo-Controlled Interventions for Relapse Prevention in BN

Source	N	Treatment	Medication prevented relapse?	Comments
Romano et al. (2002)	150	FLX vs. PBO, OP	Mixed results	Both groups worsened on all measures, but FLX group had significantly smaller mean increases in purging, binge eating, total eating disorder behavior, rituals, preoccupations, and symptom severity compared to PBO. With FLX, relapse occurred significantly less frequently in the first 3 months of a 52-week extended treatment period.
Fichter et al. (1996, 1997)	72	FLV vs. PBO, OP	Mixed results	Individuals treated with FLV experienced a significantly higher binge abstinence rate, reduced clinical severity, and lower relapse rate compared to PBO. FLV associated with significantly lower increases in bulimic behavior (urge to binge, vomiting), global eating disorder symptoms (SIAB total), EDI bulimia scores, fear of losing control, obsessive–compulsive symptoms, and global severity during relapse prevention phase.

Note. Studies presented include those initiated with 30 or more patients who were followed for a minimum of 3 months and met the criteria of Shapiro et al. (2007). *N*, sample size; FLX, fluoxetine; PBO, placebo; OP, outpatient; FLV, fluvoxamine; SIAB, Structured Inventory for Anorexia and Bulimia; EDI, Eating Disorder Inventory.

intensive psychotherapy (Fichter et al., 1991), and the studies with the largest sample sizes (Fluoxetine Bulimia Nervosa Collaborative Study Group, 1992; Goldstein et al., 1995) were those that found significant reductions in binge-eating and purging behaviors (see Table 21.1 and Figure 21.1). Additionally, results from one trial that included CBT nonresponders indicate that fluoxetine may be a useful intervention for patients with BN who have not responded adequately to psychotherapeutic treatment (Walsh et al., 2000), though another study of CBT nonresponders was less optimistic about patients' ability to respond either to medication or a change in psychotherapy type (Mitchell et al., 2002).

The side effect profile of fluoxetine is relatively benign in comparison to other psychotropic agents. Most side effects present in the initial 1–4 weeks of treatment and often subside (Schatzberg, Cole, & DeBattista, 2003). The emergence of side effects before full therapeutic effects (2 weeks or longer) can be a potential issue in treatment compliance, and patients should be adequately counseled that they may experience the side effects before the positive response, and that many of the side effects can be expected to be transient. These nuisance side effects include nausea, insomnia or somnolence, dizziness, and headache (Schatzberg et al., 2003). Side effects that are possibly less likely to subside include emergence of sexual deficits (delayed or absent orgasm), excessive sweating, and increased vividness of dreams (Schatzberg et al., 2003). Finally, a very small but statistically significant increase in rates of suicidal ideation in SSRI-treated adolescents and adults up to 25 years of age has been reported in meta-analyses of antidepressant trials (Hetrick, Merry, McKenzie, Sindahl, & Proctor, 2007) and has currently led to a Food and Drug Administration (FDA) warning about this possible effect, though at this time the precise clinical significance of these data remain controversial among experts in the field.

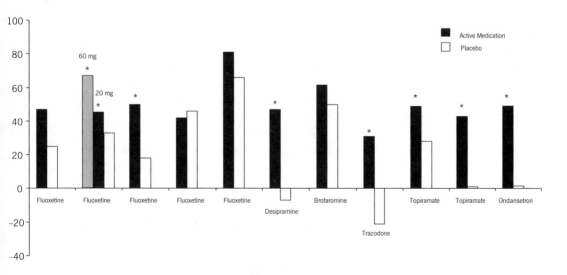

FIGURE 21.1. Percent reduction in frequency of binge eating. Note that in the depicted trials of trazodone and desipramine, frequency of binge eating increased in the placebo groups. Trials represented are those listed (in the same order) in Table 21.1. Asterisks denote a significant difference between medication and placebo.

Other Antidepressant Treatment Strategies

The remaining controlled antidepressant medication trials in BN meeting criteria roughly equivalent to the criteria for a "good" rating of Shapiro and colleagues have included trials of fluvoxamine (Fichter, Kruger, Rief, Holland, & Dohne, 1996; Fichter, Leibl, Kruger, & Rief, 1997), citalopram (fluoxetine-controlled; Leombruni et al., 2006), trazodone (at a dose of 400 mg/day; Pope, Keck, McElroy, & Hudson, 1989), desipramine (Walsh, Hadigan, Devlin, Gladis, & Roose, 1991), and brofaromine, a monoamine oxidase inhibitor (Kennedy et al., 1993). All of these trials were considered positive controlled trials, although another study conducted with fluvoxamine but not meeting the Shapiro and colleagues criteria was negative (Schmidt et al., 2004). As with the trials of fluoxetine, the precise mechanisms of action by which these various medications reduce symptoms of BN are unknown.

Some of these trials of other agents have notable features. The trial of fluvoxamine (Fichter et al., 1996, 1997) was for maintenance of symptom reduction, as medication was started toward the end of inpatient treatment for BN. A larger sustained reduction of BN symptoms was observed in the fluvoxamine group. The positive trial of desipramine (Walsh et al., 1991) was followed by an interesting secondary analysis demonstrating that medication response at just 2 weeks predicted efficacy of symptom reduction at the end of the trial. Therefore, these data call into question the long-held assumption that a patient should be maintained on an antidepressant medication for several weeks in the event of an initial lack of response—a clinical management strategy commonly practiced, albeit without empirical support (Taylor, Freemantle, Geddes, & Bhagwagar, 2006), in the use of antidepressants for the treatment of major depressive illness.

In addition to the small number of controlled trials, the side effect profile of many non-SSRI antidepressant medications (e.g., tricyclic antidepressants, monoamine oxidase inhibitors [MAOIs]) renders them less useful in comparison to the SSRI medications. Side effects of tricyclic antidepressants include various anticholinergic reactions (dry mouth, constipation, orthostatic hypotension, and urinary hesitancy), sedation, dizziness, as well as more potentially serious effects, including potential for cardiac toxicity in overdose. Management of patients taking MAOIs involves maintenance of patients on a tyramine-free diet, which includes several restrictions on foods (e.g., aged cheeses, smoked meats) in order to avert dangerously high blood pressure levels ("hypertensive crises") (Schatzberg et al., 2003). Use of MAOIs may therefore be particularly complicated for patients struggling with disturbances of eating behavior.

Nonantidepressant Psychopharmacological Interventions

Topiramate and ondansetron, medications without conclusive antidepressant efficacy, have also been investigated as treatments for BN. Topiramate is an anticonvulsant medication that pharmacologically acts as a GABA/glutamate receptor antagonist. Through an unclear mechanism of action, topiramate has demonstrated some potential efficacy in the treatment of obesity (Eliasson et al., 2007; McElroy et al., 2007) and in some psychiatric disorders (Schatzberg et al., 2003). The rationale for utilizing topiramate in the treatment of BN stems from the medication's apparent interaction with appetite regulation (as suggested by its effect in patients with obesity) as well as its possible regulation of impulsive behavior (as suggested by its potential utility in some psychiatric disorders). Two controlled trials have indicated efficacy of topiramate in the treatment of BN (Hedges et al., 2003; Hoopes et al., 2003; Nickel et al., 2005). However, topiramate is associated with several side effects. Cognitive side effects are most common, including difficulties in concentration, somnolence, memory impairment, and language/speech impairment. Other rare but potentially more serious side effects with use of topiramate include anion-gap metabolic acidosis, the potential for kidney stone formation, and a risk of glaucoma (Schatzberg et al., 2003). Finally, an issue unique to use of topiramate in patients with BN is the side effect of weight loss, the mechanism of which is unknown. To the extent that the side effect of weight loss may be mediated in part by enhancement of dietary restraint, it is a theoretical concern that such an effect may not be desirable in this specific patient group. Overall, the higher side effect profile of topiramate, relative to SSRIs, and limited controlled studies indicate that this medication should not be viewed as a first-line choice for the treatment of BN. When used in clinical practice, periodic blood monitoring, for example, monitoring of bicarbonate and other electrolytes every 3–6 months during treatment, is recommended.

The trial of ondansetron (Faris et al., 2000), a 5-HT$_3$ antagonist used primarily for treatment of nausea and emesis in the medical/surgical setting, differed from trials of the other medications in that patients were instructed to administer ondansetron only upon symptom flare-up (i.e., when faced with an urge to binge-eat or vomit), and as such represents an innovative treatment strategy. However, no additional studies have been conducted of this treatment option, and ondansetron is not currently routinely prescribed for the treatment of BN.

Medications with Less Empirical Support

Several other agents have been evaluated in randomized controlled studies that do not fully meet the criteria of Shapiro et al., including imipramine, amitriptyline, phenelzine, moclobemide, isocarboxazid, mianserin, and bupropion (Carruba et al., 2001; Horne et al., 1988; Kennedy et al., 1988; Mitchell & Groat, 1984; Pope et al., 1983; Rothschild et al., 1994; Sabine, Yonace, Farrington, Barratt, & Wakeling, 1983; Walsh et al., 1988). The side effect/tolerability profile of these agents, especially when compared to SSRIs, may limit any further interest in their continued investigation as treatment options for BN.

The use of bupropion in patients with BN, for both the treatment of the BN as well as comorbid depression, merits particular mention due to the question of increased risk of seizure with use of this agent. In the single trial of women with BN (55 on bupropion, 26 on placebo), bupropion (up to 450 mg/day) was effective at reducing symptoms of BN (Horne et al., 1988). The study was terminated prematurely, however, because four women experienced grand mal seizures. Because of this association, bupropion is rarely used in treatment of BN.

Several other open-label studies have examined agents with indications of efficacy in the addictive disorders as treatments for BN. Three such agents are naltrexone, baclofen, and memantine. Naltrexone is an opioid antagonist used in the maintenance of abstinence from alcohol dependence. Two open-label studies suggested potential efficacy of naltrexone in treating BN (Alger, Schwalberg, Bigaouette, Michalek, & Howard, 1991; Jonas & Gold, 1986–1987). Mitchell and colleagues (1989) later conducted a double-blind, placebo-controlled study of a low dose of this medication (50 mg). Although no difference was found between treatment groups, it is possible that use of a lower dose range in part accounts for the negative finding, and that a replication of this trial in a higher dose range would be of interest. Baclofen, currently used clinically primarily as a muscle relaxant, is an agonist at GABA-B receptors, which, when activated, can reduce the rewarding effects of substances of abuse (Cousins, Roberts, & de Wit, 2002). A recent open-label trial suggests that baclofen may be effective for the treatment of binge-type EDs, though in this trial, only three patients with BN were included (Broft et al., 2007). Finally, in a recent small, open-label trial, Brennan and colleagues (2008) found that memantine, an N-methyl-D-aspartate (NMDA) glutamate receptor antagonist, reduced binge-eating frequency in patients with binge-eating disorder (BED) without significantly affecting body mass index (BMI) or weight. While there are no published results of such a trial at present, the potential efficacy of memantine on symptoms of binge eating may be relevant to the treatment of BN as well, and future clinical trials may be warranted.

Combination Interventions: Pharmacotherapy and Behavioral Interventions

Several controlled trials have tested medication alone versus psychotherapy alone for the treatment of BN, whereas others have investigated whether the combination of pharmacotherapy with psychological treatment is more effective than the use of either modality in isolation. Findings regarding the relative benefits of medication over psychotherapy have been mixed. Several studies have found that cognitive-behavioral therapy (CBT) without medication was superior to medication alone (Agras et al., 1992; Goldbloom et al., 1997; Walsh et al, 1997). The available studies suggest some benefit of combination treatment over medication alone, though the superiority of combination treatment over psychotherapy alone is less clear. The addition of medication to psychotherapy appears to be of benefit in reducing associated symptoms of BN (dietary restraint, associated depressed mood or anxiety), but is not as clearly useful in reducing binge eating and purging (Agras et al., 1992; Walsh et al., 1997; Wilson et al., 1999). Furthermore, one study has suggested differential outcome of combination treatment based on psychotherapy type, though this finding was a secondary outcome measure and therefore requires further study (Walsh et al., 1997).

Limitations of the Current Literature

Limitations of the existing literature on the psychopharmacological treatment of BN are numerous. Except for a few smaller studies (Milano, Petrella, Sabatino, & Capasso, 2004) and the one trial of fluvoxamine (Fichter et al., 1996, 1997), there are no trials of SSRIs other than fluoxetine (or of serotonin norepinephrine reuptake inhibitors [SNRIs]) meeting the Shapiro and colleagues criteria. Another significant gap in the empirical literature is that the length of the optimal treatment period for sustained remission of symptoms remains uncertain. There are few data describing the course of symptoms following medication discontinuation, and the few studies on maintenance of symptom relief following initial response report substantial relapse rates during 6-month medication treatment periods (Pyle et al., 1990; Walsh et al., 1991). Thus, clinical guidelines in this regard are few, and, at best, are based on recommendations from the depression clinical trials literature, in which a guideline of 6 months to 1 year of treatment is recommended as a minimum (Schatzberg et al., 2003). Future studies of medication and psychotherapy combinations should shed further light on the optimal combination of the two. Furthermore, there are only limited studies of pharmacological strategies for BN in children or adolescents at present (Couturier & Lock, 2007; Kotler, Devlin, Davies, & Walsh, 2003).

Clinical Recommendations

One reference for clinical guidelines for the psychopharmacological treatment of EDs (including BN) is the American Psychiatric Association's (2006) *Practice Guideline for the Treatment of Patients with Eating Disorders*. It is of note that, given the evidence for CBT being at least as effective as medication for the treatment of BN, that it may be appropriate to delay initiation of medication treatment of BN during the initial treatment stages.

Medication treatment for BN might therefore be initiated in event of patient preference for a medication approach. A pharmacological approach may also be appropriate in the case of poor or partial response to CBT, or when CBT is unavailable. Assuming the choice for medication treatment of BN has been made, current clinical psychopharmacological treatment for BN would usually begin with fluoxetine (or another SSRI, if fluoxetine is known to be poorly tolerated by the patient), and with a change to another SSRI or SNRI if a trial of fluoxetine is ineffective. Side effect profile has been the driving force behind the preference for SSRI/SNRI medications over the other antidepressant classes, though these other classes might be considered as well, depending on the clinical case. Topiramate could be a possible option after one or more failed antidepressant trials.

Tricyclic antidepressants and MAOIs are also not usually recommended as initial medication treatment for BN, but may be considered in the case of symptoms refractory to SSRI/SNRI, as well as in cases where there is a comorbid depression that has failed SSRI/SNRI treatment. It is recommended that bupropion be avoided when possible, although in unusual situations, treatment with this agent might be contemplated, though only after a careful discussion with the patient of the potential risks of a bupropion trial.

Clinical experience also suggests caution with medications such as stimulants (e.g., brand-name medications including Ritalin, Adderall, and others), due to their potential for appetite suppression, which can interact adversely with eating-disordered drives toward restrictive eating. Caution is also recommended with anxiolytic medications such as benzodiazepines (lorazepam, clonazepam, alprazolam, and others), which may temporarily relieve anxiety symptoms in a way that, in theory, could be helpful for affective modulation, but which also has the potential for behavioral disinhibition and potentially a worsening of binge–purge symptoms.

References

Agras WS, Rossiter EM, Arnow B, Schneider JA, Telch CF, Raeburn SD, et al. (1992). Pharmacologic and cognitive-behavioral treatment for bulimia nervosa: A controlled comparison. *American Journal of Psychiatry*, 149:82–87.

Alger SA, Schwalberg MD, Bigaouette JM, Michalek AV, & Howard LJ. (1991). Effect of a tricyclic antidepressant and opiate antagonist on binge-eating behavior in normoweight bulimic and obese, binge-eating subjects. *American Journal of Clinical Nutrition*, 53(4):865–871.

American Psychiatric Association. (2006). *Practice guideline for the treatment of patients with eating disorders* (3rd ed.). Retrieved July 25, 2008, from *www.psychiatryonline.com/pracGuide/pracGuideTopic_12.aspx.*

Bacaltchuk J, & Hay P. (2003). Antidepressants versus placebo for people with bulimia nervosa. *Cochrane Database of Systematic Reviews*, Issue 3 (Article No. CD003391), DOI: 10.1002/14651858.CD003391.

Beumont PJ, Russell JD, Touyz SW, Buckley C, Lowinger K, Talbot P, et al. (1997). Intensive nutritional counseling in bulimia nervosa: A role for supplementation with fluoxetine? *Australian and New Zealand Journal of Psychiatry*, 31:512–524.

Brennan BP, Roberts JL, Fogarty KV, Reynolds KA, Jonas JM, & Hudson JI. (2008). Memantine in the treatment of binge eating disorder: An open-label, prospective trial. *International Journal of Eating Disorders*, 41:520–526.

Broft AI, Spanos A, Corwin RL, Mayer L, Steinglass J, Devlin MJ, et al. (2007). Baclofen for binge eating: An open-label trial. *International Journal of Eating Disorders*, 40:687–691.

Carruba MO, Cuzzolaro M, Riva L, Bosello O, Liberti S, Castra R, et al. (2001). Efficacy and tolerability of moclobemide in bulimia nervosa: A placebo-controlled trial. *International Clinic of Psychopharmacology*, 16:27–32.

Colantuoni C, Rada P, McCarthy J, Patten C, Avena NM, Chadeayne A, et al. (2002). Evidence that intermittent, excessive sugar intake causes endogenous opioid dependence. *Obesity Research*, 10:478–488.

Colantuoni C, Schwenker J, McCarthy J, Rada P, Ladenheim B, Cadet JL, et al. (2001). Excessive sugar intake alters binding to dopamine and mu-opioid receptors in the brain. *NeuroReport*, 12:3549–3552.

Cousins MS, Roberts DCS, & de Wit H. (2002). GABA-B receptor agonists for the treatment of drug addiction: A review of recent findings. *Drug and Alcohol Dependence*, 65:209–220.

Couturier J, & Lock J. (2007). A review of medication use for children and adolescents with eating disorders. *Journal of the Canadian Academy of Child and Adolescent Psychiatry*, 16:173–176.

Eliasson B, Gudbjörnsdottir S, Cederholm J, Liang Y, Vercruysse F, & Smith U. (2007). Weight loss and metabolic effects of topiramate in overweight and obese Type 2 diabetic patients: Randomized double-blind placebo-controlled trial. *International Journal of Obesity*, 31:1140–1147.

Fairburn C. (1997). Eating disorders. In D Clark & C Fairburn (Eds.), *The science and practice of cognitive behaviour therapy* (pp. 209–242). Oxford, UK: Oxford University Press.

Faris PL, Kim SW, Meller WH, Goodale RL, Oakman SA, Hofbauer RD, et al. (2000). Effect of decreasing afferent vagal activity with ondansetron on symptoms of bulimia nervosa: A randomised, double-blind trial. *Lancet*, 355:792–797.

Fichter MM, Kruger R, Rief W, Holland R, & Dohne J. (1996). Fluvoxamine in prevention of relapse in bulimia nervosa: Effects on eating-specific pyschopathology. *Journal of Clinical Psychopharmacology*, 16:9–18.

Fichter MM, Leibl C, Kruger R, & Rief W. (1997). Effects of fluvoxamine on depression, anxiety, and other areas of general psychopathology in bulimia nervosa. *Pharmacopsychiatry*, 30:85–92.

Fichter MM, Leibl K, Rief W, Brunner E, Schmidt-Auberger S, & Engel RR. (1991). Fluoxetine versus placebo: A double-blind study with bulimic inpatients undergoing intensive psychotherapy. *Pharmacopsychiatry*, 24:1–7.

Fluoxetine Bulimia Nervosa Collaborative Study Group. (1992). Fluoxetine in the treatment of bulimia nervosa: A multicenter, placebo-controlled, double-blind trial. *Archives of General Psychiatry*, 49:139–147.

Gendall KA, Joyce PR, Sullivan PF, & Bulik CM. (1998). Food cravers: Characteristics of those who binge. *International Journal of Eating Disorders*, 23:353–360.

Gold MS, Frost-Pineda K, & Jacobs WS. (2003). Overeating, binge eating, and eating disorders as addictions. *Psychiatric Annals*, 33:117–122.

Goldbloom DS, Olmsted M, Davis R, Clewes J, Heinmaa M, Rockert W, et al. (1997). A randomized controlled trial of fluoxetine and cognitive behavioral therapy for bulimia nervosa: Short-term outcome. *Behaviour Research and Therapy*, 35(9):803–811.

Goldstein D, Wilson M, Thompson V, Potvin J, Rampey A, & the Fluoxetine Bulimia Nervosa Collaborative Study Group. (1995). Long-term fluoxetine treatment of bulimia nervosa. *British Journal of Psychiatry*, 166:660–666.

Grilo CM, Sinha R, & O'Malley SS. (2002). Eating disorders and alcohol use disorders. *Alcohol Research and Health*, 26:151–160.

Hedges DW, Reimherr FW, Hoopes SP, Rosenthal NR, Kamin M, Karim R, et al. (2003). Treatment of bulimia nervosa with topiramate in a randomized, double-blind, placebo-controlled trial: Part 2: Improvement in psychiatric measures. *Journal of Clinical Psychiatry*, 64:1449–1454.

Hetrick S, Merry S, McKenzie J, Sindahl P, & Proctor M. (2007). Selective serotonin reuptake inhibitors (SSRIs) for depressive disorders in children and adolescents. *Cochrane Database of Systematic Reviews*, Issue 3 (Article No. CD004851), DOI: 10.1002/1465.1858.CD004851.pub2.

Holderness CC, Brooks-Gunn J, & Warren MP. (1994). Co-morbidity of eating disorders and substance abuse review of the literature. *International Journal of Eating Disorders*, 16:1–34.

Hoopes SP, Reimherr FW, Hedges DW, Rosenthal NR, Kamin M, Karim R, et al. (2003). Treatment of bulimia nervosa with topiramate in a randomized, double-blind, placebo-controlled trial: Part 1: Improvement in binge and purge measures. *Journal of Clinical Psychiatry*, 64:1335–1341.

Horne RL, Ferguson JM, Pope HG, Hudson JI, Lineberry CG, Ascher J, et al. (1988). Treatment of bulimia with bupropion: A multicenter controlled trial. *Journal of Clinical Psychiatry*, 49:262–266.

Hsu L. (1990). Experiential aspects of bulimia nervosa: Implications for cognitive behavioral therapy. *Behavior Modification*, 14:50–65.

Hudson JI, Hiripi E, Pope HG, & Kessler RC. (2007). The prevalence and correlates of eating disorders in the National Comorbidity Survey replication. *Biological Psychiatry*, 61:348–358.

Jonas, JM, & Gold MS. (1986–1987). Treatment of antidepressant-resistant bulimia with naltrexone. *International Journal of Psychiatry in Medicine*, 16(4):305–309.

Kanerva R, Rissanen A, & Sarna S. (1995). Fluoxetine in the treatment of anxiety, depressive symptoms, and eating-related symptoms in bulimia nervosa. *Nordic Journal of Psychiatry*, 49:237–242.

Kennedy SH, Goldbloom D, Ralevski E, Davis C, D'Souza J, & Lofchy J. (1993). Is there a role for selective monoamine oxidase inhibitor therapy in bulimia nervosa?: A placebo-controlled trial of brofaromine. *Journal of Clinical Psychopharmacology*, 13:415–422.

Kennedy SH, Piran N, Warsh JJ, Prendergast P, Mainprize E, Whynot C, et al. (1988). A trial of isocarboxazid in the treatment of bulimia nervosa. *Journal of Clinical Psychopharmacology*, 8:391–396.

Kotler L, Devlin M, Davies M, & Walsh BT. (2003). An open trial of fluoxetine for adolescents with bulimia nervosa. *Journal of Adolescent Psychopharmacology*, 13:329–335.

Leibowitz S, & Alexander J. (1998). Hypothalamic serotonin in control of eating behavior, meal size, and body weight. *Biological Psychiatry*, 44:851–864.

Leibowitz S, Weiss G, & Suh J. (1990). Medial hypothalamic nuclei mediate serotonin's inhibitory effect on feeding behavior. *Pharmacological and Biochemical Behavior*, 37:735–742.

Leombruni P, Amianto F, Delsedime N, Gramaglia C, Abbate-Daga G, & Fassino, S. (2006). Citalopram versus fluoxetine for the treatment of patients with bulimia nervosa: A single blind randomized controlled trial. *Advances in Therapy*, 23:481–494.

McElroy SL, Hudson JI, Capece JA, Beyers K, Fisher AC, & Rosenthal NR. (2007). Topiramate for the treatment of binge eating disorder associated with obesity: A placebo-controlled study. *Biological Psychiatry*, 61:1039–1048.

Milano W, Petrella C, Sabatino C, & Capasso A. (2004). Treatment of bulimia with sertraline: A randomised controlled trial. *Advances in Therapy*, 21:232–237.

Mitchell JE, Chistenson G, Jennings J, Huber M, Thomas B, Pomeroy C, et al. (1989). A placebo-controlled, double-blind crossover study of naltrexone hydrochloride in outpatients with normal weight bulimia. *Journal of Clinical Psychopharmacology*, 9:94–97.

Mitchell JE, & Groat R. (1984). A placebo-controlled, double-blind trial of amitriptyline in bulimia. *Journal of Clinical Psychopharmacology*, 4:186–196.

Mitchell JE, Halmi K, Wilson GT, Agras WS, Kraemer H, & Crow S. (2002). A randomized secondary treatment study of women with bulimia nervosa who fail to respond to CBT. *International Journal of Eating Disorders*, 32:271–281.

National Institute for Health and Clinical Excellence. (2004). *Eating disorders: Core interventions in the treatment and management of anorexia nervosa, bulimia nervosa, and related eating disorders.* Retrieved on October 17, 2008, from *www.nice.org.uk/Guidance/CG9/NiceGuidance/pdf/English.*

Nickel C, Tritt K, Muehlbacher M, Pedrosa Gil F, Mitterlehner FO, Kettler C, et al. (2005). Topiramate treatment in bulimia nervosa patients: A randomized, double-blind, placebo-controlled trial. *International Journal of Eating Disorders*, 38:295–300.

Pope HG, Jr, Hudson JI, Jonas JM, & Yurgelun-Todd D. (1983). Bulimia treated with imipramine: A placebo-controlled, double-blind study. *American Journal of Psychiatry*, 140:554–558.

Pope HG, Jr, Keck PE, McElroy SL, & Hudson JI. (1989). A placebo-controlled study of trazodone in bulimia nervosa. *Journal of Clinical Psychopharmacology*, 9:254–259.

Pyle RL, Mitchell JE, Eckert ED, Hatsukami D, Pomeroy C, & Zimmerman R. (1990). Maintenance treatment and 6-month outcome for bulimic patients who respond to initial treatment. *American Journal of Psychiatry*, 147:871–875.

Romano S, Halmi K, Sarkar N, Koke S, & Lee J. (2002). A placebo-controlled study of fluoxetine in continued treatment of bulimia nervosa after successful acute fluoxetine treatment. *American Journal of Psychiatry*, 159:96–102.

Rothschild R, Quitkin HM, Quitkin FM, Stewart JW, Ocepek-Welikson K, McGrath PJ., et al. (1994). A double-blind placebo-controlled comparison of phenelzine and imipramine in the treatment of bulimia in atypical depressives. *International Journal of Eating Disorders*, 15:1–9.

Sabine EJ, Yonace A, Farrington AJ, Barratt KH, & Wakeling A. (1983). Bulimia nervosa: A placebo controlled double-blind therapeutic trial of mianserin. *British Journal of Clinical Pharmacology*, 15:195S–202S.

Salamone JD, Correa M, Farrar A., & Mingote S. M. (2007). Effort-related functions of nucleus accumbens dopamine and associated forebrain circuits. *Psychopharmacology*, 191(3):461–482.

Schatzberg A, Cole J, & DeBattista C. (2003). *Manual of clinical psychopharmacology* (4th ed.). Washington, DC: American Psychiatric Association.

Schmidt U, Cooper PJ, Essers H, Freeman CP, Holland RL, Palmer RL, et al. (2004). Fluvoxamine and graded psychotherapy in the treatment of bulimia nervosa: A randomized, double-
blind, placebo-controlled, multicenter study of short-term and long-term pharmacotherapy
combined with a stepped care approach to psychotherapy. *Journal of Clinical Psychopharmacology*, 24:549–552.

Shapiro JR, Berkman N, Brownley K, Sedway J, Lohr K, & Bulik C. (2007). Bulimia nervosa
treatment: A systematic review of randomized controlled trials. *International Journal of Eating Disorders*, 40:321–336.

Small DM, Jones-Gotman M, & Dagher A. (2003). Feeding-induced dopamine release in dorsal
striatum correlates with meal pleasantness ratings in healthy human volunteers. *NeuroImage*, 19:1709–1715.

Taylor MJ, Freemantle N, Geddes JR, & Bhagwagar Z. (2006). Early onset of selective serotonin
reuptake inhibitor antidepressant action: Systematic review and meta-analysis. *Archives of
General Psychiatry*, 63:1217–1223.

Van Ree JM, Niesink RJ, Van Wolfswinkel LV, Ramsey NF, Kornet ML, Van Furth WR, et al.
(2000). Endogenous opioids and reward. *Euopean Journal of Pharmacology*, 405:89–101.

Volkow ND, Wang GJ, Fowler JS, Logan J, Jayne M, Franceschi D, et al. (2002). "Nonhedonic"
food motivation in humans involves dopamine in the dorsal striatum and methylphenidate
amplifies this effect. *Synapse*, 44:175–180.

Walsh BT, Agras WS, Devlin MJ, Fairburn CG, Wilson GT, Kahn C, et al. (2000). Fluoxetine for
bulimia nervosa following poor response to psychotherapy. *American Journal of Psychiatry*,
157:1332–1334.

Walsh BT, Gladis M, Roose SP, Stewart JW, Stetner F, & Glassman AH. (1988). Phenelzine vs
placebo in 50 patients with bulimia. *Archives of General Psychiatry*, 45:471–475.

Walsh BT, Hadigan CM, Devlin MJ, Gladis M, & Roose SP. (1991). Long-term outcome of antidepressant treatment for bulimia nervosa. *American Journal of Psychiatry*, 148:1206–1212.

Walsh BT, Wilson GT, Loeb KL, Devlin MJ, Pike KM, Roose SP, et al. (1997). Medication and
psychotherapy in the treatment of bulimia nervosa. *American Journal of Psychiatry*, 154:523–
531.

Wilson GT, Loeb KL, Walsh BT, Labouvie E, Petkova E, Liu X, et al. (1999). Psychological versus
pharmacological treatments of bulimia nervosa: Predictors and processes of change. *Journal of Consulting and Clinical Psychology*, 67:451–459.

CHAPTER 22

Pharmacotherapy for Binge-Eating Disorder

Lindsay P. Bodell and Michael J. Devlin

Although the phenomenon of binge eating was initially recognized in the late 1950s (Stunkard, 1959), binge eating disorder (BED) was first conceptualized as a distinct diagnosis only in the early 1990s, and it is currently included in the DSM-IV-TR under the umbrella category of eating disorder not otherwise specified (EDNOS). Following the formulation of BED as an eating disorder (ED) came the exploration for effective treatments, including new pharmacological interventions. In light of the behavioral overlap between BED and bulimia nervosa (BN), with binge eating characterizing both groups of individuals, initial medication trials for BED drew upon established medication treatments for BN, primarily antidepressants, which were known to effectively reduce binge-eating frequency in BN. In addition, since many patients with BED were also obese, appetite suppressants were explored as potential treatments for this newly identified disorder. Although obesity is not a diagnostic criterion for BED as defined in DSM-IV-TR, much of the treatment literature has focused specifically on the subject of overweight or obese patients with BED. This focus may reflect both a competing model of BED as a behavioral subtype of obesity (Devlin, Goldfein, & Dobrow, 2003), as well as the greater frequency with which obese individuals with BED present for treatment compared to nonobese individuals with BED. Thus, studies of medications for BED often targeted behavioral (binge eating), somatic (obesity), and psychological (comorbid depression) aspects of the disorder.

With regard to the pharmacological treatment of BN, several classes of medications have been investigated, but antidepressants appear to be the most established pharmacological treatment in reducing bulimic symptoms (i.e., binge eating and purging). Notably, these positive effects of antidepressants in reducing binge eating in patients with BN have been demonstrated regardless of patients' level of depression. This finding suggested that antidepressant treatment might lead to decreased binge eating in patients with BED, including in those without comorbid depression. Although a variety of antidepressants has been studied in the treatment of BED, the class of antidepressants studied most extensively is the selective serotonin reuptake inhibitors (SSRIs). Based on the BN literature, the presence of comorbid affective symptoms was not expected to be a prerequisite for the successful treatment of BED. Nonetheless, it was thought that, for those patients who did suffer from comorbid depression, antidepressant treatment might lead to an amelioration of such symptoms, either as an indirect benefit of a reduction in binge-eating frequency, or due to a direct effect of treatment on mood symptoms. Furthermore, it was thought to be likely that binge-eating cessation would be accompanied by weight loss, and this was often a primary or secondary outcome variable in clinical trials. That this expectation has largely not been borne out by experience has been one of the more interesting and frustrating findings to emerge from the initial generation of BED treatment studies.

In addition to exploring the use of antidepressants in patients with BED, investigators have turned to the obesity treatment literature for potential treatments to reduce appetite and facilitate weight loss. Several trials of Food and Drug Administration (FDA)–approved medications for obesity and other medications known to affect appetite or weight, such as anticonvulsants, have been conducted to specifically examine whether such medications might be particularly effective in helping obese patients with BED to not only decrease or stop their binge eating but also lose weight.

The initial generation of medication studies for BED focused on medication as a single treatment. As psychotherapy for BED, particularly cognitive-behavioral therapy (CBT), became more established, a second generation of studies has focused on questions regarding the benefits of adding medication to psychotherapy for patients with BED. Specifically, investigators have hypothesized that medication might augment the response to psychotherapy, specifically target particular symptoms such as depressive symptoms, help particular subgroups of patients, or yield a better clinical response in psychotherapy partial or nonresponders. This chapter reviews the results of controlled medication trials for primarily obese individuals with BED, including trials using medication as a sole intervention and those using medication in the context of psychosocial interventions.

Theoretical Models

Figure 22.1 illustrates putative relationships among behavioral, somatic, and psychological aspects of BED and mechanisms by which antidepressant and antiobesity medications are hypothesized to have beneficial effects. To the degree that binge eating reflects a state of nonhomeostasis in which eating is driven by forces other than a normal appetitive drive to maintain adequate nutrition and healthy weight, it may give rise to weight gain and obesity. Antiobesity medication may suppress appetite and binge eating, thereby facilitating weight loss, or may directly facilitate weight loss by other means—for example, increased energy expenditure or, in the case of orlistat, via fat malabsorption. Improvements in binge eating and weight loss may both lead secondarily to reductions in psychological symptoms. Not reflected in the diagram is the fact that some antidepressants may promote weight gain, thereby exerting a negative effect.

The figure also suggests a bidirectional relationship between binge eating and psychological symptoms. Binge eating is often described as a coping mechanism for unpleasant emotional states, yet it can in turn give rise to emotional distress either directly or via its effects on weight. Antidepressants may ameliorate depressive symptoms and thereby secondarily relieve binge eating, or may exert a direct antibinge effect.

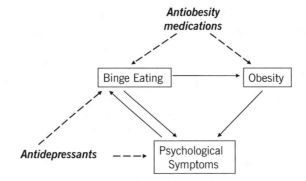

FIGURE 22.1. Theoretical model of medication action for BED.

Treatment Literature

The pharmacological treatment of BED has been the subject of several recent high-quality reviews, most notably that of Reas and Grilo (2008). This chapter is intended to summarize, contextualize, and update these reviews.

Are Antidepressants Superior to Placebo in the Treatment of BED?

SSRI antidepressants that have been studied as possible treatments for BED include fluoxetine, fluvoxamine, sertraline, citalopram, and escitalopram (see Table 22.1). Although no single SSRI has been recognized as an established treatment for BED, several studies have demonstrated SSRI medications to be at least statistically significantly superior to placebo in decreasing BED symptoms in the short term. However, these benefits are not consistent throughout the literature. Other non-SSRI antidepressants, such as desipramine and reboxetine, have been investigated in the treatment of obese patients with BED, but these medications have not been studied in controlled trials and therefore are excluded from this summary. In general, dosages of SSRI antidepressants used in these studies are higher than those used in the treatment of depression and similar to those used for BN.

Fluoxetine

Two placebo-controlled trials of fluoxetine (Arnold et al., 2002; Grilo, Masheb, & Wilson, 2005) present mixed findings regarding the efficacy of fluoxetine in the reduction of binge eating. Arnold and colleagues (2002) suggested that fluoxetine was associated with a reduction in binge-eating episodes per week, modest weight loss, and moderate improvement in symptoms of depression. In contrast, Grilo and colleagues (2005) did not find that fluoxetine was superior to placebo on any outcome measure, including binge eating, ED and associated psychopathology, and depression.

Fluvoxamine

Although one controlled trial of fluvoxamine (Hudson et al., 1998) found that it was associated with improvements in binge-eating frequency and illness severity, a more

TABLE 22.1. Placebo-Controlled Trials of SSRI Antidepressants for BED

Study	Sample	Intervention[a]	Binge/ED symptoms[b]	Weight loss[c]	Psychological symptoms
Arnold et al. (2002)	$N = 60$	FLX (71.3 mg) vs. PLA, 6-week trial	**FLX (−70%)** > PLA (−55.7%) ($p = 0.033$)	**FLX (−3.9 kg)** > PLA (+0.7 kg) ($p = .001$)	Depressive symptoms measured by HAMD: FLX = PLA ($p = .061$)
Grilo, Masheb, & Wilson (2005)	$N = 54$	FLX (60 mg) vs. PLA, 16-week trial	FLX (−42%) = PLA (−45%) ($p = $ NS)	FLX (−0.7 BMI) = PLA (−0.0 BMI) ($p = $ NS)	Depressive symptoms measured by BDI ($p = $ NS)
Hudson et al. (1998)	$N = 85$	FLV (260 mg) vs. PLA, 9-week trial	**FLV (−79.3%)** > PLA (−39.8%) ($p < .001$)	**FLV (−2.7 lb)** > PLA (−0.3 lb) ($p = .04$)	Depressive symptoms measured by HAMD ($p = $ NS)
Pearlstein et al. (2003)	$N = 20$	FLV (239 mg) vs. PLA, 12-week trial	FLV (−78.9%) = PLA (−63.5%) ($p = $ NS)	FLV (−1 lb) > PLA (+4 lb) ($p = $ NS)	Depressive symptoms measured by BDI, HAMD ($p = $ NS)
McElroy et al. (2000)	$N = 34$	SERT (187 mg) vs. PLA, 6-week trial	**SERT (−85.5%)** > PLA (−45.8%) ($p < .01$)	**SERT (−12.3 lb)** > PLA (−5.3 lb) ($p < .01$)	Depressive symptoms measured by HAMD ($p = $ NS)
McElroy, Hudson, et al. (2003)	$N = 38$	CIT (57.9 mg) vs. PLA, 6-week trial	**CIT (−63.7%)** > PLA (−40.3%) ($p = .003$)	**CIT (−0.2 BMI)** > PLA (+1.5 BMI) ($p < .001$)	Depressive symptoms measured by HAMD **CIT > PLA** ($p = .05$)
Guerdjikova et al. (2007)	$N = 44$	ESCIT (26.5 mg) vs. PLA, 12-week trial	ESCIT (−81.6%) = PLA (−66.7%) ($p = $ NS)	**ESCIT (−1.0 kg)** > PLA (+0.6 kg) ($p = .037$)	Depressive symptoms measured by HAMD ($p = $ NS)

Note. NS, not significant; HAMD, Hamilton Depression Rating Scale; BDI, Beck Depression inventory; FLX, fluoxetine; PLA, placebo; FLV, fluvoxamine; SERT, sertraline; CIT, citalopram; ESCIT, escitalopram.
[a]Dosage expressed as end mean dosage (mg/day) unless otherwise indicated.
[b]Results expressed as percent decrease in binge episodes unless otherwise indicated.
[c]Mean weight loss or mean decrease in body mass index (BMI).

recent controlled trial (Pearlstein et al., 2003) did not find fluvoxamine to be superior to placebo on any treatment outcome variable. It is important to note that in the former trial, the dropout rate was significantly greater in the fluvoxamine group due to adverse events related to medication (Hudson et al., 1998).

Sertraline

One randomized controlled trial (McElroy et al., 2000) suggested that sertraline was associated with a greater decrease in binge-eating frequency and weight than placebo, as well as improvement in illness severity.

Citalopram

One randomized placebo-controlled trial of citalopram indicated that it may be helpful in reducing BED symptoms (McElroy, Hudson, et al., 2003). Compared to placebo, citalopram was associated with greater weight loss and decrease in binge eating days per week; however, the frequency of binge-eating episodes per week did not differ between the groups at the end of the 6-week trial (McElroy, Hudson, et al., 2003).

Escitalopram

In the single placebo-controlled trial of escitalopram in the treatment of BED, it was superior to placebo in decreasing body mass index (BMI) but not binge-eating frequency over the 12-week trial. A secondary endpoint analysis suggested a modest effect of escitalopram on binge-eating frequency (Guerdjikova et al., 2007).

Although some studies suggest that the SSRI class of antidepressants has positive effects in treating BED, no definitive conclusions regarding the effectiveness of SSRI antidepressants can be drawn because of the limited number of controlled trials to date and inconsistent findings. Additionally, no studies have investigated follow-up outcomes, so the maintenance of any improvements is largely unknown. As is the case throughout the BED treatment literature, there is a substantial placebo response rate, underscoring clinical reports that binge eating is often unstable and can be suppressed in the short term by a variety of specific and nonspecific interventions. Furthermore, despite some improvements in binge eating compared to placebo, many patients were not abstinent from binge eating at the end of treatment and no a priori factors have been identified that reliably predicted overall or differential treatment response.

Are Antiobesity Medications Superior to Placebo in the Treatment of BED?

Sibutramine is the only FDA-approved medication for weight loss that has been tried in placebo-controlled trials using medication as a sole intervention for BED (see Table 22.2). Orlistat, a non-CNS-acting medication approved by the FDA for weight loss, has been studied as a treatment for BED, but only in conjunction with other forms of treatment (i.e., dietary restriction or CBT), and therefore is not included in this section.

Three randomized controlled trials comparing sibutramine to placebo in the treatment of BED have been conducted. In all three trials sibutramine was associated with both a decrease in the frequency of binge-eating episodes and significant weight loss compared to placebo. Although not consistent throughout this literature, there is

TABLE 22.2. Placebo-Controlled Trials of Antiobesity Medications for BED

Study	Sample	Intervention[a]	Binge/ED symptoms[b]	Weight loss	Psychological symptoms
Appolinario et al. (2003)	N = 60	SIB (15 mg) vs. PLA, 12-week trial	SIB (−65.8%) > PLA (−41%) ($p = .03$)	SIB (−7.4 kg) > PLA (+1.4 kg) ($p < .001$)	Depressive symptoms measured by BDI: SIB > PLA ($p < .001$)
Milano et al. (2005)	N = 20	SIB (10 mg) vs. PLA, 12-week trial	SIB (−75.6%) > PLA (−6.38%) ($p < .01$)	SIB (−4.5 kg) > PLA (−059 kg) ($p < .01$)	Psychological symptoms measured by BES: SIB > PLA ($p < .001$)
Wilfley et al. (2008)	N = 304	SIB (15 mg) vs. PLA, 24-week trial	SIB (−81.8%) > PLA (−64.7%) ($p < .01$)	SIB (−1.6 BMI) > PLA (−0.4 BMI) ($p < .001$)	Depressive symptoms (p = NR)

Note. NR, not reported; BDI, Beck Depression Inventory; BES, Body Esteem Scale; SIB, sibutramine.
[a]Dosage expressed as end mean dosage (mg/day) unless otherwise indicated.
[b]Results expressed as percent decrease in binge episodes.

some evidence to suggest that sibutramine may also be associated with improvements in self-reported depression (Appolinario et al., 2003). Of note, sibutramine has been associated with several adverse events, including dry mouth, constipation, insomnia, and dizziness. In the obesity literature, sibutramine has also been associated with increased heart rate and is not recommended in patients with uncontrolled hypertension or a history of cardio- or cerebrovascular disease. For those able to tolerate these adverse reactions, sibutramine may be effective in reducing the frequency of binge-eating episodes as well as facilitating weight loss for up to 6 months of treatment (Wilfley et al., 2008).

Are Other Medications Superior to Placebo in the Treatment of BED?

Topiramate and Zonisamide

Due to their known side effect of weight loss, the anticonvulsants topiramate and zonisamide have also been studied as treatments for obese individuals who binge-eat (see Table 22.3). The results of two controlled trials of topiramate versus placebo (McElroy, Arnold, et al., 2003; McElroy, Hudson, et al., 2007) indicate that topiramate is superior to placebo in reducing the frequency of binge-eating episodes as well as facilitating weight loss. Topiramate was not associated with improvements in psychological symptoms; however, it was associated with overall improvement in illness severity in both studies. Despite these potential benefits, several adverse events were reported by patients taking topiramate, including paresthesias, dry mouth, headache, taste perversion, and cognitive problems (McElroy et al., 2004). Additionally, McElroy and colleagues (2004) conducted a 42-week open-label extension trial of topiramate, in which only 32% of participants who entered the study completed the trial. The main reasons for dropout were nonadherence to the protocol and adverse events. Among those able

TABLE 22.3. Placebo-Controlled Trials of Other Medications for BED

Study	Sample	Intervention[a]	Binge/ED symptoms[b]	Weight loss	Psychological symptoms
McElroy, Arnolt, et al. (2003)	$N = 61$	TOP (212 mg)[c] (TOP) vs. PLA, 14-week trial	**TOP (−94%)** > PLA (−46%) ($p < .001$)	**TOP (−5.9 kg)** > PLA (−1.2kg) ($p < .001$)	Depressive symptoms measured by HAMD (p = NS)
McElroy, Hudson, et al. (2007)	$N = 394$	TOP (300 mg) vs. PLA, 16-week trial	**TOP (−80.3%)** > PLA (−55.5%) > ($p < .001$)	**TOP (−4.5 kg)** > PLA (+0.2 kg) ($p < .001$)	Depressive symptoms measured by MADRS (p = NS)
McElroy et al. (2006)	$N = 60$	ZON (436 mg) vs. PLA, 16-week trial	ZON (−75%) = PLA (−72%) (p = NS)[d]	**ZON (−4.8 kg)** > PLA (−1.0 kg) ($p < .001$)[d]	Depressive symptoms measured by HAMD (p = NS)
McElroy, Guerdjikova, et al. (2007)	$N = 40$	ATX (106 mg) vs. PLA, 10-week trial	**ATX (−90%)** > PLA (−78%) ($p < .001$)	**ATX (−2.7 kg)** > PLA (−0.0 kg) ($p < .05$)	Depressive symptoms measured by HAMD (p = NS)

Note. NS, not significant; HAMD, Hamilton Depression Scale; MADRS, Montgomery–Asberg Depression Rating Scale; TOP, topiramate; ZON, zonisamide; ATX, atomoxetine.
[a]Dosage expressed as end mean dosage (mg/day) unless otherwise indicated.
[b]Results expressed as percent decrease in binge episodes.
[c]Median end dosage (mg/day).
[d]Results based on endpoint analysis.

to complete the trial, binge-eating frequency was significantly reduced; however, this finding may be overshadowed by the fact that topiramate was not well tolerated by a majority of the patients (McElroy et al., 2004).

A single controlled trial suggested that zonisamide may be helpful in decreasing binge eating and weight (McElroy et al., 2006). Similar to topiramate, however, zonisamide was relatively poorly tolerated by patients. Although superior to placebo in one controlled trial, further research is needed to determine the efficacy of zonisamide in treating BED, especially compared to more established or better tolerated interventions.

Atomoxetine

Atomoxetine, a norepinephrine reuptake inhibitor indicated for the treatment of attention-deficit/hyperactive disorder (ADHD), has been used in the treatment of BED due to its known appetite suppressant effects (see Table 22.3). In initial investigations, atomoxetine appears superior to placebo in decreasing binge-eating frequency as well as increasing weight loss; however, it does not appear to be effective in improving psychological symptoms of depression (McElroy, Guerdjikova, et al., 2007).

Do Antidepressants Enhance Treatment Benefits of Psychosocial Interventions for BED?

Combining medication with psychosocial interventions, such as psychotherapy or behavioral weight loss counseling, to treat BED may theoretically help, hinder, or have no effect in targeting the multiple domains of the disorder: eating, weight, and psychological symptoms; as previously mentioned, evidence concerning the utility of medication as a sole intervention is mixed. Potential benefits of medication in combination with psychosocial interventions include converting partial to full response, broadening the range of response (i.e., response in a separate domain, such as mood) or extending the duration of response. In addition to potential benefits of medication treatment, potential risks and costs should be considered. Ideally, future studies will identify subgroups of patients for whom the addition of medication is of particular benefit. To date, such differential predictors of response have not been identified.

The studies listed in Table 22.4 explore the question of whether antidepressants, most notably fluoxetine and fluvoxamine, enhance the benefit of behavior weight loss (BWL) treatment as well as traditional psychotherapies on frequency of binge eating, weight loss, and psychological symptoms. Because CBT is the most established form of psychotherapy in treating BED, most controlled trials have focused on the addition of medication to CBT specifically.

Selective Serotonin Reuptake Inhibitors

Three controlled trials have been conducted specifically examining the value of the addition of fluoxetine or fluvoxamine to psychotherapy (Devlin et al., 2005; Grilo, Masheb, & Wilson, 2005; Ricca et al., 2001). The results of all three trials suggest that these medications do not add to the effectiveness of psychotherapy on primary outcome measures, including binge-eating frequency and weight loss. Although one study

TABLE 22.4. Controlled Trials of Antidepressants plus Psychosocial Interventions for BED

Study	Sample	Intervention	Binge/ED symptoms[a]	Weight loss	Psychological symptoms
Ricca et al. (2001)	$N = 108$	CBT vs. CBT + FLX vs. CBT + FLV vs. FLX vs. FLV, 24-week trial, 1-year follow-up	CBT (−55.5%) = CBT + FLX (58.8%) = CBT + FLV (55.5%) (p = NS)	CBT (−2 BMI) = CBT + FLV (−2 BMI) = CBT + FLX (−3 BMI) (p = NS)	Depressive symptoms measured by BDI (p = NS)
Devlin et al. (2005)	$N = 116$	FLX vs. PLA vs. CBT + FLX vs. CBT + PLA (all in addition to BWL), 16-week trial, 2-year follow-up	BWL/CBT + FLX (−77.8%) = BWL/CBT + PLA (−69.2%) (p = NS)[b]	BWL/CBT + FLX (−2.93 kg) = BWL/CBT + PLA (−2.14 kg) (p = NS)[b]	Depressive symptoms measured by BDI: **BWL/CBT + FLX** > BWL/CBT + PLA (p < .05)[b]
Grilo, Masheb, & Wilson (2005)	$N = 108$	FLX vs. PLA vs. CBT + FLX vs. CBT + PLA, 16-week trial	CBT + FLX (−69%) = CBT + PLA (−89%) (p = NS)	CBT + FLX (−0.8 BMI) = CBT + PLA (−0.4 BMI) (p = NS)	Depressive symptoms measured by BDI: CBT + FLX = CBT + PLA (p = NS)
Agras et al. (1994)	$N = 108$	BWL vs. CBT followed by BWL vs. CBT/BWL + DMI, 9-month treatment, 3-month follow-up	**CBT/BWL + DMI (32% abst)** > CBT/BWL (28% abst) (p = NS)[d]	**CBT/BWL + DMI (−4.8 kg)** > CBT/BWL (−0.0 kg) (p = < .05)[e]	Depressive symptoms measured by BDI (p = NS)
Laederach-Hofmann et al. (1999)	$N = 31$	IMI vs. PLA (in addition to DCST), 8-week trial, 6-month open phase without continued medication treatment	**DCST + IMI (−72.7%)** > DCST + PLA (−28.3%) (p = .02)	**DCST + IMI (−2.2 kg)** > DCST + PLA (+ .02 kg) (p < .05)	Depressive symptoms measured by HAMD: **DCST + IMI** > DCST + PLA (p < .02)

Note. NS, not significant; BWL, behavioral weight loss; BDI, Beck Depression Inventory; HAMD, Hamilton Depression Scale; CBT, cognitive-behavioral therapy; FLX, fluoxetine; FLV, fluvoxamine; DMI, desipramine; IMI, imipramine; PLA, placebo; DCST, diet counseling and supportive therapy; BMI, body mass index; abst, abstinent.
[a]Results expressed as percent decrease in binge episodes unless otherwise indicated.
[b]Main effect of fluoxetine added to psychotherapy, including patients receiving BWL only and BWL with CBT.
[c]Baseline binge-episode frequency not reported.
[d]Results expressed as percent abstinent from binge eating at 3-month follow-up.
[e]Mean weight loss at 3-month follow-up.

found the addition of fluoxetine to BWL treatment to be associated with a greater improvement of depressive symptoms (Devlin et al., 2005), this finding has not been consistent in this literature.

Other Antidepressants

The tricyclic antidepressants desipramine and imipramine have also been studied in combination with psychosocial interventions for the treatment of BED in controlled trials (Agras et al., 1994; Laederach-Hofman et al., 1999). Based on the results of these two trials, evidence is mixed regarding the additive effect of tricyclic antidepressants on reduction in binge-eating frequency during treatment. However, both studies suggest that the addition of imipramine or desipramine during treatment may be helpful in increasing the amount of weight loss in the short term following treatment, interestingly, even after medication is discontinued.

Do Antiobesity or Other Medications Enhance Treatment Benefits of Psychosocial Interventions for BED?

In addition to the controlled trials of antidepressants, trials of antiobesity and other medications have also been conducted in conjunction with psychosocial interventions (see Table 22.5). Overall, findings suggest that orlistat and topiramate may add additional weight loss benefits to psychosocial interventions, but their effect on reducing binge eating remains unclear.

Orlistat

Based on the results from two controlled trials of the addition of orlistat to CBT guided self-help or mildly reduced caloric diet (Golay et al., 2005; Grilo, Masheb, & Salant, 2005), orlistat appears superior to placebo in decreasing weight. Additionally, Grilo, Masheb, and Salant (2005) found this weight loss to be maintained at 3-month follow-up. Although orlistat does appear to enhance weight loss, it did not significantly improve binge eating compared to placebo in either study (Grilo, Masheb, & Salant, 2005; Golay et al., 2005).

Topiramate

One controlled trial of CBT plus topiramate (M end daily dosage 205.8 mg) suggested that when added to CBT, topiramate may be beneficial in enhancing both remission

TABLE 22.5. Controlled Trials of Antiobesity and Other Medications plus Psychosocial Interventions for BED

Study	Sample	Intervention	Binge/ED symptoms[a]	Weight loss	Psychological symptoms
Grilo, Masheb, & Salant (2005)	$N = 50$	CBT + ORL vs. CBT + PLA, 12-week trial, 3-month follow-up	CBT + ORL (−77.7%) = CBT + PLA (−78.1%) (p = NS)[b]	CBT + ORL (−3.4 kg) = CBT + PLA (−1.3 kg) (p = .09)[b]	Depressive symptoms measured by BDI (p = NS)
Golay et al. (2005)	$N = 89$	Mildly hypocaloric diet + ORL vs. diet + PLA, 24-week trial	diet + ORL (−81.5%) = diet + PLA (−72.6%) (p = NS)	**Diet + ORL** (−7.4%) > diet + PLA (−2.3%) (p < .0001)	Depressive symptoms measured by BDI, HAD (p = NS)
Claudino et al. (2007)	$N = 73$	CBT + TOP vs. CBT + PLA, 21-week trial	Remission rates **CBT + TOP (84%)** > CBT + PLA (61%) (p = .03)	**CBT + TOP (−6.8 kg)** > CBT + PLA (−.9 kg) (p < .001)	Depressive symptoms measured by BDI (p = NS)

Note. RCT, randomized controlled trial; NS, not significant; BDI, Beck Depression Inventory; HAD, Hospital Anxiety and Depression; EDI, Eating Disorder Inventory; CBT, cognitive-behavioral therapy; ORL, orlistat; TOP, topiramate; PLA, placebo.
[a]Results expressed as percent decrease in binge episodes unless otherwise indicated.
[b]Results based on intent-to-treat analysis.

from binge eating and weight loss for at least 5 months (Claudino et al., 2007). Interestingly, in this trial, topiramate was somewhat better tolerated than in previous trials, with only 1 of 37 participants discontinuing topiramate due to adverse events.

Conclusion

Based on initial trials of antidepressants, antiobesity medications, and other medications known to effect appetite or weight, there is significant evidence suggesting that medication as a sole treatment may be superior to placebo in reducing the frequency of binge eating. As indicated by Reas and Grilo (2008), pharmacological treatments yielded significantly greater remission rates from binge eating as compared to placebo in the short term (48.7 vs. 28.5%). However, to the degree that efficacy in reducing binge eating is the primary factor driving clinical decision making, there is little to suggest that medication, as opposed to CBT, should be considered the treatment of choice for BED (Wilson, Grilo, & Vitousek, 2007). In fact, two controlled trials indicate that when compared, CBT alone is more effective in reducing BED symptoms than medication alone (Grilo, Masheb, & Wilson, 2005; Ricca et al., 2001). Nonetheless, medication treatment might be chosen for reasons of availability, cost, preference, or alternative treatment goals, such as weight reduction or improvement in comorbid psychiatric disorders. As with all interventions, potential benefits must be weighed against risks, including adverse short-term effects, long-term effects of continued treatment, and effects of discontinuation.

The evidence that antidepressant, antiobesity, or other medications may improve psychological symptoms in patients with BED is extremely limited. In contrast, there is significant evidence that antiobesity and anticonvulsant medications, in particular, may have a beneficial effect on weight in obese patients with BED. Longer-term study of this phenomenon is needed; however, based on the obesity literature, the likely long-term outcome is that lost weight will be regained following medication cessation, even if benefits on binge eating are maintained.

Limiting enthusiasm for the apparent short-term benefits of antidepressants, antiobesity, and other medications on binge eating is the fact that few controlled trials have been conducted with any particular medications, and no studies have reported follow-up information. Although there is some evidence that medications are more effective than placebo alone in reducing binge-eating frequency, the current literature suggests that medications do not add to the effectiveness of CBT or other psychosocial interventions in reducing binge eating or psychological symptoms. For patients receiving psychosocial treatment, there is some indication that the addition of certain medications (antiobesity, anticonvulsant) may enhance weight loss, if tolerated, but there are few hints of any additional benefits (i.e., improvements of binge eating or psychological symptoms).

As we embark on the next generation of treatment studies for BED, several potential roles for medication remain, even for patients for whom CBT or other empirically supported psychological therapies are readily available. First, it is possible that a subgroup of patients may respond preferentially to CBT augmented by medication. As yet, no predictors or moderators of response to pharmacotherapy have been identified. One recent report suggests that early response to treatment may represent a subgroup of responders that is more likely to meet response criteria at the end of the trial (Grilo,

Masheb, & Wilson, 2006). Additional findings regarding predictors of outcome, particularly *a priori* predictors, could help determine treatment and may in turn lead to better treatment success. In addition, nonresponders to initial treatment with CBT or other psychotherapies may conceivably respond to the addition of medication. Certainly, individuals who have stopped binge eating but who have not lost significant amounts of weight may benefit from considering available treatment options for obesity, including BWL, pharmacological, and surgical approaches. Finally, it is possible that medication may play a role in restoring the response of individuals who relapse following an initial favorable response to psychotherapy or behavioral counseling. Longitudinal studies with large numbers of participants will be needed to answer these questions and to fully mine the potential benefits of medications in treating the behavioral, somatic, and psychological aspects of BED.

References

Agras WS, Telch CF, Arnow B, Eldredge K, Wilfley DE, Raeburn SD, et al. (1994). Weight loss, cognitive-behavioral, and desipramine treatments in binge eating disorder: An additive design. *Behavior Therapy*, 25:225–238.

Appolinario JC, Bacaltchuck J, Sichieri R, Claudino AM, Godoy-Matos A, Morgan C, et al. (2003). A randomized, double-blind, placebo-controlled study of sibutramine in the treatment of binge-eating disorder. *Archives of General Psychiatry*, 60:1109–1116.

American Psychiatric Association. (2000). *Diagnostic and statistical manual of mental disorders* (4th ed., text rev.). Washington, DC: American Psychiatric Association.

Arnold LM, McElroy SL, Hudson JI, Welge JA, Bennett AJ, & Keck PE. (2002). A placebo-controlled, randomized trial of fluoxetine in the treatment of binge-eating disorder. *Journal of Clinical Psychiatry*, 63:1028–1033.

Claudino AM, de Oliveira IR, Appolinario JC, Cordas TA, Duchesne M, Sichieri R, et al. (2007). Double-blind, randomized, placebo-controlled trial of topiramate plus cognitive-behavior therapy in binge-eating disorder. *Journal of Clinical Psychiatry*, 68:1324–1332.

Devlin MJ, Goldfein JA, & Dobrow I. (2003). What is this thing called BED?: Current status of binge eating disorder nosology. *International Journal of Eating Disorders*, 34:2–18.

Devlin MJ, Goldfein JA, Petkova E, Jiang H, Raizman PS, Wolk S, et al. (2005). Cognitive behavioral therapy and fluoxetine as adjuncts to group behavioral therapy for binge eating disorder. *Obesity Research*, 13:1077–1088.

Golay A, Laurent-Jaccard A, Habicht F, Gachoud JP, Chabloz M, Kammer A, et al. (2005). Effect of orlistat in obese patients with binge eating disorder. *Obesity Research*, 13:1701–1708.

Grilo CM, Masheb RM, & Salant SL. (2005). Cognitive behavioral therapy guided self-help and orlistat for the treatment of binge eating disorder: A randomized, double-blind, placebo-controlled trial. *Biological Psychiatry*, 57:1193–1201.

Grilo CM, Masheb RM, & Wilson GT. (2005). Efficacy of cognitive behavioral therapy and fluoxetine for the treatment of binge eating disorder: A randomized double-blind placebo-controlled comparison. *Biological Psychiatry*, 57:301–309.

Grilo CM, Masheb RM, & Wilson GT. (2006). Rapid response to treatment for binge eating disorder. *Journal of Counseling and Clinical Psychology*, 74:602–613.

Guerdjikova AI, McElroy SL, Kotwal R, Welge JA, Nelson E, Lake K, et al. (2007). High-dose escitalopram in the treatment of binge-eating disorder with obesity: A placebo-controlled monotherapy trial. *Human Psychopharmacology*, 23:1–11.

Hudson JI, McElroy SL, Raymond NC, Crow S, Keck PE Jr, Carter WP, et al. (1998). Fluvoxamine in the treatment of binge-eating disorder: A multicenter placebo-controlled, double-blind trial. *American Journal of Psychiatry*, 155:1756–1762.

Laederach-Hofmann K, Graf C, Horber F, Lippuner K, Lederer S, Michel R, et al. (1999). Imipramine and diet counseling with psychological support in the treatment of obese binge eaters: A randomized, placebo-controlled double-blind study. *International Journal of Eating Disorders*, 26:231–244.

McElroy SL, Arnold LM, Shapira NA, Keck PE, Rosenthal NR, Karim MR, et al. (2003). Topiramate in the treatment of binge eating disorder associated with obesity: A randomized, placebo-controlled trial. *American Journal of Psychiatry*, 160:255–261.

McElroy SL, Casuto LS, Nelson EB, Lake KA, Soutullo CA, Keck PE, Jr, et al. (2000). Placebo-controlled trial of sertraline in the treatment of binge eating disorder. *American Journal of Psychiatry*, 157:1004–1006.

McElroy SL, Guerdjikova A, Kotwal R, Welge JA, Nelson EB, Lake KA, et al. (2007). Atomoxetine in the treatment of binge-eating disorder: A randomized placebo-controlled trial. *Journal of Clinical Psychiatry*, 68:390–398.

McElroy SL, Hudson JI, Capece JA, Beyers K, Fisher AC, & Rosenthal NR. (2007). Topiramate for the treatment of binge eating disorder associated with obesity: A placebo-controlled study. *Biological Psychiatry*, 61:1039–1048.

McElroy SL, Hudson JI, Malhotra S, Welge JA, Nelson EB, & Keck PE, Jr. (2003). Citalopram in the treatment of binge-eating disorder: A placebo-controlled trial. *Journal of Clinical Psychiatry*, 64:807–813.

McElroy SL, Kotwal R, Guerdjikova AI, Welge JA, Nelson EB, Lake KA, et al. (2006). Zonisamide in the treatment of binge eating disorder with obesity: A randomized controlled trial. *Journal of Clinical Psychiatry*, 67:1897–1906.

McElroy SL, Shapira NA, Arnold LM, Keck PE, Jr, Rosenthal NR, Wu SC, et al. (2004). Topiramate in the long-term treatment of binge-eating disorder associated with obesity. *Journal of Clinical Psychiatry*, 65:1463–1469.

Milano W, Petrella C, Casella A, Capasso A, Carrino S, & Milano L. (2005). Use of sibutramine, an inhibitor of the reuptake of serotonin and noradrenaline, in the treatment of binge eating disorder: A placebo-controlled study. *Advances in Therapy*, 22:25–31.

Pearlstein T, Spurell E, Hohlstein LA, Gurney V, Read J, Fuchs C, et al. (2003). A double blind, placebo-controlled trial of fluvoxamine in binge eating disorder: A high placebo response. *Archive of Women's Mental Health*, 6:147–151.

Reas DL, & Grilo CM. (2008). Review and meta-analysis of pharmacotherapy for binge-eating disorder. *Obesity*, 16:2024.

Ricca V, Mannucci E, Mezzani B, Moretti S, Di Bernardo M, Bertelli M, et al. (2001). Fluoxetine and fluvoxamine combined with individual cognitive-behaviour therapy in binge eating disorder: A one-year follow-up study. *Psychotherapy and Psychosomatics*, 70:298–306.

Stunkard AJ. (1959). Eating patterns and obesity. *Psychiatic Quarterly*, 33:284–295.

Wilfley DE, Crow SJ, Hudson JI, Mitchell JE, Berkowitz RI, Blakesley V, et al. (2008). Efficacy of sibutramine for the treatment of binge eating disorder: A randomized multicenter placebo-controlled double-blind study. *American Journal of Psychiatry*, 165:4–6.

Wilson GT, Grilo CM, & Vitousek K. (2007). Psychological treatments for eating disorders. *American Psychologist*, 62:199–216.

Special Topics in Treatment

This section includes material on a variety of treatment issues that did not fit neatly into Parts II or III of this book. However, all these topics are of great relevance to clinicians and researchers who work with and treat patients with eating disorders (EDs).

Part IV begins with a chapter that provides an overview of treating eating disorders in childhood, by Rachel Bryant-Waugh and Bryan Lask. Childhood EDs are an area of great clinical importance that has been largely neglected in the past, and the authors' summary of material in this area will be of great interest to clinicians who work with younger patients and their families.

Martina de Zwaan then discusses the treatment of obesity in patients with binge-eating disorder (BED). Since many patients seen clinically with BED also have excess weight, this chapter is of considerable importance to clinicians who work with these patients. Although several of the psychotherapeutic treatments developed thus far for BED result in significant reductions in binge eating, most do not impact significantly on weight.

Melissa A. Kalarchian, Marsha D. Marcus, and Anita P. Courcoulas offer a chapter on eating problems in bariatric surgery patients. We know from research in this area that a sizeable subgroup of bariatric surgery candidates have significant eating problems in addition to their severe obesity, including problems with binge eating and night eating. Emerging research has revealed that abnormal eating patterns can also develop or recur after bariatric surgery. This chapter summarizes what is known about the clinical significance of disordered eating pre- and postoperatively and provides important guidance to clinicians. Given the growing frequency of bariatric surgery for severe obesity, more of these patients are being seen by professionals who work with EDs.

Howard Steiger and Mimi Israel provide an overview of the treatment of psychiatric comorbidities in patients with EDs in Chapter 26. We know that comorbidities in patients with EDs, including mood disorders, anxiety disorders, substance use disorders, and personality disorders, are seen very frequently in patients with EDs. The presence of such psychiatric comorbidities raises complex questions about when and how treatments for EDs should incorporate components to address these other issues as well.

The next chapter in this section, by Kelly C. Allison and Albert J. Stunkard from the University of Pennsylvania, provides a review of night eating syndrome, which Stunkard originally described more than 50 years ago. These authors also provide detailed information about the treatment of individuals with this syndrome. Although the data here are quite limited, Allison and Stunkard suggest several useful approaches to working with these individuals.

In Chapter 28 Susan J. Paxton and Siân A. McLean provide an overview of treatment for body image disturbances. This material is relevant for patients with any form of ED. We know that body image comprises complex multidimensional constructs and represents particularly difficult-to-treat aspects of EDs.

Elizabeth Goddard, Pam MacDonald, and Janet Treasure then provide a chapter on caregiver issues in EDs, an area in which they have done some of the most important work. They have documented the tremendous psychosocial burden associated with caring for and supporting someone with an ED. This has been a relatively neglected topic and is one of great clinical importance to those working with patients with EDs and their families. This chapter provides exciting information regarding emerging interventions geared toward helping the caregivers themselves.

The final chapter in Part IV, by Scott G. Engel and Stephen A. Wonderlich, provides an overview of new technologies in ED treatment. These investigators are at the forefront of research into the use of different technologies in the treatment of EDs and they have done much work using ecological momentary assessment as a way of gathering data on patients in their natural environment. This work has great promise and may play an important role in disseminating treatments and making them readily available to many more patients.

CHAPTER 23

Treatment of Childhood Eating Difficulties and Disorders

Rachel Bryant-Waugh and Bryan Lask

We begin by defining "childhood" and "eating disorders" for the purposes of this chapter. The term "childhood" is used here to cover the age range from approximately 6 to 13 years. Such age boundaries are inevitably arbitrary to some extent. It is important, however, to be clear that this chapter does not describe the treatment of infants and young children with feeding disorders nor of adolescent-onset anorexia nervosa (AN) and bulimia nervosa (BN).

We interpret the term "eating disorders" broadly because of all children presenting with clinically significant eating disturbances, a minority will be likely to have the "true" eating disorders of AN, BN, or a related eating disorder not otherwise specified (EDNOS) presentation. Therefore, as well as including discussion of AN and BN with childhood onset (for which we use the term "eating disorders"), we also include discussion of a wider range of eating disturbances. These include presentations that are characterized by disturbed or disordered eating, and associated with clinically significant impairment in one or more areas of development or functioning, but are not accompanied by the abnormal weight and shape cognitions associated with AN/BN. We do not regard these as EDNOS presentations, but as clinical eating disturbances that remain poorly classified in current diagnostic systems. We outline the main types of childhood eating disturbances seen in clinical practice below. Systematic data on prevalence and prognosis are largely unavailable for these presentations, as this group of patients remains relatively poorly studied. Some follow-up data are available for childhood-onset AN, the outcome of which is similar to that seen in adolescence. Fuller details of these conditions can be found in Lask and Bryant-Waugh (2007).

The main types of eating disturbance/disorder in childhood are described below:

- *Selective eating (SE)* refers to when children limit their food intake to a very narrow range of preferred foods, often high in carbohydrates, as selective eaters. Many such children maintain a normal weight and height and do not have significant impairments in other areas of functioning. When the child is thriving and developing normally, treatment may not be indicated. In some children this type of eating is present in the context of clinical features of an autistic spectrum disorder. SE can reach clinical significance requiring intervention when it results in chronic nutritional inadequacies and/or a significant deleterious impact on social development or family functioning.

• *Food avoidance emotional disorder (FAED)* is characterized by limited food intake and weight loss, with associated generalized mood disturbance and/or anxiety (Higgs, Goodyear, & Birch, 1989). It should be distinguished from appetite loss secondary to depression or medical illness; in children with FAED the eating disturbance is the main presenting problem. Such children can become acutely physically compromised. They usually recognize that they are thin and express a wish to be bigger but find it extraordinarily difficult to eat. In a number of cases there is a personal or family history of medically undiagnosed physical symptoms, and there may have been previous episodes of poor eating. This presentation can initially appear very similar to AN but core cognitive disturbances in relation to weight and shape, and weight management behaviors such as excessive exercising and vomiting, are absent.

• *Restrictive eating* refers to an apparently intrinsic tendency toward having a small appetite and limited food intake in terms of quantity, but not in terms of texture or range. Again there tend to be no abnormal cognitions in relation to weight or shape and no significant mood disturbance. Weight and height tend to track lower centiles. This presentation can become clinically significant when limited intake inhibits normal growth or pubertal development, and in situations where the child's eating has had a significant negative effect on family relationships and functioning.

• *Specific fear/phobia leading to avoidance of eating.* Some children present with disturbed eating related to specific fears or phobias. Commonly encountered fears include contamination, poisoning, vomiting, and fear of swallowing or choking (functional dysphagia). The child associates the ingestion of food or specific foodstuffs with a feared outcome to be avoided. Such children can present as very underweight and physically compromised, and may be extremely distressed. None of the abnormal cognitions of AN/BN is present, and there is often a clear precipitant.

• *AN* does occur in children from around the age of 7 years upward but remains relatively rare below the age of 10. The clinical presentation is broadly similar to that of adults, with an obvious exception in relation to amenorrhea. Boys often present as being more concerned with fat avoidance for health and fitness rather than weight reasons, and frequently have comorbid obsessive–compulsive symptoms.

• *BN* is rare below age 12, and the comorbid features, such as self-harming and substance misuse, that are common in adolescents and young adults with BN are very unusual in this younger age group. Despite a number of adult patients recalling having first developed BN in childhood, there is limited evidence of full diagnostic presentations in this younger age range.

• *Pervasive refusal syndrome (PRS)* is characterized by a profound and pervasive avoidance of eating, drinking, walking, talking, and self-care accompanied by marked resistance to treatment (Lask, 2004). Refusal to eat is therefore only one of a number of refusal behaviors, but it inevitably leads to weight loss. This can be a very difficult and distressing disorder to treat; it is difficult to elicit any underlying thoughts and feelings driving the refusal behavior, as most of these children are noncommunicative. In some children there may have been preceding trauma or abuse.

Treatment Research and Evidence-Based Interventions

Robust treatment research in children (distinct from adolescents) with eating disorders (EDs) and disturbances is almost nonexistent. There are a number of reasons why this might be the case. First, there are continuing difficulties regarding the adequacy of existing diagnostic criteria for EDs to capture the developmental nuances in childhood-onset eating problems seen in clinical practice (Bravender et al., 2007). Second, and related to this first point, inconsistent terminology is used to describe clinical presentations, hampering research endeavors. Third, onset of AN below the age of 13 is relatively rare, and onset of BN below the age of 13 even rarer, thus requiring multicenter studies to ensure sufficient power. Such studies, although necessary, have not yet been conducted, not least because they are so difficult to set up. Also this group of patients is particularly difficult to recruit into research projects for a number of reasons. They are commonly in denial of their illness, miserable and frightened, resistant to authority, and antagonistic to therapeutic endeavors. Obtaining true and informed consent is a considerable challenge.

Despite the paucity of empirical evidence, however, our clinical experience suggests the utility of a number of important basic principles in guiding treatment. These are outlined in the next section.

Basic Principles of Management

Comprehensive Assessment

Comprehensive assessment is an essential component of the management of childhood EDs and disturbances. Assessment must cover different aspects of the child's current state and areas of functioning, as outlined below. Due to the multidisciplinary nature of the assessment required, we would generally recommend the involvement of more than one clinician. Inherent to the assessment of the eating disturbance is assessment of risk in relation to each of the areas outlined below. Risk may differ significantly between individual children and their families, even though there may be superficial similarities in presentation.

Physical Assessment

Physical assessment is of considerable importance given that children with eating difficulties are far more likely than adults to suffer physical decompensation, due to their relative lack of fat reserves and their need for adequate nutrition to ensure growth. Physical assessment usefully includes evaluation of weight, height, body mass index (BMI) percentile or weight-for-height (WfH) ratio adjusted for age, blood pressure and pulse rate, peripheral circulation, and state of hydration. Physical observation can sometimes detect the presence of unhealthy behaviors. For example, salivary gland enlargement, dental erosion, or Russell's sign (scarring on the knuckles or dorsum of the hand) may be present in children who are self-inducing vomiting in order to try to control shape/weight. Laboratory tests may be indicated, including a full blood count, urea, and electrolytes to include phosphate and magnesium levels. Pelvic ultrasound can be useful to assess degree of maturity of reproductive organs and menstrual status, and bone scans and assessment of bone age may assist in the evaluation of skeletal growth and bone health.

Nutritional Assessment

Nutritional assessment and detailed information about current intake should be gathered from the parents as well as from the child. It is important to consider major omissions from the current diet not just in energy terms but also in terms of nutritional adequacy. For example, in those with SE, some key nutrients/food groups may be missing. Identification of missing components of a balanced diet is important as it can help prioritize which new food types might be addressed most helpfully. As in so many other respects, prioritization of intervention should be informed via risk assessment; in this example, nutritional risk.

Psychological and Neuropsychological Assessment

Psychological and neuropsychological assessment should include mood, anxiety, behavior, thought content and form, attitudes, motivational stage, cognitive maturity, educational functioning, and social and peer group skills. Approximately 70% of children with AN have been shown to have significant neuropsychological anomalies (Brewerton, Frampton, & Lask, in press; Frampton & Hutchinson, 2007), specifically attention to detail at the cost of central coherence, weak visuospatial memory, and impaired cognitive flexibility. These anomalies, which appear to be primary (i.e., predating the illness and therefore possible risk factors) have often gone unrecognized. Such children tend to have perfectionistic tendencies and will often work excessively hard to ensure success. Indeed they are likely to be overachieving at considerable emotional cost. Recognition of these issues may inform treatment formulation and planning of interventions to improve coping and psychosocial adaptation.

Family Assessment

Family assessment is critical since the parents (and family) are vital to the child's physical and emotional well-being. It is important to assess family strengths and those areas where assistance could be helpful. Specific attention needs to be paid to the ability of the parents to work well together, to be consistent between each other and over time, to communicate well with each other, and to allow sufficient age-appropriate autonomy while providing clear and appropriate boundaries. The impact of the ED on family members, including siblings, is also helpful to assess.

Formulation and Treatment Planning

As stated above, a number of commonly seen childhood eating disturbances are difficult to formally diagnose (Nicholls, Christie, Randall, & Lask, 2001). In this patient group, diagnosis is not the primary means of determining appropriate treatment intervention. A more useful approach is to use a case formulation format to provide the link between assessment and treatment. A good formulation will include a description of the nature and severity of the presenting problem as well as a conceptualization of factors that are believed to have contributed to, and are serving to maintain, the current difficulty. Intervention is usefully guided by prioritization on the basis of areas of risk combined with consideration of maintaining factors open to change through treatment input.

Once assessment is complete and a formulation has been discussed with the family, a treatment plan should be constructed via consultation with all concerned. The treatment plan should include aims, content, roles and responsibilities, and a time frame for review and, when required, modification. The aims should be based on the outcome of the assessment, incorporating risk factors, and should be comprehensive rather than focused simply on restoration of healthy weight or of a normal eating pattern. In our view, treatment for childhood EDs and disturbances must include attention to eating issues as a primary, though not necessarily exclusive, focus. Content of treatment is individually tailored to the child's developmental, psychological, and physical status, as well as family strengths and potential. Some components of treatment that we have found to be consistently useful are discussed below.

Comprehensive Treatment

Integral to the successful implementation of any treatment plan is teamwork, wherein the team is comprised of clinicians, parents, and ultimately the children themselves, working together in a collaborative manner. The tendency of childhood eating disturbances to be associated with considerable resistance to treatment (often understandable when the child's and/or parent's anxiety regarding change is acknowledged) makes high-quality teamwork essential. Implicit in such an ethos is the importance of clarity regarding each person's roles and responsibilities, including the issue of leadership.

When the child is being treated as an outpatient, the parent or parents need to be the leaders because they are responsible for their child 24 hours a day. The clinicians should act as advisers, counselors, and consultants to the child and parent(s), their prime task being to advise and support parents, rather than dictating what should be done. If the child is hospitalized, then clearly the clinicians must take charge but should always work as collaboratively as possible with the child and parents.

Everyone involved (child, parents, and clinicians) needs to have as clear an understanding as possible of the nature of the presenting problem and any identified underlying or contributory factors. Because parents and children will be required to make informed decisions in relation to treatment, providing them with relevant information that includes possible causes, course, outcome, and treatment is essential. Information should be made available to siblings in an age-appropriate format. Also important is the matter of addressing parental anxiety. The understandable intensity of their anxiety can impair their ability to take in information, think, and act, sometimes making it difficult for them to adopt a constructive approach to treatment. Alleviating parents' anxiety, helping them to understand their child's behavior, and taking an empathic and nonpunitive approach are all essential.

Finally, successful teamwork must be based on consistency and clear communication. Consistency needs to be present between all team members, as well as over time. Inconsistency in either domain leads to confusion and splitting, and is bound to delay recovery. Regardless of the content of the treatment plan, consistency is essential.

Physical Approaches

Refeeding

Children who are significantly underweight to the extent that they are physically comprised, and/or growth and development are impaired need to return to a healthy weight range. Addressing high-risk nutritional deficiencies, dehydration, and electrolyte imbalance may need to be prioritized. Because the exact weight that constitutes a healthy weight will vary among individuals, we find it generally unhelpful to cite a specific target weight. Attaining a specific weight is less important that the return of normal, age-appropriate physical functioning and development. We would recommend that plans to increase an underweight child's intake should be formulated in liaison with parents, as much as possible, with the child's cooperation, although many children with AN are terrified and initially unable to contribute actively to their own treatment. The child's likes and dislikes and motivational stage need to be considered, and when the child is an outpatient, plans discussed for how parents will manage mealtimes in terms of amounts the child is expected to eat and how to deal with the child's distress. Parents can be supported to specify non-negotiable expectations, for example, approximate amount of calories ingested per day. When a child has eaten very little over a prolonged period, there should be a gradual buildup of caloric intake (an additional 200–300 kilocalories [kcal] every third day or so). Refeeding syndrome is a rare complication of too rapid refeeding. Avoiding this syndrome in high-risk patients includes gradual buildup of calories, administration of prophylactic phosphate, avoidance of high-carbohydrate fluids, and medical monitoring (see Hart, 2007). In general, a refeeding plan should be based on regular meals and snacks that allow for variety, flexibility, and spontaneity.

Medications

Medications have little part to play in the first-line treatment of childhood eating disturbances. There is no significant evidence that any medications or vitamin or mineral supplements truly enhance appetite, and any such deficiencies are readily overcome by adequate nutrition.

Antidepressants should be used only in children after very careful consideration and with considerable caution. The depression often associated with malnutrition is usually alleviated once nutritional health is restored. When this is not the case, or in other situations where depression is clearly evident, it is wise to use a combination of cognitive-behavioral therapy (CBT) and parental counseling in the first instance. Should these fail, then the cautious use of a low-dose selective serotonin reuptake inhibitor (SSRI) might be considered, introduced at a dose of 25% of the intended therapeutic dose and increased at intervals of 3–4 days. However, there should be close monitoring for side effects, especially suicidal thoughts or high levels of anxiety (Lask, Taylor, & Nunn, 2003). The emergence of such side effects should lead to immediate reduction of the dose to that being used prior to onset of the side effects.

Anxiolytics and atypical antipsychotics have a minimal role in the management of childhood eating disturbances. Anxiolytics may be used, but with considerable care and only for short periods, in those children with anxiety, phobias, or obsessionality.

Atypical antipsychotics should be reserved for children suffering extreme anxiety or distress associated with their ED.

Physical Activity/Exercise

Physical activity and exercise are important components of healthy everyday life and can contribute to an improved sense of well-being. Unfortunately, excessive exercise can also play a major part in unhealthy attempts to control weight and serves to alleviate anxiety in AN (it is less significant in some of the other childhood eating problems). Clinicians often become overconcerned with attempting to control the child's activity levels, with subsequent intensification of the child's resistance to treatment and a failure to appreciate the anxiety-relieving significance. Decisions about activity levels are best made within the context of the therapeutic alliance, in discussion with the parents, and with concerns about weight being balanced against consideration of the child's physical and emotional needs for exercise.

Psychological Approaches

Family Approaches

Parental (or primary carer) involvement is essential in the management of childhood eating problems. Involvement of other family members is indicated to a greater or lesser extent depending on individual circumstances. Family work might include regular sessions with the whole family, working separately with parents, or a focus on relationships between siblings. The formulation is important in identifying key areas for work. EDs and disturbances inevitably have an effect on all members of the family. However, this does not mean that the family is the cause of the problem. In general, we recommend a focus on three main domains in relation to family work: (1) supporting parents to manage their child's food intake and mealtimes; (2) addressing the "currency" of weight and shape within the family; and (3) facilitating the expression, acknowledgment, and acceptance of different emotional experiences between family members. Above all, family approaches need to encourage the appropriate exercising of parental responsibility for the child's well-being, combined with attention to key issues of independence and control.

Individual Approaches

Individual therapy with the child is not always necessary, but, when indicated, should be offered alongside or as part of the work with the family. The choice of therapy is less likely to be diagnosis driven and more likely to be problem focused. An essential early step in any successful individual work is the development of a therapeutic alliance. Because of the frequent and intense resistance to treatment, often underpinned by anxiety about change and loss of control, successful treatment of eating difficulties is especially dependent on a good therapeutic alliance between child, parents, and clinicians. Key components to creating such an alliance include a facilitative therapeutic stance, provision of clear and adequate information, avoiding coercion as much as possible, acknowledging and exploring anxieties, focusing on motivation (see below),

and utilizing a range of nonblaming, nonpathologizing techniques, such as externalization (see below). The means for achieving the therapeutic alliance is child-specific and
based on age, developmental status, personality, and motivational stage (see below).

There is no evidence at this stage that any one form of individual therapy is superior
to another and, in practice, given the range of different types of presentation as well
as differences in individual children's cognitive, social, and emotional development,
a number of different approaches might usefully be considered. In our experience,
some children respond well to a cognitive-behavioral approach; in those with restricted
eating in relation to specific phobias as well as SE, a combination of desensitization
and anxiety management strategies can be helpful. Individual interventions based on
understanding and working with presenting problem behaviors within a developmental and systemic framework can also be very useful. In this type of individual work,
the young person and the therapist seek to explore, understand, and address current
patterns of thought and behavior in relation to his/her past experiences as well as contributory factors in the child's family, school, or wider environment (Bryant-Waugh,
2006).

Cognitive remediation represents a novel, theoretically based, user-friendly (including child) approach to the management of the neuropsychological anomalies mentioned
above. The approach, which focuses on cognitive styles rather than content (the "how"
rather than the "what" of thinking), has been adapted from its use in brain injury and
schizophrenia (Delahunty & Morice, 1993). In this way it differs from more traditional
therapies such as CBT and psychodynamic psychotherapy. Cognitive remediation might
involve, for example, providing exercises to help widen a focus on fine detail at the cost
of the whole picture, or to improve impaired cognitive flexibility or poor visuospatial
memory. Session content is determined by a consideration of neuropsychological deficits and identification of subsequent strengths and weaknesses related to everyday life,
leading to the learning and practicing of new strategies and their application to everyday life (Tchanturia, Davies, & Campbell, 2007; Tchanturia et al., 2008).

Other specific techniques that may be useful include externalization and motivational interviewing. Many children with eating difficulties are seen by others as being
wilfully difficult, as choosing to behave in the way that they do for illogical or incompre-
hensible reasons. Although there is an element of choice in many such circumstances,
to some extent, it is by no means as categorical as generally considered. In other words,
the element of choice is best considered on a continuum, at one end of which the child
is in complete control of his/her eating and is making an autonomous decision not to
eat. At the other end is the child, most commonly with AN or BN, who is "in the grips"
of the illness and has little or no control of his/her eating. Most commonly children
do not fall at one end or the other of this continuum. Rather they lie between the two,
with some degree, but not complete freedom, of choice. This concept would normally
be conveyed to the child and parents during the provision of information (see above).

Externalization is the process of making a clear distinction between the child and
the disorder/illness. In this context, rather than conceptualizing the child as choosing
to behave the way that he/she does, it is possible to use wording such as, "It seems like
the AN is very demanding/controlling today." There are numerous variants on this
theme and ways of utilizing the concept. Many children can give a name to the AN, be
it "the anorexia," "my voice," and so on. When this happens the child is already using

externalization, but in any event, it is useful to incorporate the concept into the "language of treatment" and use it as often as seems helpful/appropriate.

The child's motivation—that is, readiness and willingness to overcome the eating difficulties—does, to some extent, determine the nature of treatment. Motivation is described as having five stages: (1) *precontemplation*—no insight or awareness of there being a problem and therefore extreme resistance to change; (2) *contemplation*—awareness of a problem but no wish to change; (3) *preparation*—awareness and a wish to change at some point in the future; (4) *action*—awareness and a wish to take action to overcome the problem; and (5) *maintenance*—a wish to do what is necessary to maintain the changes made (Prochaska & DiClemente, 1983). There is commonly some overlap among these stages and movement between them in either direction.

In our clinical experience children who are predominantly in the precontemplation or contemplation stage will require a different approach from those predominantly in the preparation or action stage. Children in the former group have very limited or even no insight, are only being seen because of parental concerns, and themselves resist all efforts to treat them.

In taking a motivational approach the stance adopted by the clinician is characterized by supportiveness, warmth, respect, empathy, honesty, acceptance, curiosity, humility, and flexibility. It differs, however, from many therapeutic approaches in having a primary focus on motivation rather than change. The therapist recognizes that any attempt to encourage change may be experienced as coercive, with subsequent anxiety and resistance to that change. Consequently, the therapist's agenda is devoid of efforts to change the child's behavior but rather involves exploration of the child's lack of motivation to change. This exploration, sometimes referred to as motivational interviewing, helps both the child and the therapist to understand the constraints to change. In time this process leads to the child progressing through the motivational stages to the point of wishing to change and to overcome the problem (Lask, Geller, & Srikameswaran, 2007).

Techniques used in motivational interviewing include:

- *Open questioning*—asking questions that do not lead to a "yes" or "no" answer, but rather allow for a wide range of answers and subsequently a broader discussion
- *Reflective listening*—reflecting back to the child what he/she has said, using slightly different words, thus helping the child to feel listened to and understood
- *Affirming*—warm and respectful validation of the child's perspective, consequently helping the child to feel accepted
- *Tracking*—following and responding to the child's thoughts and feelings, with no attempt to set or follow an agenda, accordingly helping the child to feel safe enough to set his/her own agenda
- *Exploring ambivalence*—acknowledging the mixed feelings the child might have about his/her problem(s), thus helping the child to feel less confused and better understood, and to weigh the pros and cons of change
- *Summarizing*—a more complex form of reflective listening, in which the therapist summarizes not only what has just been said but attempts to capture the essence of all that has been said in the session, thus providing a reflection of the bigger picture

- *Draining*—a detailed and exhaustive exploration of the advantages of staying ill/not changing, the purpose being to gain a joint understanding of how the problems may actually be helpful to the child.
- *Transferring*—exploring other areas of the child's life to which the advantages of staying ill might be applied, for example, feeling special and in control, consequently helping him/her to consider how she might achieve the good feelings without having to endanger her health

Parents can usually be included in the sessions, providing that their presence does not inhibit the child. Their participation allows parents to better understand their child's motivation to resist change. Motivational interviewing is not an exclusive treatment but rather complementary to other approaches. It can be utilized as a treatment in its own right, with or without other treatments. It can also be used in everyday conversations with the child. Its primary focus is to enhance motivation rather than to reduce symptoms, so that the wish for change comes from within the child rather than being imposed upon him/her. Motivational interviewing is in keeping with the creation and maintenance of a therapeutic alliance and is likely to lead to more complete and sustained change.

Schooling

It is important to assess whether the child is well enough to attend school and, if so, how much work and physical activity are appropriate for him/her. Many children with AN are desperate to continue their schoolwork, despite being far too ill to do so, and manage to convince their parents to allow them to do so. Such children are also usually perfectionistic and are driven to achieve at very high levels, often in the face of cognitive difficulties (see above). Peer-group pressures in many areas are common, especially around weight and shape. These pressures are particularly problematic for children with EDs. All these issues require careful consideration by the parents and clinical team.

Conclusions

We have described the common clinical presentations of EDs and disturbances in children and discussed some basic management principles and strategies. In our view it is essential to conduct a detailed comprehensive assessment, as there are no diagnosis-linked evidence-based treatments for this patient group. We have recommended the use of risk assessment and formulation to inform the content and prioritization of treatment efforts and described some techniques for working with young people that have been found to be useful. The central tenets of successful management of these young patients are collaborative and consistent teamwork, the promotion of effective parenting, and the establishment of noncoercive relationships with children that acknowledge and address motivation and anxiety.

References

Bravender T, Bryant-Waugh R, Herzog D, Katzman D, Kreipe RD, Lask B, et al. (2007). Classification of child and adolescent eating disturbances: Workgroup for classification of eating disorders in children and adolescents (WCEDCA). *International Journal of Eating Disorders*, 40:117–122.

Brewerton T, Frampton I, & Lask B. (in press). The neurobiology of anorexia nervosa. *European Review of Psychiatry*.

Bryant-Waugh R. (2006). Pathways to recovery: Promoting change within a developmental systemic framework. *Clinical Child Psychology and Psychiatry*, 2:213–224.

Delahunty A, & Morice R. (1993). *A training programme for the remediation of cognitive deficits in schizophrenia*. Albury, NSW, Australia: Department of Health.

Frampton I, & Hutchinson A. (2007). Eating disorders and the brain. In B Lask & R Bryant-Waugh (Eds.), *Eating disorders in childhood and adolescence* (3rd ed., pp. 125–148). London: Routledge.

Hart M. (2007). Nutrition and refeeding. In B Lask & R Bryant-Waugh (Eds.), *Eating disorders in childhood and adolescence* (3rd ed., pp. 199–214). London: Routledge.

Higgs J, Goodyer I, & Birch J (1989). Anorexia nervosa and food avoidance emotional disorder. *Archives of Disease in Childhood*, 64:346–351.

Lask B. (2004). Pervasive refusal syndrome. *Advances in Psychiatric Treatment*, 10:153–159.

Lask B, & Bryant-Waugh R. (Eds.). (2007). *Eating disorders in childhood and adolescence* (3rd ed.). London: Routledge.

Lask B, Geller J, & Srikameswaran S. (2007). Motivational approaches. In B Lask & R Bryant-Waugh (Eds.), *Eating disorders in childhood and adolescence* (3rd ed., pp. 177–198). London: Routledge.

Lask B, Taylor S, & Nunn K. (2003). *Practical child psychiatry: The clinician's guide*. Oxford, UK: Blackwell.

Nicholls D, Christie D, Randall L, & Lask B. (2001). Selective eating: Symptom, disorder or normal variant. *Clinical Child Psychology and Psychiatry*, 6:257–270.

Prochaska J, & DiClemente C. (1983). Stages and processes of self-change of smoking: Towards an integrative model of change. *Journal of Counseling and Clinical Psychology*, 51:390–295.

Tchanturia K, Davies H, & Campbell I. (2007). Cognitive remediation therapy for patients with anorexia nervosa: Preliminary findings. *Annals of General Psychiatry*, 10:1186–1214.

Tchanturia K, Davies H, Lopez C, Schmidt U, Treasure J, & Wykes T. (2008). Neuropsychological task performance before and after cognitive remediation in anorexia nervosa: A pilot case series. *Psychological Medicine*, 38:1371–1373.

CHAPTER 24

Obesity Treatment
for Binge-Eating Disorder in the Obese

Martina de Zwaan

The treatment of binge-eating disorder (BED) poses a special problem relative to other eating disorders (EDs), given that obesity is a major comorbidity in BED patients. In the National Cormobidity Survey Replication 27.6% of the participants with BED had a body mass index (BMI) between 30 and 39.9 kg/m^2 and 14.8% $\geq$40 kg/m^2 (Hudson, Hiripi, Pope, & Kessler, 2007). Although BED does occur in normal-weight and even underweight individuals, individuals with BED who present for treatment are usually obese. Normal-weight individuals with BED may not be sufficiently distressed to seek treatment, which might explain the selection bias toward obese samples in clinical studies. The prevalence of binge eating also increases with increasing levels of obesity. Consequently, those in the BED subgroup of obese are among those at highest risk for medical complications of obesity. In addition, the presence of binge eating in obese individuals appears to be associated with both medical and psychiatric conditions independent of the effect of obesity (Reichborn-Kjennerud, Bulik, Sulivan, Tambs, & Harris, 2004).

Devlin, Goldfein, and Dobrow (2003) described four theoretical models of BED, two of which are related to obesity. First, BED might be a meaningful behavioral subtype of obesity. Even though there is evidence that binge eating may contribute to the development of obesity, there is no evidence that the available treatments for binge eating bring about significant weight loss. The second model posits BED as an epiphenomenon that emerges when obesity co-occurs in those with psychopathology (general or eating-related). Psychopathology might be the mediator in the relationship between obesity and BED. Accordingly, BED would not be a disorder in its own right—which would have implications for the targets in treatment.

Clinicians working with patients with BED who are obese are faced with the challenge of encouraging weight loss or at least preventing additional weight gain. In treating obese patients with BED there are several potential goals for treatment, including cessation of binge eating, weight loss or prevention of further weight gain, improvement of physical health, and reduction of psychological disturbances. Goals must be prioritized, preferably without impacting negatively on other goals. Combining treatment for binge eating with the treatment of obesity, with the goal of reducing both binge eating and excess weight, may be useful. However, since treatment trials for weight reduction have generally not produced sustained weight loss outcomes, and weight fluctuations are thought to have some potential adverse consequences, "anti-diet" or "non-diet" approaches have received considerable publicity. Such an approach targets the improvement of physical and psychological health by nondieting interventions, such as increasing exercise and normalizing food intake, as well as qualitative changes in diet composition and modifications of negative body image and poor self-esteem. Alternatively, one can conceptualize obesity as a chronic disease requiring ongoing treatment for extended periods of time. Even though clinicians often wish to focus on the binge-eating behavior, the clinical reality is that these patients primarily want and usually seek treatment for weight loss.

This chapter begins with a short overview of weight loss and weight loss maintenance findings in samples of obese patients. I then provide an overview of data on the effects of weight loss treatments on obese patients with and without binge-eating behaviors, and also summarize the findings regarding weight loss in treatments targeting the binge-eating behaviors.

Weight Loss, Weight Loss Maintenance, and Weight Regain in Obese Persons

In a clinical review Jain (2005) concluded that even effective dietary and exercise treatments for adult obesity produce only modest weight loss, usually resulting in a mean loss of about 3–5 kg, which is 5–10% of initial body weight. Weight loss medications also produce, on average, 3–5 kg of weight loss, but the effects often do not last after the medication is stopped. Such modest amounts of weight loss, if maintained, are associated with physical and psychosocial benefits for some obese people. For example, a 5–10% reduction of excess body weight, maintained for at least 1 year, reduces risk factors for diabetes and cardiovascular disease in some persons. However, standard weight loss interventions based on promoting lifestyle changes and increased physical activity are difficult to sustain, and the weight losses are almost always regained over time (Curioni, & Lourenço, 2005; Shaw, Gennat, O'Rourke, & Del Mar, 2006). Patients treated with lifestyle modification generally regain 30–35% of their lost weight in the year after treatment and will have regained the majority, if not all, of the lost weight by 5 years (Jeffery et al., 2000). Furthermore, once weight gain occurs, further weight loss is challenging (Wing & Phelan, 2005). Jain (2005) concluded that despite the high prevalence of obesity, there is a surprising lack of high-quality clinical weight loss trials, dropout rates are usually high, and that intention-to-treat analyses are rarely conducted. In addition, with few exceptions (Franz et al., 2007), participants in weight loss programs are usually followed for only 1 year or less after their initial weight loss, which is an inadequate duration to properly assess weight loss maintenance.

It has become increasingly clear that some weight loss is achievable by adults, but that long-term weight maintenance is very rare. In an effort to learn more about those individuals who have been successful at long-term weight loss, Wing and Hill established the National Weight Control Registry (NWCR) in 1994 (*www.nwcr.ws*; Wing & Phelan, 2005). There is considerable variety in how NWCR members maintain their weight loss long term. Most reported continuing to maintain a low-calorie, low-fat diet and doing high levels of activity; 78% report eating breakfast every day; 75% weigh themselves at least once a week; 62% watch less than 10 hours of TV per week; and 90% exercise, on average, about 1 hour per day. Further predictors of successful weight loss maintenance were lower levels of dietary inhibition and of objective binge eating as well as lower levels of depressive symptoms. Medical reasons for initiating weight loss were associated with better weight loss maintenance. Finally, individuals who had kept their weight off for 2 years or more were more likely to continue to maintain their weight. Only a few people recovered from even minor lapses of 1–2 kg. Other factors that were positively related to long-term weight loss maintenance were reaching a self-determined goal weight, internal motivation to lose weight, social support, and the use of better coping strategies (Elfhag & Rössner, 2005). The issue of how to prevent, or at least minimize, the weight regain that follows treatment for obesity has become a research priority.

The Effect of Weight Loss Treatments in Obese Individuals with BED

Estimates of the prevalence of BED among patients seeking weight loss treatments vary markedly, depending on recruitment and assessment methods, and frequently range up to roughly 30%. Interview-based studies usually produce lower rates of BED, with rates sometimes less than 5% in obesity treatment samples, although as many as 10–25% in weight loss samples report binge eating without meeting full diagnostic criteria for BED (Mitchell, Devlin, de Zwaan, Crow, & Peterson, 2008).

Obese patients who binge-eat have been found to respond to weight loss programs similarly to non-binge-eating obese patients. Reviews of the literature on weight loss programs have concluded that binge eating apparently does not affect short-term weight loss or attrition rate (American Psychiatric Association, 2006; de Zwaan & Mitchell, 2001; Wonderlich, de Zwaan, Mitchell, Peterson, & Crow, 2003). No difference in weight loss between obese patients with and without BED have been found in behavior weight loss therapy (Marcus, Wing, & Hopkins, 1988). Also, in a large-scale study using telephone- and mail-based behavioral weight control for obesity in managed care samples, binge-eating status at baseline was not associated with outcome (Linde et al., 2004). This study suggested that level of depression and low-weight self-efficacy may be more powerful predictors of weight loss than binge eating, particularly for obese women. The authors recommended considering mood management in obesity interventions.

Short-term weight loss with a very-low-calorie diet (VLCD) is usually excellent, with about 20% of initial body weight lost (Yanovski, Gormally, Leser, Gwirtsman, & Yanovski, 1994); however, many patients rapidly regain any weight lost, and weight regain may be accompanied by a return of binge-eating behavior. Yanovski and colleagues (1994) reported that patients with BED were more likely than non-binge-eaters to experience larger lapses in adherence during fasting and during refeeding as well as early weight regain of lost weight. The overall amount of weight lost and regained, however, did not differ between patients with and without BED. de Zwaan and colleagues

(2005) reported no difference in rate and amount of weight loss and regain between subjects with and without BED participating in a VLCD program; both groups regained approximately three-quarters of the lost weight in a 1-year follow-up. It is important to note that weight regain is common in all general medical and psychological treatments for obesity and not only for obesity associated with BED (American Psychiatric Association, 2006). Interestingly, VLCD programs are even effective in reducing binge-eating frequency. Fifty-six percent of the VLCD participants who met criteria for BED at baseline did not meet diagnostic criteria 1 year after the end of a VLCD diet (Raymond, de Zwaan, Mitchell, Ackard, & Thuras, 2002). The absence of a BED diagnosis at 1-year follow-up after the VLCD diet was associated with less weight gain at 1-year follow-up, regardless of baseline diagnosis. Thus, binge eating may pose a risk for weight regain (Elfhag & Rössner, 2005).

A few studies have reported a negative influence of BED on weight loss. For example, Pagoto and colleagues (2007) reported that only 16% of the participants with BED achieved a 7% weight reduction in a hospital-based weight loss program, as opposed to 38% of the participants without BED. Furthermore, a recent matched-study meta-analysis (Blaine & Rodman, 2007) concluded that in weight loss treatments, non-BED samples lost on average 10.7 kg, whereas BED samples lost 1.5 kg, corresponding to average percent weight losses of 2 and 11%. However, the rather unusual methodology of this meta-analysis calls the results into question.

It is important to keep in mind that most of the above studies included individuals who were primarily interested in weight loss, and they may represent a different group of individuals than those who present specifically for treatment of binge eating. A few studies have specifically compared the effect of a behavior weight loss treatment (BWLT) with moderate caloric restriction to cognitive-behavioral therapy (CBT) targeting BED in obese individuals with BED (Agras et al. 1994; Devlin et al., 2005; Goodrick et al., 1998; Grilo & Masheb, 2005; Grilo, Masheb, Brownell, Wilson, & White, 2007; Munsch et al., 2007). Overall, BWLT generally resulted in somewhat more weight loss, but overall the amount of weight lost and maintained was low, whereas at the end of treatment CBT usually was significantly superior in reducing binge-eating frequency. Nauta, Hospers, Kok, and Janssen (2000) reported that cognitive therapy (CT) was more effective than behavior therapy (BT) in terms of abstinence from binge eating, but BT resulted in greater weight loss than CT. It might be expected that weight loss treatment will, by encouraging increased dietary restraint, promote the onset of binge eating. However, caloric restriction does not appear to exacerbate binge eating among obese patients with BED. In fact, in recent studies there is even some evidence that, in the long run, BWLT can be as effective as CBT for BED in reducing binge eating (Grilo et al., 2007; Munsch et al., 2007). Many of the behavioral components of BWLT overlap with those of CBT for BED, and it may be that the inclusion of strategies such as the encouragement of regular meals and snacks, the promotion of self-acceptance, and the use of stimulus control is effective in reducing binge eating in patients with BED.

Bariatric Surgery

Conventional approaches to the management of obesity generally have proven unsuccessful for the morbidly obese (BMI ≥ 40 kg/m^2), encouraging the development of effective surgical treatments. The Swedish Obese Subjects study demonstrated that during an average of 10.9 years of follow-up after bariatric surgery, long-term weight loss, reduced comorbidity, and decreased overall mortality was seen (Sjöström et al., 2007). The most commonly used procedures in the United States are gastric bypass and gastric banding. On average, patients maintain a weight loss of 25–40% of their preoperative body weight after these procedures. BED appears to be common among the morbidly obese presenting for bariatric surgery, with prevalence rates ranging from 1.4 to 49% (median 20%) (de Zwaan, 2005), depending on the means of assessment. In a recent study in which the Structured Clinical Interview for DSM-IV Axis I Disorders (SCID) was conducted to assess presurgery comorbidity, the lifetime prevalence of BED was 27.1% and the current prevalence was 16.0% (Kalarchian et al., 2007). In most studies baseline BED presurgery was not associated with poorer postoperative weight loss (Burgmer et al., 2005; de Zwaan, 2005; White, Masheb, Rothschild, Burke-Martindale, & Grilo, 2006). There is consensus that bariatric surgery reduces or eliminates binge eating at least in the short-term postsurgical period. This is probably attributable to the fact that most patients are unable to consume objectively large amounts of food after such a procedure, given the mechanical limitations on food intake.

There is growing evidence that non-normative eating behavior may reemerge following surgery. The emergence or reemergence after surgery of binge-eating problems, including loss of control and "grazing," might be related to poorer results with regard to weight loss or greater weight regain (Burgmer et al., 2005; Colles, Dixon, & O'Brien, 2008; de Zwaan, 2005; Niego, Kofman, Weiss, & Geliebter, 2007, Scholz et al., 2007). In a group of 59 gastric bypass patients 2 years, on average, after gastric bypass, 25% reported subjective bulimic episodes (SBEs; i.e., loss of control while eating quantities of food that are not unusually large) and more than half reported at least weekly episodes. SBEs were significantly more common in participants with a presurgical ED and were associated with less weight loss (de Zwaan et al., 2009). These findings are consistent with data from Colles and colleagues (2008), who reported that 20% of patients, 1 year after gastric banding, were identified as both "uncontrolled eaters" and "grazers" and exhibited poorer weight loss and a poorer psychological outcome. However, in most studies the amount of weight lost in "uncontrolled eaters," or those who experience loss of control or grazing, was still statistically and clinically significant.

Summary

Obese binge-eating subjects have been found to respond to weight loss programs similarly to non-binge-eating subjects. Most studies on the use of weight loss programs found that binge eating did not affect weight loss, adherence to diet, or attrition. There is even some evidence for lower attrition rates in binge-eating subjects. However, there is also some evidence for greater weight regain when binge eating reemerges after treatment. Weight loss treatments do not exacerbate binge-eating problems and, in fact, are associated with short-term reductions in binge eating. Consequently, there is little empirical evidence to suggest that those obese individuals who binge-eat and who are primarily seeking weight loss should receive a different treatment than obese individuals who do not binge-eat. However, in focusing on weight reduction, we are confronted with the well-known problem that obesity treatment is associated with a poor long-term maintenance of weight reduction, and binge eating may recur when weight is regained. The American Psychiatric Association Guidelines (2006) suggest that patients with a history of repeated weight loss followed by weight gain ("yo-yo" dieting) or patients with an early onset of binge eating might benefit from programs that focus on decreasing binge eating rather than losing weight. However, there is no research evidence to support this opinion.

Weight Loss
and Weight Loss Maintenance in BED Treatments

Psychological Treatment

In clinical studies as well as in routine clinical work most patients with BED present with some degree of overweight and obesity. Psychological approaches (e.g., CBT, interpersonal psychotherapy, dialectical behavior therapy) to BED treatment have resulted in little weight loss at the end of treatment and at follow-up, with no substantial differences between treatment approaches (Wilson, Grilo, & Vitousek, 2007). This finding seems somewhat counterintuitive since the reduction or cessation of binge-eating episodes would seem to lead to an overall reduction in calorie consumption, which should promote weight loss. It might be that calories previously consumed during binge-eating episodes become distributed over nonbinge meals after treatment, which would contribute to the lack of weight change in BED treatment (Brownley, Berkman, Sedway, Lohr, & Bulik, 2007). Thus, although specific psychological approaches to BED treatment have demonstrated efficacy for reducing binge eating and enhancing psychological functioning, excess weight continues to be a problem for most patients with BED.

It must be kept in mind that binge eating may increase the risk of obesity (Neumark-Sztainer et al., 2006). Although non-weight-focused therapy approaches may not promote significant weight loss, they may be associated with less weight gain. Hence, successful BED treatment might play a role in the prevention of obesity.

Pharmacotherapy

In a recent meta-analysis of pharmacotherapy for BED, Reas and Grilo (2008) also examined the effect of pharmacotherapy on weight loss. They reported a significant weight reduction of 3.4 kg for medication compared to placebo, with modest effects for selective serotonin reuptake inhibitors (SSRIs; fluoxetine, fluvoxamine, sertralin, citalopram, escitalopram) and larger effects for antiepileptic (topiramate, zonisamide) and antiobesity (sibutramine) medications. However, topiramate has several adverse central nervous system (CNS) side effects, the most disturbing being cognitive impairment and paresthesias, which raises serious questions regarding the utility of this drug in patients with BED. The average mean weight loss for medication was 3.5 kg versus 0.08 kg for placebo across the 14 trials. The observed percent weight loss achieved with medication equaled 3.2% of baseline body weight. The authors also provided a review of eight studies combining pharmacotherapy with psychotherapy interventions. There was evidence that the addition of topiramate and orlistat to CBT and the addition of imipramine or orlistat to diet and behavioral treatments enhanced weight loss outcomes, whereas SSRIs did not improve weight loss outcome. The lack of follow-up data, especially with regard to weight maintenance after withdrawal of medication, raises serious questions about the importance of these results. In addition, a weight loss of 3 kg or 3% of baseline weight is not substantial; in fact, this amount falls in the lower range of what is achieved with most weight loss programs. Lastly, since medications exert their effect only during active treatment, there is little reason to expect that weight loss would be maintained following medication discontinuation, and rebound weight gain after termination of the drug is common. Also for medication trials there is some evidence that patients who stop binge-eating entirely lose significantly more weight than those who are not abstinent at the end of treatment (Agras et al., 1994; Devlin et al., 2005; Grilo, Masheb, & Wilson, 2005).

Summary

Even though certain therapies, particularly CBT, are successful in reducing binge-eating frequency in the short term, this reduction results in only modest weight loss, if any. Patients seeking psychotherapy treatment should be informed that all psychological treatments for BED have a limited effect on body weight. Concurrent or consecutive interventions focusing on the management of comorbid obesity should be considered. There is evidence that patients who stop binge-eating lose more weight and are usually more successful in maintaining their weight loss than those who do not stop binge-eating.

References

Agras WS, Telch CF, Arnow B, Eldredge K, Wilfley DE, Reaburn SD, et al. (1994). Weight loss, cognitive-behavioral, and desipramine treatments in binge-eating disorder: An additive design. *Behavior Therapy*, 25:225–238.

American Psychiatric Association. (2006). *Practice guidelines for the treatment of patients with eating disorders* (3rd ed.). Washington, DC: Author. Available online at *www.psych.org/psych–pract/*.

Brownley KA, Berkman ND, Sedway JA, Lohr KN, & Bulik C.M. (2007). Binge-eating disorder treatment: A systematic review of randomized controlled trials. *International Journal of Eating Disorders*, 40:337–348.

Burgmer R, Grigutsch K, Zipfel S, Wolf AM, de Zwaan M, Husemann B, et al. (2005). The influence of eating behavior and eating pathology on weight loss after gastric restriction operations. *Obesity Surgery*, 15:684–691.

Colles SL, Dixon JB, & O'Brien PE. (2008). Grazing and loss of control related to eating: Two high-risk factors following bariatric surgery. *Obesity*, 16:615–622.

Curioni CC, & Lourenço PM. (2005). Long-term weight loss after diet and exercise: A systematic review. *International Journal of Obesity*, 29:1168–1174.

de Zwaan M. (2005). Weight and eating changes after bariatric surgery. In JE Mitchell & M de Zwaan (Eds.), *Bariatric surgery: A guide for mental health professionals* (pp. 77–100). New York: Routledge.

de Zwaan M, Hilbert A, Swan-Kremeier L, Simonich H, Lancaster K, Howell LM, et al. (2009). *A comprehensive interview assessment of eating behavior 2 years after gastric bypass surgery for morbid obesity.* Manuscript submitted for publication.

de Zwaan M, & Mitchell JE. (2001). Binge eating disorder. In JE Mitchell (Ed.), *The outpatient treatment of eating disorders: A guide for therapists, dietitians, and physicians* (pp. 59–96). Minneapolis: University of Minnesota Press.

Devlin MJ, Goldfein JA, & Dobrow I. (2003). What is this thing called BED?: Current status of binge eating disorder nosology. *International Journal of Eating Disorders*, 34:S2–S18.

Devlin MJ, Goldfein JA, Petkova E, Jiang H, Raizman PS, Wolk S, et al. (2005). Cognitive behavioral therapy and fluoxetine as adjuncts to group behavioral therapy for binge eating disorder. *Obesity Research*, 13:1077–1088.

Elfhag K, & Rössner S. (2005). Who succeeds in maintaining weight loss?: A conceptual review of factors associated with weight loss maintenance and weight regain. *Obesity Review*, 6:67–85.

Franz MJ, VanWormer JJ, Crain AL, Boucher JL, Histon T, Caplan W, et al. (2007). Weight-loss outcomes: A systematic review and meta-analysis of weight-loss clinical trials with a minimum 1-year follow-up. *Journal of the American Dietetic Association*, 107:1755–1767.

Goodrick GK, Wadden TA, Poston WSC, Kimball KT, Reeves RS, & Foreyt JP. (1998). Nondieting versus dieting treatment for overweight binge-eating women. *Journal of Consulting and Clinical Psychology*, 66:363–368.

Grilo CM, & Masheb RM. (2005). A randomized controlled comparison of guided self-help cognitive behavioral therapy and behavioral weight loss for binge eating disorder. *Behaviour Research and Therapy*, 43:1509–1525.

Grilo CM, Masheb RM, Brownell KD, Wilson GT, & White MA. (2007). *Randomized comparison of cognitive behavioral therapy and behavioral weight loss treatments for obese patients with binge eating disorder: 12-month outcomes.* Paper presented at the World Congress of Behavioral and Cognitive Therapy, Barcelona, Spain.

Grilo CM, Masheb RM, & Wilson GT. (2005). Efficacy of cognitive behavioural therapy and fluoxetine for the treatment of binge eating disorder: A randomized double-blind placebo-controlled comparison. *Biological Psychiatry*, 57:301–309.

Hudson JI, Hiripi E, Pope HG, & Kessler RC. (2007). The prevalence and correlates of eating disorders in the National Comorbidity Survey Replication. *Biological Psychiatry*, 61:348–358.

Jain A. (2005). Treating obesity in individuals and populations. *British Medical Journal*, 331:1387–1390.

Jeffery RW, Drewnowski A, Epstein LH, Stunkard AJ, Wilson GT, Wing RR, et al. (2000). Long-term maintenance of weight loss: Current status. *Health Psychology*, 19:5–16.

Kalarchian MA, Marcus MD, Levine MD, Courcoulas AP, Pilkonis PA, Ringham RM, et al. (2007). Psychiatric disorders among bariatric surgery candidates: Relationship to obesity and functional health status. *American Journal of Psychiatry*, 164:328–334.

Linde JA, Jeffery RW, Levy RL, Sherwood NE, Utter J, Pronk NP, et al. (2004). Binge eating disorder, weight control self-efficacy, and depression in overweight men and women. *International Journal of Obesity and Related Metabolic Disorders*, 28:418–425.

Marcus MD, Wing RR, & Hopkins J. (1988). Obese binge eaters: Affect, cognitions, and response to behavioural weight control. *Journal of Consulting and Clinical Psychology*, 56:433–439.

Mitchell JE, Devlin MJ, de Zwaan M, Crow SJ, & Peterson CB. (Eds.). (2008). *Binge eating disorder: Clinical foundation and treatment.* New York: Guilford Press.

Munsch S, Biedert E, Meyer A, Michael T, Schlup B, Tuch A, et al. (2007). A randomized comparison of cognitive behavioral therapy and behavioral weight loss treatment for overweight individuals with binge eating disorder. *International Journal of Eating Disorders*, 40:102–113.

Nauta H, Hospers H, Kok G, & Jansen A. (2000). A comparison between a cognitive and a behavioral treatment for obese binge eaters and obese non-binge eaters. *Behavior Therapy*, 31:441–461.

Neumark-Sztainer D, Wall M, Guo J, Story M, Haines J, & Eisenberg M. (2006). Obesity, disordered eating, and eating disorders in a longitudinal study of adolescents: How do dieters fare 5 years later? *Journal of the American Dietetic Association*, 106:559–568.

Niego SH, Kofman MD, Weiss JJ, & Geliebter A. (2007). Binge eating in the bariatric surgery population: A review of the literature. *International Journal of Eating Disorders*, 40:349–359.

Pagoto S, Bodenlos JS, Kantor L, Gitkind M, Curtin, C, & Ma Y. (2007). Association of major depression and binge eating disorder with weight loss in a clinical setting. *Obesity*, 15:2557–2559.

Porzelius LK, Houston C, Smith M, Arfken C, & Fisher E. (1995). Comparison of a standard behavioral weight loss treatment and a binge eating weight loss treatment. *Behavioral Therapy*, 26:119–134.

Raymond NC, de Zwaan M, Mitchell JE, Ackard D, & Thuras P. (2002). Effect of a very low calorie diet on the diagnostic category of individuals with binge eating disorder. *International Journal of Eating Disorders*, 31:49–56.

Reas DL, & Grilo CM. (2008). Review and meta-analysis of pharmacotherapy for binge-eating disorder. *Obesity*, 16:2024–2038.

Reichborn-Kjennerud T, Bulik CM, Sulivan P, Tambs K, & Harris JR. (2004). Psychiatric and medical symptoms in binge eating in the absence of compensatory behaviors. *Obesity Research*, 12:1445–1454.

Scholz S, Bidlake L, Morgan J, Fiennes A, El-Etar A, Lacey JH, et al. (2007). Long-term outcome following laparoscopic adjustable gastric banding: Postoperative psychological sequelae predict outcome at 5-year follow-up. *Obesity Surgery*, 17:1220–1225.

Shaw K, Gennat H, O'Rourke P, & Del Mar C. (2006). Exercise for overweight or obesity. *Cochrane Database of Systematic Reviews*, Issue 4 (Article No. 003817), DOI: 10.1002/14651858.CD003817.pub3.

Sjöström L, Narbro K, Sjöström CD, Karason K, Larsson B, Wedel H, et al. (2007). Swedish obese subjects study: Effects of bariatric surgery on mortality in Swedish obese subjects. *New England Journal of Medicine*, 357:741–752.

White MA, Masheb RM, Rothschild BS, Burke-Martindale CH, & Grilo CM. (2006). The prognostic significance of regular binge eating in extremely obese gastric bypass patients: 12-month postoperative outcomes. *Journal of Clinical Psychiatry*, 67:1928–1935.

Wilson GT, Grilo CM, & Vitousek KM. (2007). Psychological treatment of eating disorders. *American Psychologist*, 62:199–216.

Wing RR, & Phelan S. (2005). Long-term weight loss maintenance. *American Journal of Clinical Nutrition*, 82(Suppl.):222–225.

Wonderlich SA, de Zwaan M, Mitchell JE, Peterson C, & Crow S. (2003). Psychological and dietary treatments of binge eating disorder: Conceptual implications. *International Journal of Eating Disorders*, 34:S58–S73.

Yanovski SZ, Gormally JF, Leser MS, Gwirtsman HE, & Yanovski JA. (1994). Binge eating disorder affects outcome of comprehensive very-low-calorie diet treatment. *Obesity Research*, 2:205–212.

CHAPTER 25

Eating Problems and Bariatric Surgery

Melissa A. Kalarchian, Marsha D. Marcus, and Anita P. Courcoulas

The acceptance and popularity of bariatric surgery have grown due to increases in the prevalence of obesity, advances in surgical technique, and mounting evidence of the benefits of the procedures. In this chapter we begin with an overview of the history of bariatric surgery for the mental health professional. We then provide information on eating problems in patients before and after the operation, concluding with treatment recommendations and stressing the need for careful monitoring for the postsurgical onset or recurrence of disordered eating.

Overview of Bariatric Surgery

Early surgical operations for weight loss, such as intestinal (jejuno-ileal) bypass, resulted in significant morbidity and mortality and were all but eliminated by about 1980 (Benotti & Forse, 1995). Although the health implications of obesity were established during the 1980s, questions about the surgical treatment of this condition remained. In 1991 a National Institutes of Health Consensus Development Conference on Gastrointestinal Surgery for Severe Obesity brought together a multidisciplinary panel of experts who reviewed the evidence. The panel recommended that bariatric surgery be considered for well-informed, motivated, severely obese individuals (body mass index [BMI] ≥40) with acceptable operative risks and for moderately obese individuals (BMI ≥35) with high-risk comorbid medical conditions such as severe sleep apnea or diabetes mellitus (National Institutes of Health Consensus Development Panel, 1992). The panel endorsed the two surgical procedures that dominated practice at that time: gastric bypass (GBP) and vertical banded gastroplasty (VBG).

Of these two procedures, studies documented superior weight loss following GBP versus VBG (Hall et al., 1990; Sugerman, Starkey, & Birkenhauer, 1987). The use of VBG decreased, and GBP became the most common weight loss operation performed in the United States in the 1990s. Laparoscopic surgery also became commonplace, and the laparoscopic adjustable gastric band (LAGB; Lap-Band®) was approved by the Food and Drug Administration (FDA) in 2001. At present, GBP and LAGB represent the vast majority of weight loss procedures performed in the United States. However, there are several other options, such as biliopancreatic diversion (BPD) with or without duodenal switch, as well as gastric sleeve resection with or without future conversion to GBP or BPD. The future of bariatric surgery will likely see the approval and development of new techniques such as intragastric balloon placement and endoluminal surgery.

Meta-analyses indicate that patients experience significant weight loss after bariatric surgery, averaging 61% of excess weight loss across diverse procedures (Buchwald et al., 2004) or 20–30 kg (Maggard et al., 2005). In addition, most individuals experience resolution or improvement in obesity-related comorbid conditions such as diabetes, hyperlipidemia, hypertension, and obstructive sleep apnea. These health benefits are weighed against the risks associated with a major abdominal surgery, including a small possibility (less than 0.5%) of death.

The primary mechanism for weight loss following surgery is restriction with or without intestinal malabsorption. Some procedures limit caloric intake by gastric restriction alone. For example, LAGB involves surgical placement of an adjustable silicone band near the top of the stomach, just below the esophagus, that permits the surgeon to adjust the diameter of the opening through which food passes. As a result, patients consume less solid food at each eating episode, losing weight gradually over a 2- to 3-year period. Other procedures combine gastric restriction with malabsorption, such as Roux-en-Y GBP. This procedure creates a small gastric "pouch" near the top of the stomach and also bypasses most of the stomach, the duodenum, and a portion of the remainder of the small intestine to create a degree of intestinal malabsorption. As compared to procedures involving restriction only, weight loss is more rapid after GBP, continuing for about 18 months. Across various procedures, approximately 20% of patients will experience inadequate weight loss or significant weight regain (Benotti & Forse, 1995).

Many research studies in bariatric surgery are limited by small sample sizes, cross-sectional and retrospective designs, and nonstandardized assessments (Bocchieri, Meana, & Fisher, 2002; Herpertz et al., 2003). When utilizing the extant literature to inform clinical practice, one must consider the type of operation investigated and whether the study sample includes individuals who have undergone diverse procedures. Procedures involving restriction of gastric capacity may differ in their impact on eating relative to those combining restriction and malabsorption. Additionally, it is important to consider the time point relative to operation. That is, the prevalence and clinical significance of eating problems may change as patients progress from the presurgery to the postsurgery period. In addressing the topic of eating problems and bariatric surgery, we draw on our clinical expertise as well as the research literature in this area.

Eating Disorders and Psychopathology among Candidates for Weight Loss Surgery

Most work on eating problems and bariatric surgery has focused specifically on binge eating, or recurrent objective bulimic episodes, a relatively common eating pattern among obese patients (Hudson, Hiripi, Pope, & Kessler, 2007). A review of studies with bariatric surgery candidates and patients documented estimates of binge eating ranging from 1.4 to 49% (de Zwaan, 2005). The difference in prevalence rates across studies is likely due to differences in patient samples and research methodology.

Studies using semistructured clinical interviews suggest that binge eating is common among candidates for bariatric surgery. In a broad assessment of psychopathology, Rosenberger, Henderson, and Grilo (2006) administered the Structured Clinical Interview for DSM-IV Axis I Disorders (SCID; First, Spitzer, Gibbon, & Williams, 1997) to 174 bariatric surgery candidates. In this study 13.8% of participants received eating disorder (ED) diagnoses (4.6% had binge-eating disorder [BED] and 9.2% had eating disorder not otherwise specified [EDNOS]), 22.4% mood disorder diagnoses, and 22.4% anxiety disorder diagnoses. These rates are similar to those reported in nationally representative surveys. However, these data were derived from psychological evaluations required as part of the bariatric surgery candidacy procedure, which may have affected patients' willingness to disclose problems they perceived could affect their approval for surgery.

Kalarchian and colleagues (2007) administered the SCID to a sample of 288 candidates for weight loss surgery independently of the preoperative screening and approval process. In this study 66.3% of participants reported a lifetime history of an Axis I disorder, including eating, mood, anxiety, and substance use disorders. With respect to EDs specifically, 3.5% reported a lifetime history of bulimia nervosa (BN; including 0.3% who met criteria at the time of evaluation), and 27.1% reported a lifetime history of BED (including 16% who met criteria at the time of evaluation). Moreover, presence of at least one Axis I disorder was related to greater severity of obesity and poorer functional health status.

Less is known about disordered eating among youths who seek surgery; binge eating may have a youth-specific presentation in which loss of control over eating is the most salient feature (Tanofsky-Kraff et al., 2007). In one study of adolescents undergoing bariatric surgery (Kim et al., 2008), depression and aberrant eating behaviors were very common, including binge eating (48%), rapid eating (44%), guilt over eating (36%), eating until uncomfortably full (36%), loss of control (24%), and eating alone (20%). Available findings suggest that psychiatric disorders, including but not limited to EDs, are a major concern for this patient population.

Night Eating
among Bariatric Surgery Patients

Night-eating syndrome (NES) is marked by morning anorexia, evening hyperphagia, and insomnia (Stunkard & Allison, 2003). However, research on NES has been hampered by a lack of consensus on diagnostic criteria. Furthermore, NES frequently co-occurs with BED, raising questions as to what extent these are distinctive syndromes (Adami, Meneghelli, & Scopinaro, 1999). Although there have been considerable inconsistencies in the characterization of night eating among bariatric surgery samples (Colles & Dixon, 2006), research suggests that night eating and binge eating are only partially overlapping syndromes (Allison et al., 2006). Future studies will determine whether night eating constitutes a distinct clinical syndrome, and, if so, help to identify the key behavioral features.

Relationship of Preoperative Disordered Eating to Postoperative Outcomes

The literature that has examined the relationship of preoperative EDs to postoperative weight outcomes is limited and contradictory. Prospective studies using standardized assessments provide some information, but longer-term studies are lacking. In a short-term prospective study, we examined the relationship of Axis I psychiatric disorders to 6-month outcomes among 207 GBP patients (Kalarchian et al., 2008). After adjusting for demographic factors, patients diagnosed with at least one lifetime Axis I disorder upon interview prior to operation exhibited significantly less weight loss after the operation. Specifically, mood and anxiety, but not substance disorders or EDs, accounted for a modest but significant amount of the variability in short-term weight outcomes. In a separate study of the relationship of preoperative binge eating to outcomes 12 months after GBP (N = 139), self-report of regular binge eating prior to surgery was not associated with poor outcomes after surgery (White, Masheb, Rothschild, Burke-Martindale, & Grilo, 2006). Thus, these two prospective studies, which utilized different assessment methods, failed to find a relationship between preoperative disordered eating and weight loss at 6 and 12 months after surgery.

Although patients are commonly screened for eating problems prior to weight loss surgery (Devlin, Goldfein, Flancbaum, Bessler, & Eisenstadt, 2004), there is no clear evidence that presurgery disordered eating affects postoperative weight loss, at least over the short term. Therefore, preoperative EDs should not be used to exclude patients from surgery, especially considering the lack of alternate treatments for severe obesity (Kalarchian & Marcus, 2003). However, further prospective study is warranted, including long-term follow-up of patients who have undergone diverse surgical procedures.

Impact of Bariatric Surgery on Disordered Eating

Binge eating is reduced after surgery in part due to patients' restricted gastric capacity, which inhibits the consumption of objectively large amounts of food. In a prospective study documenting the short-term impact of GBP on EDs, 50 patients were administered the Eating Disorder Examination (EDE; Fairburn & Cooper, 1993) before and about 4 months after the procedure (Kalarchian, Wilson, Brolin, & Bradley, 1999). Following the operation, no subjects reported recurrent binge eating, loss of control over eating, or use of inappropriate compensatory behaviors (e.g., self-induced vomiting) to influence shape and weight. In a prospective study of 139 patients followed for 1 year, White and colleagues (2006) reported that 24% self-reported weekly binge eating preoperatively, but that only 0.7% reported weekly binge eating at follow-up. Similar improvements in binge eating have been documented after LAGB (Larsen et al., 2004) and BPD (Adami, Gandolfo, Meneghelli, & Scopinaro, 1996). Thus, short-term improvements in binge eating have been documented across diverse surgical procedures.

Impact of Bariatric Surgery on Body Image

In addition to improvements in disordered eating, body image tends to improve after bariatric surgery. For example, in a prospective study utilizing standardized questionnaires, female patients ($N = 180$) experienced significant reductions in body image dissatisfaction, as measured by the questionnaire version of the Eating Disorder Examination (EDE-Q) and Body Shape Questionnaire (BSQ) at 6 and 12 months after GBP (Hrabosky et al., 2006). Furthermore, over 80% of participants had body image scores comparable to published norms at follow-up. Interestingly, changes in BMI and body image were only weakly associated, indicating that weight loss does not fully account for the improvements reported by patients. A similar pattern of results has been reported after BPD (Adami, Meneghelli, Bressani, & Scopinaro, 1999).

Despite overall improvements, some patients do experience body image concerns after surgery. After significant weight loss, many individuals are concerned about excess skin in the abdomen and other areas. Loose skin is not only considered unattractive but also can be associated with development of chafing, rashes, or infection, and can interfere with physical activity. Such concerns lead many patients to consider corrective body contouring surgery (Sarwer, Thompson, Mitchell, & Rubin, 2008), and there are even some clinical reports suggesting that a minority of patients resist further weight loss or try to regain weight (Rusch & Andris, 2007). Gusenoff, Messing, O'Malley, and Langstein (2008) found that 84.5% of 926 bariatric surgery patients who responded to a survey were considering body contouring. Mitchell and colleagues (2008) reported that 33 of 70 patients who responded to a survey had undergone a total of 38 body contouring procedures 6–10 years after GBP. Despite the additional procedures, many patients continued to have body image concerns. However, other data suggest that body contouring after bariatric surgery is associated with overall improvements in body image and quality of life (Song et al., 2006). The reader is referred to Sarwer and colleagues (2008) for a review and current recommendations for the psychosocial assessment of body contouring patients.

Other Eating Problems after Bariatric Surgery

The onset of threshold-level EDs after surgery appears to be uncommon, but case reports do appear in the literature (Atchison, Wade, Higgins, & Slavotinek, 1998; Scioscia, Bulik, Levenson, & Kirby, 1999). However, EDs may manifest differently in patients with a reduced gastric capacity after weight loss surgery. A number of aberrant eating patterns are described below that may not meet full diagnostic criteria for EDs, but that can be nonetheless associated with clinically significant distress and impaired weight management.

Nausea and Vomiting

Nausea and vomiting tend to occur most often during the initial months after surgery. Patients may vomit after eating too fast, not chewing well, or overeating. Some individuals will learn to self-induce vomiting to alleviate the discomfort associated with overeating, or the feeling that food has become stuck in the upper digestive tract or "pouch," which is known as plugging. In a long-term follow-up 13–15 years after GBP, 69% of patients reported involuntary vomiting and 43% reported plugging (Mitchell et al., 2001).

Nausea and vomiting tend to improve over time as patients learn to use bariatric surgery as a tool to help them eat less. Eventually, most patients are able to consume a diet that includes a fairly wide range of healthy foods, with the exception of frequent intolerance to red meats and soft white breads. Nonetheless, a minority of patients may develop severe or persistent problems with vomiting. Although uncommon, some individuals may self-induce vomiting to counteract the effects of eating on body weight and shape.

Nutritional Problems

Nutritional problems after bariatric surgery may include protein-calorie malnutrition or vitamin or mineral deficiencies, especially vitamin B_{12}, calcium, folate, and iron. Patients who have persistent vomiting or poor food intake in the postoperative period are at higher risk for acute nutritional deficiencies. These deficiencies are most common after procedures involving intestinal malabsorption, such as GBP, and less common following a procedure in which the digestive tract remains intact, such as LAGB. One serious complication is the development of acute thiamine (B_1) deficiency post GBP. If not recognized and treated early, thiamine deficiency can result in Wernicke–Korsakoff syndrome, with symptoms including nystagnus, memory loss, and personality changes (Juhasz-Pocsine, Rudnicki, Archer, & Harik, 2007). Multivitamin supplementation reduces the chance of developing nutritional deficiencies, but does not eliminate it (Gasteyger, Suter, Gaillard, & Giusti, 2008).

Dumping Syndrome

One consequence of procedures associated with malabsorption is a reaction called "dumping syndrome," characterized by lightheadedness, sweating, flushing, palpitations, cramps, and diarrhea. This usually occurs when patients consume too much sugary or carbohydrate-rich food at one time, such as ice cream or cake, after GBP. Early dumping occurs 30–60 minutes following a meal and is believed to result from the accelerated gastric emptying of hyperosmolar contents from the stomach, leading to fluid shifts, gastric distension, and associated symptoms. Late dumping occurs 1–3 hours following a meal and is likely due to a hyperinsulinemic response and resulting hypoglycemia. Fortunately, dumping syndrome can be reduced or eliminated with dietary changes to avoid high-sugar and -carbohydrate foods (Sugerman et al., 1987). Thus, some patients view this complication favorably because it deters them from making poor food choices, whereas for others it is considered problematic.

Excessive Caloric Intake

Patients with greater adherence to the recommended postoperative reduced-calorie eating plan exhibit a greater weight loss after GBP (Sarwer, Wadden, et al., 2008). In contrast, the adoption of aberrant eating patterns makes it possible for patients to consume a large amount of calories despite a reduced gastric capacity. For example, an eating pattern of frequent consumption of smaller amounts of food throughout the day after operation ("grazing") can contribute to inadequate weight loss or significant weight regain (Saunders, 2004). Additionally, because gastric restriction does not limit the intake of softer foods and liquids, regular consumption of high-calorie foods like ice cream and drinks like soda and juice has been associated with poorer weight outcomes (Sugerman et al., 1987).

Loss of Control or Subjective Binge Eating

A growing body of evidence documents that weight loss and eating behavior patterns shift around 2 years post GBP, a time when recurrent loss of control over eating has been associated with poor weight outcomes (Niego, Kofman, Weiss, & Geliebter, 2007). For example, retrospective and cross-sectional studies have linked loss of control over eating or subjective binge eating to weight regain at longer-term follow-up (Kalarchian et al., 2002; Mitchell et al., 2001). The relationship between postoperative loss of control over eating and weight regain is further substantiated in recent prospective studies. Among 361 GBP patients, presurgery loss of control over eating did not predict postoperative outcomes (White, Kalarchian, Masheb, Marcus, & Grilo, in press). In contrast, postsurgery loss of control was associated with poorer weight loss at 12 months and 24 months postsurgery. In another study of 129 LAGB patients, postoperative loss of control over eating and "grazing" showed high overlap and were associated with less weight loss 12 months after the operation (Colles, Dixon, & O'Brien, 2008).

In summary, current evidence suggests that surgery has a positive impact on eating behavior, such that many patients with preoperative binge eating do not resume this eating pattern after surgery. However, postoperative loss of control has been associated with longer-term weight regain. Therefore, it appears that the resumption (or onset) of loss of control or subjective binge eating after postsurgery, as opposed to binge eating prior to surgery, may be a clinically important target for intervention.

Treating Eating Problems after Surgery

Most postoperative eating problems are transient and related to the effects of the operation. All patients require lifelong medical monitoring after weight loss surgery, including intervention when clinically significant eating problems are detected. Psychiatrists, psychologists, and nutritionists must work in consultation with the surgical team to rule out physiological and surgical causes. A full diagnostic workup for eating problems or inadequate weight loss may include laboratory testing, a nutritional evaluation, psychological evaluation, and an upper gastrointestinal (GI) series to assess the anatomy and functionality of the altered GI tract. Self-monitoring of dietary intake (including any episodes of vomiting) along with the associated circumstances (including both external factors, such as the type and quantity of food consumed or interpersonal context, and internal factors, such as thoughts and feelings) may serve as the foundation for developing an individualized cognitive-behavioral treatment plan. In extreme cases, a patient may benefit from an inpatient hospitalization for observation of his/her problematic eating behavior, or referral for specialty care in a center experienced in the treatment of eating and weight problems.

Summary

Bariatric surgery is recommended for treatment of severe obesity. Eating problems such as binge eating and night eating are relatively common among individuals seeking obesity treatment and should not be considered a contraindication to surgery. The positive effects of surgery include not only weight loss but also short-term reductions in binge eating and improvements in body image. However, aberrant eating patterns can develop postsurgery. These can include persistent vomiting, nutritional deficiencies, dumping syndrome, excessive caloric intake, and recurrent loss of control over eating. Postoperative eating problems may be mild for some but severe for others. All patients should be monitored carefully after the operation for the onset or recurrence of disordered eating. Multidisciplinary interventions are needed to help patients both prepare for bariatric surgery and achieve optimal weight loss and psychosocial adjustment after the operation.

References

Adami GF, Gandolfo P, Meneghelli A, & Scopinaro N. (1996). Binge eating in obesity: A longitudinal study following biliopancreatic diversion. *International Journal of Eating Disorders*, 20:405–413.

Adami GF, Meneghelli A, Bressani A, & Scopinaro N. (1999). Body image in obese patients before and after stable weight reduction following bariatric surgery. *Journal of Psychosomatic Research*, 46:275–281.

Adami GF, Meneghelli A, & Scopinaro N. (1999). Night eating and binge eating disorder in obese patients. *International Journal of Eating Disorders*, 25:335–338.

Allison KC, Wadden TA, Sarwer DB, Fabricatore AN, Crerand CE, Gibbons LM, et al. (2006). Night eating syndrome and binge eating disorder among persons seeking bariatric surgery: Prevalence and related features. *Surgery for Obesity and Related Diseases*, 2:153–158.

Atchison M, Wade T, Higgins B, & Slavotinek T. (1998). Anorexia nervosa following gastric reduction surgery for morbid obesity. *International Journal of Eating Disorders*, 23:111–116.

Benotti PN, & Forse RA. (1995). The role of gastric surgery in the multidisciplinary management of severe obesity. *American Journal of Surgery*, 169:361–367.

Bocchieri LE, Meana M, & Fisher BL. (2002). A review of psychosocial outcomes of surgery for morbid obesity. *Journal of Psychosomatic Research*, 52:155–165.

Buchwald H, Avidor Y, Braunwald E, Jensen MD, Pories W, Fahrbach K, et al. (2004). Bariatric surgery: A systematic review and meta-analysis. *Journal of the American Medical Association*, 292:1724–1737.

Colles SL, & Dixon JB. (2006). Night eating syndrome: Impact on bariatric surgery. *Obesity Surgery*, 16:811–820.

Colles SL, Dixon JB, & O'Brien PE. (2008). Hunger control and regular physical activity facilitate weight loss after laparoscopic adjustable gastric banding. *Obesity Surgery*, 18:833–840.

de Zwaan M. (2005). Weight and eating changes after bariatric surgery. In JE Mitchell & M de Zwaan (Eds.), *Bariatric surgery: A guide for mental health professionals* (pp. 77–100). New York: Taylor & Francis.

Devlin MJ, Goldfein JA, Flancbaum L, Bessler M, & Eisenstadt R. (2004). Surgical management of obese patients with eating disorders: A survey of current practice. *Obesity Surgery*, 14:1252–1257.

Fairburn CG, & Cooper Z. (1993). The eating disorder examination. In CG Fairburn & GT Wilson (Eds.), *Binge eating: Nature, assessment, and treatment* (pp. 317–360). New York: Guilford Press.

First MB, Spitzer RL, Gibbon M, & Williams JBW. (1997). *User's guide for the Structured Clinical Interview for DSM-IV Axis 1 disorders (SCID-I)*. Washington, DC: American Psychiatric Press.

Gasteyger C, Suter M, Gaillard RC, & Giusti V. (2008). Nutritional deficiencies after Roux-en-y gastric bypass for morbid obesity often cannot be prevented by standard multivitamin supplementation. *American Journal of Clinical Nutrition*, 87:1128–1133.

Gusenoff JA, Messing S, O'Malley W, & Langstein HN. (2008). Temporal and demographic factors influencing the desire for plastic surgery after gastric bypass surgery. *Plastic and Reconstructive Surgery*, 121:2120–2126.

Hall JC, Watts JM, O'Brien PE, Dunstan RE, Walsh JF, Slavotinek AH, et al. (1990). Gastric surgery for morbid obesity: The Adelaide study. *Annals of Surgery*, 211:419–427.

Herpertz S, Kielmann R, Wolf AM, Langkafel M, Senf W, & Hebebrand J. (2003). Does obesity surgery improve psychosocial functioning?: A systematic review. *International Journal of Obesity and Related Metabolic Disorders*, 27:1300–1314.

Hrabosky JI, Masheb RM, White MA, Rothschild BS, Burke-Martindale CH, & Grilo CM. (2006). A prospective study of body dissatisfaction and concerns in extremely obese gastric bypass patients: 6- and 12-month postoperative outcomes. *Obesity Surgery*, 16:1615–1621.

Hudson JI, Hiripi E, Pope HG, Jr, & Kessler RC. (2007). The prevalence and correlates of eating disorders in the national comorbidity survey replication. *Biological Psychiatry*, 61:348–358.

Juhasz-Pocsine K, Rudnicki SA, Archer RL, & Harik SI. (2007). Neurologic complications of gastric bypass surgery for morbid obesity. *Neurology*, 68:1843–1850.

Kalarchian MA, & Marcus MD. (2003). Management of the bariatric surgery patient: Is there a role for the cognitive behavioral therapist? *Cognitive and Behavioral Practice*, 10:112–119.

Kalarchian MA, Marcus MD, Levine MD, Courcoulas AP, Pilkonis PA, Ringham RM, et al. (2007). Psychiatric disorders among bariatric surgery candidates: Relationship to obesity and functional health status. *American Journal of Psychiatry*, 164:328–334; quiz 374.

Kalarchian MA, Marcus MD, Levine MD, Soulakova JN, Courcoulas AP, & Wisinski MS. (2008). Relationship of psychiatric disorders to 6-month outcomes after gastric bypass. *Surgery and Obesity Related Disorders*, 4:544–549.

Kalarchian MA, Marcus MD, Wilson GT, Labouvie EW, Brolin RE, & LaMarca LB. (2002). Binge eating among gastric bypass patients at long-term follow-up. *Obesity Surgery*, 12:270–275.

Kalarchian MA, Wilson GT, Brolin RE, & Bradley L. (1999). Effects of bariatric surgery on binge eating and related psychopathology. *Eating and Weight Disorders*, 4:1–5.

Kim RJ, Langer JM, Baker AW, Filter DE, Williams NN, & Sarwer DB. (2008). Psychosocial status in adolescents undergoing bariatric surgery. *Obesity Surgery*, 18:27–33.

Larsen JK, van Ramshorst B, Geenen R, Brand N, Stroebe W, & van Doornen LJ. (2004). Binge eating and its relationship to outcome after laparoscopic adjustable gastric banding. *Obesity Surgery*, 14:1111–1117.

Maggard MA, Shugarman LR, Suttorp M, Maglione M, Sugarmen HJ, Livingston EH, et al. (2005). Meta-analysis: Surgical treatment of obesity. *Annals of Internal Medicine*, 142:547–559.

Mitchell JE, Crosby RD, Ertelt TW, Marino JM, Sarwer DB, Thompson JK, et al. (2008). The desire for body contouring surgery after bariatric surgery. *Obesity Surgery*, 18:1308–1312.

Mitchell JE, Lancaster KL, Burgard MA, Howell LM, Krahn DD, Crosby RD., et al. (2001). Long-term follow-up of patients' status after gastric bypass. *Obesity Surgery*, 11:464–468.

National Institutes of Health Consensus Development Panel. (1992). Gastrointestinal surgery for severe obesity: National institutes of health consensus development conference statement. *American Journal of Clinical Nutrition*, 55:615S–619S.

Niego SH, Kofman MD, Weiss JJ, & Geliebter A. (2007). Binge eating in the bariatric surgery population: A review of the literature. *International Journal of Eating Disorders*, 40:349–359.

Rosenberger PH, Henderson KE, & Grilo CM. (2006). Psychiatric disorder comorbidity and association with eating disorders in bariatric surgery patients: A cross-sectional study using structured interview-based diagnosis. *Journal of Clinical Psychiatry*, 67:1080–1085.

Rusch MD, & Andris D. (2007). Maladaptive eating patterns after weight-loss surgery. *Nutrition in Clinical Practice*, 22:41–49.

Sarwer DB, Thompson JK, Mitchell JE, & Rubin JP. (2008). Psychological considerations of the bariatric surgery patient undergoing body contouring surgery. *Plastic and Reconstructive Surgery*, 121:423e–434e.

Sarwer DB, Wadden TA, Moore RH, Baker AW, Gibbons LM, Raper SE, et al. (2008). Preoperative eating behavior, postoperative dietary adherence, and weight loss after gastric bypass surgery. *Surgery and Obesity Related Disorders*, 4:640–646.

Saunders R. (2004). "Grazing": A high-risk behavior. *Obesity Surgery*, 14:98–102.

Scioscia TN, Bulik CM, Levenson J, & Kirby DF. (1999). Anorexia nervosa in a 38-year-old woman 2 years after gastric bypass surgery. *Psychosomatics*, 40:86–88.

Song AY, Rubin JP, Thomas V, Dudas JR, Marra KG, & Fernstrom MH. (2006). Body image and quality of life in post massive weight loss body contouring patients. *Obesity (Silver Spring)*, 14:1626–1636.

Stunkard AJ, & Allison KC. (2003). Two forms of disordered eating in obesity: Binge eating and night eating. *International Journal of Obesity and Related Metabolic Disorders*, 27:1–12.

Sugerman HJ, Starkey JV, & Birkenhauer R. (1987). A randomized prospective trial of gastric bypass versus vertical banded gastroplasty for morbid obesity and their effects on sweets versus non-sweets eaters. *Annals of Surgery*, 205:613–624.

Tanofsky-Kraff M, Goossens L, Eddy KT, Ringham R, Goldschmidt A, Yanovski SZ, et al. (2007). A multisite investigation of binge eating behaviors in children and adolescents. *Journal of Consulting and Clinical Psychology*, 75:901–913.

White MA, Kalarchian MA, Masheb RM, Marcus MD, & Grilo CM. (in press). Loss of control over eating predicts outcomes in bariatric surgery: A prospective 24-month follow-up study. *Journal of Clinical Psychiatry*.

White MA, Masheb RM, Rothschild BS, Burke-Martindale CH, & Grilo CM. (2006). The prognostic significance of regular binge eating in extremely obese gastric bypass patients: 12-month postoperative outcomes. *Journal of Clinical Psychiatry*, 67:1928–1935.

CHAPTER 26

Treatment of Psychiatric Comorbidities

Howard Steiger and Mimi Israel

Anorexia nervosa (AN), bulimia nervosa (BN), and binge-eating disorder (BED) co-occur frequently with mood, anxiety, impulse-control, and substance use disorders. This chapter provides guidelines for the clinical management of psychiatric comorbidity in patients with eating disorders (EDs). We aim for broad coverage, but also constrain our discussion to recommendations for which there is reasonable empirical support.

Mood Disorders

Many patients with EDs will experience a mood disorder (MD; i.e., major depressive disorder, dysthymic disorder, or bipolar disorder) in their lifetimes. A recent U.S. National Comorbidity Survey estimated lifetime prevalence of MD to be 42% in AN, 71% in BN, and 46% in BED (Hudson, Hiripi, Pope, & Kessler, 2007). Although MDs frequently co-occur with EDs, some care is required to avoid overdetection, as malnutrition can produce dysphoria, fatigue, poor concentration, insomnia, and other symptoms that mimic a MD syndrome (Keys, Brozek, Mickelsen, & Taylor, 1950). Likewise, guilt, indecisiveness, and social withdrawal may arise in eating-disordered individuals, without implying depression. Unlike mood symptoms attributable to a MD, mood symptoms that are secondary to the ED tend to improve rapidly with nutritional stabilization (Meehan, Loeb, Roberto, & Attia, 2006) and without specific MD treatment. In contrast, symptoms such as psychomotor retardation, anhedonia, and early morning awakening tend to belie a genuine major depressive disorder, except in highly emaciated patients (in whom such symptoms can reflect effects of advanced starvation). An implication of the preceding is that, when working with patients who have EDs, it is important to distinguish "depression as a symptom" (likely to improve with ED-focused treatments) from "depression as a syndrome" (likely to require specific management). Careful attention to phenomenology and the patient's response to a nutritionally focused therapy will often help make the needed determination.

Many treatment practices that are recommended for the treatment of ED symptoms are well suited to the treatment of mood disturbances—and such points of crossover help indicate techniques that can be applied in treating a patient with an ED and a comorbid MD. Cognitive-behavioral therapy (CBT), which has demonstrated efficacy for the treatment of ED symptoms—especially for BN and BED (Wilson, Grilo, & Vitousek, 2007)—is also a standard part of the evidence-based repertoire of treatments for depression (National Institute for Health and Clinical Excellence [NICE], 2007). CBT helps patients acquire cognitive reappraisal skills, and hence to challenge dysfunctional beliefs that maintain maladaptive responses and symptoms. An informed psychotherapist can adjust the focus of cognitive interventions to assist patients in modifying irrational beliefs that support mood disturbances (at one moment) and eating symptoms (at another)—and often it is possible to isolate shared thinking errors (e.g., "dichotomous" or "black-and-white" thinking) that simultaneously support negative moods (e.g., "I wasn't the best, so I'm no good") and maladaptive weight control behaviors ("I'm not the thinnest, so I must be fat"). Similarly, interpersonal psychotherapy (IPT), which addresses interpersonal issues (conflicts, losses, role transitions, social skills deficits) that are believed to maintain eating and mood disturbances, has proven efficacy for BN, BED (NICE, 2007; Wilfley, MacKenzie, Welch, Ayres, & Weissman, 2000; Wilson et al., 2007), and depression (NICE, 2007).

Given that they have many shared neurobiological substrates, EDs and MDs can often be treated with common pharmacotherapeutic agents. For eating symptoms in BN and BED, most classes of antidepressants have been found to be effective (NICE, 2004b; Reas & Grilo, 2008), although selective serotonin reuptake inhibitors (SSRIs) are preferred because of their favorable side effect profile. It is noteworthy that antibulimic effects of antidepressants appear to occur regardless of the presence or absence of concurrent depression. Available evidence shows a more limited utility of pharmacotherapy in AN (Walsh et al., 2007; Wilson et al., 2007). Nonetheless, it is common clinical practice to attempt to relieve depression in the depressed patient with AN by using adjunctive antidepressant therapy. Neurobiological alterations in severely malnourished patients, however, tend to limit therapeutic responses to antidepressants so that, with low-weight patients who have AN, weight restoration often needs to be a first goal, with antidepressants introduced only once patients have achieved some degree of nutritional rehabilitation. Pointing to an alternative adjunctive treatment in patients with BN and seasonal mood fluctuations, data indicate that light therapy benefits both bulimic and depressive symptoms (Lam, Lee, Tam, Grewal, & Yatham, 2001).

Studies document elevated rates of bipolar disorder (BD) in people with EDs— especially those in the bulimia spectrum. In the National Comorbidity Survey, Hudson and colleagues (2007) estimated the lifetime prevalence of BD to be 3% in AN, 18% in BN, and 12.5% in BED. We add two caveats: (1) The presence of BD may be difficult to ascertain in patients with EDs, particularly younger ones in whom a dormant BD may not yet have declared itself. (2) Affective instability, common in many patients with EDs, can confound (and inflate) diagnostic determinations related to BD prevalence in those who have EDs.

BD has such devastating potentials that it invariably becomes a treatment priority when present. Pharmacotherapy of BD in patients with EDs requires special provisos. Mood stabilizers and antipsychotics have been associated with weight gain and overeating (Aronne & Segal, 2003), both of which can result in nonadherence. Use of lithium, the oldest and best known of mood stabilizers, is risky in individuals who purge or severely restrict food intake, as both behaviors increase susceptibility to lithium toxicity by promoting dehydration and metabolic disturbances. As an incidental note on the pharmacological treatment of patients with EDs and bipolarity, it is worthwhile remembering that SSRIs, although the drug treatment of choice in bulimic syndromes, can trigger mania or hypomania in patients with an underlying BD (Goodwin et al., 2008).

The preferred pharmacological treatment of the patient with an ED and a comorbid BD is often one that is simultaneously therapeutic for eating and affective problems. For instance, the antipsychotic olanzapine, already used in the treatment of mania, has recently been shown to facilitate weight restoration in AN (Bissada, Tasca, Barber, & Bradwejn, 2008), and would thus warrant consideration when treating patients with AN and BD. Likewise, the mood stabilizer topiramate, proven to be effective in the treatment of BN (Hoopes et al., 2003) and BED (McElroy et al., 2007), might be considered as an adjunctive treatment for comorbid BD in an individual with a bulimia-spectrum disorder.

Suicidality

Suicidality is relatively common in patients with EDs. However, rates of suicidality vary considerably in function of ED subtype: 25–35% of patients with BN make suicide attempts, whereas only 3–20% of those with AN do so (Franko & Keel, 2006). Paradoxically, rates of completed suicides are actually higher in AN (Franko et al., 2006)—owing, in part, to the fact that the attempts of patients with AN tend toward very lethal means (Bulik et al., 2008). In the EDs suicidality does not always arise in the context of a MD. For instance, Bulik and colleagues found that, in AN, after controlling for MD, purging behaviors, impulsive behaviors, substance abuse, panic disorder, post-traumatic stress disorder, and severe ED symptoms conferred additional risk. A similar study in BN linked suicidality to substance use and impulse-control disorders (Corcos et al., 2002). Given these observations, suicide potential should be carefully evaluated in all patients with EDs, even in the absence of a comorbid MD. For those deemed to be at risk, early incorporation of treatments for impulse and affect regulation problems (see the section on personality traits, to follow) may help reduce tendencies that confer suicidal risk.

Anxiety Disorders

Anxiety disorders (ADs) are common in eating-disordered individuals and often declare themselves prior to the onset of the ED (Kaye, Bulik, Thornton, Barbarich, & Masters, 2004). Although rates of individual AD diagnoses differ among ED subtypes, higher-than-expected rates of social phobia, obsessive–compulsive disorder, panic disorder, agoraphobia, and generalized anxiety disorder have been reported in all subtypes (Hudson et al., 2007; Kaye et al., 2004). For diagnostic purposes, it is necessary to differentiate anxiety that is limited to an ED-specific theme (e.g., fear of weight gain) from anxiety that has a nonspecific focus (e.g., fear of failure, fear that loved ones may come to harm). Conversely, anxiety sometimes influences eating and weight without being indicative of an ED (e.g., weight loss resulting from a fear of choking).

As with MDs, ADs often implicate similar cognitive errors to those structuring EDs—and this creates opportunities for the conjoint psychotherapeutic management of common components of disturbance. For example, EDs generally implicate phobic elements (e.g., the fear of weight gain), obsessive preoccupations (e.g., overattention to body shape), and compulsive reactions (e.g., the felt need to compensate after eating). This being so, it becomes feasible to frame and work with eating symptoms as variants of anxiety-driven behaviors, applying the concepts of "phobias," "obsessions," and "compulsions" to weight gain fears, bodily preoccupations, and driven weight loss strategies. Patients often need to reappraise their problem: Is it a "problem of body weight" or a "phobia of weight gain"? Likewise, is the felt necessity of compensating for calories eaten (through exercise, purging, or later caloric restraint) part of a "sensible weight control strategy" or the "enactment of a compulsive ritual"? Basic tenets of cognitive-behavioral management of anxiety apply—including altering antecedent cognitive appraisals, preventing emotional avoidance, and facilitating adaptive action patterns (see Barlow, Allen, & Choate, 2004).

In a similar vein, it is possible to take aim at eating and anxiety disturbances concurrently using common pharmacological interventions. SSRIs, currently recommended in the pharmacological treatment of BN and BED (NICE, 2004b), are also recommended for panic disorder, generalized anxiety disorder, and obsessive–compulsive disorder (NICE, 2004a). Evidence does not, however, support the notion that simply treating the AD suffices as a treatment for the ED. Likewise, studies have failed to demonstrate that drugs that decrease anxiety, such as fluoxetine, are sufficient to prevent relapse following weight restoration in AN (Walsh et al., 2007).

Posttraumatic Stress Disorder

Clinical evidence associates the EDs, and specifically those variants characterized by bulimic symptoms (e.g., BN, BED, or AN binge–purge subtype), with prior exposure to traumatic stress. Modal figures suggest that about 30% of adults with BN report unwanted sexual experiences during childhood, whereas over half of such adults report physical maltreatment during childhood (Steiger & Bruce, 2004, 2008). Likewise, findings have associated BN and BED with such experiences as rape or assault (Brewerton, 2008). Correspondingly, the recent National Comorbidity Survey (Hudson et al., 2007) reported lifetime posttraumatic stress disorder (PTSD) in 45% of individuals with BN and 26% of those with BED, but in only 12% of those with AN.

Although bulimic ED variants are associated with prior traumatization, rates of trauma exposure and of PTSD in BN and BED do not consistently exceed those observed in appropriate comparison groups—for example, in women showing other psychiatric problems (Steiger & Bruce, 2008). Furthermore, even though prior traumata emerge as consistent predictors of comorbid psychiatric symptoms in BN (e.g., depression, self-mutilation, or substance abuse), findings do not strongly associate a traumatic history with severity of ED symptoms. Such tendencies suggest that, if posttraumatic stress has an etiological role in the EDs, the role is an indirect one. This is not, however, to minimize the clinical importance of a traumatic history. Aside from an association with more-pronounced psychiatric symptoms, past trauma may predict unfavorable treatment response or increased recidivism and relapse (Anderson, LaPorte, Brandt, & Crawford, 1997).

Very few data are available to guide the treatment of concurrent PTSD in patients with EDs. In the absence of a disorder-specific empirical base, informed ED practitioners have tended to incorporate general PTSD treatment techniques into their ED treatments (see Brewerton, 2008). In the section to follow, we draw liberally from the American Psychiatric Association (2004) guidelines for the treatment of PTSD, and those of Brewerton (2008), both of which are supported by empirical evidence and expert consensus.

As with other forms of comorbidity, when there is comorbid PTSD in a patient with an ED, it is generally advisable to "work" the ED first (or at least concurrently). This recommendation runs contrary to a common clinical intuition—that severely traumatized patients will be unable to achieve normal eating until posttraumatic reactions are resolved—or even that the early introduction of structured eating can be retraumatizing. Not only are such views unfounded, they neglect two important realities of ED treatment (that prevail in the presence and absence of prior trauma): (1) Psychological and physiological effects of starvation, dieting, or regular purging, if unchecked, exacerbate the mental status. (2) Overcoming intense emotional reactions to eating invariably implicates reexposure to normal varieties and quantities of food.

Evidence from the PTSD literature suggests that a key component of the psychotherapeutic management of posttraumatic symptoms is the objective review of traumatic experiences in a state of relative calm. Various empirically supported interventions—including stress inoculation training, cognitive restructuring, imaginal exposure, and eye movement desensitization and reprocessing (EMDR)—involve some variant of this technique, and many clinicians advocate such specialized interventions as treatment adjuncts in the management of patients with EDs and comorbid PTSD (Brewerton, 2008). The actual treatment of dissociation remains controversial. We advocate the normalization of dissociative symptoms (in preference to their further elaboration). In other words, our preference is to integrate rather than to dis-integrate. Therapy should also help build capacities for emotional integration, to limit the triggering of dissociative reactions. With this goal in mind, it is usually necessary to help patients revise cognitive appraisals of their experiences ("Should you really have been able to stop him?") and the values they associate with them (e.g., "Are you 'weak' or 'to blame' or someone who was confronted with an experience she should never have had to face?"). Finally, given the typical interpersonal sequelae of abuse (affecting the ability to trust, to tolerate intimacy, to allow others influence, etc.), close attention to the implications of disclosure of traumatic memories to a therapist is warranted.

Various pharmacological agents yield benefits in PTSD, including the SSRIs, tricyclic antidepressants, and monoamine oxidase inhibitors (MAOIs). Use of the latter two medications, however, is complicated with patients with EDs due to side effects, potential lethality in overdose, and (in the case of MAOIs) dangerousness unless used while on a well-controlled diet. Importantly, benzodiazepines are reported to have limited or even countertherapeutic effect in PTSD. In contrast, recent findings point to potentials of the antihypertensive agent (which has specific antianxiety properties) propranolol—in that it reduces cardiac reactivity and anxiety during scripted review of traumatic experiences in patients with chronic PTSD (Brunet et al., 2008).

Substance Use Disorders

Co-occurrence of substance use disorders (SUDs) with EDs has been observed in clinical and community samples. A lifetime history of SUDs is reported in up to 27% of individuals with AN, 55% of those with BN, and 23% of those with BED (Holderness, Brooks-Gunn, & Warren, 1994; Hudson et al., 2007). Prospective studies have shown that, in patients with EDs, substance abuse problems develop at various stages of illness (Franko et al., 2008)—a reminder to clinicians to remain attentive to the possible emergence of SUDs in patients who do not initially endorse substance use or abuse. In addition, it is useful to be aware that, in the EDs, drug abuse is sometimes motivated by an attraction to appetite-suppressing substances (e.g., cocaine, amphetamines). However, abuse of other drugs, some that potentially stimulate appetite (e.g., cannabis), occurs quite commonly (Franko et al., 2008). Substance abuse presents various risks in patients with EDs: It amplifies impulsivity and affective instability and increases risk of parasuicidal and other self-destructive behaviors. Moreover, alcohol abuse has adverse nutritional, hepatic, and gastrointestinal consequences. Stimulant abuse can cause cardiovascular and neurological complications.

The impact of SUDs upon ED treatment outcome has not been studied extensively. However, contrary to clinical lore, recent findings suggest that the substance-abusing patient need not necessarily receive a specialized treatment for chemical dependence before accruing benefits from ED treatment. Indeed, evidence suggests that a comorbid SUD has surprisingly little influence upon outcome of ED-focused treatment (Franko et al., 2008; Grilo, Sinha, & O'Malley, 2002). Furthermore, recent evidence suggests that psychotherapy aimed at substance abuse may incidentally improve eating symptoms (O'Malley et al., 2007). In a related vein, logic dictates that treatments that bolster motivation for change and adherence to therapy (e.g., motivational enhancement techniques) or that improve coping skills and mood regulation (e.g., dialectical behavior therapy) may similarly benefit eating and substance abuse in patients exhibiting problems in these areas (Grilo et al., 2002).

Research on pharmacological agents that could concurrently reduce eating disturbances and substance abuse is scanty. Ondansetron, a $5-HT_3$ antagonist, has been shown to be beneficial in the treatment of alcohol dependence (Johnson, 2008) and BN (Faris et al., 2000), but has not been evaluated in patients with comorbid BN and alcohol use disorders. Similarly, antibulimic potentials of naltrexone, an opioid antagonist approved for the treatment of alcohol and opioid dependence, have not been adequately investigated (Grilo et al., 2002). One caveat about pharmacotherapy is needed: When medicating substance-abusing patients, clinicians should be cognizant that interactions between prescription medications and substances of abuse can increase cardiovascular, gastrointestinal, and neurological risks.

Personality Traits and Personality Disorders

Patients with EDs are consistently found to be more likely to display comorbid personality disorders (PDs) than are individuals in the general population (Bruce & Steiger, 2005; Cassin & von Ranson, 2005; Grilo, 2002; Lilenfeld, Wonderlich, Riso, Crosby, & Mitchell, 2006; Steiger & Bruce, 2004). Restrictive AN coincides relatively "neatly" with anxious-fearful PDs (typically obsessive–compulsive or avoidant variants), and binge–purge ED subtypes coincide with heterogeneous Axis II disturbances—dramatic-erratic PDs (often borderline PD) occurring in 30–45% of such cases and anxious-fearful variants being present in another third (or more). Such findings are consistent with the general view that PDs are common in patients with EDs, and that different ED diagnoses are characterized by different patterns of PD comorbidity (Grilo, 2002).

Although clinical impressions have associated PD comorbidity with unfavorable outcome, empirical data suggest that this notion needs to be carefully nuanced. In AN, data are quite consistent in linking severe obsessive–compulsive PD, and corresponding traits of perfectionism, harm avoidance, and preference for sameness, with unfavourable prognosis (see Bruce & Steiger, 2005). Likewise, findings in BN and BED associate Axis-II comorbidity—and especially dramatic-erratic PDs, borderline PD, and corresponding traits (e.g., impulsivity)—with adverse global outcomes (see Bruce & Steiger, 2005). However, several sources suggest that, in BN, predictive effects of personality pathology may apply more to general psychopathological dimensions, such as mood disturbances or suicidality, than to eating-specific ones, such as bingeing or purging (Bruce & Steiger, 2005; Grilo, 2002). The preceding implies that eating symptoms can improve independently of improvements on personality dimensions (and vice versa) and, in turn, that individuals with comorbid personality disturbances may benefit from specialized interventions focused on ED symptoms. At the same time, clinical experience and empirical data dictate that, in patients with severe PDs, generalized adjustment problems often persist even if eating attitudes and behaviors improve. There is also evidence that such patients may be exceptionally prone to dropping out of therapy (see Bruce & Steiger, 2005).

Empirically validated guidelines for the treatment of patients with EDs and marked personality pathology are not yet available. However, based on recent treatments of the role of personality trait–focused interventions in ED treatment (see Bruce & Steiger, 2005; Fairburn, 2008; Sansone & Levitt, 2006; Wonderlich, Peterson, Mitchell, & Crow, 2000), and an integration of recent findings, we propose the following "dicta":

- *Prioritize problematic thoughts and behaviors around eating.* By definition, individuals with severe PDs present diverse crises and adjustment problems—repeated states of despair, parasuicidal threats or gestures, legal dilemmas, and financial binds all being common. A treatment aimed at reducing eating symptoms becomes easily sidetracked (if not fully derailed). This being the case, it is important for clinicians to keep their focus. Improving nutritional status yields demonstrable improvements on personality indices, and eating symptoms often improve despite ongoing problems of adjustment. Furthermore, it is our impression that eating-focused treatment provides skills and structures that help highly dysregulated patients. A clinical application of this knowledge is: Insofar as possible, treat eating problems from the start.
- *Adjust interventions in function of comorbid traits.* Eating-disordered individuals can be clustered into distinct, personality trait–defined subgroups—some emotionally and behaviorally "dysregulated" (i.e., showing impulsivity and affective instability), some leaning toward overregulation (compulsivity and emotional constriction), and others displaying relatively low psychopathology (e.g., Steiger & Bruce, 2004). Intuition dictates that these different groups will tend to have different treatment needs. Circumscribed

ED-centered treatments should be well suited to the needs of the subgroup displaying low concurrent psychopathology. In contrast, the group (usually bingers or purg-
ers) displaying marked dysregulation, while still requiring ED-focused interventions, is
likely to need adjunctive interventions aimed at impulse and affect regulation, whereas
the group displaying marked constriction or compulsivity (often, but not always AN
restricting subtype) is likely to benefit from adjuncts aimed at emotional, behavioral,
and interpersonal inhibition. Previously justified by clinical lore alone, findings by Fairburn and his group provide at least partial corroboration of the intuitive proposal we
have outlined. In a heterogeneous sample of patients with EDs (and BMIs above 17.5),
those with low psychiatric comorbidity responded best to a traditional CBT, whereas
those with high comorbidity showed better response to an "enhanced" CBT, with specific treatment components addressing low self-esteem, clinical perfectionism, affective
instability, and interpersonal disturbances (Fairburn et al., 2008).

• *Personality problems shape eating symptoms.* We find it useful to conceptualize eating pathology as existing independently of personality pathology—but as being closely
shaped by it. (See Lilenfeld et al., 2006; Steiger & Bruce, 2004; and Bruce & Steiger,
2005, for treatments of "pathoplastic" effects of personality pathology on eating symptoms.) The key notion here is that specific psychopathological tendencies may accen-
tuate specific components of eating disturbances—impulsivity driving high-frequency
purging, compulsivity accentuating relentless dieting and pursuit of thinness, narcis-
sism fueling overinvestments in achieving bodily (and other forms of) perfection, and
so on. Intuition argues that treatments work better when they manage the impact of
personality traits (affective instability, perfectionism, impulsivity, hostility, etc.) upon
eating symptoms. It is equally important to remember, however, that in patients with
minimal comorbidity, focal (eating-centered) treatments may work best.

There is some empirical support for the application of personality-focused, adjunctive psychotherapeutic techniques in the treatment of patients with EDs (although specific efficacy for specific areas of disturbance remains to be established). Dialectical
behavior therapy (DBT), for example, encompasses a mix of CBT and Eastern medita-
tive strategies that aim to increase patients' mindfulness of emotional experiences (i.e.,
measured experiencing of emotions), capacities for emotion regulation, and tolerance
of emotional distress (Linehan, 1993; Marcus & Levine, 2004). DBT has shown at least
initial promise in the treatment of all ED variants, yielding benefits in terms of reduced
eating symptoms, affective problems, and other symptoms. In addition, there is support
for the use, in treating concurrent disturbances in patients with EDs, of techniques
that focus on interpersonal functioning—such as ED-adapted forms of interpersonal
therapy (Wilfley et al., 2000). Likewise, preliminary support has become available for
the use of techniques that target clinical perfectionism (Riley, Lee, Cooper, Fairburn,
& Shafran, 2007).

Aside from psychotherapeutic techniques, adjuncts for pronounced mood and
impulse dysregulation seen in patients with comorbid PDs often include judiciously
applied SSRIs, mood stabilizers, or atypical antipsychotics (Duggan, Husband,
Smailagic, Ferriter, & Adams, 2008). Where there is emotional and behavioral constriction, adjunctive medications may include use of SSRIs or atypical antipsychotics such as
olanzapine (Bissada et al., 2008).

Conclusions

Several basic tenets can be gleaned from the literature on the interface between eating disturbances and comorbid psychopathology. To start, it is often true that eating and generalized disturbances are separately responsive to treatment, meaning that it is usually worthwhile tackling eating disturbances independently of symptoms in other areas. Likewise, in a general hierarchy of treatment goals, aside from management of problems that overtly jeopardize patients' safety (e.g., active suicidality), it is often indicated to target eating symptoms first. This is because ED-symptom sequelae exacerbate functioning in many collateral areas and, consequently, many generalized gains can be accrued through an initial phase of nutritional stabilization. In contrast, numerous mutual influences between "eating-specific" and "generalized" disturbances are observed in the EDs, such that eating disturbances influence the course and expression of various co-occurring psychopathological symptoms, and psychopathological symptoms (particularly personality traits), in turn, impact the expression and course of eating symptoms. It is in the latter area that much work remains to be done before we can claim to have developed an empirically informed practice guideline for treating patients with EDs and comorbid psychopathology. For instance, we still need to more fully differentiate those problems that indicate recourse to a sequential approach (treating comorbidity prior to eating symptoms, or vice versa) from those in which comorbidity should be treated concurrently with the ED, from those in which comorbidity is best "left alone." We also need to develop more fully the repertoire of interventions that will enable clinicians to more optimally manage the set of behavioral, affective, and interpersonal repercussions that psychiatric comorbidity can have upon the treatment process.

References

American Psychiatric Association. (2004). Practice guideline for the treatment of patients with acute stress disorder and posttraumatic stress disorder. *American Journal of Psychiatry*, 162:3–31.

Anderson KP, LaPorte DJ, Brandt H, & Crawford S. (1997). Sexual abuse and bulimia: Response to inpatient treatment and preliminary outcome. *Journal of Psychiatric Research*, 31:621–633.

Aronne LJ, & Segal KR. (2003). Weight gain in the treatment of mood disorders. *Journal of Clinical Psychiatry*, 64:22–29.

Barlow DH, Allen LB, & Choate ML. (2004). Toward a unified treatment for emotional disorders. *Behavior Therapy*, 35:205–230.

Bissada H, Tasca GA, Barber AM, & Bradwejn J. (2008). Olanzapine in the treatment of low body weight and obsessive thinking in women with anorexia nervosa: A randomized, double-blind, placebo-controlled trial. *American Journal of Psychiatry*, 165:1281–1288.

Brewerton TD. (2008). The links between PTSD and eating disorders. *Psychiatric Times*, 25:1–3.

Bruce K, & Steiger H. (2005). Treatment implications of Axis-II comorbidity in eating disorders. *Eating Disorders*, 13:93–108.

Brunet A, Orr SP, Tremblay J, Robertson K, Nader K, & Pitman RK. (2008). Effect of post-retrieval propranolol on psychophysiologic responding during subsequent script-driven traumatic imagery in post-traumatic stress disorder. *Journal of Psychiatric Research*, 42:503–506.

Bulik CM, Thornton L, Pinheiro AP, Plotnicov K, Klump KL, Brandt H. et al. (2008). Suicide attempts in anorexia nervosa. *Psychosomatic Medicine*, 70:378–383.

Cassin SE, & von Ranson KM. (2005). Personality and eating disorders: A decade in review. *Clinical Psychology Review*, 25:895–916.

Corcos M, Taieb O, oit-Lamy S, Paterniti S, Jeammet P, & Flament MF. (2002). Suicide attempts in women with bulimia nervosa: Frequency and characteristics. *Acta Psychiatrica Scandinavica*, 106:381–386.

Duggan C, Husband N, Smailagic N, Ferriter M, & Adams C. (2008). The use of pharmacological treatments for people with personality disorder: A systematic review of randomized controlled trials. *Personality and Mental Health*, 2:119–170.

Fairburn CG. (2008). *Cognitive behavior therapy and eating disorders*. New York: Guilford Press.

Fairburn CG, Cooper Z, Doll HA, O'Connor ME, Bonn R, Hawker DM, et al. (2009). Transdiagnostic cognitive behavioral therapy for patients with eating disorders: A two-site trial with 60-week follow-up. *American Journal of Psychiatry*, 166:311–319.

Faris PL, Kim SW, Meller WH, Goodale RL, Oakman SA, Hofbauer RD. et al. (2000). Effect of decreasing afferent vagal activity with ondansetron on symptoms of bulimia nervosa: A randomised, double-blind trial. *Lancet*, 355:792–797.

Franko DL, Dorer DJ, Keel PK, Jackson S, Manzo MP, & Herzog DB. (2008). Interactions between eating disorders and drug abuse. *Journal of Nervous and Mental Disease*, 196:556–561.

Franko DL, & Keel PK. (2006). Suicidality in eating disorders: Occurrence, correlates, and clinical implications. *Clinical Psychology Review*, 26:769–782.

Goodwin GM, Anderson I, Arango C, Bowden CL, Henry C, Mitchell PB. et al. (2008). ECNP consensus meeting: Bipolar depression. *European Neuropsychopharmacology*, 18:535–549.

Grilo CM. (2002). Recent research on relationships among eating disorders and personality disorders. *Current Psychiatry Reports*, 4:18–24.

Grilo CM, Sinha R, & O'Malley SS. (2002). Eating disorders and alcohol use disorders. *Alcohol Research and Health*, 26:151–160.

Holderness CC, Brooks-Gunn J, & Warren MP. (1994). Eating disorders and substance use: A dancing vs. a nondancing population. *Medicine and Science in Sports and Exercise*, 26:297–302.

Hoopes SP, Reimherr FW, Hedges DW, Rosenthal NR, Kamin M, Karim R. et al. (2003). Treatment of bulimia nervosa with topiramate in a randomized, double-blind, placebo-controlled trial: Part 1. Improvement in binge and purge measures. *Journal of Clinical Psychiatry*, 64:1335–1341.

Hudson JI, Hiripi E, Pope HG, & Kessler RC. (2007). The prevalence and correlates of eating disorders in the national comorbidity survey replication. *Biological Psychiatry*, 61:348–358.

Kaye WH, Bulik CM, Thornton L, Barbarich N, & Masters K. (2004). Comorbidity of anxiety disorders with anorexia and bulimia nervosa. *American Journal of Psychiatry*, 161:2215–2221.

Keys A, Brozek J, Mickelsen O, & Taylor HL. (1950). *The biology of human starvation* (Vols. 1 and 2). Minneapolis: University of Minnesota Press.

Lam RW, Lee SK, Tam EM, Grewal A,, & Yatham LN. (2001). An open trial of light therapy for women with seasonal affective disorder and comorbid bulimia nervosa. *Journal of Clinical Psychiatry*, 62:164–168.

Lilenfeld LRR, Wonderlich S, Riso LP, Crosby R, & Mitchell J. (2006). Eating disorders and personality: A methodological and empirical review. *Clinical Psychology Review*, 26:299–320.

Linehan MM. (1993). *Cognitive-behavioral treatment of borderline personality disorder*. New York: Guilford Press.

Marcus MD, & Levine MD. (2004). Use of dialectical behavior therapy in the eating disorders. In TD Brewerton (Ed.), *Clinical handbook of eating disorders* (pp. 473–488). New York: Marcel Dekker.

McElroy SL, Hudson JI, Capece JA, Beyers K, Fisher AC, & Rosenthal NR. (2007). Topiramate for the treatment of binge eating disorder associated with obesity: A placebo-controlled study. *Biological Psychiatry*, 61:1039–1048.

Meehan KG, Loeb KL, Roberto CA, & Attia E. (2006). Mood change during weight restoration in patients with anorexia nervosa. *International Journal of Eating Disorders*, 39:587–589.

National Institute for Health and Clinical Excellence (NICE). (2004a). *Anxiety: Management of anxiety (panic disorder, with or without agoraphobia, and generalised anxiety disorder) in adults in primary, secondary and community care* (Clinical Guideline No. 22). Available online at *www. nice.org.uk/CG022*.

National Institute for Health and Clinical Excellence (NICE). (2004b). *Eating disorders: Core interventions in the treatment and management of anorexia nervosa, bulimia nervosa and related eating disorders* (Clinical Guideline No. 9). Available online at *www.nice.org.uk/guidance/CG9*.

National Institute for Health and Clinical Excellence (NICE). (2007). Depression: Management of depression in primary and secondary care (Clinical Guideline No. 23). Available online at *www.nice.org.uk/CG023*.

O'Malley SS, Sinha R, Grilo CM, Capone C, Farren CK, Mckee SA. et al. (2007). Naltrexone and cognitive behavioral coping skills therapy for the treatment of alcohol drinking and eating disorder features in alcohol-dependent women: A randomized controlled trial. *Alcoholism: Clinical and Experimental Research*, 31:625–634.

Reas DL, & Grilo CM. (2008). Review and meta-analysis of pharmacotherapy for binge-eating disorder. *Obesity*, 16:2024–2038.

Riley C, Lee M, Cooper Z, Fairburn CG, & Shafran R. (2007). A randomised controlled trial of cognitive-behaviour therapy for clinical perfectionism: A preliminary study. *Behaviour Research and Therapy*, 45:2221–2231.

Sansone RA, & Levitt JL. (Eds.). (2006). *Personality disorders and eating disorders: Exploring the frontier*. New York: Routledge.

Steiger H, & Bruce K. (2004). Personality traits and disorders in anorexia nervosa, bulimia nervosa, and binge eating disorder. In TD Brewerton (Ed.), *Clinical handbook of eating disorders: An integrated approach* (pp. 207–228). New York: Marcel Dekker.

Steiger H, & Bruce K. (2008). Eating disorders: Anorexia nervosa and bulimia nervosa. In T Millon, PH Blaney, & RD Davis (Eds.), *Oxford textbook of psychopathology* (2nd ed.). New York: Oxford University Press.

Walsh BT, Kaplan AS, Ahia E, Olmsted M, Parides M, Carter JC, et al. (2006). Fluoxetine after weight restoration in anorexia nervosa. *Journal of the American Medical Association*, 295:2605–2612.

Wilfley DE, MacKenzie KR, Welch RR, Ayres VE, & Weissman MM. (2000). *Interpersonal therapy for groups*. New York: Basic Books.

Wilson GT, Grilo CM, & Vitousek KM. (2007). Psychological treatment of eating disorders. *American Psychologist*, 62:199–216.

Wonderlich SA, Peterson C, Mitchell JE, & Crow S. (2000). Integrative approaches to treating eating disorders. In KJ Miller & JS Mizes (Eds.), *Comparative treatments of eating disorders* (pp. 173–195). New York: Springer.

CHAPTER 27

Treatment for Night-Eating Syndrome

Kelly C. Allison and Albert J. Stunkard

Night-eating syndrome (NES) was originally described over 50 years ago as a disorder characterized by morning anorexia, evening hyperphagia (eating 25% of the daily food intake after 6:00 P.M.), and insomnia (Stunkard, Grace, & Wolff, 1955). NES was thought to be associated with stress and was reported among obese persons who had difficulty losing weight (Stunkard et al., 1955). In the late 1990s, during the rise in the prevalence of obesity in the United States and other developed countries, there was renewed interest in NES. Studies of treatment for NES are still limited, with more pharmacotherapy trials than psychotherapy trials. We review these treatment approaches and outline the cognitive-behavioral therapy (CBT) program that has been developed for the treatment of NES.

Clinical Description and Characterization

NES is characterized by a delay in the circadian pattern of eating. It is not included in the DSM-IV-TR (American Psychiatric Association, 2000), and in the past its criteria have varied considerably across studies. Recently, a consensus was reached on a set of diagnostic criteria (First International Night Eating Symposium, April 26, 2008; Allison et al., in press), which is summarized in Table 27.1. One of the two core criteria must be present: (a) consumption of at least 25% of intake after the evening meal (i.e., evening hyperphagia), and/or (b) nocturnal ingestions at least two times per week (defined as waking up during the main sleep period to eat). Additionally, three of five associated features must be present, including lack of morning hunger or breakfast, a strong desire to eat after dinner and/or during the night, sleep onset or sleep maintenance insomnia, a belief that one must eat to fall asleep or resume sleep, and depressed mood. These criteria should help raise awareness about the syndrome and promote further research on the characteristics and treatment of NES.

TABLE 27.1. Proposed Research Diagnostic Criteria for NES

I. The daily pattern of eating demonstrates a significantly increased intake in the evening and/or nighttime, as manifested by one or both of the following:
   A. At least 25% of food intake is consumed after the evening meal
   B. At least two episodes of nocturnal eating per week

II. Awareness and recall of evening and nocturnal eating episodes are present.

III. The clinical picture is characterized by at least three of the following features:
   A. Lack of desire to eat in the morning and/or breakfast is omitted on four or more mornings per week
   B. Presence of a strong urge to eat between dinner and sleep onset and/or during the night
   C. Sleep onset and/or sleep maintenance insomnia are present four or more nights per week
   D. Presence of a belief that one must eat in order to initiate or return to sleep
   E. Mood is frequently depressed and/or mood worsens in the evening

IV. The disorder is associated with significant distress and/or impairment in functioning.

V. The disordered pattern of eating has been maintained for at least 3 months.

VI. The disorder is not secondary to substance abuse or dependence, medical disorder, medication, or another psychiatric disorder.

NES versus Other Sleep-Related Disorders

A disorder that must be distinguished from NES is sleep-related eating disorder (SRED) (American Academy of Sleep Medicine, 2005). SRED is characterized by episodes of involuntary eating during the sleep period or arousal from nighttime sleep, typically while sleepwalking (Howell, Schenk, & Crow, 2008). Persons with SRED often consume nonfood items and may injure themselves during these episodes by bumping into walls and furniture, or by burning or cutting themselves while preparing food in their sleep. Thus, their level of awareness of their nocturnal ingestions is very low, and there is typically little to no recall of the events.

Howell and colleagues (2008) suggest that SRED and NES are at opposite ends of an eating disorders (EDs) spectrum, but no studies have examined this suggestion systematically to date. Our clinical experience suggests that a small minority of patients who present for NES treatment describe having SRED initially, but then gain more awareness of their nocturnal eating over the course of several years. Additionally, another small minority of persons with NES who experience repetitive nocturnal ingestions with awareness report occasional episodes of sleepwalking and eating. It is possible that those occasional sleepwalking episodes are influenced by the use of sleep medications, such as zolpidem (see Howell et al., 2008), but no systematic descriptions of these cases in an NES population have been published.

NES versus Other Forms of Disordered Eating

Other forms of disordered eating may co-occur with NES. The overlap between NES and binge-eating disorder (BED) is modest, with most studies finding rates of 7–25% (Allison et al., 2006, 2007; Allison, Grilo, Masheb, & Stunkard, 2005; Powers, Perez, Boyd, & Rosemurgy, 1999; Stunkard et al., 1996). An important difference between NES and BED is that nocturnal ingestions in NES typically are not objectively large, with one study reporting an average of about 300 calories consumed per episode (Birketvedt et al., 1999). It is worth noting that nighttime eating without the other features required for NES, such as the circadian abnormalities in eating patterns, are not uncommon in BED, particularly among men (Grilo & Masheb, 2004). Even if binge episodes occur in the late evening or nighttime hours before sleep onset, the underlying reasons for the eating appear to differ from those of persons with NES. Among patients with NES, nocturnal eating has been correlated with nocturnal anxiety, but among patients with BED there is no significant correlation between their nocturnal eating behavior and their nocturnal anxiety (Sassaroli et al., 2009).

Persons with BED and those with NES share similar psychopathology in relation to their disordered eating, but to differing degrees (Allison et al., 2005). They report similar, elevated levels of depressed mood and dietary restraint and eating concerns, as measured by the Eating Disorder Examination (EDE). Participants with NES also reported higher levels of several other aspects of disordered eating than non-eating-disordered control participants (i.e., shape and weight concerns on the EDE, and disinhibition and hunger on the Eating Inventory), but participants with BED scored significantly higher than both the NES and control groups. Thus, persons with NES show elevated levels of disordered eating pathology, but not always or to the same extent as those with BED.

NES and Obesity

The evidence for a relationship between NES and obesity has been mixed. In the population-based Danish MONICA study (1,051 women, 1,061 men), the report of nocturnal ingestions was linked with greater weight gain among obese women (5.2 kg vs. 0.9 kg), but not among men, over a 6-year period (Anderson, Stunkard, Sorensen et al. 2004). Among outpatient psychiatric patients, obese patients were 5.2 times more likely to have NES than normal-weight patients (Lundgren et al., 2006). Two additional studies have described a positive relationship between NES prevalence and body mass index (BMI) (Aranoff, Geliebter, & Zammit, 2001; Colles, Dixon, & O'Brien, 2007). However, two nationally based epidemiological studies have not supported this relationship (Striegel-Moore et al., 2005; Striegel-Moore, Franko, Thompson, Affenito, & Kraemer, 2006), suggesting that more work is needed in this area.

Preliminary evidence suggests that persons with NES have been less successful at weight loss attempts than those without NES (Gluck, Geliebter, & Zammit, 2001; Stunkard et al., 1955). Gluck and colleagues (2001) reported that, after controlling for BMI, participants with NES lost less weight (4.4 kg) than the non-night eaters (7.3 kg, p = .003), suggesting that pure weight loss efforts may be difficult for night eaters, without addressing evening and nocturnal eating behaviors.

Cognitive Features of NES

Allison and colleagues (Allison, Stunkard, & Thier, 2004) examined the specific content of cognitions associated with eating by persons with NES. In this study patients with NES were asked to record their thoughts before and after evening and nighttime eating episodes. Among the most common dysfunctional thoughts were (1) food cravings (for specific foods), (2) anxiety or agitation, (3) distress about sleep disruption, and (4) feeling compelled to eat (needing to feel full to sleep). Less common themes were feeling stressed, depressed, or bored. These dysfunctional thoughts can be identified in treatment with the Nighttime Eating Assessment (NEA; Allison & Stunkard, 2007), which consists of visual analog scales used to identify and target those themes that are most salient for an individual in treatment.

Neurobiological Aspects of NES

There is growing knowledge about the neurobiological aspects of NES. In light of initial promising findings for SSRI treatment (described below), a pilot imaging study using single photon emission computerized tomography (SPECT) examined the uptake ratio of the serotonin transporter (SERT) among persons with NES as compared to control participants and persons with major depressive disorder (Lundgren, Amsterdam, Newberg, Allison, & Stunkard, 2009; Lundgren, Newberg, et al., 2008). Those with NES showed significantly higher levels of SERT in the midbrain than controls, whereas patients with depression showed markedly decreased levels of SERT. Increased reuptake of serotonin by the elevated SERT leads to impaired postsynaptic serotonin transmission and may thereby contribute to NES. Since serotonin receptors modulate both food intake and circadian rhythms, the impaired transmission of serotonin may underlie the delayed circadian rhythms of both food intake and neuroendocrine measures (Goel et al., 2009). Such impaired function suggests that improvement of serotonergic function, precisely the effects of SSRIs, may alleviate NES.

Clinical Presentation

Now that we have reviewed the features of NES, we present the case of Stephanie, a woman who has suffered with NES for many years. Her case and its associated distress and embarrassment are typical of many persons seeking help for NES. Stephanie is a 50-year-old middle school teacher with a BMI of 28 kg/m² who presented for treatment of NES. She describes being consumed by thoughts of food in the evening before bedtime. She typically "grazes" throughout the evening until she goes to bed, and it takes her about 30 minutes to fall asleep. After Stephanie falls asleep, she wakes up about 1–2 hours later to eat and repeats this one to two additional times during the night. During these episodes, she eats a variety of foods, depending on what she has available in the house. Some nights she may eat only fruit, but on other occasions she will have some cake and other sweets. Upon awakening in the morning, she says she still feels full from her nighttime snacks.

Stephanie remembers eating at night as a teenager and that her father also had NES. She began dieting after the night eating emerged, and across her lifetime has tried many structured diet programs. She reached her highest weight of over 250 pounds when she was 46 years old, and proceeded to lose 100 pounds through a 12-step program and private counseling. During this time, she gained control of her nocturnal ingestions and eating during the evening. However, after 2 years, her night-eating symptoms reemerged, and she became very distressed at her inability to control them. She began regaining some weight, which increased her distress and anxiety. Stephanie continued to eat well during the day and exercised twice each day in the summer when she was not teaching. She presented for treatment in tears, feeling as though others could not understand how difficult it was to stop her eating at night.

Treatment Literature

The treatment literature for NES is still small, so much of the available data are from open-label, pilot, and case studies. We present what is available with the caveat that additional randomized trials in pharmacotherapy and psychotherapy are needed.

Pharmacotherapy

One case-series report and two open-label trials have suggested the potential usefulness of SSRIs for NES. Miyaoka and colleagues (2003) described a case series of four patients successfully treated with paroxetine or fluvoxamine. Contemporaneously, an open-label 12-week trial of sertraline with 17 night eaters yielded significant reductions in the number of nocturnal awakenings (60% decrease) and ingestions (67% decrease) and percentage of caloric intake after dinner (50% decrease) (O'Reardon, Stunkard, & Allison, 2004). Weight decreased by 4.8 kg in those whose NES remitted, but increased modestly in the remaining 12 participants by 0.6 kg. Dosing was flexible, starting at 50 mg and increasing up to 200 mg as needed. Finally, similar outcomes were reported in a long-distance treatment trial of 50 persons with NES who received treatment from their own physicians while being assessed and monitored by our research team (Stunkard et al., 2006). This group achieved a 66% reduction in calories consumed after the evening meal, 70% reduction in nocturnal ingestions, and a 2.2 kg weight loss among overweight and obese participants.

To date, only one randomized double-blind controlled pharmacotherapy trial has investigated a treatment for NES (O'Reardon et al., 2006). O'Reardon and colleagues (2006) randomized 34 patients with NES to 8 weeks either of sertraline ($n = 17$) or placebo ($n = 17$). Again, dosing began at 50 mg and was titrated, as needed, up to 200 mg. The sertraline group had significantly greater percent reductions than the placebo group in number of awakenings (74 vs. 14%), nocturnal ingestions (81 vs. 14%), and the Night Eating Symptom Scale (NESS) total score (57 vs. 16%). Percent of calories consumed after dinner decreased significantly in the sertraline group and approached normative levels (from 47.3 to 14.8% of total daily intake), but it was not significantly different from the placebo group after Bonferroni correction. The majority of those in the sertraline group (71%) reached "responder" status, according to the Clinical Global Impression of Improvement Scale (CGI-I ≤2) (Guy, 1976), and 41% of the sample was classified as "remitters" (CGI-I = 1). Only 18% of the placebo group attained responder status. Overweight and obese participants on sertraline lost significantly more weight (-2.9 ± 3.8 kg) as compared to those on placebo (-0.3 ± 2.7 kg, $p < .01$). As sertraline has not resulted in weight loss among obese persons without NES, this weight loss seems specifically related to the reductions in night eating.

Case reports of topiramate have also shown some promise in treating NES, although they are more commonly reported among patients with SRED (see Howell et al., 2008). Winkelman (2003) reported decreases in nocturnal ingestions and weight in two patients with NES and two patients with SRED. Additionally, a case series of six sertraline nonresponders showed that topiramate produced significant reductions on the NESS, percentage of calories consumed after dinner, and weight (-4.6 kg over 12 weeks, $p < .05$), accompanied by nonsignificant decreases in nocturnal awakenings and ingestions (Allison, 2005). Side effects leading to discontinuation of treatment with topiramate are more common than with SSRIs. Nevertheless, these initial findings suggest the need for controlled trials to test topiramate for NES.

An important contraindication to treatment for NES should be noted. Health care providers often seek to treat the insomnia related to NES and SRED. However, treatment with benzodiazapines and hypnotics, particularly zolpidem, seems to worsen or even induce nocturnal ingestions (see Howell et al., 2008, for a review). Specifically, those persons with NES who typically have awareness of their nighttime eating become less aware of their actions or experience episodes of frank sleepwalking with eating after taking hypnotics. They report that they have even less control over their actions and eat more than they typically would without those medications.

Psychosocial Approaches

Early attempts at behavioral treatment in cases of NES were reported with mixed success (Coates, 1978; Williamson, Lawson, Bennett, & Hinz, 1989). The only controlled psychosocial treatment trial was conducted by Pawlow, O'Neil, and Malcolm (2003). They compared a 1-week abbreviated progressive muscle relaxation (PMR) versus a control condition of sitting quietly. Morning hunger was increased and evening hunger ratings decreased significantly among the PMR group; consequently there was a trend for more breakfasts to be consumed and less nighttime eating. As expected, levels of stress, anxiety, and depression were also significantly reduced in the PMR group. As NES has been described as a stress-related disorder (Allison et al., 2004; Stunkard et al., 1955), these results are promising, but need to be tested more rigorously.

Cognitive-Behavioral Therapy for NES

Building on our earlier exploration of cognitions related to nighttime eating, we developed and tested a CBT program for NES (Allison, Martino, O'Reardon, & Stunkard, 2005). This CBT for NES was based partly on manuals designed for the treatment of binge eating (Fairburn, Marcus, & Wilson, 1993) and behavioral weight loss (Brownell, 2004) and modified for the specific features of NES. This treatment focused on shifting the circadian pattern of food intake to earlier in the day, while simultaneously uncoupling the habituated response of eating in order to fall asleep initially or to resume sleep during the night. Persons with NES do not eat regular meals throughout the day, but instead eat more frequently without specific meals (Boston, Moate, Allison, Lundgren, & Stunkard, 2008), as shown schematically in Figure 27.1. Although prescribing regular meals and snacks throughout the daytime hours seems necessary to break the night-eating pattern, this is often not sufficient. Thus, significant attention must also be paid to cognitions related to the eating episodes, behavioral strategies such as stimulus control, and the implementation of physical barriers to food.

In our initial pilot study (Allison, Martino, O'Reardon, & Stunkard, 2005), 25 participants with NES enrolled in the CBT intervention and 14 completed treatment. Significant reductions in four major outcome measures were noted at treatment end, using last observation carried forward (LOCF) analyses, including the NESS (O'Reardon et al., 2004), percent of caloric intake consumed after dinner, number of awakenings, and number of nocturnal ingestions. Completers showed greater improvements than the LOCF results, decreasing their nocturnal ingestions from 5.6 to 0.5 per week

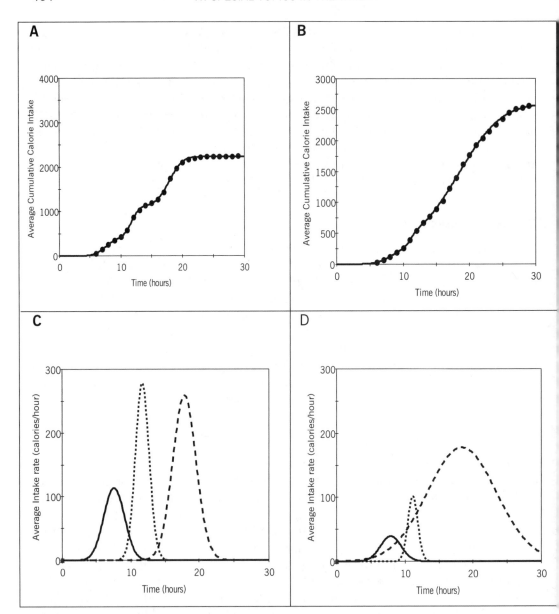

FIGURE 27.1. Use of the sum of three Gaussian curves to describe the average cumulative caloric intake of control participants (panel A) and NES participants (panel B). Panel C (control participants) and panel D (NES participants) depict the individual Gaussian curves that describe the average rate of eating during each of three separate meals. Note the distinct meals, represented by bumps in the curves, for controls in panel A, as opposed to the more variable eating pattern without pronounced meals shown for NES participants in panel B. From Boston, Moate, Allison, Lundgren, and Stunkard (2008). Copyright 2008 by the American Society for Nutrition. Reprinted by permission.

($p < .01$) and reducing the percentage of calories consumed after dinner from 36 to 22% ($p < .05$). Both the LOCF and completers analyses showed significant weight losses, with deficits of 1.6 kg ($p < .01$) and 2.8 kg ($p < .001$), respectively. These results are promising and demonstrate the need for a larger, randomized controlled trial of CBT.

Mini-Manual for CBT of NES

Ten individual therapy sessions are conducted over 12 weeks, weekly during the first 8 weeks and biweekly for sessions 9 and 10. In the first phase of treatment, the therapeutic alliance must be developed, and the key aspects of the CBT treatment are explained. Clinical experience suggests that the effort involved in keeping sleep and food logs 24 hours per day is much more work than many persons expect treatment to entail, so discussing this up front is useful. Not having a full appreciation of the time commitment may increase dropout rates. The early sessions (1–4) are largely focused on behavioral techniques and modifications. This includes keeping a food and sleep log every day and completing assessments of hunger, cravings, and emotions before eating at night, using the NEA (Allison & Stunkard, 2007). As is typical of CBT, each session begins with a review of the previous session's homework, including such tasks as food and sleep logs, NEAs, and thought records.

In the first session, the clinician and patient review the patient's typical eating pattern. Ideally, patients should complete a food and sleep log before beginning therapy to help with this review and so that the therapist can calculate the baseline proportion of calories typically consumed after the evening meal. If eating does not begin until midafternoon, then lunch will be encouraged; if lunch is the first meal eaten, a mid-morning snack is encouraged. This goal setting continues until three meals and two to three snacks are consumed throughout the day. In the evening, patients are encouraged to pick a "kitchen is closed" time that fits in their lifestyle (e.g., after the dishes have been washed and they have enjoyed their planned evening snack). After this time, behavioral techniques are used to provide obstacles and discouragement to eating (e.g., locks on cabinets or brushing teeth immediately after the evening snack).

The clinician helps the patient complete a behavioral chain in the second session to highlight each step in the process of evening and/or nighttime eating and to assess the "weakest links" of the chain needed to break the cycle (Allison et al., 2004). It is important for the clinician to raise the patient's awareness that the process is not as automatic as it is often described, and that persons with NES do make active decisions about food choices during the night. Caloric restriction is introduced at the third session for those with a weight loss goal. The clinician continues to focus on eliminating or reducing caloric intake between dinner and bedtime and during nocturnal ingestions by changing the food environment and creating physical barriers and meaningful signs (e.g., "I don't need to eat to fall back to sleep!" or "What is the worst thing that would happen if I didn't eat right now?"). Dysfunctional thought records are also introduced in Session 3 and further explained in Session 4 with the help of salient experiences from the previous week. This tool helps challenge the underlying stimuli for the evening and nighttime eating, whether it is resisting cravings or dealing with anxiety or insomnia. As stressful events throughout the day often influence nighttime eating, it is appropriate to examine thoughts from any distressing situation that impact and tax a patient's emotional resources and to propose alternative thoughts and solutions for those situations. An example of a thought record is included in Figure 27.2.

Sessions 5–8 continue to focus on the interplay of cognitions, emotions, and behaviors. Other topics addressed in these middle sessions include sleep hygiene (e.g., no sleeping with television on all night, no food in the bedroom, set standard bedtime and morning awakening times), stress reduction through deep breathing and progressive muscle relaxation (practiced in session), and the importance of an appropriate amount of exercise.

The final two sessions focus on increasing self-efficacy in patients so that they feel mastery on their own regarding their progress in reducing their night-eating behaviors. Additionally, troubleshooting anticipated stressors or cues for night eating and relapse prevention are covered. Additional sessions can be continued as needed, and booster sessions may also be desired to continued relapse prevention efforts.

The Importance of Weight Status

In our studies and communications with many different persons with night eating over the years, we have found that weight status is an important factor that impacts the focus of treatment. Lundgren, Allison, and colleagues (2008) reported that those of normal

Situation Where were you and what was happening when you felt the urge to eat or were in an upsetting situation (include date and time)?	Emotions What emotions (sad, angry, anxious, etc.) did you feel at the time?	Automatic Thoughts What thoughts and/or images went through your mind?	Alternative Responses Propose responses to the automatic thoughts.	Outcome Reevaluate your emotions and belief in your automatic thoughts.
Friday night, 9:30 P.M.: Bought favorite dessert and was scared I would eat it in the night, so I ate it while cleaning up from dinner, since I was still hungry.	I was anxious and felt that I set myself up.	I pictured wanting the dessert in the night. I am out of control. I will probably gain more weight.	I could have sat down and had it as part of my dinner when I felt more control. I was hungry, it was okay to eat it and enjoy it. If I eat enough during my meals and snacks in the day, I will be better able to control my eating during the night.	No nocturnal ingestions that night. Felt relieved and that I have more control over this than I thought.

FIGURE 27.2. Example of Dysfunctional Thought Record for NES. Thought record form adapted from Beck (1995). Copyright 1995 by Judith S. Beck. Adapted with permission from The Guilford Press.

weight who eat at night reported more daytime caloric restriction and more compulsive exercise than normal-weight control participants. We have also noted this distinction in treatment. Overweight and obese patients typically do not have as much deliberate daytime restriction of calories and engage in less physical activity than do the normal-weight night eaters who present to us for treatment. Normal-weight night eaters often show anxiety when asked to shift their eating earlier in the day, for fear of gaining weight. Weighing during sessions becomes important evidence that if the clinician and patient work together on reducing nighttime intake while simultaneously increasing daytime intake, there will not be a significant weight gain, and perhaps even a small weight loss.

Overall, CBT for NES is promising, but the manual needs to be refined for these differences in treating night eaters of different weight categories (i.e., focus on weight loss vs. reducing daytime restriction and compulsive exercise). Randomized controlled trials are needed to test CBT for NES and to compare its efficacy to that of SSRIs or other medications. We know that many persons with NES are suffering in silence because their health care providers may not know how to treat it. Goncalves and colleagues (2009) recently reported that, among patients with night eating, only 27% of their doctors had definitely heard of NES. It is our hope that these words will help those professionals better identify and treat this distressing disorder.

Forms and Worksheets

- *Night Eating Questionnaire (NEQ)*. A 14-item screening tool for NES (Allison, Lundgren, et al., 2008).
- *Night Eating Symptom Scale (NESS)*. Similar to the NEQ, the NESS assesses NES symptoms with more specificity and using a time frame of the previous week that is useful for tracking progress in treatment (O'Reardon et al., 2004).
- *Night Eating Syndrome History and Inventory (NESHI)*. Assessment interview based on the NEQ. Unpublished interview available from the authors (Allison, Lundgren, O'Reardon, & Stunkard).
- *Night Eating Assessment (NEA)*. A series of visual analog scales used to assess the feelings and behavioral states associated with evening and nighttime eating (published in Devlin, Allison, Goldfein, & Spanos, 2007).

Resources for Treatment

The CBT for NES manual is largely outlined in the following references:

- Allison KC, Stunkard AJ, & Thier SL. (2004). *Overcoming night eating syndrome: A step-by step guide to breaking the cycle.* Oakland, CA: New Harbinger.
- Allison KC, & Stunkard AJ. (2007). Self-help for night eating syndrome. In J Latner & GT Wilson (Eds.), *Self-help for obesity and binge eating* (pp. 310–324). New York: Guilford Press.
- Devlin MJ, Allison KC, Goldfein JA, & Spanos A. (2007). Management of EDNOS (eating disorder not otherwise specified). In J Yager & P Powers (Eds.), *Clinical*

management of eating disorders (pp. 195–224). Washington, DC: American Psychiatric Association.

For additional training opportunities, contact Kelly C. Allison, PhD, 3535 Market Street, Suite 3021, Philadelphia, PA 19104-3309; *kca@mail.med.upenn.edu*, 215-898-7314.

References

Allison KC. (2005, September). *Treatment of the night eating syndrome.* Symposium talk presented at the annual meeting of the Eating Disorders Research Society, Toronto, Canada.

Allison KC, Ahima RS, O'Reardon JP, Dinges DF, Sharma V, Cummings DE, et al. (2005). Neuroendocrine profiles associated with energy intake, sleep, and stress in the night eating syndrome. *Journal of Clinical Endocrinology and Metabolism,* 90:614–6217.

Allison KC, Crow SJ, Reeves RR, West DS, Foreyt JP, DiLillo VG, et al. (2007). The prevalence of binge eating disorder and night eating syndrome in adults with Type 2 diabetes mellitus. *Obesity,* 15:185–1291.

Allison KC, Grilo CM, Masheb RM, & Stunkard AJ. (2005). Binge eating disorder and night eating syndrome: A comparative study of disordered eating. *Journal of Consulting and Clinical Psychology,* 73:1107–1115.

Allison KC, Lundgren JD, O'Reardon JP, Martino NS, Sarwer DB, Wadden TA, et al. (2008). The Night Eating Questionnaire (NEQ): Psychometric properties of a measure of severity of the night eating syndrome. *Eating Behaviors,* 9:62–72.

Allison KC, Martino N, O'Reardon J, & Stunkard A. (2005). CBT treatment for night eating syndrome: A pilot study. *Obesity Research,* 13:A83.

Allison KC, & Stunkard AJ. (2007) Self-help for night eating syndrome. In JD Latner & GT Wilson (Eds.), *Self-help approaches for obesity and eating disorders: Research and practice* (pp. 310–324). New York: Guilford Press.

Allison KC, Stunkard AJ, & Thier SL. (2004). *Overcoming night eating syndrome: A step-by step guide to breaking the cycle.* Oakland, CA: New Harbinger.

Allison KC, Wadden TA, Sarwer DB, Fabricatore AN, Crerand C, Gibbons L, et al. (2006). Night eating syndrome and binge eating disorder among persons seeking bariatric surgery: Prevalence and related features. *Obesity,* 14:77S–82S.

American Academy of Sleep Medicine. (2005). *International classification of sleep disorders: Diagnostic and coding manual* (2nd ed.). Westchester, IL: Author.

American Psychiatric Association. (2000). *Diagnostic and statistical manual of mental disorders* (4th ed., text rev.). Washington, DC: Author.

Aronoff NJ, Geliebter A, & Zammit G. (2001). Gender and body mass index as related to the night eating syndrome. *Journal of the American Dietetic Association,* 101:102–104.

Beck JS. (1995). *Cognitive therapy: Basics and beyond.* New York: Guilford Press.

Birketvedt GS, Florholmen J, Sundsfjord J, Osterud B, Dinges D, Bilker W, et al. (1999). Behavioral and neuroendocrine characteristics of the night-eating syndrome. *Journal of the American Medical Association,* 282:657–663.

Boston RC, Moate PJ, Allison KC, Lundgren JD, & Stunkard AJ. (2008). Modeling circadian rhythms of food intake by means of parametric deconvolution: Results from studies on the night eating syndrome. *American Journal of Clinical Nutrition,* 87:1672–1677.

Brownell KD. (2004). *The LEARN program for weight management* (10th ed.). Dallas: LEARN.

Coates TJ. (1978). Successive self-management strategies towards coping with night eating. *Journal of Behavior Therapy and Experimental Psychiatry,* 9:181–183.

Colles SL, Dixon JB, & O'Brien PE. (2007). Night eating syndrome and nocturnal snacking:

Association with obesity, binge eating and psychological distress. *International Journal of Obesity*, 31:1722–1730.

Devlin MJ, Allison KC, Goldfein JA, & Spanos A. (2007). Management of EDNOS (eating disorder not otherwise specified). In J Yager & P Powers (Eds.), *Clinical management of eating disorders* (pp. 195–224).Washington, DC: American Psychiatric Association.

Fairburn CG, Marcus MD, & Wilson GT. (1993). Cognitive-behavioral therapy for binge eating and bulimia nervosa: A comprehensive treatment manual. In CG Fairburn & GT Wilson (Eds.), *Binge eating: Nature, assessment, and treatment* (pp. 361–404). New York: Guilford Press.

Gluck ME, Geliebter A, & Zammit G. (2001). Night eating syndrome is associated with depression, low self-esteem, reduced daytime hunger, and less weight loss in obese outpatients. *Obesity Research*, 9:264–267.

Goel N, Stunkard AJ, Rogers NL, Van Dongen HPA, Allison KC, O'Reardon JP, et al. (2009). Circadian rhythm profiles in women with night eating syndrome. *Journal of Biological Rhythms*, 24:85–94.

Goncalves MD, Moore RH, Stunkard AJ, & Allison KC. (2009). The treatment of night eating: The patient's perspective. *European Eating Disorders Review*, 17:184–190.

Grilo CM, & Masheb RM. (2004). Night-time eating in men and women with binge eating disorder. *Behaviour Research and Therapy*, 42:397–407.

Guy W. (1976). *ECDEU assessment manual for psychopharmacology*. Rockville, MD: National Institute of Mental Health.

Howell MJ, Schenck CH, & Crow SJ. (2008). A review of nighttime eating disorders. *Sleep Medicine, 13*(1), 23–34.

Lundgren JD, Allison KC, Crow S, O'Reardon JP, Berg KC, Galbraith J, et al. (2006). Prevalence of the night eating syndrome in a psychiatric population. *American Journal of Psychiatry*, 163:156–158.

Lundgren JD, Allison KC, O'Reardon JP, & Stunkard AJ. (2008). A descriptive study of nonobese persons with night eating syndrome and a weight-matched comparison group. *Eating Behaviors*, 9:352–359.

Lundgren JD, Amsterdam J, Newberg A, Allison KC, Wintering N, & Stunkard AJ. (in press). Differences in serotonin transporter binding affinity in patients with major depressive disorder and night eating syndrome. *Eating and Weight Disorders*.

Lundgren JD, Newberg AB, Allison KC, Wintering NA, Ploessl K, & Stunkard AJ. (2008). [123]ADAM SPECT imaging of serotonin transporter binding in patients with night eating syndrome: A preliminary report. *Psychiatry Research: Neuroimaging*, 162:214–220.

Miyaoka T, Yasukawa R, Tsubouchi K, Miura S, Shimizu Y, Sukegawa T, et al. (2003). Successful treatment of nocturnal eating/drinking syndrome with selective serotonin reuptake inhibitors. *International Clinical Psychopharmacology*, 18:175–177.

O'Reardon JP, Allison KC, Martino NS, Lundgren JD, Heo M, & Stunkard AJ. (2006). A randomized placebo controlled trial of sertraline in the treatment of the night eating syndrome. *American Journal of Psychiatry*, 163:893–898.

O'Reardon JP, Stunkard AJ, & Allison KC. (2004). A clinical trial of sertraline in the treatment of the night eating syndrome. *International Journal of Eating Disorders*, 35:16–26.

Pawlow LA, O'Neil PM, & Malcolm RJ. (2003). Night eating syndrome: Effects of brief relaxation training on stress, mood hunger and eating patterns. *International Journal of Obesity and Related Metabolic Disorders*, 27:970–978.

Powers PS, Perez A, Boyd F, & Rosemurgy A. (1999). Eating pathology before and after bariatric surgery: A prospective study. *International Journal of Eating Disorders*, 25:293–300.

Sassaroli S, Ruggiero GM, Vinai P, Cardetti S, Carpegna G, & Ferrato N. (2009). Daily and nightly anxiety among patients affected by night eating syndrome and binge eating disorder. *Eating Disorders: The Journal of Treatment and Prevention*, 17:140–145.

Striegel-Moore RH, Dohm FA, Hook JM, Schreiber GB, Crawford PB, & Daniels SR. (2005). Night eating syndrome in young adult women: Prevalence and correlates. *International Journal of Eating Disorders*, 37:200–206.

Striegel-Moore RH, Franko DL, Thompson D, Affenito S, & Kraemer HC. (2006). Night eating: Prevalence and demographic correlates. *Obesity Research*, 14:139–147.

Stunkard AJ, Allison KC, Lundgren JD, Martino NS, Heo M, Etemad B, et al. (2006). A paradigm for facilitating pharmacotherapy at a distance: Sertraline treatment of the night eating syndrome. *Journal of Clinical Psychiatry*, 67:1568–1572.

Stunkard AJ, Berkowitz R, Wadden T, Tanrikut C, Reiss E, & Young L. (1996). Binge eating disorder and the night eating syndrome. *International Journal of Obesity*, 20:1–6.

Stunkard AJ, Grace WJ, & Wolff HG. (1955). The night-eating syndrome: A pattern of food intake among certain obese patients. *American Journal of Medicine*, 19:78–86.

Williamson DA, Lawson OD, Bennett SM, & Hinz L. (1989). Behavioral treatment of night bingeing and rumination in an adult case of bulimia nervosa. *Journal of Behavior Therapy and Experimental Psychiatry*, 20:73–77.

CHAPTER 28

Treatment for Body-Image Disturbances

Susan J. Paxton and Siân A. McLean

Body image is a multidimensional construct with perceptual, affective, and cognitive components (Thompson, Heinberg, Altabe, & Tantleff Dunn, 1999). Thus, body image includes perception of size and shape, satisfaction with appearance, body esteem, acceptance or self-loathing of one's body, body anxiety, and salience of weight and shape (Ben-Tovim & Walker, 1991; Thompson et al., 1999). An individual's body image focus may be directed toward his/her body in general or toward a specific aspect of the body or body part. Body image may be positive and a source of pleasure, enjoyment, and satisfaction. However, all too often, perceptions of the body are distorted, and the body is associated with extremely negative emotions, anxiety, distress, and disparagement. While recognizing the multidimensional nature of body image and consequently the multidimensional nature of treatment, we refer to the wide range of negative body image experiences in a generic way as "body dissatisfaction."

Body dissatisfaction affects both females and males, although it is reported more frequently by females. Body dissatisfaction in females tends to be directed toward being larger than desired, while in males the focus is frequently on being insufficiently muscular (e.g., Smolak & Stein, 2006). In adolescents, body dissatisfaction has been reported by 24–46% of girls and 12–26% of boys (Narring et al., 2004; Neumark-Sztainer, Story, Hannan, Perry, & Irving, 2002; Presnell, Bearman, & Stice, 2004). In adulthood, body image appears to improve slightly in females but continues to decline in males (Eisenberg, Neumark-Sztainer, & Paxton, 2006).

Body dissatisfaction can be conceptualized as falling along a continuum from none to extreme (Thompson et al., 1999). At the extreme of body dissatisfaction is body dysmorphic disorder (BDD), which is characterized by a preoccupation with an imagined or slight defect in physical appearance that causes significant impairment in social, occupational, or other functioning (American Psychiatric Association, 2000) and affects 1–2% of the population (Otto, Wilhelm, Cohen, & Harlow, 2001). Treatment for body dissatisfaction is clearly indicated when it causes distress and interferes with role functioning.

Prevention, early intervention, and treatment for body dissatisfaction are also warranted due to its role as a risk factor for other significant psychological problems. Body dissatisfaction is a risk factor for the development of depressive symptoms and low self-esteem (Holsen, Kraft, & Roysamb, 2001; Paxton, Neumark-Sztainer, Hannan, & Eisenberg, 2006). Importantly, body dissatisfaction is a risk factor for the use of behaviors intended to change body shape. Body dissatisfaction predicts use of extreme weight loss behaviors such as crash dieting, fasting, self-induced vomiting, laxative misuse, and excessive exercise in both males and females (Neumark-Sztainer, Paxton, Hannan, Haines, & Story, 2006). In males, body dissatisfaction is associated with the use of steroids and other substances to increase muscle bulk (e.g., Cafri et al., 2005).

Importantly, body dissatisfaction is frequently treated in the context of eating disorders (EDs) for two major reasons. First, it is one of the most reliably observed risk factors for the development of disordered eating and clinical EDs in Western cultures (Jacobi, Hayward, de Zwaan, Kraemer, & Agras, 2004; Neumark-Sztainer et al., 2006; Stice, 2002) and developing countries (e.g., Jackson & Chen, 2008). Stice (2002) has also identified body dissatisfaction as an important maintaining factor once an ED has been established. Furthermore, continued body dissatisfaction in patients treated for anorexia nervosa (AN) and bulimia nervosa (BN) is associated with higher risk of relapse (Rosen, 1990).

Second, a disturbance in body image is a key diagnostic feature of AN and BN (American Psychiatric Association, 2000) and has also been observed as an important aspect of binge-eating disorder (BED), although it is not a required diagnostic criterion for the diagnosis of BED (Masheb & Grilo, 2000). It is worth noting that the body image disturbances that characterize EDs are specific forms of intense body dissatisfaction. Although many persons have body dissatisfaction, only a minority has the intense fear of fatness or perceptual distortions that define AN or the overvaluation of shape or weight that characterizes BN and is viewed as the central cognitive disturbance of EDs and a critical maintaining factor of disordered eating behaviors (Fairburn, Cooper, & Shafran, 2003; Hrabosky, Masheb, White, & Grilo, 2007). Thus, in addition to body dissatisfaction (a common problem in Western cultures), persons with EDs usually suffer from specific cognitive-evaluative problems tied to body image. This important distinction has been demonstrated in studies showing that overvaluation of shape and weight is more closely tied to self-esteem than is body dissatisfaction (Masheb & Grilo, 2003) and that overvaluation better differentiates persons with EDs from those without EDs (Goldfein, Walsh, & Midlarsky, 2000; Grilo et al., 2008). Thus, alleviating body dissatisfaction and related perceptions and cognitions is essential for optimal outcomes in the treatment of EDs.

In light of the negative impact of body dissatisfaction described above, treatment for body image problems is frequently indicated in clinical practice. When considering appropriate targets for treatment, it is valuable to understand risk and maintaining factors that underpin body dissatisfaction on the grounds that eliminating these factors will reduce body dissatisfaction itself. The following section describes key risk and maintaining factors identified in the research literature as a means of identifying targets for treatment that are appropriate for patients.

Identifying Intervention Targets:
Risk and Maintaining Factors for Body Dissatisfaction

Numerous factors have been identified as contributing to the development and main-tenance of body dissatisfaction as well as a number for which evidence is still in the early stages. These factors can be considered broadly in three categories: sociocultural, individual temperament, and physical factors (Wertheim, Paxton, & Blaney, 2009). It is widely recognized that Western societies promote a thin body ideal for females and a lean and muscular ideal for males through many avenues, including media, popular culture, toys, and family, peer, and school subcultures (Wertheim et al., 2009). Thus, there are pervasive sociocultural pressures to aspire to an idealized thin body that, by its very nature, is very difficult to achieve and thus likely to result in a perceived discrepancy between the ideal and reality, or perceived reality, and subsequent body dissatisfaction. Greater risk for body dissatisfaction appears to be conveyed by greater exposure to these pressures. Higher frequency of viewing appearance-oriented tele-vision is associated with greater body dissatisfaction during childhood—a formative period of body image (Dohnt & Tiggemann, 2006), although a risk factor role for more frequent exposure to idealized images in later years has not been conclusively demon-strated. Exposure to a more intense peer appearance–related culture, in which friends are frequently dieting or talking about appearance, also contributes to body dissatisfac-tion (Dohnt & Tiggemann, 2006; Jones, 2004; Paxton, Neumark-Sztainer, et al., 2006; Paxton, Schutz, Wertheim, & Muir, 1999). Furthermore, exposure to appearance teas-ing consistently predicts body dissatisfaction and associated dieting behaviors (Wade & Lowes, 2002; Wertheim, Koerner, & Paxton, 2001). However, when considering treat-ment, these environmental factors are not necessarily under patient control. In this situation, treatments may focus on management of these external pressures.

It has been proposed that sociocultural pressures influence body image by increas-ing the value placed on achieving the appearance ideal by the individual (Thompson et al., 1999; Wertheim et al., 2009)—that is, increasing internalization of the thin body ideal (Keery, van den Berg, & Thompson, 2004). Discrepancy between these strongly held ideals and perceived reality are proposed to result in body dissatisfaction (Thomp-son et al., 1999). Research demonstrates that internalization of appearance ideals is a risk factor for body dissatisfaction in girls (Clark & Tiggemann, 2008), strongly asso-ciated with body dissatisfaction in adolescence and adulthood in both females and males (e.g., Knauss, Paxton, & Alsaker, 2007; Smolak, Levine, & Thompson, 2001), and a predictor of a negative impact on body image following exposure to idealized media images in females and males (e.g., Durkin & Paxton, 2002; Humphreys & Pax-ton, 2004). The overevaluation of appearance ideals becomes an integral characteristic of patients with EDs. Unlike the sociocultural environment that may contribute to their development, these attitudes, beliefs, and schemas can be challenged in therapy.

The tendency to compare one's body with others in person or in media images, and especially to make upward comparisons that result in a negative evaluation of one's own body, has also been identified as a risk factor for the development of body dissatisfac-tion, and there is a strong association between body comparison and body dissatisfac-tion (Jones, 2004; van den Berg et al., 2007). The process of comparing in this manner is likely to highlight perceived physical inadequacies and thus contribute to, and maintain, body dissatisfaction. Research suggests that, particularly in females, body comparison tendency mediates relationships between sociocultural pressures to be thin and also low self-esteem and body dissatisfaction (Durkin, Paxton, & Sorbello, 2007; van den Berg et al., 2007). Thus, treatments to reduce body comparison, especially in relation to particularly disliked body parts, can play an important part in reducing body dissatisfaction and related disordered behaviors.

Two variables that are regarded as behavioral expressions of body dissatisfaction and may also contribute to its development and maintenance are body avoidance and body checking (Shafran, Fairburn, Robinson, & Lask, 2004; Shafran, Lee, Payne, & Fairburn, 2007). "Body avoidance" refers to behaviors that are designed to prevent or sidestep situations that provoke concern about physical appearance, such as not weighing, ignoring or covering mirrors, wearing baggy clothes, and not going into situations in which there may be physical scrutiny (Rosen, Srebnik, Saltzberg, & Wendt, 1991; Shafran et al., 2004). "Body checking" relates to "critical scrutiny of one's body size, shape and weight ... including examining oneself in the mirror, using the fit of clothes to judge whether size has changed, feeling for bones, seeking reassurance about shape, and making negative comparisons with others" (Shafran et al., 2007, p. 113).

Body avoidance and body checking have consistently been observed to be elevated in people with EDs (Reas, Grilo, Masheb, & Wilson, 2005; Shafran et al., 2004). Body avoidance may prevent patients from disconfirming their irrational beliefs surrounding their weight and shape (Reas et al., 2005). Although causal pathways have not been clarified, in non-eating-disordered women body checking has been shown to temporarily increase body dissatisfaction, feelings of fatness, and body-related self-critical thinking (Shafran et al., 2007), suggesting that body checking may contribute to body dissatisfaction by increasing attention to disliked parts of the body (Williamson, Muller, Reas, & Thaw, 1999). Body checking may also serve to reinforce dietary restraint (Mountford, Haase, & Waller, 2006). Although mechanisms of action are not well understood, the evidence is building to suggest that treatments that reduce these behaviors will be valuable in alleviating body dissatisfaction. Mountford and colleagues (2006) propose that challenging underlying beliefs that maintain body avoidance and body checking, using behavioral experiments, should enable patients to become aware of the inaccuracies of their beliefs. Mirror exposure, described further below, is one such experiment that has been shown to reduce body dissatisfaction (Delinsky & Wilson, 2006).

Higher body mass index (BMI) is consistently observed to be a prospective risk factor for body dissatisfaction in females (Jones, 2004; Paxton, Eisenberg, & Neumark-Sztainer, 2006) and typically (e.g., Paxton, Eisenberg, et al., 2006; Ricciardelli, McCabe, Lillis, & Thomas, 2006) but not always (Barker & Galambos, 2003) in boys. This finding is not surprising in social environments that value thinness. Thus, managing the discrepancy between the sociocultural body ideal and the reality for many women may also become a focus of treatment, either by teaching healthy weight management or by assisting patients to accept the body they have, despite social pressures to do otherwise. Notably, at extremes, the philosophies behind these approaches differ considerably. On one hand, weight management approaches may be seen to be endorsing the social ideal and capitulating to social pressures, while at the other extreme accepting any size may be seen as ignoring health risks associated with obesity. In the middle ground, treatment that facilitates improved eating patterns as well as increased acceptance of the reality of one's own body shape is important in intervention approaches for body dissatisfaction.

One aspect of body image, body size perception, and particularly body size overestimation has frequently been associated with ED symptomatology (Farrell, Lee, & Shafran, 2005). A review of the somewhat inconsistent research literature suggests that patients with EDs do not have a sensory deficit contributing to body size distortion, but that compared to healthy controls, patients with AN or BN do tend to overestimate their body size (Farrell et al., 2005). Evidence is building that body size overestimation is a manifestation of, rather than a contributor to, body dissatisfaction (Mussap, McCabe, & Ricciardelli, 2008). Thus, it may be anticipated that overestimation would decrease with improvement in ED symptoms (Farrell et al., 2005). However, to date, the role of body size overestimation remains very unclear, and it is possible that it contributes to the development of disordered eating. In this context, beneficial treatments have been explored to reduce body image distortion in patients for whom body size distortion is high, especially in patients with AN (Rushford & Ostermeyer, 1997).

Finally, general psychological characteristics and temperament have been linked to the development or maintenance of body dissatisfaction. Low self-esteem and depressive symptoms increase risk of body dissatisfaction, possibly as a result of increasing the likelihood of a generalized negative view of the self, including a negative view of one's appearance (Paxton, Eisenberg, et al., 2006). A perfectionistic temperament has also been shown to be associated with body dissatisfaction and disordered eating, but the nature of these relationships remains to be clarified (Downey & Chang, 2007; Wade & Lowes, 2002). In light of relationships between perfectionism, low-self esteem, and depressive mood and body image dissatisfaction (Dunkley & Grilo, 2007), interventions that address these characteristics can also be valuable in improving body image.

Treatment Strategies

The treatment for body dissatisfaction outlined in the next section broadly follows a cognitive-behavioral therapy (CBT) approach, with cognitive, behavioral, and perceptual risk and maintaining factors addressed separately. Strategies to be used are discussed explicitly with the patient, and the rationale underlying each treatment approach is carefully explained. Although the different techniques are presented separately here, a combination of components would typically be used in treatment for any one patient. CBT programs incorporating cognitive, behavioral, and perceptual interventions produce clinically meaningful reductions in body dissatisfaction (e.g., Butters & Cash, 1987; Heinicke, Paxton, McLean, & Wertheim, 2007; Jarry & Ip, 2005; Paxton, McLean, Gollings, Faulkner, & Wertheim, 2007; Rosen, Saltzberg, & Srebnik, 1989).

Sociocultural Pressures

Engaging patients in questioning the realism and purpose of the portrayal of women in the media—that is, developing their "media literacy"—is the main approach for dealing with sociocultural pressures. This approach has been shown to reduce thin-ideal internalization in adolescent boys and girls in prevention research (Wilksch, Tigge-mann, & Wade, 2006). To facilitate media literacy work the patient can be asked to bring particular examples of media portrayals of men or women to the session. The clinician can use a Socratic questioning approach to help the patient recognize that (1) in the majority of cases only women who fit within a limited appearance range are presented in the media, (2) media images are not real and are subject to a high degree of manipulation before the final product is complete, and, (3) advertising deliberately presents unattainable images in tandem with desirable characteristics such as wealth, popularity, and fun. One purpose of advertising is to entice people not only to buy the product but to also buy the image and desirable characteristics that are presented alongside the product.

Examples of Socratic questions to elicit the patient's understanding are:

"What do the men/women you see in the media typically look like? What are the similarities in these images?"

"What processes have been undertaken before the model has his/her photo taken? What sort of manipulation is done after the photo is taken?"

"What message is the advertiser sending you when the product is presented along-side an ideal image of this model in a successful situation?"

To reinforce the new perception of media images as "not real" and the narrow depiction of women in media images, patients can be encouraged to consider the attributes that are missing from media images and how these attributes are important in the relationships they have with people in their lives. Such attributes might include diversity in appearance, such as ethnic and age differences, as well as personality characteristics such as warmth, humor, and caring.

There may be sources of social pressure to be thin or muscular other than media, such as peer and family pressures, that play an important role in sustaining patients' body dissatisfaction. Identification of these sources of pressure and exploring and questioning the motives and validity of them may also be a valuable intervention strategy.

Internalization of the Thin Ideal

Challenging attitudes and beliefs that maintain internalization of the thin ideal can alleviate sociocultural pressures to be thin. One approach that has gained support in ED prevention programs is the use of cognitive dissonance (e.g., Becker, Bull, Schaumberg, Cauble, & Franco, 2008; Boivin, Polivy, & Herman, 2008; Stice, Shaw, Burton, & Wade, 2006). In this approach, patients develop arguments against unrealistic expectations of attaining the thin ideal (e.g., "I will be happier/have more energy/be more successful") and generate thoughts about the costs and unreality of pursuing such an ideal. These counterarguments create cognitive dissonance, that is, inconsistencies between the patient's existing beliefs and the stated counterargument. Dissonance creates psychological discomfort and the patient is motivated to try to reduce the dissonance by changing his/her behavior or cognitions (Festinger, 1962). Reappraising the costs and benefits of pursuing the thin ideal will reduce the extent to which the patient holds the ideal as a personal standard.

For cognitive dissonance to be evoked in the therapeutic setting, the patient must believe that he/she is voluntarily taking the position of arguing against prevailing attitudes, rather than being coerced. Patients can be told that discussing how to help other people think critically about the thin ideal can help them to address their own body dissatisfaction. Following the elicitation of arguments examining the costs and benefits of the thin ideal, engaging the patient in a role play can help to reinforce the gains made in the dissonance task. The clinician takes the role of a person with a high degree of thin-ideal internalization, and the role of the patient is to convince the person to let go of the thin ideal, using arguments developed earlier. Discussing the benefits that would be obtained from not being preoccupied with the thin ideal can also help to reinforce the attitude shift away from internalization of the thin ideal.

Body Comparisons

The treatment for appearance comparisons aims to reduce the frequency of comparisons by facilitating a shift from upward (i.e., with people who have more of the desired quality) to downward (i.e., with people who have less of the desired quality) comparisons, selecting realistic comparison targets, and altering the negative affective consequences of comparisons through cognitive restructuring. Gaining detailed information, through the use of monitoring sheets, about the patient's comparison behavior, including the situation, comparison targets, attribute for comparison, and consequences of the comparison, is the first step. From the monitoring task, patients recognize that the comparisons in which they engage are selective both for the attribute about themselves on which they compare—usually one that they do not like—and for the target with whom they choose to compare—usually a target superior on the chosen attribute. This selective targeting results in upward, rather than downward, comparisons, thus leading to a negative evaluation of one's body and subsequently body dissatisfaction. This approach has reduced comparisons in an experimental intervention (Posavac, Posavac, & Weigel, 2001).

The second process consists of an *in vivo* behavioral experiment in which the patient evaluates the outcome of two sets of comparisons. For the experiment, the patient monitors the details of the comparison as indicated for the monitoring task above. First, the patient engages in his/her usual comparisons and chooses any 10 people with whom to compare him- or herself. For the second set of comparisons, the instruction is to compare him- or herself with 10 consecutive people of the same gender who pass by, but without being selective for the target. The patient will realize that he/she does not compare unfavorably with all people, and that he/she tends to be unaware of people with whom he/she would compare positively. The clinician reinforces the perception that the patient has control over the comparison process and can therefore choose to make upward comparisons, with the consequent negative outcomes, or downward comparisons, which are more likely to preserve self-esteem and positive feelings about his/her body.

Cognitive restructuring also can be used to reduce negative affective consequences of comparisons by diminishing the evaluative or comparative component of the behavior. For example, an alternative for the negative thought "He has great muscle definition—my muscles are nowhere near as big" might be "He has great muscle definition, good for him." Cognitive restructuring can also be implemented to sever the connection between appearance and the possession of other desirable characteristics; for example, "She has great legs, she must be really popular" becomes "She has great legs but that doesn't make her more fun to be with than I am."

Avoidance of Mirrors and Reflections

The approach to treating avoidance of mirrors and looking at one's reflection is similar to the use of graded exposure hierarchies for phobias, and has been shown to be effective for body dissatisfaction and BDD (e.g., Delinsky & Wilson, 2006; Hilbert & Tuschen-Caffier, 2004; McKay, Todaro, Neziroglu, & Campisi, 1997). In relation to body dissatisfaction, the phobia is the patient's own appearance, which has come to be associated with severely negative cognitive and emotional consequences. The negative response to his/her body is reinforced by avoiding or ignoring any reflective surfaces.

Patients are first presented with psychoeducation to explain the CBT model, including a rationale for exposure therapy. A graded exposure hierarchy list related to looking at their reflection is developed with patients. As with hierarchies for phobias, patients assign ratings of distress to each of these situations, and they are placed in rank order. Some of these may be imaginal, and the exposure would be directed by the clinician, such as imagining trying on new clothes in a dressing room with three-sided mirrors. Other situations are *in vivo* and conducted either in session, with the aid of a mirror, or as homework exercises, such as looking in a full-length mirror wearing underwear. Patients begin by addressing the situations from the list in order from those that provoke the least distress to those that provoke the most.

Patients begin the exposure procedure in as relaxed and comfortable state as possible. A short relaxation exercise, such as deep breathing or progressive muscle relaxation, may be helpful. For imaginal exposure, patients imagine the phobic stimulus by thinking about it or describing it to the clinician in sufficient detail to provoke anxiety, and continue to think about it for as long as it takes for the anxiety to subside. Similarly, for *in vivo* exposure, patients look at themselves in a mirror and remain in the situation while concentrating on their reflection until the anxiety subsides. It is important that each exposure exercise is prolonged so that the anxiety or distress diminishes before patients move out of the situation. Each step on the hierarchy is repeated until patients can place themselves in that situation comfortably, without experiencing anxiety, before moving on to the next step. Throughout each of the steps in the exposure process, the rationale for the approach is revisited, reinforcing patients' understanding of the process and enhancing their self-efficacy for changing their behavior and body image–related distress.

Avoidance of Behaviors and Situations

Treating other forms of avoidance, such as avoidance of social situations, people, or places, is undertaken in a similar fashion to mirror avoidance, using the exposure technique. Patients are presented with a similar rationale, emphasizing how avoidance contributes to the maintenance of their body-related distress. In conjunction with the clinician, patients develop a list of graded exposure tasks for the relevant avoided behavior. It is important to focus on activities in which patients want to engage and can practically do so at the time of treatment. For example, it is not helpful to undertake a beach-related exposure procedure in the middle of winter or if, regardless of body concerns, patients have no intention or desire to visit the beach.

The mechanism of action for successful exposure to situations, people, and places requires that, in addition to experiencing initial distress or anxiety in the avoided situation, patients must also recognize that the anticipated negative consequences of exposure, such as embarrassment or humiliation, do not occur to the extent that they had predicted. Careful monitoring and recording of each exposure task will highlight the discrepancy between the expected and actual outcomes.

Exposure to situations involving other people can be more complicated than mirror exposure, as unforeseen factors may influence the exposure process. Prior to exposure, patients must prepare for unpredictable incidents and not attribute failure to themselves if changing circumstances prevented the exposure from being carried out as they had planned.

Finding the motivation to continually expose oneself to distressing situations can be difficult to maintain. To assist with motivation the clinician can help patients recognize that they are enjoying participation in previously avoided activities, despite the initial anxiety or distress.

Checking

Behavioral techniques such as stimulus control and exposure and response prevention are used to reduce checking behaviors, following modification of treatments for BDD (Grant & Phillips, 2005; Rosen, Reiter, & Orosan, 1995). Stimulus control is a short-term strategy that addresses the conditioning component inherent in checking behaviors. To reduce checking behaviors the environment is altered, removing objects that facilitate checking. This may include putting away scales that are a requisite for frequent weighing or throwing away a particular article of clothing, the fit of which is used to determine a "fat" or "thin" day, and subsequently a "good" or "bad" day. Exposure and response prevention involves purposeful exposure to triggers for distress, such as thoughts, images, or situations, and prevention of accompanying rituals and checking behaviors that are conducted to diminish distress.

A rationale similar to that for exposure work with avoidance behavior is presented to patients with additional information conveying the importance of stopping checking behaviors. The following is an example for a patient who checks the prominence of her hip bones after eating to assuage concerns about gaining weight following food intake:

> "Although you may at first feel reassured when you feel your hip bones, doing so is a problem because it maintains your body distress by focusing attention onto your abdomen—the part of your body that you do not like. By using the exposure and response prevention technique, we are going to break the vicious circle between your trigger thoughts about gaining weight after eating, imagining that your stomach is bloated after eating and feeling distress, and carrying out your body checking behavior."

For this patient, a clinician-directed exposure and response prevention session would be scheduled directly after a meal, allowing a naturalistic provocation of weight gain concerns. With prompting from the clinician for information about cognitions, physical feelings, and perceptions of her body, the patient would describe in detail her worries about gaining weight after eating, her current image of herself in relation to her body size, and the level of distress she was feeling. The patient would be instructed not to check the feel of her hip bones during this procedure, and to comply with the response prevention instruction she may keep her hands on the chair, or by her side, or engage in some other behavior to keep her hands occupied. To assess the level of distress evoked by the exposure, the clinician would check with the patient every 10 minutes and wait for it to diminish. The clinician would continue to prompt the patient to focus on her triggers for body concerns until the distress decreased by about 50% from the highest level. Exposure and response prevention tasks would be planned for the patient to conduct out of session so that the effects occur more rapidly, and the patient would be able to engage in *in vivo* exposure that would not be possible to simulate within the therapy session.

Additional strategies advocated by Cash (2008) can be planned in advance to help decrease the occurrence of the rituals or checking, leading to a gradual cessation of the behavior. These include delay tactics such as introducing graduated increases in time between the trigger and the checking or ritual; giving oneself permission to spend a particular amount of time, but no more, on rituals or checking; limiting of the number of episodes of checking behaviors performed each day; and making appointment times for checking whereby all checking must be done by appointment only and not outside of appointments made in advance.

Distorted Body Perception

Distorted body perception, usually manifest as size overestimation, can be addressed with size estimation feedback. Video feedback procedures have improved body image distortion in patients with AN (Rushford & Ostermeyer, 1997).

Patients are provided with a rationale for the exercise:

> "Women who are dissatisfied with their bodies sometimes perceive themselves to be larger than they actually are. When that happens, it is hard for them to feel okay about their bodies. I sense that something similar is going on for you. To help you to look at your body more accurately, I would like to take a video recording of you wearing tight-fitting clothes, like sports gear, and we will look at the video together and talk about the way that you perceive your body. I know this might seem like a really uncomfortable thing to do, but I think it will be helpful for you to reduce the negative feelings you have about your body."

The patient must be assured that this process will be completely private, and the video will be viewed only by herself and her clinician.

During the video recording the patient is asked to turn slowly so that she is viewed from the front, back, and both sides, to allow each aspect of her distorted perception of her body to be addressed during the feedback component of the exercise. For the review of the recording the patient is asked to try to view the shape on the screen as though she were seeing someone for the first time and to describe her appearance. This frame strengthens the objectivity of the process (Rushford & Ostermeyer, 1997).

The patient's description is discussed with the clinician, pausing when necessary to highlight particular aspects. The clinician's role is to highlight discrepancies between the patient's perception of her body and the reality of the image on the screen. For example, if the patient reports that she has a "fat stomach," the clinician can show the disputing evidence from the side view on the video. Discussion of how the patient's body size and shape are similar to, or different from, similar-age women of normal weight is also helpful.

Healthy Weight Management and Self-Care

Healthy weight management, similar to nondiet approaches that encompass balanced, regular eating in conjunction with regular physical activity, has been shown to improve body image (Bacon et al., 2002; Stice et al., 2006; Stice, Trost, & Chase, 2003). Fears of weight gain are reduced with the acquisition of stable eating patterns, and there is a concomitant decrease in unhealthy weight loss practices such as fasting, restrictive dieting, purging, and excessive exercise.

The healthy weight approach begins with a reconceptualization of the body ideal from thin to healthy. The costs and benefits of these ideals can be explored in a similar manner to the critical analysis of thin-ideal internalization presented above. Adopting the healthy ideal as a personal standard helps the patient to embrace the rationale for regular eating and can reduce fears of weight gain that typically accompany eating regularly.

Planning and scheduling meals and snacks in advance and committing to eat only at scheduled times, which prevents nonhungry eating (e.g., grazing), establishes a regular pattern of eating and reduces fluctuations in hunger. Patients gradually learn to respond to hunger cues rather than having body concerns dictate when they will and will not eat. Care must be taken to ensure that eating patterns do not become too rigid. To assist with this, once the eating schedule is stable, patients can start to broaden the types of foods that they eat and introduce flexibility into their eating pattern to account for normal contextual influences on eating, such as celebrations. Exposure can be used to introduce feared forbidden foods and break rigid rules surrounding eating. This process allows patients to feel less out of control as they experience fewer cycles of restriction and overeating. Subsequently, worry about weight gain is reduced.

Engaging in body-related self-care and moving the body for pleasure (e.g., dancing) enhances positive feelings toward the body. Conversely, attitudes that act as barriers to self-care must be addressed to increase the patient's involvement in these activities. Frequently, patients with body dissatisfaction experience guilt from doing something for themselves or believe they are not deserving of self-care or nurturance. Cognitive restructuring to challenge these types of thoughts is indicated in these instances.

Increasing self-care behaviors can be achieved through activity scheduling, such as making regular appointments for nurturing activities like relaxation, and stimulus control to manage cues for self-care, such as placing scented hand cream in a conspicuous place. Patients are actively encouraged to not put off engaging in activities until reaching what they perceive to be an acceptable size to do so. Reinforcing experiences of enjoying one's body at any size can foster self-acceptance and enhancement of positive feelings toward one's body.

General Psychology

Depressed mood and low self-esteem within the context of dissatisfaction with one's body often center on beliefs and assumptions that self-worth is reliant upon meeting strict expectations and standards of appearance. As proposed by Shafran and colleagues (e.g., Riley, Lee, Cooper, Fairburn, & Shafran, 2007; Shafran, Cooper, & Fairburn, 2002) in their conceptualization of clinical perfectionism, "perceived failure to meet those standards results in self-criticism and negative self-evaluation" (Shafran et al., 2002, p. 778), contributing to depressed mood and low self-esteem. Treatment aims are to reduce the high expectations placed on appearance and to expand the sources from which the patient derives self-worth. This is achieved through cognitive restructuring of negative thoughts and beliefs. Beliefs related to perfectionism, black-and-white thinking, and "shoulds" can be targeted. Socratic questioning can draw from the patient alternate sources of self-esteem so that self-appraisal is shifted from a singular focus on appearance to encompass other factors, including achievements, relationships, intellectual abilities, etc. Activity scheduling to enhance accomplishment and enjoyment of activities can also improve mood and contribute to a change in focus away from the appearance of the body.

Conclusions

Interventions for body dissatisfaction may be required when body image problems occur alone, but they are essential when treating most EDs because body dissatisfaction, extreme cognitive-evaluative concerns, and perceptual distortions frequently underpin ED symptoms. A careful analysis of factors that maintain body dissatisfaction in each patient will help to highlight specific behaviors, cognitions, and perceptions that should be targeted. Interventions can then be matched to the needs of the patient to maximize treatment outcomes. In addition, it is imperative that further clinical research be conducted to increase the techniques currently available.

References

American Psychiatric Association. (2000). *Diagnostic and statistical manual of mental disorders* (4th ed., text rev.). Washington, DC: Author.

Bacon L, Keim N, Van Loan M, Derricote M, Gale B, Kazaks A, et al. (2002). Evaluating a "non-diet" wellness intervention for improvement of metabolic fitness, psychological well-being and eating and activity behaviors. *International Journal of Obesity*, 26:854–865.

Barker ET, & Galambos NL. (2003). Body dissatisfaction of adolescent girls and boys: Risk and resources factors. *Journal of Early Adolescence*, 23:141–165.

Becker CB, Bull S, Schaumberg K, Cauble A, & Franco A. (2008). Effectiveness of peer-led eating disorders prevention: A replication trial. *Journal of Consulting and Clinical Psychology*, 76:347–354.

Ben-Tovim DI, & Walker M. (1991). The development of the Ben-Tovim Walker Body Attitudes Questionnaire (BAQ), a new measure of women's attitudes towards their own bodies. *Psychological Medicine*, 21:775–784.

Boivin MK, Polivy J, & Herman C. (2008). An intervention to modify expectations of unrealistic rewards from thinness. *Eating Disorders: The Journal of Treatment and Prevention*, 16:160–179.

Butters JW, & Cash TF. (1987). Cognitive behavioral treatment of women's body-image dissatisfaction. *Journal of Consulting and Clinical Psychology*, 55:889–897.

Cafri G, Thompson J, Ricciardelli L, McCabe M, Smolak L, & Yesalis C. (2005). Pursuit of the muscular ideal: Physical and psychological consequences and putative risk factors. *Clinical Psychology Review*, 25:215–239.

Cash TF. (2008). *The body image workbook. An sight-step program for learning to like your looks.* Oakland, CA: New Harbinger.

Clark L, & Tiggemann M. (2008). Sociocultural and individual psychological predictors of body image in young girls: A prospective study. *Developmental Psychology*, 44:1124–1134.

Delinsky SS, & Wilson G. (2006). Mirror exposure for the treatment of body image disturbance. *International Journal of Eating Disorders*, 39:108–116.

Dohnt H, & Tiggemann M. (2006). The contribution of peer and media influences to the development of body satisfaction and self-esteem in young girls: A prospective study. *Developmental Psychology*, 42:929–936.

Downey CA, & Chang EC. (2007). Perfectionism and symptoms of eating disturbances in female college students: Considering the role of negative affect and body dissatisfaction. *Eating Behaviors*, 8:497–503.

Dunkley DM, & Grilo CM. (2007). Self-criticism, low self-esteem, depressive symptoms, and over-evaluation of shape and weight in binge eating disorder patients. *Behaviour Research and Therapy*, 45:139–149.

Durkin SJ, & Paxton SJ. (2002). Predictors of vulnerability to reduced body image satisfaction and psychological wellbeing in response to exposure to idealized female media images in adolescent girls. *Journal of Psychosomatic Research*, 53:995–1005.

Durkin SJ, Paxton SJ, & Sorbello M. (2007). An integrative model of the impact of exposure to idealized female images on adolescent girls' body satisfaction. *Journal of Applied Social Psychology*, 37:1092–1117.

Eisenberg ME, Neumark-Sztainer D, & Paxton SJ. (2006). Five-year change in body satisfaction among adolescents. *Journal of Psychosomatic Research*, 61:521–527.

Fairburn CG, Cooper Z, & Shafran R. (2003). Cognitive behaviour therapy for eating disorders: A "transdiagnostic" theory and treatment. *Behaviour Research and Therapy*, 41:509–528.

Farrell C, Lee M, & Shafran R. (2005). Assessment of body size estimation: A review. *European Eating Disorders Review*, 13:75–88.

Festinger L. (1962). *A theory of cognitive dissonance.* Palo Alto, CA: Stanford University Press.

Goldfein JA, Walsh B, & Midlarsky E. (2000). Influence of shape and weight on self-evaluation in bulimia nervosa. *International Journal of Eating Disorders*, 27:435–445.

Grant JE, & Phillips KA. (2005). Recognizing and treating body dysmorphic disorder. *Annals of Clinical Psychiatry*, 17:205–210.

Grilo CM, Hrabosky JI, White MA, Allison KC, Stunkard AJ, & Masheb RM. (2008). Overvaluation of shape and weight in binge eating disorder and overweight controls: Refinement of a diagnostic construct. *Journal of Abnormal Psychology*, 117:414–419.

Heinicke BE, Paxton SJ, McLean SA, & Wertheim EH. (2007). Internet-delivered targeted group intervention for body dissatisfaction and disordered eating in adolescent girls: A randomized controlled trial. *Journal of Abnormal Child Psychology*, 35:379–391.

Hilbert A, & Tuschen-Caffier B. (2004). Body image interventions in cognitive-behavioural therapy of binge-eating disorder: A component analysis. *Behaviour Research and Therapy*, 42:1325–1339.

Holsen I, Kraft P, & Roysamb E. (2001). The relationship between body image and depressed mood in adolescence: A 5-year longitudinal panel study. *Journal of Health Psychology*, 6:613–627.

Hrabosky JI, Masheb RM, White MA, & Grilo CM. (2007). Overvaluation of shape and weight in binge eating disorder. *Journal of Consulting and Clinical Psychology*, 75:175–180.

Humphreys P, & Paxton SJ. (2004). Impact of exposure to idealised male images on adolescent boys' body image. *Body Image*, 1:253–266.

Jackson T, & Chen H. (2008). Predicting changes in eating disorder symptoms among Chinese adolescents: A 9-month prospective study. *Journal of Psychosomatic Research*, 64:87–95.

Jacobi C, Hayward C, de Zwaan M, Kraemer HC, & Agras W. (2004). Coming to terms with risk factors for eating disorders: Application of risk terminology and suggestions for a general taxonomy. *Psychological Bulletin*, 130:19–65.

Jarry JL, & Ip K. (2005). The effectiveness of stand-alone cognitive-behavioural therapy for body image: A meta-analysis. *Body Image*, 2:317–331.

Jones CD. (2004). Body image among adolescent girls and boys: A longitudinal study. *Developmental Psychology*, 40:823–835.

Keery H, van den Berg P, & Thompson J. (2004). An evaluation of the tripartite influence model of body dissatisfaction and eating disturbance with adolescent girls. *Body Image*, 1:237–251.

Knauss C, Paxton SJ, & Alsaker FD. (2007). Relationships amongst body dissatisfaction, internalisation of the media body ideal and perceived pressure from media in adolescent girls and boys. *Body Image*, 4:353–360.

Masheb RM, & Grilo CM. (2000). Binge eating disorder: A need for additional diagnostic criteria. *Comprehensive Psychiatry*, 41:159–162.

Masheb RM, & Grilo CM. (2003). The nature of body image disturbance in patients with binge eating disorder. *International Journal of Eating Disorders*, 33:333–341.

McKay D, Todaro J, Neziroglu F, & Campisi T. (1997). Body dysmorphic disorder: A preliminary evaluation of treatment and maintenance using exposure with response prevention. *Behaviour Research and Therapy*, 35:67–70.

Mountford V, Haase A, & Waller G. (2006). Body checking in the eating disorders: Associations between cognitions and behaviors. *International Journal of Eating Disorders*, 39:708–715.

Mussap AJ, McCabe MP, & Ricciardelli LA. (2008). Implications of accuracy, sensitivity, and variability of body size estimations to disordered eating. *Body Image*, 5:80–90.

Narring F, Tschumper A, Inderwildi L, Jeannin A, Addor V, & Bütikofer A. (2004). *Gesundheit der Jugendlichen in der Schweiz (2002) [SMASH Swiss multicenter adolescent study on health (2002)]*. Switzerland: Bern, Institut für Psychologie.

Neumark-Sztainer D, Paxton SJ, Hannan PJ, Haines J, & Story M. (2006). Does body satisfaction matter?: Five-year longitudinal associations between body satisfaction and health behaviors in adolescent females and males. *Journal of Adolescent Health*, 39:244–251.

Neumark-Sztainer D, Story M, Hannan PJ, Perry C, & Irving LM. (2002). Weight-related concerns and behaviors among overweight and non-overweight adolescents: Implications for preventing weight-related disorders. *Archives of Pediatrics and Adolescent Medicine*, 156:171–178.

Otto MW, Wilhelm S, Cohen LS, & Harlow BL. (2001). Prevalence of body dysmorphic disorder in a community sample of women. *American Journal of Psychiatry*, 158:2061–2063.

Paxton SJ, Eisenberg ME, & Neumark-Sztainer D. (2006). Prospective predictors of body dissatisfaction in adolescent girls and boys: A five-year longitudinal study. *Developmental Psychology*, 42:888–899.

Paxton SJ, McLean SA, Gollings EK, Faulkner C, & Wertheim EH. (2007). Comparison of face-to-face and Internet interventions for body image and eating problems in adult women: An RCT. *International Journal of Eating Disorders*, 40:692–704.

Paxton SJ, Neumark-Sztainer D, Hannan PJ, & Eisenberg ME. (2006). Body dissatisfaction prospectively predicts depressive mood and low self-esteem in adolescent girls and boys. *Journal of Clinical Child and Adolescent Psychology*, 35:539–549.

Paxton SJ, Schutz HK, Wertheim EH, & Muir SL. (1999). Friendship clique and peer influences on body image concerns, dietary restraint, extreme weight-loss behaviors, and binge eating in adolescent girls. *Journal of Abnormal Psychology*, 108:255–266.

Posavac HD, Posavac SS, & Weigel RG. (2001). Reducing the impact of media images on women at risk for body image disturbance: Three targeted interventions. *Journal of Social and Clinical Psychology*, 20:324–340.

Presnell K, Bearman SK, & Stice E. (2004). Risk factors for body dissatisfaction in adolescent boys and girls: A prospective study. *International Journal of Eating Disorders*, 36:389–401.

Reas DL, Grilo CM, Masheb RM, & Wilson GT. (2005). Body checking and avoidance in overweight patients with binge eating disorder. *International Journal of Eating Disorders*, 37:342–346.

Ricciardelli LA, McCabe MP, Lillis J, & Thomas K. (2006). A longitudinal investigation of the development of weight and muscle concerns among preadolescent boys. *Journal of Youth and Adolescence*, 35:177–187.

Riley C, Lee M, Cooper Z, Fairburn CG, & Shafran R. (2007). A randomised controlled trial of cognitive-behaviour therapy for clinical perfectionism: A preliminary study. *Behaviour Research and Therapy*, 45:2221–2231.

Rosen JC. (1990). Body image disturbance in eating disorders. In T. F. Cash & T. Pruzinsky (Eds.), *Body image: A handbook of theory, research and clinical practice* (pp. 190–214). New York: Guilford Press.

Rosen JC, Reiter J, & Orosan P. (1995). Cognitive-behavioral body image therapy for body dysmorphic disorder. *Journal of Consulting and Clinical Psychology*, 63:2263–2269.

Rosen JC, Saltzberg E, & Srebnik D. (1989). Cognitive behavior therapy for negative body image. *Behavior Therapy*, 20:393–404.

Rosen JC, Srebnik D, Saltzberg E, & Wendt S. (1991). Development of a body image avoidance questionnaire. *Psychological Assessment*, 3:32–37.

Rushford N, & Ostermeyer A. (1997). Body image disturbances and their change with videofeedback in anorexia nervosa. *Behaviour Research and Therapy*, 35:389–398.

Shafran R, Cooper Z, & Fairburn CG. (2002). Clinical perfectionism: A cognitive-behavioural analysis. *Behaviour Research and Therapy*, 40:773–791.

Shafran R, Fairburn CG, Robinson P, & Lask B. (2004). Body checking and its avoidance in eating disorders. *International Journal of Eating Disorders*, 35:93–101.

Shafran R, Lee M, Payne E, & Fairburn CG. (2007). An experimental analysis of body checking. *Behaviour Research and Therapy*, 45:113–121.

Smolak L, Levine MP, & Thompson J. (2001). The use of the Sociocultural Attitudes Towards Appearance Questionnaire with middle school boys and girls. *International Journal of Eating Disorders*, 29:216–223.

Smolak L, & Stein JA. (2006). The relationship of drive for muscularity to sociocultural factors, self-esteem, physical attributes, gender role, and social comparison in middle school boys. *Body Image*, 3:121–129.

Stice E. (2002). Risk and maintenance factors for eating pathology: A meta-analytic review. *Psychological Bulletin*, 128:825–848.

Stice E, Shaw H, Burton E, & Wade E. (2006). Dissonance and healthy weight eating disorder prevention programs: A randomized efficacy trial. *Journal of Consulting and Clinical Psychology*, 74:263–275.

Stice E, Trost A, & Chase A. (2003). Healthy weight control and dissonance-based eating disorder prevention programs: Results from a controlled trial. *International Journal of Eating Disorders*, 33:10–21.

Thompson JK, Heinberg LJ, Altabe M, & Tantleff Dunn S. (1999). *Exacting beauty: Theory, assessment, and treatment of body image disturbance*. Washington, DC: American Psychological Association.

van den Berg P, Paxton SJ, Keery H, Wall M, Guo J, & Neumark-Sztainer D. (2007). Body dissatisfaction and body comparison with media images in males and females. *Body Image*, 4:257–268.

Wade TD, & Lowes J. (2002). Variables associated with disturbed eating habits and overvalued ideas about the personal implications of body shape and weight in a female adolescent population. *International Journal of Eating Disorders*, 32:39–45.

Wertheim EH, Koerner J, & Paxton SJ. (2001). Longitudinal predictors of restrictive eating and bulimic tendencies in three different age groups of adolescent girls. *Journal of Youth and Adolescence*, 30:69–81.

Wertheim EH, Paxton SJ, & Blaney S. (2009). Body image in girls. In L Smolak & JK Thompson (Eds.), *Body image, eating disorders and obesity in youth* (2nd ed., pp. 47–76). Washington, DC: American Psychological Association.

Wilksch SM, Tiggemann M, & Wade TD. (2006). Impact of interactive school-based media literacy lessons for reducing internalization of media ideals in young adolescent girls and boys. *International Journal of Eating Disorders*, 39:385–393.

Williamson DA, Muller SL, Reas DL, & Thaw JM. (1999). Cognitive bias in eating disorders: Implications for theory and treatment. *Behavior Modification*, 23:556–577.

CHAPTER 29

Caring for Someone with an Eating Disorder

Elizabeth Goddard, Pam Macdonald, and Janet Treasure

There is increasing recognition that the carers of someone with an eating disorder (ED) can be valuable resources in the process of recovery (Eliot & Baker, 2000; Le Grange, 1999). This chapter examines some of the caregiving issues and specific needs of those who find themselves confronted with this role, and how these may be incorporated into intervention programs.

We begin by considering a theoretical model that can help to shape interventions and support for carers of someone with an ED. This model includes consideration of carer distress and burden, effects of high expressed emotion in the home and its consequences, as well as those family factors that may accommodate, maintain, or enable symptoms to persist. We then discuss the importance of family work along with recent interventions developed from research in this field. Skills-based training research, for example, has evolved in response to specific requirements of the carer, as ongoing studies and training inform different approaches to interventions. Finally, we consider the manner in which motivational enhancement is utilized in a DVD and manual skills-based training project, offering examples from excerpts in response to potentially problematic areas.

Carer Burden and Distress

Carers are usually the first individuals to guide their loved one toward treatment and remain a constant presence throughout the illness and into recovery. Research has shown that carers of someone with an ED provide high levels of emotional and practical support and that this role often leads the carers themselves to have high levels of distress and unmet needs (e.g., Haigh & Treasure, 2003). Living with a loved one with an ED can have a considerable impact on both the physical and mental health of the carer and is associated with poor quality of life (Treasure et al., 2001; Whitney, Haigh, Weinman, & Treasure, 2007; Whitney et al., 2005). The burden and distress can be interpersonally challenging, producing a clear disruption in family life. In addition, carers frequently report that they lack the skills and resources required to care for their loved one with an ED.

Broadly, the term "caregiver burden and appraisal" refers to the extent to which a carer perceives the impact of the illness upon the normal routines or daily functioning in his/her life (Platt, 1985; Szmukler et al., 1996). Research has found that carers of someone with an ED experience high levels of caregiver burden and negative appraisals of caregiving (Haigh & Treasure, 2003; Kyriacou, Treasure, & Schmidt, 2008a; Sepulveda, Lopez, Macdonald, & Treasure, 2008; Sepulveda, Lopez, Todd, Whitaker, & Treasure, 2008; Whitney et al., 2007; Winn, Perkins, Murray, Murphy, & Schmidt, 2004).

In addition to high levels of burden, carers of someone with an ED frequently report high levels of general health concerns, distress, and anxiety (Haigh & Treasure, 2003; Sepulveda, Lopez, Macdonald, et al., 2008; Sepulveda, Lopez, Todd, et al., 2008; Treasure et al., 2001; Whitney et al., 2007; Winn et al., 2007). In one study, 36% of 115 carers had scores that reflected poor mental health. This finding indicates the seriousness of the toll that caring for someone with an ED can take on a carer's psychological well-being (Kyriacou, Treasure, & Schmidt, 2008b). Whitney and colleagues (2005) carried out a qualitative study in which letters from 40 carers were analyzed. All but one letter expressed negative emotions such as sadness, distress, fear, anger, and hostility, as well as self-blaming emotions such as guilt, failure, and inadequacy. Mothers in this study, in particular, reported an increased emotional response that included sleep deprivation and feelings of helplessness.

When comparing ED populations with controls, ED carers report elevated levels of negative appraisal compared to parents of someone without an ED (Kyriacou et al., 2008a). ED carers, particularly mothers, also have higher levels of depression and anxiety relative to healthy control comparisons (Espina, 2003; Kyriacou et al., 2008a). In another study family members of a person with anorexia nervosa (AN) reported higher burden than family members caring for a person with bulimia nervosa (BN) (Santonastaso, Saccon, & Favaro, 1997).

A Model Describing the Factors That Contribute to Carer Distress and Burden

In a study on parental experience and roles in the recovery from AN, Sharkey-Orgnero (1999) found that carers were able to recognize, with hindsight, that their own emotional arousal hindered their ability to cope effectively. A carer stress model (see Figure 29.1) conceptualizes the difficulties faced by carers that contribute to their elevated levels of distress and anxiety.

• *Unmet needs.* A lack of clear understanding of ED, including causes and consequences, contributes to distress. Therefore, there is a need for carers to acquire a deeper knowledge about ED in order to be able to cope effectively and to contribute to the recovery process. Furthermore, carers of adult patients are often excluded from treatment programs and thus can feel helpless and isolated. Involving carers in support and training programs may increase their feelings of self-efficacy.

• *Stigma.* Stigma about the illness and toward families who have a member with a mental illness can contribute to the burden and distress felt by carers, leading them to feel isolated and withdrawn in an attempt to avoid facing stigma.

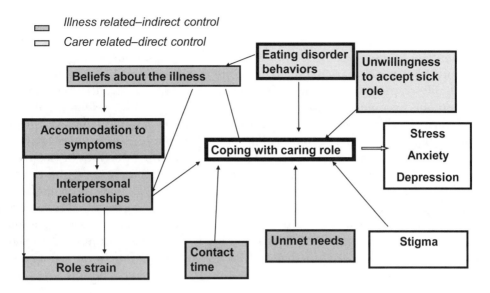

FIGURE 29.1. Areas that can contribute to maladaptive coping and lead to carer stress. The boxes in light shading illustrate the domains that are primarily relevant for the carer. The boxes in darker shading represent the disorder-related problems. In interventions developed for carers, they are encouraged to tackle the lightly shaded issues (i.e., those that they have control over) first.

- *Beliefs about the illness.* A lack of accurate information about the illness allows unhelpful beliefs to develop, which can impact on every role.
- *ED behaviors.* Symptoms and behaviors that are associated with the illness can be a cause of stress and anxiety to carers. Obsessive–compulsive behaviors, abnormal eating patterns, social isolation, and decreased work and leisure opportunities can cause carers to worry and feel anxiety about the impact of the ED on their loved one.
- *Unwillingness to accept the sick role.* Confusion about the illness is compounded by the fact that the affected individuals themselves do not see that they have a problem. Thus, parent–offspring appraisals relating to the illness are in conflict.
- *Role strain.* A lack of clear understanding about aspects of any mental illness contributes to uncertainties about how best to help. Because meals are at the core of family life and contribute a great deal to social bonds, ED symptoms disrupt many relationships. Siblings are exposed to high levels of anger and stress, and the family becomes isolated. The time and energy needed for caregiving interferes with other familial roles.
- *Interpersonal relationships.* The stress and strain associated with the illness may fuel unhelpful behaviors such as hostility, criticalness, and overprotection (so-called high expressed emotion, described below). This reaction is commonly seen in response to all forms of psychiatric illness and has a moderate-to-strong adverse impact on patient outcome (Butzlaff & Hooley, 1998). Unhelpful caregiving appraisals contribute to these undesirable patterns of relating, and a vicious cycle develops (Barrowclough & Hooley, 2003).
- *Contact time.* The number of contact hours a carer has with the individual with the ED may impact upon the degree of stress felt by a carer.
- *Accommodation to symptoms.* Individuals with ED characteristically display

obsessive–compulsive traits such as rigidity, ritualism, perfectionism, perseveration, compulsiveness, and meticulousness in their behaviors and attitudes (Bastiani et al., 1996). Families of people with EDs interface with these rule-bound eating, weight, and shape control behaviors that characterize the illness and so can inadvertently accommodate to the symptoms, for example, by offering constant reassurance. Accommodating to symptoms becomes a common response when faced with the visible and distressing symptoms of an ED. Carers may also become emotionally bullied by the individual with an ED. Family members report colluding with the individual's rules related to eating, such as accepting the use of kitchen scales for weighing portions or the precise measurement of liquids, the cutting of solid food into minuscule pieces, and the allocation of the patient's daily ration into small containers. They may also collude with shape and body concern rituals such as body checking, providing repeated reassurance to alleviate unfounded fears or accept compulsive exercise routines. Carers may allow their home to become cluttered with hoarded foods or exercise equipment. In short, families can be drawn into organizing their lives around the ED behaviors and accommodate to, or enable, some of the core symptoms (Treasure et al., 2008).

The Role of Carers in the Maintenance of EDs

Misperceptions and misunderstandings of the illness and disturbed interpersonal relationship patterns are seen as key factors in a maintenance model of ED (Schmidt & Treasure, 2006). Carer distress and uncertainty over the caregiving role can impact on the interactions between the carer and the individual with the ED. Illness misperceptions and fear of the consequences of the illness, for example, are associated with overprotecion, particularly in mothers (Whitney et al., 2005). Carer patterns of behavior in response to the illness, such as overprotection, criticalness, hostility (expressed emotion), or accommodation to symptoms, can be viewed as a consequence of the illness rather than a cause and can thus be understood within a maintenance framework.

Expressed Emotion

Expressed emotion (EE) is a construct that includes criticalness, hostility, warmth, positive comments, and emotional overinvolvement or overprotectiveness (Wearden, Tarrier, Barrowclough, Zastowny, & Rahill, 2000). These emotions constitute key aspects of interpersonal relationships and are found to impact upon outcome in a number of psychiatric disorders, including EDs (Butzlaff & Hooley, 1998; Hodes & Le Grange, 1993; Wearden et al., 2000). Research into EE originated primarily in the context of patients with schizophrenia and the interpersonal relationships with their families. In a classic study Brown, Carstairs, and Topping (1958) found that patients were more likely to experience a relapse of schizophrenic symptoms if they returned to live with parents or wives than if they went to live in lodgings or with siblings, and that the quality of the relationship between the relative and patient appeared to be related to outcome. High levels of criticism and emotional overinvolvement have been found in carers of young adults with ED relative to healthy comparison groups where the proband was living at home (Kyriacou et al., 2008a). High levels of EE influence both the engagement with, and outcome of, therapy for people with EDs (Szmukler et al., 1996; van Furth et al.,

1996). The main aim of van Furth's study was to evaluate the contribution that family factors make to the perpetuation of ED in a sample of adolescents. The authors showed that a substantial amount of outcome variance (28–34%) could be explained by EE variables, in particular maternal criticalness. They also demonstrated that maternal criticalness can predict changes in psychiatric status over a treatment period.

Clinical Implications of Carers' Needs and the Role of Carers in the Maintenance of EDs

Rolland (1999) suggested that a primary developmental challenge for a family is to create a meaning for the illness experience that promotes a sense of competency and mastery. Families adapt best when their representation of the illness is empowering, sustains hope, and affirms relationships. In order to equip carers with feelings of empowerment and efficacy, professionals should regard carers as a resource within the treatment and help them to feel included and valued (McMaster, Beale, Hillege, & Nagy, 2004; Winn et al., 2004). Promoting beliefs that sustain hope and empower families, and encouraging families to take "safe risks" by possibly changing some of their behaviors, may be an important step in reducing carers' feelings of helplessness and interrupting unhelpful interactions within the family (Treasure, Whitaker, Whitney, & Schmidt, 2005). Figure 29.2 illustrates how specifically tailored interventions can target areas of difficulty for carers in a bid to minimize their distress as well improve outcome for the affected individual.

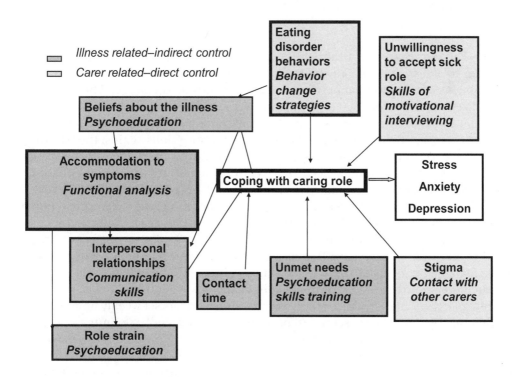

FIGURE 29.2. How interventions are used to target specific areas of difficulty for the carer.

Psychoeducation for Carers of Someone with an ED

Providing information and correcting misperceptions about the illness may be of value both for the carers and for the person with an ED. This can be delivered in various forms, such as books, websites, and support groups. Self-help organizations such as B-eat (United Kingdom) and the National Eating Disorders Association (United States) play an important role in the dissemination of this knowledge. Furthermore, interventions that target factors and change behaviors that maintain ED symptoms within the family context may improve the outcome for the affected individual.

Psychoeducation has been delivered by clinicians in a variety of ways. Uehara, Kawashima, Goto, Tasaki, and Someya (2001) developed a multifamily group method to deliver psychoeducation to carers of people with an ED disorder. Sessions included information on epidemiology, history, treatment, diagnosis, symptoms, etiology, course, and complications. The purpose of the group was to provide knowledge of ED and mutual support, rebuild the family network, reduce anxiety, and to discover and enhance positive features of the families and patients themselves. The intervention included a mixture of information delivery via lectures/talks and group discussion work. Uehara and colleagues reported a reduction of EE (especially emotional overinvolvement), carer distress, and family burden. Although objective ED symptoms did not significantly decrease over time, social functioning and interpersonal activities increased, and other (non-ED) psychiatric symptoms decreased in patients after the psychoeducation sessions.

Skills Training for Carers of Someone with an ED

Group Parent Training Program

Zucker, Ferriter, Best, and Brantley (2005) devised a Group Parent Training (GPT) program to assist caregivers in the management of their child's ED and facilitate the development of a healthy home environment for sustained change. The authors conceptualized ED in terms of (1) the symptoms and (2) the way in which the illness helps the individual to cope with his/her environment. Consequently, the program targets decreasing ED symptoms and increasing adaptive skills against the backdrop of ambivalence. In addition to providing strategies to address the acute disorder, this program included reflection on aspects of caregiver functioning that could enhance task implementation, such as making environmental and attitudinal changes (Zucker et al., 2005). Thus, this program encourages carers themselves to make changes to enhance social support and the self-efficacy of the individual with the ED.

Group material was disseminated in 16 weekly, 90-minute sessions. Caregivers could repeat this sequence as often as deemed necessary. Emotion regulation in disorder management was at the core of skills training. Content from this section was repeated every fourth session for the benefit of any new caregivers; that is, new caregivers join an established group. To increase adherence, carers set weekly homework tasks for themselves that were presented to other members for feedback on the relevance of the chosen goals. Goals, for example, included decreasing problematic behavior such as an ED behavior, increasing adaptive behavior, role modeling an adaptive behavior, and engaging in a self-care behavior (i.e., doing something good for themselves).

Zucker and colleagues (2005) identified several major themes in qualitative data from focus group transcriptions. The key theme to emerge regarding content was the need for background psychoeducational material to complement the group parent training skills component. Parents desired a specific approach: information on basic nutrition, medication management, and bodily changes associated with weight regain. When asked to identify essential skills learned in GPT, parents listed behavior modification and emotion regulation skills as critical. With respect to the format, a two-tier system for new carers and established carers was favored—that is, a group established for those new to the program along with an "alumni" group for those who continued to need support and information but who had mastered the basic skills. Finally, a "buddy system" was endorsed whereby caregivers arranged to connect with one another for support outside of group meetings.

Collaborative Care Workshops

The content of the workshops is described in Treasure, Sepulveda, and colleagues (2007). Training methods include role-play demonstrations on how to implement those skills required to instigate behavior change using the transtheoretical model of change (Prochaska & Velicer, 1997) and the principles of motivational interviewing (Rollnick, Miller, & Butler, 2008).

The initial aim of the workshops is to help participants work together toward moderating EE. Carers are encouraged to reflect on their emotional reactions to the illness and to use this information in guiding their goal setting and action planning. Lighthearted animal metaphors are used to promote thoughts on maladaptive relationship patterns and can be used by both professionals and carers. Carers often fall into extreme patterns of emotional responses, reacting in an overly emotional manner (jellyfish) or denying their emotions (ostrich). In terms of directedness, they can also be overprotective (kangaroo) or overdirective (rhinoceros). The most important step is for carers to recognize that they may need to change those patterns of behavior that may be aggravating the symptoms in order to cultivate a more constructive relationship with their family member with the ED. The goal is to utilize a "dolphin- and St. Bernard–like" approach in an atmosphere of warmth, gentle nudging, and negotiation.

Carers are taught how to listen to and analyze their emotional responses while reflecting upon what they might need to change in their own situation, giving them both the opportunity and permission to explore their own needs as individuals. By reflecting upon their own difficulties with change, carers may also develop more compassion toward sufferers in their struggle for change. The acronym OARS is introduced to demonstrate the value of using open questioning, affirmations, reflective listening, and summarizing. By communicating in this nonconfrontational manner with the person with the ED, it is hoped that the carer will elicit a degree of commitment toward change. Later sessions concentrate on advanced communication skills, such as empathy and sidestepping ED talk, to try and avoid confrontation and arguments. Carers are taught to concentrate on the bigger picture by contextualizing the situation within a longer-term scenario. Throughout the sessions, the final aim for carers is to help their daughters identify any ambivalence they may have about their ED and to try and increase the discrepancy between their current situation and their goals and desires for their future.

Research suggests that the Collaborative Care Workshops are effective in reducing caregiver distress and burden and were highly acceptable to caregivers (Sepulveda, Lopez, Todd, Whitaker, & Treasure, 2008). Recent data suggests that patients with AN also benefit from their caregivers taking part in the workshops (Goddard, Macdonald, & Treasure, 2009). This qualitative study found that patients experienced positive effects of the workshops, specifically discussing direct positive effects on the ED, improved communication, and moderated expression of emotions of their caregivers, a more positive family environment, and improved relationships with caregivers. Negative themes highlighted the patronizing nature of their caregivers' implementation of the skills learned and their tendency to generalize the information gathered from the workshops. Despite this, the results overall suggest that the workshops have beneficial effects for those with AN, although future research needs to investigate this further.

Self-Help Interventions for Carers

Self-help interventions overcome some of the problems of accessibility to treatment. A variety of methods has been developed using tools such as self-help books (Treasure, Smith, & Crane, 2007), the Web, and DVDs in order to reach out to a wider audience and to address issues of high demand, scarce treatment resources, and various constraints, including geographical, financial, and time limitations. The Web-based and DVD programs include role-play scenarios that illustrate communication, assessment, and motivational skills. The impact of these is under investigation (Sepulveda, Lopez, Macdonald, et al., 2008).

A form of guided self-help has been developed that includes a self-help book and a set of DVDs (Treasure, Smith, & Crane, 2007), using telephone coaching. The content of intervention materials resembles that of Collaborative Care workshops, discussed previously. Carers receive a specified number of coaching sessions, whereby they are encouraged to use their own creativity and resources to identify manageable target behaviors, both their own and the sufferer's, using the strategies and techniques illustrated in the intervention materials. The coach essentially uses the same principles in guiding the carers as those taught to carers in the materials. Examples of excerpts from coaching sessions follows.

Promoting Communication

> COACH: In our last session you wanted to try and think of new ways of opening up communication. How did you get on with that? [Reflective listening + open question]

> CARER: Not very well, really. I was trying to encourage her to talk about looking at the pros and cons of things. I think I've been struggling a bit as well ... it's not easy.

> COACH: It's tough ... fantastic that you've been trying, though. Sounds like you're still a bit stuck with the communication problem. [Empathy + affirmation + complex reflection]

> CARER: Yeah, definitely, certainly ... she's hoping to go to university. That's what we're all kind of aiming for and trying to support her, but, you know ... well we were in town the other day ... and she said "oh, my whole life is always going to be a mess" ... just like kind of shouted at me.

> COACH: So she said "my whole life is always going to be a mess." That sounds to me like communication. [Simple reflection + complex reflection]

CARER: It is ... it is ... isn't it? (laugh) but it was only a few sentences ...

COACH: But still communication (pause) and a pretty powerful communication. [Complex reflection]

CARER: But what would you answer? I mean, I struggled with that one when we were walking along. I thought, "I don't want to miss this opportunity, but ... "

COACH: It's difficult when you're put on the spot. How could you use reflective listening and open questions to a similar response next time around? [Affirmation + open question]

CARER: I guess ... "your whole life is a mess? Can you tell me a bit more why you think like that?"

COACH: Wonderful use of OARS*! [Affirmation] [*Note*: OARS is an acronym that stands for the some of the principles used in motivational interviewing: O, open questions; A, affirmation; R, reflections; S, summary.]

Promoting Change Talk

Animal metaphors are used as a playful way of discussing patterns of interaction that are commonly present (Treasure, Sepulveda, et al., 2007). The interactions typically seen with high EE are likened to specific animals. The kangaroo is used to represent overprotection (keeping the child in the pouch); a rhinoceros represents criticism and hostility (charging relentlessly on with one's own agenda); the jellyfish represents a highly anxious carer (transparent emotions that sting); and an ostrich represents an avoidant carer. The optimal form of caring is described as a combination of a dolphin (an intelligent, hands-off, guiding approach) and St. Bernard dog (warm, loyal, and nurturing).

COACH: What were your feelings on the animal analogies? [Open question]

CARER: Well, I can see very much where I fit in ... I'm overly protective and, you know, I need to change my approach to be more like the dolphin and less like ... is it the kangaroo?

COACH: The kangaroo. What examples of kangaroo behavior can you think of right now? [Simple reflection + open question]

CARER: Well, always sort of fretting, always making her feel that she can't make decisions on her own anymore, about all sorts of things, not just about food but particularly about food, you know? I have to be the one who decides what she's going to eat. If, on the rare occasion, we do go out and she's faced with a menu, she can't make a choice of her own. She has to ask me. I have to, you know, decide for her, and I think what I've got to do is try and stop doing that ... sort of say to her, "Well, you've got to decide for yourself."

COACH: That's extremely self-reflective of you, J. It can be tough examining our own behavior and approach at times. You said you tend to make decisions in all areas of her life. What ways can you think of that would allow her to make decisions without the food talk? [Affirmation + empathy + simple reflection + open question]

CARER: Well, because she's not really doing very much, it's quite hard to see how I can ... but I suppose, really, it's just a way of encouraging her to try and get more involved in things outside the home and the illness ... and try and make arrangements to actually go out and see people and to do things. I mean, the exercising thing is a big problem for us because she goes mad with it and that's all she really ever wants to do, so I need to try and encourage her to do other things.

COACH: Sounds like you've got a good grasp of where you want to go next. How important do you think it is for you to tackle the kangaroo behaviors? [Complex reflection + open question]

CARER: Well, I can see that if I want her to change her attitude, then I probably need to change mine ...

These examples illustrate how the cascade of change is taught. High levels of anxiety can disrupt communication, and teaching carers to listen and reflect can beneficial, as the individual with an ED feels understood and cared for. Also, the illness and high anxiety can produce unhelpful patterns of interaction. Individuals with the EDs appreciate the changes in their family members that these forms of interventions produce. Below are examples of two patients who have shared their perspective on the effectiveness and helpfulness of this type of work.

SUFFERER 1: Well, it is almost like they are in my head kind of thing, where as before it was just *eat* and that is the answer. I think they understand the difficulty in my doing that, whereas before they didn't.

INTERVIEWER: So they understand that you find it really tough.

SUFFERER 1: Yeah, and I think talking to the other parents, finding it was really similar, I think that probably helped.

SUFFERER 2: Mealtimes were obviously always the hardest, and there would always be a big scene and before I would just end up storming out. But now, they would just kind of sit there and talk me through it. Rather than getting angry with me, they'd sit there and stay calm with me and try and calm me down and ... rather than just getting upset, they'd say, you know, "Take your time, do what you want to do," and it was sort of making it less of a big deal ... just "here's your dinner, there you go" and not making a fuss about it.

Table 29.1 provides a summary of the interventions that have been developed for carers of people with ED. These studies suggest that psychoeducation and skills training for carers is helpful and has potential for reducing the risk of relapse and minimizing ED symptoms.

Conclusion

In this chapter we have considered some of the caregiving issues that can arise when supporting a loved one with an ED. We have explored the background research that has informed recent interventions for working with the family. In general, carers of people with EDs are highly motivated partners in collaborative caring programs. It is important that they are equipped with the necessary skills and resources in an approach that includes both professionals *and* family members. This approach should include sharing

TABLE 29.1. Psychoeducational and Skills-Based Family Interventions for EDs

Intervention	Population	Multistructure	Description	Results
Psychoeducation for carers (Uehara, Kawashima, Goto, Tasaki, & Someya, 2001).	Outpatients and inpatients	5 × 2-hour monthly meetings	Multifamily psychoeducation groups to reduce carer expressed emotion (EE) and enhance coping.	Reduction in EE, especially emotional overinvolvment; reduction in observation of patient symptoms (by relatives) and family distress.
Group parent training, (Zucker, Ferriter, Best, & Brantley, 2005).	Outpatient program	16 × 90-minute sessions	Targets three domains: (1) disorder management, (2) caregiver characteristics (perfectionism, self-efficacy), and expressed emotion), and (3) healthy home environment.	Acceptable to carers. Qualitative analysis suggested need for psychoeducation to complement group skills training approach.
Collaborative care workshops (Treasure, Sepulveda, et al., 2007).	Outpatient setting	6 × 3-hour workshops	Address maintaining interpersonal factors of ED, including carer distress, misattributions of illness, carers accommodation to the illness, and EE by improving emotional intelligence and communication, problem-solving, and behavior change skills.	Quantitative results suggest reduced distress and burden. Qualitative results suggest carers learned new and helpful skills and were able to put them into practice, even if they found it difficult at times. Overall this intervention was acceptable to carers.
Manual and DVD intervention (Sepulveda, Lopez, Macdonald, et al., 2008).	All settings; distance learning	5 DVDs and telephone coaching sessions accompanied by a skills training book	Addresses interpersonal maintaining factors, including carer stress, misattributions, accommodation, and EE. DVDs illustrate complex skills and behaviors. Telephone coaching sessions follow a topic guide to encourage goal setting.	Depression, anxiety, burden, and EE reduced, but results were not significant due to small sample sizes. Qualitative feedback suggests high acceptability and usefulness of most aspects of DVDs. Telephone coaching enhanced carer ability to commit to change and develop skills. Enables carers to develop their skills and access resources from their home.

information and teaching carers the same basic skills as those taught to professionals. It is important to help carers recognize those self-behaviors that may be maintaining or accommodating to the symptoms as well as techniques that help them break out of this vicious cycle. The common enemy is the ED. Carers are the solution, not the problem, and it is vital that the approach to treatment reflects this basic reality.

Acknowledgments

This work was part of the ARIADNE programme (Applied Research into Anorexia Nervosa and Not Otherwise Specified Eating Disorders), funded by a Department of Health National Institute of Health Research (DH/NIHR) Programme Grant for Applied Research (No. RP-PG-

0606-1043) to U. Schmidt, J. Treasure, K. Tchanturia, H. Startup, S. Ringwood, S. Landau, M. Grover, I. Eisler, I. Campbell, J. Beecham, M. Allen, and G. Wolff. The views expressed herein are not necessarily those of DH/NIHR.

References

Barrowclough C, & Hooley JM. (2003). Attributions and expressed emotion: A review. *Clinical Psychology Review*, 23:849–880.

Bastiani AM, Altemus M, Pigott TA, Rubenstein C, Weltzin TE, & Kaye WH. (1996). Comparison of obsessions and compulsions in patients with anorexia nervosa and obsessive compulsive disorder. *Biological Psychiatry*, 39:966–969.

Brown GW, Carstairs GM, & Topping G. (1958). Post-hospital adjustment of chronic mental patients. *Lancet*, 2:685–689.

Butzlaff RL, & Hooley JM. (1998). Expressed emotion and psychiatric relapse: A meta-analysis. *Archives of General Psychiatry*, 55:547–552.

Eliot AO, & Baker CW. (2000). Maternal stressors and eating-disordered adolescent girls. *Family Therapy*, 27:165–178.

Espina A. (2003). Alexithymia in parents of daughters with eating disorders: Its relationship with psychopathological and personality variables. *Journal of Psychosomatic Research*, 55:553–560.

Goddard E, Macdonald P, & Treasure J. (2009). *An examination of the impact of the Maudsley eating disorder collaborative care skills workshops on patients with anorexia nervosa: A qualitative study.* Unpublished manuscript.

Haigh R, & Treasure J. (2003). Investigating the needs of carers in the area of eating disorders: Development of the Carer's Needs Assessment Measure (CaNAM). *European Eating Disorders Review*, 11:125–141.

Hodes M, & Le Grange D. (1993). Expressed emotion in the investigation of eating disorders: A review. *International Journal of Eating Disorders*, 13:279–288.

Kyriacou O, Treasure J, & Schmidt U. (2008a). Expressed emotion in eating disorders assessed via self-report: An examination of factors associated with expressed emotion in carers of people and anorexia nervosa in comparison to control families. *International Journal of Eating Disorders*, 41:37–46.

Kyriacou O, Treasure J, & Schmidt U. (2008b). Understanding how parents cope with living with someone with anorexia nervosa: Modelling the factors that are associated with carer distress. *International Journal of Eating Disorders*, 41:233–242.

Le Grange D. (1999). Family therapy for adolescent anorexia nervosa. *Psychotherapy in Practice*, 55:727–739.

McMaster R, Beale B, Hillege S, & Nagy S. (2004). The parent experience of eating disorder: Interactions with health professionals. *International Journal of Mental Health Nursing*, 13:67–73.

Platt S. (1985). Measuring the burden of psychiatric illness on the family: An evaluation of some rating scales. *Psychological Medicine*, 15:383–393.

Prochaska JM, & Velicer WF. (1997). The transtheoretical model of health behavior. *American Journal of Health Promotion*, 12(1):38–48.

Rolland JS. (1999). Parental illness and disability: A family systems framework. *Journal of Family Therapy*, 27:144–146.

Rollnick S, Miller, WR, & Butler CC. (2008). *Motivational interviewing in health care: Helping patients change behavior.* New York: Guilford Press.

Santonastaso P, Saccon D, & Favaro A. (1997). Burden and psychiatric symptoms of key relatives of patients with eating disorders: A preliminary study. *Eating and Weight Disorders*, 2:44–48.

Schmidt U, & Treasure J. (2006). Anorexia nervosa: Valued and visible—a cognitive–interpersonal maintenance model and its implications for research and practice. *British Journal of Clinical Psychology*, 45:343–366.

Sepulveda AR, Lopez C, Macdonald P, & Treasure J. (2008). Feasibility and acceptability of DVD and telephone coaching-based skills training for carers of people with an eating disorder. *International Journal of Eating Disorders*, 41:318–325.

Sepulveda AR, Lopez C, Todd G, Whitaker W, & Treasure J. (2008). An examination of the impact of the Maudsley eating disorder collaborative care skills workshops on the well-being of carers: A pilot study. *Social Psychiatry and Psychiatric Epidemiology*, 43:584–591.

Sharkey-Orgnero MI. (1999). Anorexia nervosa: A qualitative analysis of parents' perspectives on recovery. *Eating Disorders: The Journal of Treatment and Prevention*, 7:269–283.

Szmukler GI, Burgess P, Herrmman H, Benson A, Colusa S, & Bloch S. (1996). Caring for relatives with serious mental illness: The development of the Experience of Caregiving Inventory. *Social Psychiatry and Psychiatric Epidemiology*, 31:137–148.

Treasure J, Murphy T, Szmukler G, Todd G, Gavan K, & Joyce J. (2001). The experience of caregiving for severe mental illness: A comparison between anorexia nervosa and psychosis. *Social Psychiatry and Psychiatric Epidemiology*, 36:343–347.

Treasure J, Sepulveda AR, Macdonald P, Whitaker W, Lopez C, Zabala M, et al. (2008). The assessment of the family of people with eating disorders. *European Eating Disorders Review*, 16:247–255.

Treasure J, Sepulveda AR, Whitaker W, Todd G, Lopez C, & Whitaker W. (2007). Collaborative care between professionals and non-professionals in the management of eating disorders: A description of workshops focused on interpersonal maintaining factors. *European Eating Disorders Review*, 15:24–34.

Treasure J, Smith G, & Crane A. (2007). *Skills-based learning for caring for a loved one with an eating disorder: The new Maudsley method*. East Sussex, UK: Routledge.

Treasure J, Whitaker W, Whitney J, & Schmidt U. (2005). Working with families of adults with anorexia nervosa. *Journal of Family Therapy*, 27:158–170.

Uehara T, Kawashima Y, Goto M, Tasaki SI, & Someya T. (2001). Psychoeducation for the families of patients with eating disorders and changes in expressed emotion: A preliminary study. *Comprehensive Psychiatry*, 42:132–138.

van Furth EF, van Strien DC, Martina LML, van Son MJM, Hendrickx JJP, & van Engeland H. (1996). Expressed emotion and the prediction of outcome in adolescent eating disorders. *International Journal of Eating Disorders*, 20:19–31.

Wearden AJ, Tarrier N, Barrowclough C, Zastowny TR, & Rahill AA. (2000). A review of expressed emotion research in health care. *Clinical Psychology Review*, 20:633–666.

Whitney J, Haigh R, Weinman J, & Treasure J. (2007). Caring for people with eating disorders: Factors associated with psychological distress and negative caregiving appraisals in carers of people with eating disorders. *British Journal of Clinical Psychology*, 46:413–428.

Whitney J, Murray J, Gavan K, Todd G, Whitaker W, & Treasure J. (2005). Experience of caring for someone with anorexia nervosa: Qualitative study. *British Journal of Psychiatry*, 187:444–449.

Winn S, Perkins S, Murray J, Murphy R, & Schmidt U. (2004). A qualitative study of the experience of caring for a person with bulimia nervosa: Part 2. Carers' needs and experience of services and other support. *International Journal of Eating Disorders*, 36:269–279.

Winn S, Perkins S, Walwyn R, Schmidt U, Eisler I, Treasure J, et al. (2007). Predictors of mental health problems and negative caregiving experiences in carers of adolescents with bulimia nervosa. *International Journal of Eating Disorders*, 40:171–178.

Zucker NL, Ferriter C, Best S, & Brantley A. (2005). Group parent training: A novel approach for the treatment of eating disorders. *Eating Disorders*, 13:391–405.

CHAPTER 30

New Technologies in Treatments for Eating Disorders

Scott G. Engel and Stephen A. Wonderlich

Clinicians delivering mental health services obviously want their treatments to be effective, accessible, and cost-effective. There has been increased interest in the employment of new technologies as tools to enhance the likelihood of reaching these goals, and this literature has grown dramatically over the last decade. A recent review summarizes the large number of psychiatric disorders for which treatment by computer and Internet-based interventions has been described: obsessive–compulsive disorder, posttraumatic stress disorder, insomnia, schizophrenia, phobias, alcohol and drug problems, panic disorders, smoking, pain, encopresis, asthma, depression, and eating disorders (Marks, Cavanagh, & Grega, 2007). In addition to computer and Internet-based treatments, a number of other technology-based interventions and/or adjuncts to treatment has also been piloted and/or evaluated. CD-ROM, e-mail, text messaging, telemedicine, and virtual reality have received attention regarding their potential benefit in the treatment of various forms of psychopathology (Powers & Emmelkamp, 2008).

In an effort to make care more accessible to patients and provide cost-effective interventions, clinicians and researchers in the eating disorder (ED) field have also begun to make use of technology-based options in the treatment of their patients (Myers, Swan-Kremeier, Wonderlich, Lancaster, & Mitchell, 2004). This chapter provides a selective overview of some of the new technologies that have been used in the treatment of patients with EDs and reviews the available information on their utility.

The Internet and ED Treatment

There are a number of reasons to make use of the Internet in treating patients. For example, most patients with EDs report that the Internet is easy to use, readily accessible, convenient, and efficient (regarding cost and time; Bauer, Golkaramnay, & Kordy,

2005). Furthermore, most patients who have used the Internet as a component of treatment report that they experienced high levels of support and acceptance, were able to disclose important information, and generally experienced positive feelings related to the endeavor (Kordy, Golkaramnay, Wolf, Haug, & Bauer, 2006). Emerging research on Internet-based applications for patients with EDs has yielded promising preliminary findings (Newton & Ciliska, 2006).

Early Studies

A few studies made use of technologies that laid the groundwork for the Internet studies reviewed below. Gleason (1995), for example, created a campus-wide electronic bulletin board that allowed students to interact with each other about issues such as body image, food, and eating. Similarly, Winzelberg (1997) found that individuals who were in an electronic support group employed similar helping strategies to those used by individuals in face-to-face treatment. Another report from Zabinski and colleagues (2001) found that four patients with EDs provided very positive feedback on the use of an Internet chat room, which allowed them to interact with each other about ED-related issues.

Interapy

Lange and colleagues (2003) have developed an Internet-based treatment of bulimia nervosa (BN) called "Interapy" (see also Ruwaard, Lange, Bouwman, Broeksteeg, & Schrieken, 2007). Interapy patients are allowed to proceed at their own pace through the protocol, with a typical treatment duration lasting approximately 25 weeks. Patients are thoroughly screened on the Internet with validated psychiatric and psychological measures that have established cutoff scores. The BN treatment consists of 10 sequential modules that are based on previous work by this research group (e.g., Lange, Vries, de Gest, & van Oostendorp, 1994). Each of the 10 treatment modules follows a common format, including components of psychoeducation, homework assignments, and feedback from a clinician that is provided via the Internet. The 10 treatment modules cover topics that include increasing awareness of the ED, setting up a behavioral self-control plan, challenging dysfunctional thoughts, addressing concerns about shape and weight, improving self-image, discussing the ED with other people, and relapse prevention.

Lange and colleagues are currently conducting a treatment study comparing three conditions: Interapy, self-help (Vanderlinden, 2002), and a wait-list control. Preliminary findings ($N = 63$; A. Lange, personal communication, August 9, 2008) suggest that the completers of self-help and Interapy improved more than wait-list participants on a wide range of dependent measures (e.g., BN symptoms, general psychopathology, self-esteem). The Interapy completers improved slightly more than the self-help completers for most dependent measures. However, the self-help group had a dropout rate of 50%, whereas the Interapy group had a dropout rate of only 33%. Intention-to-treat analyses suggest clinically relevant differences in outcome between self-help and the Interapy treatment. Finally, patients report very high levels of satisfaction with the Interapy treatment. This study, when completed, will provide a fairly rigorous test of the efficacy of an Internet-based treatment.

ES[S]PRIT

Although largely designed as a prevention program, ES[S]PRIT (Bauer, Moessner, Wolf, Haug, & Kordy, in press) can also be conceptualized as an Internet-based stepped-care treatment for patients with EDs who are mildly symptomatic. Individuals are included if they are considered to be at risk for an ED, but excluded if they are currently in treatment for EDs or report ED symptoms that are severe. Individuals who qualify for the program are given access to the ES[S]PRIT website, where they receive general information about EDs. All accepted patients also gain access to the ES[S]PRIT Internet forum, where they can exchange information with other participants and discuss whatever topics interest them. Patients who register for the ES[S]PRIT program also receive supportive monitoring feedback through an Internet-based message delivery system. Monitoring and feedback are focused on four dimensions: body dissatisfaction, overconcern with weight and shape, unbalanced nutrition and dieting, and binge eating and compensatory behaviors. Assessments are completed by participants online on a weekly basis, and feedback is computer generated by the ES[S]PRIT program based on the participant's self-reported status in the assessments.

Studies of the ES[S]PRIT treatment have been conducted with 44 patients enrolled by the end of April 2007. Unfortunately, efficacy data are not yet available, but preliminary findings suggest that the patients enjoy the anonymity and flexibility of the treatment. Most patients also report that they would recommend the treatment to a friend and that the individual monitoring and feedback is a "good concept."

Internet-Based Self-Help for BN and BED

Ljotsson and colleagues (2007) compared a self-help CBT approach (Fairburn, 1995) combined with online support ($n = 37$) to a wait-list control condition ($n = 36$) in a study of participants with BN or BED. The online support consisted of participation in a private discussion forum in which patients could discuss their treatment with each other. The authors found that the majority of the patients (77%) used the online discussion forum, and most contributed a considerable amount of information to it. Additionally, 87% of the patients made use of e-mail to contact treatment staff at least once per week. Patients in the self-help CBT plus online support treatment condition improved significantly on most outcome measures (e.g., binge eating and purging frequency, Eating Disorder Examination Questionnaire [EDE-Q]), whereas patients in the wait-list condition did not change. Patients in the treatment group reported improvements in ED symptoms, including levels of restraint; concern over eating, weight, and shape; as well as other areas. Furthermore, at 6-month follow-up patients in the treatment group continued to maintain improvements.

Internet-Based Treatment of BN

Another Internet-based treatment protocol for BN was examined by Carrard and colleagues (2006). This treatment protocol includes a CBT-based self-help manual that was developed by the Psychiatric Liaison Unit of the University Hospitals of Geneva (Rouget, Carrard, & Archinard, 2003). The treatment is comprised of seven sequential steps: (1) motivation, (2) self-observation, (3) modification of behavior, (4) observation and modification of automatic thoughts, (5) problem solving, (6) self-affirmation, and (7) conclusion and relapse prevention. Forty-five patients were enrolled in a pilot study testing the Internet-based self-help treatment. The 45 patients were allowed to proceed through the protocol at their own pace. Each patient was assigned a coach who monitored participant progress over the study period. After 4 months of Internet-based self-help treatment, 17.2% of the participants reported abstaining completely from binge eating and vomiting. Additionally, 68.9% of participants reported a reduction in binge eating, and 58.6% reported a reduction in vomiting. Finally, at 2-month follow-up, abstinence levels were well maintained at 65.2% for binge eating and 60.8% for vomiting.

Internet-Based Social Support for Parents of Patients with EDs

The Internet has also been used as a method to provide support for the families of patients with EDs. Hopf (2007) used clinician-guided Internet-based chat groups to provide support for parents of patients with EDs. The program was based on the principles of family-based treatment (Le Grange, Crosby, Rathouz, & Leventhal, 2007). Given the proficiency of the Heidelburg group with Web-based interventions, they pursued a multicountry implementation of family chat rooms, providing services to U.S. families from the lab in Germany. Hopf noted that social support provided via Internet chat rooms can allow parents to (1) reduce their level of isolation, (2) share experiences with others, and (3) receive and give advice and reassurance. Preliminary results presented at a conference appear encouraging, although formal outcome data are not yet available.

Internet-Based Treatment of Binge Eating and Overweight in Adolescents

Two recent randomized controlled trials evaluated the use of an Internet-facilitated intervention for the treatment of overweight and binge-eating behavior in adolescents. Jones and colleagues (2008) compared an Internet-facilitated intervention ($n = 52$) with a wait-list control condition ($n = 53$). The Internet-facilitated intervention (StudentBodies2) was a 16-week semistructured program that primarily incorporated cognitive-behavioral principles. Retention rates were comparable across groups, and the majority of the intervention participants made use of the Internet-based components of the intervention. Participants in the intervention group had greater reductions in body mass index (BMI), fewer reported objective and subjective binge episodes, and reported significantly reduced weight and shape concerns at follow-up compared to the wait-list control group. Doyle and colleagues (2008) compared participants in the same StudentBodies2 Internet-facilitated condition ($n = 42$) to a treatment-as-usual condition ($n = 41$). Both groups experienced significant reductions in BMI immediately following the intervention and at 4-month follow-up, but the groups did not differ in this regard. Additionally, the Internet-facilitated group reported significantly greater increases in dietary restraint, but less improvement on shape concerns than the treatment-as-usual group at follow-up. Collectively, these findings suggest that although this specific Internet-facilitated treatment is superior to a wait-list control, it is not more effective than treatment as usual.

E-Mail and Text Messaging in ED Treatment

E-mail and text messaging have commonly been thought of as different forms of communication. However, the popularity of "smartphones" (portable phones that offer access to both text messaging as well as the Internet and e-mail accounts), has blurred the lines between e-mail and text messaging as adjuncts to ED treatments. Accordingly, we review e-mail and text messaging together below.

E-mail and text messaging can be used to monitor patient status as well as enhance therapy sessions (Yager, 2001). Other potential advantages are that these forms of communication increase patient–clinician contact, result in patients spending more time on treatment-related content, and require relatively little of the clinician's time. Some of the potential disadvantages of e-mail and text messaging are that some e-mails or text messages may contain inappropriate or ethically challenging content (e.g., suicide threat), patients may be frustrated with slow responses from the clinician (compared to face-to-face sessions), inadequate responses by the clinician, and there are concerns related to confidentiality, including, for example, that messages may be read by someone other than the patient (Yager, 2003). Nevertheless, Yager (2003) reported two case studies suggesting the potential utility of e-mail as an adjunct to standard treatment.

E-Mail Therapy for Patients with BN, BED, and EDNOS

In response to promising pilot work (Robinson & Serfaty, 2001, 2003), Robinson and Serfaty (2008) randomly assigned 97 patients with EDs (mixed ED patient group comprising BN, BED, or EDNOS) to one of three groups: self-directed writing, a wait-list control group, or e-mail therapy. Patients randomized to the wait-list control group waited 3 months and were reassessed before being placed in treatment. Patients in the self-directed writing condition were asked to write about "current difficulties" twice per week. Finally, patients in the e-mail therapy condition wrote about their feelings and thoughts related to their diet. Clinicians also challenged their automatic negative thoughts and cognitive styles. They were encouraged to eat regular meals and to examine potential predisposing and triggering factors to their disordered eating behaviors. A total of 61 patients completed the follow-up assessments: 20 patients completed the wait-list control condition, 22 finished the self-directed writing condition, and 19 completed the e-mail therapy condition. Analyses revealed that the e-mail therapy and the self-directed writing group conditions had significantly higher remission (i.e., no ED diagnosis) rates at 3-month follow-up than the wait-list control group. Both active treatments had a significant effect on diagnostic outcomes (ED diagnosis vs. none).

E-m@il Bridge

Wolf and colleagues (2007) tested the potential utility of e-mail for enhancing the aftercare of psychiatric inpatients. Following inpatient psychiatric treatment (not ED-specific), Wolf and colleagues randomly assigned patients to either a treatment-as-usual condition or an e-mail aftercare condition, which they named "E-m@il Bridge." Of the 91 clinical patients who completed the study, only 10 were diagnosed with an ED. E-mail aftercare patients were sent individual e-mails from their clinicians and were given writing assignments to be completed during the 8- to 12-week aftercare period. Patients in the e-mail aftercare condition did as well as, or significantly better than, patients in the treatment-as-usual condition on virtually all dependent measures.

Text Messaging in the Treatment of BN

In addition to using e-mail, Bauer and Kordy (2007) have implemented text messaging (TM) for the treatment of BN following hospital discharge. Bauer and Kordy randomly assigned 65 patients to a control condition and 67 patients to a TM aftercare condition. Patients provided symptom ratings on a weekly basis through a TM assessment system. TM used for automated replies to patients were semirandomly chosen from a collection of computer-selected responses that were appropriate to patients' specific symptom reports as well as their level of improvement, deterioration, or maintenance of symptoms. Patients rated the experience very positively, and indicated that they would recommend the program to others and would participate again if given the opportunity. To date, however, no data have been presented or published on the efficacy of this treatment adjunct.

Robinson and colleagues (Robinson et al., 2006) also tested TM in the outpatient treatment of BN. In this study patients received aftercare via TM following 10–20 sessions of self-help, cognitive behavior therapy (CBT), or cognitive analytic therapy. Twenty-one patients completed a pilot study intended to test the feasibility of TM aftercare. Unfortunately, 57% (12 of 21) patients dropped out by the end of the 6-month follow-up. Of the nine remaining patients, none sent the minimum expected one TM per week. Approximately half of the patients indicated that they viewed the lack of personal contact as positive, whereas about half of the patients viewed this feature of the aftercare as negative. Conclusions one can draw from this study are limited due to the small sample size and high dropout rate. However, findings suggest that TM may have limited utility in providing aftercare to patients with BN. Interestingly, this system appeared to be less favorably received in London (outpatients) than in Germany (inpatients).

Telehealth and ED Treatment

The delivery of high-quality treatment to patients with BN in rural areas represents a challenge because the typical mental health provider rarely has specific training in ED treatment. Mitchell and colleagues (2008) were interested in applying treatment via television with a "live" therapist (i.e., telemedicine or telehealth). They performed a randomized controlled clinical trial to evaluate the effectiveness of "telemedicine" as a medium for the delivery of specialized CBT for BN. This study provided a comparison of face-to-face CBT ($n = 66$) to CBT delivered via telemedicine ($n = 62$). Face-to-face and telemedicine CBT conditions did not differ significantly in retention (treatment completion) rates or abstinence rates at 12-month follow-up. Substantial clinical improvements in binge-eating frequency, global eating pathology, and depression scores were observed at posttreatment and at 12-month follow-up, and these outcomes did not differ significantly between the two delivery methods. Additionally, a second set of analyses from these data were completed to determine predictors of outcome using receiver operating characteristics (ROC) analysis. Analyses revealed that the best predictor of response to treatment at 1-year follow-up for the telemedicine CBT group was a 26.8% reduction in binge eating at week 4, whereas the best predictor of response to treatment in the face-to-face CBT group was 82.9% reduction in binge eating at week 6 (Marrone, Mitchell, Crosby, Wonderlich, & Jollie-Trottier, in press). In summary, early symptom reductions predict abstinence rates following treatment, and CBT delivered via telemedicine is rated favorably and is generally comparable in efficacy to traditional CBT delivered face to face.

Personal Digital Assistants and ED Treatment

Personal digital assistants (PDAs) have already been in use for over a decade to study a wide variety of problems and concerns. For example, Shiffman, Fischer, Paty, and Gnys (1994) employed PDAs to study the interplay between smoking and drinking behaviors. Although a large number of studies has now been conducted using PDAs in psychological research, PDAs generally have been applied as an assessment tool in studies using what is commonly called ecological momentary assessment (EMA; Stone & Shiffman, 1994) to gather ecologically valid, "real-time" data. Recently, there has been preliminary work using PDAs as treatment devices.

PDAs and the Treatment of BED

Le Grange, Gorin, Dymek, and Stone (2002) performed the first study using PDAs in the treatment of EDs. Forty-one patients with BED were randomly assigned to CBT ($n = 22$) or CBT with EMA ($n = 19$). The CBT with EMA group received the same treatment as the CBT group, plus they monitored their eating behaviors and binge eating using PDAs during the first 2 weeks of treatment. Findings revealed that the CBT with EMA group did not report greater levels of improvement than the pure CBT group on binge-eating frequency reduction (the primary outcome variable), or reduction in a general measure of eating pathology, self-esteem, or depression.

PDAs and the Treatment of BN

Another recent application of PDAs was developed by Wonderlich, Mitchell, Peterson, and Crow (2001) as a component of a new treatment being developed for BN called integrative cognitive–affective therapy (ICAT). ICAT employs PDAs to present coping modules and skill sets in an attempt to help patients overcome high-risk situations in the natural environment. Patients can select coping modules on the PDA that cover such areas as interpersonal problems, feeling of hopelessness, skipping meals, dealing with bulimic urges, and body image concerns. Additionally, the PDAs provide reminders and detailed information about the core skill sets of ICAT, which the patients have previously learned in treatment. Wonderlich and colleagues have piloted the PDAs on 17 participants with BN in a preliminary test of ICAT. Early evidence has provided support for the ICAT treatment, and a larger investigation of the treatment is currently underway.

Conclusions

Several new-technology-based interventions are being used to treat EDs and preliminary findings are now available for the use of the internet, e-mail, text messaging, telehealth, and PDAs. These interventions make use of new technologies and show promise in pilot studies, but much of this work is limited by relatively small sample sizes and/or reliance on clinical anecdotes about potential effectiveness. As noted by Newton and Ciliska (2006), although more data for technology-based research on the prevention of EDs is increasingly available (e.g., Taylor et al., 2006), there clearly is a paucity of empirical data on these types of treatment interventions. However, with the high level of interest in technology-based interventions, a considerable amount of data will soon be available on the topic.

One final thought focuses on the ever-changing nature of technology—and therefore technology-based interventions. Technology is always in flux; most cutting-edge technologies of today are typically nothing more than tomorrow's outdated and obsolete methods (keep in mind that the sun dial, abacus, and eight-track cassette players were all "cutting edge" at one time). We have seen many of these changes in our work: For example, modems that we once used with PDAs have become obsolete due to cellular phones and digital phone lines, the Internet has dramatically changed the way telehealth treatments are being delivered, and some of our older PDAs are not compatible with newer computer operating systems. Technologies will inevitably continue to change, and with these changes will come additional opportunities for new applications to the treatment of EDs.

References

Bauer S, Golkaramnay V, & Kordy H. (2005). E-mental-health-Neue medien in der psychosozialen versorgung. *Psychotherapeut*, 50:7–15.

Bauer S, & Kordy H. (2007, December). *The use of text messaging in the second level treatment of bulimia nervosa.* Paper presented at the Symposium Expert Meeting (INTACT), Heidelberg, Germany.

Bauer S, Moessner M, Wolf M, Haug S, & Kordy H. (in press). ES[S]PRIT: An Internet-based program for the prevention and early intervention of eating disorders in college students. *British Journal of Guidance and Counseling.*

Carrard I, Rouget P, Fernandez-Aranda F, Volkart A, Damoiseau M, & Lam T. (2006). Evaluation and deployment of evidence based patient self-management support program for bulimia nervosa. *International Journal of Medical Informatics*, 75:101–109.

Doyle AC, Goldschmidt A, Huang C, Winzelberg AJ, Taylor CB, & Wilfley DE. (2008). Reduction of overweight and eating disorder symptoms via the Internet in adolescents: A randomized controlled trial. *Journal of Adolescent Health*, 43:172–179.

Fairburn CG. (1995). *Overcoming binge eating.* New York: Guilford Press.

Gleason N. (1995). A new approach to disordered eating: Using an electronic bulletin board to confront social pressure on body image. *Journal of American College Health*, 44:78–80.

Hopf (2007, December). *Internet support groups for parents in FBT for adolescent EDs.* Paper presented at the Symposium Expert Meeting (INTACT), Heidelberg, Germany.

Jones M, Luce KH, Osborne MI, Taylor K, Cunning D, Doyle AC, et al. (2008). Randomized controlled trial of an Internet-facilitated intervention for reducing binge eating and over-weight in adolescents. *Pediatrics*, 121:453–462.

Kordy H, Golkaramnay V, Wolf M, Haug S, & Bauer S. (2006). Internetchatgruppen in Psychotherapie und Psychosomatik: Akzeptanz und Wirksamkeit einer Internet-Brücke zwischen Fachklinik und Alltag. *Psychotherapeut*, 51:144–153.

Lange A, Rietdijk D, Hudcovicova M, Van de Ven J-P, Schrieken B, & Emmelkamp PMG. (2003). Interapy: A controlled randomized trial of the standardized treatment of posttraumatic stress through the Internet. *Journal of Consulting and Clinical Psychology*, 71:901–909.

Lange A, Vries M, de Gest A, & van Oostendorp E. (1994). A self-management program for bulimia nervosa: The elements, the rationales and a case study. *Eating Disorders*, 2:329–340.

Le Grange D, Crosby RD, Rathouz PJ, & Leventhal BL. (2007). A randomized controlled comparison of family-based treatment and supportive psychotherapy for adolescent bulimia nervosa. *Archives of General Psychiatry*, 64:1049–1056.

Le Grange D, Gorin A, Dymek M, & Stone A. (2002). Does ecological momentary assessment improve cognitive behavioral therapy for binge eating disorder?: A pilot study. *European Eating Disorders Review*, 10:1–13.

Ljotsson B, Lundin C, Mitsell K, Carlbring P, Ramklint M, & Ghaderi A. (2007). Remote treatment of bulimia nervosa and binge eating disorder: A randomized trial of Internet-assisted cognitive behavioral therapy. *Behaviour Research and Therapy*, 45:649–661.

Marks IM, Cavanagh K, & Grega L. (2007). Hands-on help: Computer-aided psychotherapy. *American Journal of Psychiatry*, 165:142–143.

Marrone S, Mitchell JE, Crosby R, Wonderlich S, & Jollie-Trottier T. (in press). Predictors of response to cognitive behavioral treatment for bulimia nervosa delivered via telemedicine versus face-to-face. *International Journal of Eating Disorders*.

Mitchell JE, Crosby RD, Wonderlich SA, Crow S, Lancaster K, Simonich H, et al. (2008). A randomized trial comparing the efficacy of cognitive-behavioral therapy for bulimia nervosa delivered via telemedicine versus face-to-face. *Behaviour Research and Therapy*, 46:581–592.

Myers T, Swan-Kremeier L, Wonderlich S, Lancaster K, & Mitchell JE. (2004). The use of alternative delivery systems and new technologies in the treatment of patients with eating disorders. *International Journal of Eating Disorders*, 36:123–143.

Newton MS, & Ciliska D. (2006). Internet-based innovations for the prevention of eating disorders: A systematic review. *Eating Disorders: The Journal of Treatment and Prevention*, 14:365–384.

Powers P, & Emmelkamp MB. (2008). Virtual reality exposure therapy for anxiety disorders: A meta-analysis. *Journal of Anxiety Disorders*, 22:561–569.

Robinson PH, & Serfaty MA. (2001). The use of e-mail in the identification of bulimia nervosa and its treatment. *European Eating Disorders Review*, 9:182–193.

Robinson PH, & Serfaty MA. (2003). Computers, e-mail and therapy in eating disorders. *European Eating Disorders Review*, 11:210–221.

Robinson S, Perkins S, Bauer S, Hammond N, Treasure J, & Schmidt U. (2006). Aftercare intervention through text messaging in the treatment of bulimia nervosa: A feasibility pilot. *International Journal of Eating Disorders*, 39:633–638.

Rouget P, Carrard I, & Archinard M. (2003). *La boulimie: Un guide pour s'en sortir.* Unpublished manuscript.

Ruskin PE, Silver-Aylaian M, Kling MA, Reed SA, Bradham DD, Hebel JR, et al. (2004). Treatment outcomes in depression: Comparison of remote treatment through telepsychiatry to in-person treatment. *American Journal of Psychiatry*, 161:1471–1476.

Ruwaard J, Lange A, Bouwman M, Broeksteeg J, & Schrieken B. (2007). E-mailed standardized cognitive behavioural treatment of work-related stress: A randomized controlled trial. *Cognitive Behaviour Therapy*, 36:179–192.

Shiffman S, Fischer LA, Paty JA, & Gnys M. (1994). Drinking and smoking: A field study of their association. *Annals of Behavioral Medicine*, 16:203–209.

Stone A, & Shiffman S. (1994). Ecological momentary assessment (EMA) in behavioral medicine. *Annals of Behavioral Medicine*, 16:199–202.

Stricker G. (2002). Patient–therapist matching: A good start. *Journal of Psychotherapy Integration*, 12:143–146.

Taylor CB, Bryson S, Luce KH, Cunning D, Doyle AC, Abascal LB, et al. (2006). Prevention of eating disorders in at-risk college-age women. *Archives of General Psychiatry*, 63:881–888.

Vanderlinden J. (2002). *Boulimie en eetbuien overwinnen*. Lannoo, Germany: Tielt.

Winzelberg AJ. (1997). An analysis of an electronic support group for individuals with eating disorders. *Computers in Human Behavior*, 13:393–407.

Wolf M, Kordy H, Arikan M, Maurer W, & Dogs P. (2007, December). *E-mail treatment*. Paper presented at the Symposium Expert Meeting (INTACT), Heidelberg, Germany.

Wonderlich SA, Mitchell JE, Peterson CB, & Crow S. (2001). Integrative cognitive therapy for bulimic behavior. In RH Striegel-Moore & L Smolak (Eds.), *Eating disorders: Innovative directions in research and practice* (pp. 173–196). Washington, DC: American Psychological Association.

Yager J. (2001). Using e-mail to support the outpatient treatment of anorexia nervosa. In RL Hsiung (Ed.), *e-therapy: Case studies, guiding principles, and the clinical potential of the Internet* (pp. 39–68). New York: Norton.

Yager J. (2003). E-mail therapy for anorexia nervosa: Prospects and limitations. *European Disorder Review*, 11:198–209.

Zabinski M, Wilfley D, Ping M, Winzelberg A, Celio A, & Taylor C. (2001). An Internet-based intervention for women at risk of eating disorders: A pilot study. *International Journal of Eating Disorders*, 29:401–408.

Zhang Z, Qing-Rong T, Tong Y, Li O, Kang W, Zheng X, et al. (2008). The effectiveness of carbamezapine in unipolar depression: A double-blind, randomized, placebo-controlled study. *Journal of Affective Disorders*, 109:91–97.

PART V

Research Issues

The final section of the book includes five chapters addressing research issues on the treatment of eating disorders (EDs). Although these chapters are framed as "research" chapters, their content is certainly relevant for clinicians as well. As consumers of the treatment literature, it is important that clinicians consider the various issues covered in these chapters as context to help them critically evaluate and make decisions based on the literature. Moreover, astute clinical observations are often the best impetus for stimulating new and meaningful research. The reality in the treatment of EDs, like most other clinical areas, is that much clinical practice needs to occur before unequivocal empirical evidence exists to guide many clinical decisions. Much progress has been made in advancing our knowledge regarding the nature and treatment of EDs during the past two decades. This section addresses important challenges that must be met in order for the field to continue to move forward in the challenge of meeting the needs of our patients.

Chapter 31, by Ross D. Crosby and Scott G. Engel discusses research design and statistical issues essential to the evaluation of the efficacy of treatments for EDs. The authors present a cogent and highly readable overview of complex methodological issues that is essential reading for researchers and clinicians alike.

Chapter 32 by Carol B. Peterson addresses assessment issues essential to the evaluation of the efficacy of treatments. Solid assessment is a basic requirement and essential component of *both* good clinical work and research. Peterson provides an overview of the major issues and technologies for assessing patients with EDs and practical guidance for integrating these methods into clinical practice and treatment research.

This section closes with three chapters offering overviews of what treatment research is needed. W. Stewart Agras and Athena Hagler Robinson address research needs for anorexia nervosa (AN). This chapter cogently addresses the special challenges and barriers to doing treatment research with patients who have AN, such as recruitment problems and poor adherence, and offers a number of potential strategies for overcoming them. G. Terence Wilson addresses research needs for bulimia nervosa (BN). In contrast to the limited advances for AN, treatment research with BN has yielded much progress during the past two decades. This chapter highlights the need for treatment research to examine processes and mechanisms of therapeutic change. Wilson also highlights the pressing need for wider dissemination and better training in evidence-based treatments that have been identified for BN. The final chapter, by Carlos M. Grilo, addresses research needs for binge-eating disorder (BED) and eating disorder not otherwise specified (EDNOS). These two broad categories of EDs are the most prevalent yet most poorly understood. This chapter highlights a number of priorities for treatment research, including the need for improved characterization and assessment methods, longer treatment studies with follow-ups after discontinuation of treatments, and the need to find ways to help patients with BED also lose excess weight. Grilo, like Wilson in his chapter for BN, emphasizes that the identification of predictors and moderators is needed to improve treatment planning. The identification of possible mediators of change will provide clues for experimental studies to test putative mechanisms by which treatments work.

CHAPTER 31

Evaluating the Efficacy
of Eating Disorder Treatments
Research Design and Statistical Issues

Ross D. Crosby and Scott G. Engel

A variety of psychotherapeutic and pharmacological treatments for eating disorders (EDs) has been evaluated, and the efficacy of some treatments for anorexia nervosa (AN) (Bulik, Berkman, Brownley, Sedway, & Lohr, 2007), bulimia nervosa (BN) (Shapiro, Berkman, Brownley, Sedway, Lohr, & Bulik, 2007), and binge-eating disorder (BED) (Brownley, Berkman, Sedway, Lohr, & Bulik, 2007) have been empirically supported. However, few would argue with the contention that more effective treatments for EDs are needed (Wilson, Grilo, & Vitousek, 2007). In establishing the efficacy of ED treatments, sound methodological and statistical approaches are essential. The purpose of this chapter is to provide an overview of some of the key methodological and statistical issues related to conducting ED treatment research. Given that randomized controlled trials (RCTs) are currently the optimal method for establishing treatment efficacy, much of the overview focuses on issues central to RCTs. We focus on issues specific to the conduct of ED research wherever possible. Readers interested in a more general discussion are referred to an excellent volume by Meinert (1986), covering many of the methodological issues pertaining to RCTs and to the statistical guidelines for clinical trials developed by the International Committee of Harmonisation (1999).

Issues Related to Research Design

RCT Design

The most common research design for an RCT evaluating the efficacy of ED treatments is the *parallel-groups design*, wherein patients are randomized to receive only one of several possible treatments. The parallel-groups design is less complex than other designs described below and avoids many of the confounding factors associated with these designs (e.g., carryover effects, biases associated with multiple treatments). Many ED treatments involve a treatment period extending across many months and possibly years. The parallel-groups design is ideally suited to study these long-term treatments. Results of parallel-groups studies are generally considered to be more externally valid (i.e., generalizable) in that they do not involve the potential biases associated with multiple treatments (Campbell & Stanley, 1963). This is not meant to imply, however, that parallel-groups designs are not without their own limitations. These designs typically require more patients than crossover designs to achieve comparable statistical power. Recruitment can often be a limiting factor when evaluating relatively rare disorders such as AN. Other issues, such as dropout, covariate adjustment, and repeated assessments over time, can also increase the complexity of conducting parallel-groups studies.

In a *crossover design*, patients receive a sequence of two or more treatments in random order. In the simplest 2×2 crossover design, patients are randomized to receive two treatments in one of two sequences (Treatment A followed by Treatment B, or vice versa), often separated by a "washout" period of no treatment. One advantage of crossover designs is that each patient serves as his/her own control, thereby increasing statistical power and reducing the number of subjects required to achieve adequate statistical power. However, there are limitations associated with crossover studies that may limit their applicability to ED treatment research. One problem associated with crossover studies is the potential for carryover: that is, the residual influence of treatments in subsequent treatment periods. Whereas a washout period may be effective for minimizing carryover effects for pharmacological treatments, it is doubtful whether washout periods eliminate the residual effects of psychological treatments. Although there are a number of statistical approaches for addressing the potential biases associated with carryover (e.g., Cotton, 1989), these approaches are often quite complex and may not ultimately be adequate for completely removing this confound. Another question concerning crossover studies is the generalizability of the findings when patients receive multiple treatments. It is unclear whether the outcome of patients receiving a given treatment in a crossover study as part of a sequence of treatments is representative of the outcome of patients receiving that same treatment in isolation.

A third research design that has been used in ED treatment research is the *factorial design*, wherein patients receive combinations of two (or more) factors simultaneously, each with discrete levels (e.g., doses of medication, presence/absence of a treatment). An example of a factorial design is the study reported by Mitchell and colleagues (1993), who conducted a 2×2 study of cognitive-behavioral therapy (CBT) in patients with BN. Patients received one combination of treatments varying in intensity (high vs. low) and emphasis on early abstinence (high vs. low). Factorial designs are often ideal to study combinations of psychotherapy and pharmacotherapy (e.g., Grilo, Masheb, & Wilson, 2005; Walsh, Fairburn, Mickley, Sysko, & Parides, 2004) and are particularly useful for evaluating interactions between treatments. Factorial designs also have the advantage of evaluating two treatments simultaneously, thereby reducing the number of required patients, in comparison to designs where these treatments are evaluated separately in comparison to a control condition. However, factorial designs may require additional patients to provide adequate power to detect interactions between treatments. In addition, as in crossover designs, the generalizability of results from factorial designs is open to some debate, given that patients receive multiple treatments simultaneously.

Randomization

The process of randomization assigns patients to treatments on the basis of chance occurrence, thereby removing potential biases arising from the predictability of treatment assignments. Randomization tends to produce treatment groups in which the distributions of prognostic factors, both measured and unmeasured, tend to be similar. Any differences between treatment groups assigned via randomization are due solely to chance and are unrelated to the treatment to which they are assigned.

There are two general approaches to randomization. *Fixed randomization* schemes are distinguished by assignment probabilities that remain constant over the course of the trial. In *adaptive* (also referred to as *dynamic*) *randomization* schemes, the assignment probabilities for treatments change over the course of the study as a function of the distribution of previous assignments, observed baseline characteristics, or observed outcomes. As the vast majority of RCTs conducted in the ED field involve fixed randomization, they are described below. Those readers interested in learning more about adaptive randomization are referred to a review by Kalish and Begg (1985) and a comprehensive book by Rosenberger and Lachin (2002).

All fixed randomization procedures can be characterized in terms of three properties: allocation ratio, allocation strata, and block size. The *allocation ratio* describes the relative probability of assignment to each treatment. Most ED studies employ a uniform allocation ratio, wherein the probability of assignment is equal for all treatments (i.e., 1:1 for a two-group study; 1:1:1 for a three-group study, etc.). There may be some circumstances (e.g., cost concerns, safety, prior data, anticipated variability in response) in which a nonuniform allocation ratio is specified (e.g., 2:1; 2:1:1), thereby resulting in a greater number of patients assigned to some treatments. Indeed, in RCTs comparing three or more interventions, researchers are often most interested in post hoc pairwise comparisons between specific treatments. Since expected effect sizes can be larger for some treatment pairs (e.g., medication vs. placebo) than for others (e.g., two different active medications), statistical power varies for the different comparisons. Woods and colleagues (1998) described an efficient method for estimating required sample sizes for RCTs with three or more conditions and demonstrated that considerable efficiency might be achieved by allocating fewer patients to a placebo condition. An example of this strategy can be found in a RCT conducted by Grilo and Masheb (2005) in which patients with BED were randomly allocated following an unequal (5:5:2) ratio to one of three conditions (two specific treatments and one control). It is worth emphasizing that nonuniform allocation methods are not without risk. If one of the treatment cells has relatively few patients, factors such as different effect sizes (e.g., smaller effect for active treatment, higher placebo, or control response) or greater attrition than expected can pose serious problems.

The *allocation strata* refer to the number of predefined groups into which patients are placed prior to randomization. The purpose of stratification is to reduce or eliminate variation in the outcome due to the stratification variables. Stratification has the potential to increase the statistical efficiency of the design, but will do so only when the stratification variable is strongly associated with outcome. The greatest gains resulting from stratification involve small trials of 20 or fewer patients per treatment group (Meier, 1981). The increased statistical efficiency resulting from stratification is minimal for designs involving 50 or more patients per group. Stratification increases the complexity of the randomization process and the chances for randomization errors. It is impractical to control for more than two or three variables via stratification.

The *block size* refers to the number of patients that is randomized in a given sequence. For example, a block size of six in a two-group trial comparing Treatments A and B would result in six patients being randomized in a given sequence, three to Treatment A and three to Treatment B (assuming a uniform allocation ratio). Block randomization should be used when enrollment is likely to occur over an extended period (months or years) or the patient population is expected to change over the course of the enrollment period. Block randomization achieves a relative balance of patients assigned to treatments over time, thereby removing a potential source of bias. In simple randomization there is a uniform allocation ratio, a single stratum (i.e., all patients in the study), and the block size is equal to the sample size. Large multisite RCTs evaluating ED treatments will likely stratify randomization by site (and quite possibly other variables), and most will use block randomization to ensure comparability of treatment groups over time.

Statistical Power and Sample Size

Statistical power in ED treatment research deals with the probability of obtaining a significant difference between treatments in a study, given that there is a real difference in the efficacy of the treatments being compared. Statistical power is determined by three factors, described below: the significance level (alpha), the effect size, and the sample size (Cohen, 1988).

The *significance level* is the probability that the observed differences between treatment groups in a study are the result of chance alone. When that probability is at or below some predefined cutoff, typically .05, we identify those treatments as being "significantly different." Thus the significance level expresses the probability of a false-positive (or Type I) error. When multiple tests of significance are conducted, the probability of making at least one Type I error increases. Consequently, researchers often decrease the significance level (e.g., to .01) if multiple comparisons are being conducted. Other things being equal (i.e., sample size, effect size), decreasing the significance level decreases statistical power, thus reducing the probability of identifying a difference between treatments that is actually there.

The *effect size* is the magnitude of difference between treatments. Other things being equal (i.e., significance level, sample size), the larger the effect size, the greater the statistical power. Typically, when planning a study, the anticipated effect size is not known but must be estimated. This estimate can often be based on previous research, but should also take into account the magnitude of difference between treatments that would be considered clinically meaningful. Kraemer, Mintz, Noda, Tinklenberg, and Yesavage (2006) have cautioned against estimating effect size solely on the basis of a small pilot study, as this estimate is likely to be unreliable and frequently overestimates the "true" effect. Whereas pilot studies may be useful for demonstrating the feasibility of a larger project, conducting them for the sole purpose of generating effect size estimates to plan larger studies is not advised.

The *sample size* is the final factor that determines statistical power. The larger the sample size, the greater the statistical power. One crucial point to remember in calculating power is that most ED treatment studies involve some attrition (i.e., dropout, loss of participants) over time. For a variety of reasons (e.g., ineffective treatment, adverse events, relocation), not all enrolled patients will complete the trial. Power analysis must take into account the anticipated rate of attrition.

A variety of resources is available for calculating statistical power and determining the sample size necessary to achieve adequate power. Given the complexity of this task, it is beyond the scope of this chapter to provide the necessary information to calculate power. Resources available for calculating power include textbooks (Cohen, 1988; Kraemer & Thiemann 1987; Meinert, 1986) and stand-alone software programs (e.g., G-Power, PASS). Dedicated statistical analysis software programs, including SAS and SPSS, also include modules for performing power analysis.

A few final comments regarding power analysis are warranted. First, it is important that, whenever possible, the method for determining statistical power must match the actual analyses to be performed. For example, it is not appropriate to determine statistical power for a one-way analysis of variance (ANOVA) when a hierarchical linear model will be used to compare treatment groups. Second, the power analysis that was conducted in planning the study should be reported in the publication of the results (see the recommendations from the APA Task Force on Statistical Inference; Wilkinson, 1999). If the actual study deviates from the original plan used to perform the power analysis (e.g., lower sample size, higher rate of attrition), this information should be reported, since it is crucial in interpreting the results of the study. Finally, we are often asked what constitutes an adequate level of power. A frequently cited value for a minimal acceptable level of power is .80, although many methodologists would recommend a power of .90. If statistical power is .95 or higher for the primary comparison, this would suggest to some methodologists that the study is "overpowered" and has an unjustifiably large sample size. Given the very high costs associated with doing clinical trials of ED treatments and the difficulties in recruiting certain patient groups, especially those with AN, a balance between controlling costs and achieving adequate statistical power is often warranted.

Schedule of Assessments

A few comments are also relevant here regarding the planned schedule of assessments. The first concerns the importance of doing follow-up assessments after the completion of treatments. It is vital in evaluating the efficacy of treatments to know the outcome at intervals beyond the end of formal treatment. Some treatments may have effects that are delayed. Failing to include follow-up assessments would miss these delayed effects. Similarly, treatments may differ in the durability of their outcomes. Follow-up assessments are essential for determining how well treatment effects are maintained after treatment is discontinued as well as whether treatments differ in relapse rates, including time to relapse. Thus, it is recommended that several follow-up assessments be conducted, if at all possible. Follow-up assessments at 6 months, 1 year, and 2 years after treatment are often ideal. In general, longer-term follow-up periods are highly desirable for treatment studies in AN, where distal relapse and gradual improvement are both likely outcomes.

A second recommendation involves the frequency of assessment of outcome and potential mediating variables. Many studies include an assessment of outcome only at baseline (i.e., pretreatment) and at the end of treatment. The problem with this approach is that no outcome data are available for any patients dropping out of the treatment portion of the study for any reason. The methods available for including these patients in (pre- vs. post-only) comparisons of treatment efficacy (e.g., last observation carried forward, baseline observation carried forward) are limited and problematic for a variety of statistical and conceptual reasons (Crosby, 2006). A much better approach is to schedule more frequent assessments of the primary outcome measure. Although patients dropping out of the study may not complete all assessments of the primary outcome, any assessments they do complete provide important data that can contribute to the overall determination of treatment efficacy. Thus, more frequent assessments of the primary outcome measure will result in a more efficient trial. This ultimately may have some bearing on whether the efficacy of a treatment is identified in a given clinical trial. Furthermore, failure to assess potential mediating variables at multiple time points throughout a protocol may limit an investigator's ability to identify the mechanisms by which a treatment may have a therapeutic effect (see discussion of mediation below).

Patient Recruitment and Retention

Another key issue in the design of ED treatment research is that of patient recruitment and retention. This topic is covered here under research design because developing a sound recruitment plan prior to the initiation of the study is a key to conducting a successful clinical trial. A recruitment plan should specify the anticipated rate of recruitment (i.e., number of patients over a specified interval of time) and if that rate is expected to change over time (e.g., it may be more difficult to recruit patients later in the trial). The recruitment plan should also specify the recruitment methods to be used. These methods may include various combinations of direct (e.g., clinic contacts, screenings, direct mailings) and indirect (e.g., clinical referrals, retrospective record reviews, community advertisements, Web postings) patient contacts. Different recruitment methods may produce different samples. The specific recruitment methods to be used can be tailored to the specific study questions and design. It is important during the course of the trial to monitor the current rate of recruitment in relation to the recruitment plan. It is also vital during enrollment to track how many patients are successfully recruited by each of the methods being used. This information may be useful if modifications of the original recruitment plan are necessary. However, in the event that a change is made in recruitment methods during the course of the trial, an investigator should evaluate whether these different methods are in some way differentially associated with outcome.

Patient retention is also a key to a successful study. A variety of factors can help to increase retention and enhance interest and participation. These can include various aspects of the research facilities themselves, including pleasant physical surroundings, a secure and comfortable environment, convenient parking, and access to public transportation. Retention can also be increased by limiting the amount of time and inconvenience in making research visits. The payment of parking and travel fees may help to mitigate some of the costs associated with clinic visits. Scheduling research appointments during hours that are convenient for patients (e.g., evenings, lunch hours, weekends) may also serve to increase retention. Finally, increased contact with patients between scheduled clinic visits may help to increase retention. This can include written or phone contacts from study personnel, newsletters, or cards sent to patients on special occasions such as Christmas, birthdays, and anniversaries. Such strategies have particular utility during the follow-up, when contact is diminished and retention may be particularly problematic.

Issues Related to Statistical Analysis

Analysis Plan

All RCTs conducted to evaluate ED treatments should have a completely developed analysis plan prior to the initiation of the trial. This plan serves to ensure that the design of the trial will allow the investigators to address their primary questions of interest. This analysis plan should include power analysis and sample size estimation, the primary and secondary hypotheses to be evaluated, a specification of the primary and secondary outcome measures, and specific details on all of the descriptive and inferential analyses to be conducted, including the significance level to be used in evaluating hypotheses. This plan should provide the details necessary to conduct all of the initial analyses for the clinical trial. In many cases, results from the original analysis plan will lead to additional analyses that address further questions of interest. However, this should not detract from the overall importance of developing a detailed analysis plan prior to the initiation of the trial.

Trial Monitoring

One of the essential tasks in the conduct of an RCT is the ongoing monitoring of the trial. Although this is not a statistical task per se (although it is frequently conducted by the statistical staff), it does have profound implications for the statistical analyses to be conducted and, as such, is considered here. The goal of trial monitoring is to ensure the overall quality of the study, and it includes monitoring actual recruitment rates in relation to the recruitment goals, verifying that all enrolled patients meet inclusion/exclusion criteria and have provided written informed consent, ensuring that the protocol is being followed (e.g., the correct assessments are being completed at each study visit), monitoring the demographic and clinical characteristics of enrolled patients, monitoring the integrity and completeness of the collected data (i.e., are all items being completed?), verifying the data entry procedure, monitoring retention and follow-up rates, monitoring the integrity of the treatments being provided (e.g., number of sessions completed, number of doses taken), and monitoring adverse events. In the event of multisite trials, monitoring should be performed separately at each site.

Data monitoring reports summarizing all of the above information should be prepared at regular intervals (e.g., monthly) and provided to principal investigators and relevant study personnel. In some circumstances these reports can also be distributed to relevant oversight committees, such as a data safety monitoring board (DSMB) that is now required for NIH-sponsored trials. For multisite trials, monitoring information should be provided both separately by site and combined across sites.

Interim Analysis

"Interim analysis," as defined here, refers to any analysis of data during the patient enrollment or treatment stages of a trial for the purposes of assessing treatment effects with respect to efficacy or safety. Because interim analyses may have a substantial impact upon the conduct, analysis, and interpretation of the trial, all interim analyses should be included as part of the original analysis plan.

The appropriateness of using an interim analysis to make decisions about terminating a clinical trial has spurred considerable debate (see Meinert, 1986, pp. 208–216).

The goal of such an interim analysis is to stop the trial early if the efficacy of the treatment under study has been clearly established, if a lack of superiority of the treatment under study has been clearly demonstrated, or if unacceptable rates of adverse events are experienced. Those favoring the use of interim analysis in this manner argue that it would be unethical (and cost-prohibitive) to continue the trial once one of these milestones has been reached (i.e., efficacy, lack of efficacy, or treatment not well tolerated). Those opposed to the use of interim analysis for the purposes of terminating a study early raise concerns about such analyses influencing or changing the conduct of the study in some way. For example, knowledge that an interim analysis has been conducted and that the study is continuing may influence the expectations of the study personnel. Ideally, all research personnel should be blinded to the interim analysis plan. Whether this approach is practical for most ED treatment studies is unclear. A number of statistical concerns has also been raised about interim analysis relating to the problem of multiple comparisons and the adjustment of significance levels (see Meinert, 1986).

Missing Data

As noted above, all precautions should be taken to minimize the extent of missing data in ED treatment studies. Unfortunately, most longitudinal studies and treatment studies have some missing data. A variety of approaches is available for handling missing data (see Schafer & Graham, 2002, for an excellent review). Most (but not all) of these methods assume that missing data (e.g., dropouts) are missing randomly (termed "missing at random," or MAR), an assumption that is almost always untenable. Case deletion (e.g., complete case analysis) and single imputation (e.g., mean substitution, last observation carried forward) methods are discouraged in favor of hierarchical linear models (e.g., Raudenbush & Bryk, 2002), maximum likelihood imputation (e.g., expectation-maximization algorithm), and multiple imputation methods (Rubin, 1987). Several methods are available for handling "non-ignorable" (Rubin, 1976) missing data, including propensity scores (Rosenbaum & Rubin, 1983) and pattern mixture models (Little, 1993), although their applicability to ED treatment research is still unclear. Regardless of the approach, when too much data are missing, the ability of the study to provide useful information about the efficacy of ED treatments is severely compromised.

Significance Levels

Two issues are considered related to significance levels: directional versus nondirectional hypothesis testing and Type I error rates. *Directional tests* (i.e., one-tailed; Treatment A > Treatment B) provide a less stringent criterion for determining statistical significance than *nondirectional tests* (i.e., two-tailed; Treatment A ≠ Treatment B), thereby increasing the chances of finding differences in efficacy between ED treatments. Investigators may be tempted to use directional tests because, in comparison to nondirectional tests, a smaller difference between treatments is required to reach statistical significance. On the other hand, directional tests preclude the possibility of unexpected results (e.g., Treatment B > Treatment A when testing the directional hypothesis that Treatment A > Treatment B). In most circumstances, directional tests are not appropriate for comparing ED treatments and should be avoided.

In an ED treatment trial, a *Type I error* involves concluding that there is a differ-ence in efficacy between treatments (i.e., rejecting the null hypothesis of no difference between treatments) when no difference in efficacy between treatments actually exists. The probability of making a Type I error for a single hypothesis test is referred to as the *comparison-wise error rate*. When multiple hypothesis tests are performed, the chances of making *at least* one Type I error (referred to as the *experiment-wise error rate*) increase. For example, assuming a comparison-wise error rate of .05, the chances of making at least one Type I error when two hypothesis tests are performed is .0975, and is .226 when five hypothesis tests are performed. Quite obviously, the probability of making a Type I error increases dramatically as a function of the number of tests that is performed.

A number of statistical approaches are available for addressing the problem of multiple comparisons. A description of these methods is beyond the scope of the cur-rent chapter, but interested readers are referred to reviews of the various approaches by Toothaker (1993) and Hsu (1996). A strong argument can be made that the problem of multiple comparisons and alpha control is as much a matter of research design as it is a statistical issue. Investigators are encouraged to limit the number of primary outcome variables to a reasonable number (perhaps three or less), thereby limiting the number of hypothesis tests conducted to determine treatment efficacy.

Predictors, Moderators, and Mediators

Kraemer and colleagues (Kraemer, Wilson, Fairburn, & Agras, 2002) have argued that RCTs can provide important information about who is most likely to improve (i.e., pre-dictors of outcome), for whom a particular treatment may work (i.e., moderators of treatment), and the mechanisms through which a treatment may achieve its aims (i.e., mediators of treatment). This information serves a dual purpose in that it informs clini-cal practice while, at the same time, provides a guide for future studies. Kraemer and colleagues (2002) provide precise terminology for defining predictors, moderators, and mediators and an analytic framework for evaluating them in the context of RCTs. *Predictors* are defined as pretreatment variables that are not associated with treatment (by definition of random assignment) and have a main effect relationship to outcome. Predictor variables in RCTs are typically evaluated after controlling for the effects of treatment. *Moderators* are defined as pretreatment variables that are not associated with treatment (again, by definition) and have an interactive effect with treatment on out-come. *Mediators* are defined as during-treatment variables that are associated with treat-ment and have either a main effect or an interactive effect with treatment on outcome. Predictors always precede what they predict; moderators always precede treatment, which in turn precedes outcome; mediators always come temporally between what they mediate (i.e., treatment) and outcome (Kraemer et al., 2002). Analyses of mediators require that repeated assessments be performed during the course of treatment to cap-ture fluctuations or changes in the variables hypothesized to effect change in addition to the outcome variables. Recent research has highlighted the importance of planning repeated assessments starting early in the treatment process (Grilo, Masheb, & Wilson, 2006). Research has recently started to utilize this methodology for identifying predic-tors, moderators, and mediators in various ED treatments (Le Grange, Crosby, & Lock, 2008; Lock, Le Grange, & Crosby, 2008; Masheb & Grilo, 2007; Stice, Presnell, Gau, & Shaw, 2007).

Conclusions

As outlined here, there are many complicated methodological and statistical issues relating to the conduct of RCTs for the purpose of evaluating ED treatments. We have attempted to highlight and discuss some of the key issues. Given that RCTs are currently considered the best method for establishing the efficacy of ED treatments, we believe that these issues are important and will help to better inform the field about more efficacious treatments in the future.

References

Brownley KA, Berkman ND, Sedway JA, Lohr KN, & Bulik CM. (2007). Binge eating disorder treatment: A systematic review of randomized controlled trials. *International Journal of Eating Disorders*, 40:337–348.

Bulik CM, Berkman ND, Brownley KA, Sedway JA, & Lohr KN. (2007). Anorexia nervosa treatment: A systematic review of randomized controlled trials. *International Journal of Eating Disorders*, 40:310–320.

Campbell DT, & Stanley JC. (1963). *Experimental and quasi-experimental designs for research.* Boston: Houghton-Mifflin.

Cohen J. (1988). *Statistical power analysis for the behavioral sciences* (2nd ed.). Hillsdale, NJ: Erlbaum.

Cotton JW. (1989). Interpreting data from two-period crossover design (also termed the replicated 2×2 Latin Square design). *Psychological Bulletin*, 106:503–515.

Crosby RD. (2006, September). *Longitudinal data analysis for eating disorders research: Moving beyond LOCF.* Paper presented at the 12th annual meeting of the Eating Disorders Research Society, Port Douglas, Australia.

Grilo CM, & Masheb RM. (2005). A randomized controlled comparison of guided self-help cognitive behavioral therapy and behavioral weight loss for binge eating disorder. *Behaviour Research and Therapy*, 43:1509–1525.

Grilo CM, Masheb RM, & Wilson GT. (2005). Efficacy of cognitive behavioral therapy and fluoxetine for the treatment of binge eating disorder: A randomized double-blind placebo-controlled comparison. *Biological Psychiatry*, 57:301–309.

Grilo CM, Masheb RM, & Wilson GT. (2006). Rapid response to treatment for binge eating disorder. *Journal of Consulting and Clinical Psychology*, 74:602–613.

Hsu JC. (1996). *Multiple comparisons: Theory and methods.* London: Chapman & Hall.

International Committee of Harmonisation. (1999). ICH harmonized tripartite guideline: Statistical guidelines for clinical trials. *Statistics in Medicine*, 18:1905–1942.

Kalish LA, & Begg CB. (1985). Treatment allocation methods in clinical trials: A review. *Statistics in Medicine*, 4:129–144.

Kraemer HC, Mintz J, Noda A, Tinklenberg J, & Yesavage JA. (2006). Caution regarding the use of pilot studies to guide power calculations for study proposals. *Archives of General Psychiatry*, 63:484–489.

Kraemer HC, & Thiemann S. (1987). *How many subjects?: Statistical power analysis in research.* Newbury Park, CA: Sage.

Kraemer HC, Wilson GT, Fairburn CG, & Agras WS. (2002). Mediators and moderators of treatment effects in randomized clinical trials. *Archives of General Psychiatry*, 59:877–883.

Le Grange D, Crosby RD, & Lock J. (2008). Predictors and moderators of outcome in family-based treatment for adolescent bulimia nervosa. *Journal of the American Academy of Child and Adolescent Psychiatry*, 47:464–470.

Little RJA. (1993). Pattern-mixture models for multivariate incomplete data. *Journal of the American Statistical Association*, 88:125–134.

Lock J, Le Grange D, & Crosby RD. (2008). Exploring possible mechanisms of change in family-based treatment for adolescent bulimia nervosa. *Journal of Family Therapy*, 30:260–271.

Masheb RM, & Grilo CM. (2007). Examination of predictors and moderators for self-help treatments of binge eating disorder. *Journal of Consulting and Clinical Psychology*, 76:900–904.

Meier P. (1981). Stratification in the design of a clinical trial. *Controlled Clinical Trials*, 1:355–361.

Meinert CL. (1986). *Clinical trials: Design, conduct, and analysis.* New York: Oxford University Press.

Mitchell JE, Pyle RL, Eckert ED, Pomeroy C, Zollman M, Crosby RD, et al. (1993). Cognitive behavioral group psychotherapy of bulimia nervosa: Importance of logistical variables. *International Journal of Eating Disorders*, 14:277–287.

Raudenbush SW, & Bryk AS. (2002). *Hierarchical linear models: Applications and data analysis methods.* London: Sage.

Rosenbaum PR, & Rubin DB. (1983). The central role of the propensity score in observation studies for causal effects. *Biometrika*, 70:41–55.

Rosenberger WF, & Lachin JM. (2002). *Randomization in clinical trials: Theory and practice.* New York: Wiley.

Rubin DB. (1976). Inference and missing data. *Biometrika*, 63:581–592.

Rubin DB. (1987). *Multiple imputation for nonresponse in surveys.* New York: Wiley.

Schafer JL, & Graham JW. (2002). Missing data: Our view of the state of the art. *Psychological Methods*, 7:147–177.

Shapiro JR, Berkman ND, Brownley KA, Sedway JA, Lohr KN, & Bulik CM. (2007). Bulimia nervosa treatment: A systematic review of randomized controlled trials. *International Journal of Eating Disorders*, 40:321–336.

Stice E, Presnell K, Gau J, & Shaw H. (2007). Testing mediators of intervention effect in randomized controlled trials. *Journal of Consulting and Clinical Psychology*, 75:20–32.

Toothaker LE. (1993). *Multiple comparison procedures.* Newbury Park, CA: Sage.

Walsh BT, Fairburn CG, Mickley D, Sysko R, & Parides MK. (2004). Treatment of bulimia nervosa in a primary care setting. *American Journal of Psychiatry*, 161:556–561.

Wilkinson L, and the APA Task Force on Statistical Inference. (1999). Statistical methods in psychology journals: Guidelines and explanations. *American Psychologist*, 54:594–604.

Wilson GT, Grilo CM, & Vitousek KM. (2007). Psychological treatment of eating disorders. *American Psychologist*, 62:199–216.

Woods SW, Sholomskas DE, Shear MK, Gorman JM, Barlow DH, Goddard AW, et al. (1998). Efficient allocation of patients to treatment cells in clinical trials with more than two treatment conditions. *American Journal of Psychiatry*, 155:1446–1448.

CHAPTER 32

Assessment of Eating Disorder Treatment Efficacy

Carol B. Peterson

Accurate assessment of eating disorders (EDs), including careful characterization of ED psychopathology and associated problems, is a fundamental cornerstone of treatment research. In order to test an intervention's efficacy, the measurement of targeted symptoms must be both precise and comprehensive. Reliable and valid assessment data in treatment efficacy research are essential for the accurate interpretation of empirical findings. In ED treatment studies, questionnaires and interviews are typically administered to assess ED symptoms, co-occurring psychopathology, and other relevant variables.

The assessment of EDs and the associated features of these disorders poses a number of challenges (Anderson & Paulosky, 2004; Couturier & Lock, 2006; Peterson, 2005; Pike, Wolk, Gluck, & Walsh, 2000; Vitousek, Daly, & Heiser, 1991; Vitousek & Stumpf, 2005). Although issues such as cognitive recall bias affect all self-reported data (Schacter, 1999), accurate assessment of patients with EDs can be especially challenging. Some treatment-seeking individuals may exaggerate their symptoms to ensure that they will receive care. Alternatively, in some cases, potential patients may minimize or deny the existence of some problems for various reasons (e.g., to avoid treatment in those with anorexia nervosa [AN], to be eligible for certain treatments, to avoid mandated treatment). In addition, many ED symptoms and features can be difficult to assess because of their complexity. For example, variables such as body image are multidimensional in nature and may require multiple measures to assess different components (Thompson, 2004; Thompson Roehrig, Cafri, & Heinberg, 2005). Other behaviors, including binge eating, may be defined differently by patients than they are by clinicians and researchers. Some aspects of EDs, such as severe malnutrition, may make assessment of other domains, such as depression, personality, or cognition, difficult.

Treatment outcome assessment requires a series of related steps: formulating hypotheses, selecting and defining variables, prioritizing variables to be measured, selecting assessment instruments, and monitoring quality. Although these sequential procedures are typically utilized in research settings, they are equally important for clinicians who are delivering treatment and wish to systematically track areas of improvement and problems over time in order to inform treatment decisions (Anderson, Lundgren, Shapiro, & Paulosky, 2004).

Forming Hypotheses

The first step in conducting assessment in research settings is to specify hypotheses. In treatment outcome studies, these hypotheses usually focus on the efficacy of a specific treatment relative to a comparison condition. For example, a researcher may hypothesize that a given treatment will be helpful in reducing the frequency of certain ED symptoms. Empirical investigations often include hypotheses that an active treatment will be associated with greater improvement compared to comparison conditions (e.g., wait-list controls, placebo controls, or alternative treatments). Treatment outcome research can also be more complex, for example, by hypothesizing that certain variables may predict, moderate, or mediate treatment outcomes (see Kraemer, Wilson, Fairburn, & Agras, 2002; Laurenceau, Hayes, & Feldman, 2007). Typically, clinical researchers have several hypotheses that they are interested in examining in the context of treatment outcome measurement and often designate some as primary and others as secondary priorities.

The process of constructing hypotheses is an important preliminary step for several reasons. First, it helps guide the remainder of the assessment process and functions much like a road map in developing and implementing these procedures. Second, this process lowers the risk of Type I error that can occur when the investigator performs numerous analyses. With hypotheses in place, the researcher is less likely to conduct a "fishing expedition" by examining the relationships among every possible variable. Finally, hypothesis formulation helps establish the researcher's or clinician's priorities—an essential aspect of assessment to manage limited time and financial resources. Although assessment is ideally hypothesis-driven, it should also be comprehensive in scope and include measurement of prioritized primary and secondary variables as well as important outcomes to allow linkage to the relevant literature.

Selecting and Defining Variables

Although the goal of most treatment outcome research is to test whether specific treatments produce significant changes or differ significantly from comparison conditions, defining and operationalizing these variables is not always straightforward. The main treatment outcome variables (usually ED symptoms) and secondary outcome variables that are targeted by the treatment are usually a priority in this type of assessment; however, other variables should be defined, including subject selection criteria and participant characteristics.

At this stage, the researcher should specify essential variables in addition to the main outcome variables. These additional variables include potential predictor, moderator, and mediator variables. Predictor variables are prognostic of outcomes without regard for the specific treatments. Moderator variables influence the direction or intensity of an independent variable and a criterion variable. Mediator variables account for relationships between the predictor and criterion variables (Baron & Kenny, 1986).

Moderator variables tell us for whom certain treatments might work better, whereas mediator variables provide information about potential mechanisms by which a treatment works. Given recent converging findings regarding the prognostic importance of early response in various ED treatments (Grilo, Masheb, & Wilson, 2006; Wilson, Fairburn, Agras, Walsh, & Kraemer, 2002), researchers should consider measurement strategies (frequency and timing) to capture changes during the early stages of treatment. In addition, repeated assessments of relevant variables early in the treatment process can provide the necessary data to test meditational models (Strauman & Merrill, 2004). Other important variables to assess during the course of treatment may include specific measures of psychotherapeutic alliance as well as treatment fidelity and adherence (see Loeb et al., 2005).

Prioritizing Variables and Instrument Selection

Once a list of hypotheses and variables has been constructed and prioritized, the researcher or clinician should evaluate available resources (e.g., financial, time, logistic, and personnel) to determine the feasibility of the proposed plan and the best allocation of the available resources. More assessment resources should be devoted to the higher priority variables, especially those that are the main targets of the intervention.

One goal in instrument selection is to identify the best available measures for the specified variables while minimizing assessment burden on staff and participants. The risk of burdening patients with too much assessment is particularly heightened in treatment outcome research due to the repeated evaluations over time. Retention is critical but may be compromised if the patient is upset by excessive burden or by a lengthy battery of measures. Nonetheless, the data quality should not be sacrificed in the interest of reducing assessment burden. An ideal assessment protocol includes a comprehensive set of "state-of-the-art" measures that do not place excessive demands on participants or staff. Good validity and reliability, meaning that the instrument accurately measures what it intends to measure and does so in a consistent manner (Anastasi & Urbina, 1997; Anderson & Paulosky, 2004), are essential considerations in instrument selection.

Another assessment issue in ED treatment research is the uncertainty of psychometric properties of measures across different subpopulations. For example, although many instruments in the ED field have demonstrated adequate reliability and validity, much of this research was conducted with young adult females. Thus, the psychometric properties of many instruments have not yet been established with males, older and younger samples, and ethnically diverse populations. Apart from some exceptions, including the Spanish-language version of the Eating Disorders Examination (Grilo, Lozano, & Elder, 2005) and the Eating Disorder Examination—Questionnaire (Elder & Grilo, 2007), researchers should routinely consider the applicability, reliability, and validity of established measures when working with certain groups.

Multimodal Assessment

Treatment outcome assessments can include interview-based measures, questionnaire-based instruments, and a variety of other methods, including self-monitoring (Grilo et al., 2001). In addition, treatment assessment protocols often include laboratory measures to determine medical eligibility for study inclusion, and many include some repeated measures to determine changes with treatment. Although many current treatment outcome studies rely on interview-based measures of the primary outcome variables, based on the premise that they are more accurate measures of ED symptoms, utilizing multimodal assessment through the administration of questionnaire, self-monitoring, and interview-based instruments can be advantageous (Grilo et al., 2001). Questionnaires may provide some advantages over interviews, including cost and the potential for enhanced self-disclosure (see Grilo, 2005; Keel, Crow, Davis, & Mitchell, 2002).

Instruments to Assess Specific Variables

Diagnosis

Several instruments have been developed to determine diagnoses of EDs and co-occurring psychopathology (Grilo, 2005). In treatment outcome assessment, the primary purpose of these measures is usually to determine whether potential participants are eligible based on diagnostic criteria. Such diagnostic findings may also be used in predictor and moderator analyses. The Structured Clinical Interview for DSM-IV can be used to diagnose current and lifetime Axis I psychiatric disorders, including EDs (SCID-I; First, Spitzer, Gibbon, & Williams, 2002) as well as current Axis II personality disorders (SCID-II; First, Spitzer, Gibbon, & Williams, 1997). These measures have been widely used in psychiatric research and in ED research in particular, although they can also be especially valuable in clinical settings (e.g., Zimmerman, McGlinchey, Chelminksi, & Young, 2008). The main advantages of the SCID-I and SCID-II are the extent to which they provide comprehensive diagnostic information and the large base of psychometric data supporting their use (see Zanarini et al., 2000).

Several interviews have been developed as comprehensive measures of EDs that also serve as diagnostic interviews. The most widely used of these in treatment outcome research is the Eating Disorder Examination (EDE—Fairburn, 2008; Fairburn & Cooper, 1993). This investigator-based structured interview generates ED diagnoses and obtains detailed information about ED psychopathology, including behavioral features (e.g., binge eating, other weight compensatory methods including purging, and restraint) and attitudinal features (e.g., overvaluation of shape/weight, body dissatisfaction, shape/food preoccupation). The EDE has four subscales (Dietary Restraint, Eating Concern, Weight Concern, and Shape Concern) and a global severity score. Because the EDE focuses on current symptoms, it is particularly well-suited to treatment outcome measurement. In addition, a number of studies support the EDE's reliability and certain aspects of its validity (Berg, Peterson, & Crow, 2008 ; Fairburn, 2008; Fairburn & Cooper, 1993; Grilo, Masheb, Lozano-Blanco, & Barry, 2004). The fact that it is investigator-based and requires a trained interviewer to determine ratings based on established anchors is thought to enhance its psychometric features (Grilo, 2005). Its main limitation is the time required for administration, as well as interviewer training, which is usually extensive.

The Structured Interview for Anorexic and Bulimic Disorders—Expert Rating (SIAB-EX; Fichter, Herpertz, Quadflieg, & Herpertz-Dahlmann, 1998) is another interview-based ED measure that can be used to determine DSM-IV-TR and ICD-10 diagnoses. In contrast to the EDE, the SIAB-EX assesses both current and past ED and associated symptoms and for this reason can be used in descriptive and genetic studies as well as treatment outcome investigations. Several studies support the reliability and validity of the SIAB-EX; this instrument is available in several languages (Fichter et al., 1998; Fichter & Quadflieg, 2001). Like the SCID and the EDE, the main consideration in using the SIAB-EX is the time required for administration, scoring, and interviewer training.

Binge Eating

The assessment of binge eating is particularly challenging for several reasons (Peterson & Miller, 2005). First, the DSM-IV-TR definition of binge eating requires that the episode involve the consumption of a clearly large amount of food; the threshold for this amount varies depending on context and location. This context-based definition, along with a lack of consensus of what constitutes an objectively large amount, makes establishing this threshold difficult. Second, because patients often view the consumption of any amount of unplanned food as an excessive amount, they do not tend to evaluate whether their food intake is objectively large when describing their binge-eating episodes. Fortunately, providing participants with more detailed directions and examples of these types of binge-eating episodes in questionnaire administration appears to reduce this problem slightly (Celio et al., 2004; Goldfein, Devlin, & Kamenetz, 2005). A sense of lack of control during the eating episode is also a required criteria for the definition of binge eating. Although determining loss of control is arguably less difficult than determining excessive quantity, this can also sometimes be difficult to ascertain. In certain types of studies, *in vivo* assessment of eating patterns can be a particularly effective strategy (Anderson et al., 2004), including the use of human feeding laboratories (Mitchell, Crow, Peterson, Wonderlich, & Crosby, 1998).

Because investigator-based interviews such as the EDE use trained assessors to rate items according to "anchor" criteria (e.g., what is meant by a subjective loss of control or an objectively large amount of food), the EDE is particularly well suited to examining DSM-IV-TR criteria for binge eating because it specifically estimates the frequency of different types of overeating episodes (i.e., objective vs. subjective bulimic episodes). The EDE spends considerable time establishing time anchors to enhance the reliability of self-reported data, including binge eating, and the interviewer and the patient or research participant work collaboratively to estimate frequencies of different types of overeating and binge-eating episodes. Similarly, the SIAB-EX allows the interviewer to estimate the frequency of different types of overeating episodes.

The questionnaire version of the EDE (i.e., the EDE-Q; Fairburn, 2008) has been used to assess binge eating, purging, and ED psychopathology in a number of treatment studies with various ED patient groups. The EDE-Q has been found to have acceptable test–retest reliability in binge-eating disorder (BED) (Reas, Grilo, & Masheb, 2006) and is sensitive to change over time in patients with bulimia nervosa (BN) (Sysko, Walsh, & Fairburn, 2005). Because the EDE-Q is easy to use, it can be administered frequently throughout treatment to examine early treatment response and mediator effects.

Self-monitoring of eating patterns and symptoms (Grilo et al., 2001; Wilson & Vitousek, 1999) has also been used in treatment outcome studies (e.g., Grilo, Masheb, & Wilson, 2006) and has the advantage of minimizing recall bias. Self-monitoring has been found to correlate significantly with the EDE in studies of BN (Loeb, Pike, Walsh,

& Wilson, 1994) and BED (Grilo et al., 2001). More sophisticated self-monitoring meth-ods make use of ecological momentary assessment (EMA) using new electronic tech-nologies (Stone & Shiffman, 1994).

Weight Compensatory Behaviors

Weight compensatory behaviors include self-induced vomiting, misuse of laxatives and diuretics, fasting, chewing and spitting behavior, and excessive exercise. Less common but observed compensatory symptoms include insulin abuse in individuals with Type I diabetes, abuse of thyroid medication, and excessive sauna use. Interestingly, for purg-ing behaviors, the EDE-Q has been found to correlate highly with the EDE (e.g., Sysko et al., 2005).

Dietary Restricting/Restraint

Assessing dietary restraint and restriction has been complicated by inconsistent and varied definitions of these concepts. As described by Fairburn (2008), "restraint," mean-ing the attempt to eat less or modify food intake, differs from "dietary restriction," which refers to actual undereating. Several measures have been developed to assess dietary restraint, including the EDE and the EDE-Q, the Three-Factor Eating Ques-tionnaire (also known as the Eating Inventory) (TFEQ/EI; Stunkard & Messick, 1985), the Restraint Scale (Polivy, Herman, & Warsh, 1988), the Dutch Eating Behavior Ques-tionnaire (van Strien, Frijters, Bergers, & Defares, 1986), and the Dietary Intent Scale (Stice, 1998). Because observational data do not support that dietary restraint mea-sures correlate with actual food intake (Stice, Fisher, & Lowe, 2004), dietary restraint should not be used as a proxy measure of dietary intake or dietary restriction, which should be measured more directly using dietary recall (Rock, 2005)

Body Image/Attitudes toward Shape and Weight

Because body image is a multidimensional concept that cannot be incorporated into a single measure (Thompson, 2004; Thompson et al., 2005), the researcher or clini-cian must decide which aspect or aspects of body image are assessment priorities. The EDE and the EDE-Q include the Weight Concern and the Shape Concern scales, both of which contain specific items to assess the extent to which weight and shape influ-ence self-evaluation (included in the DSM-IV-TR criteria for BN and AN). The Eating Disorder Inventory–3 (Garner, 2004) is a comprehensive questionnaire that includes a body dissatisfaction subscale. The SIAB-EX also has shape and weight subscales, includ-ing weight phobia. In addition, a number of questionnaires and procedures have been developed to assess specific aspects of body image (see review by Thompson et al., 2005). These aspects include body dissatisfaction, body checking and other behaviors and attitudes, affective evaluation, and size perception.

Weight

Baseline and repeated measures of weight and body mass index (BMI) in treatment outcome studies should be based on actual weighing rather than self-reported data

(Peterson, 2005). One of the main assessment considerations is the impact of being weighed on the participant because many find the experience of being weighed and seeing their body weight to be highly distressing. For this reason, the EDE specifies that the patient should be weighed at the end of the interview rather than at the beginning, in order to minimize distress about weighing (an important issue for the well-being of the patient but also for how this distress can influence subsequent responses on interviews and questionnaires). In addition, offering blind weights or obtaining all weights as blind so that patients and participants do not see the number can also be useful in both clinical and research settings. Obtaining weights in underweight patients wearing gowns is also highly desirable to improve accuracy and minimize the likelihood of deception (Peterson, 2005). In other ED samples in which gowns are unnecessary, the measurement of weight should be standardized (e.g., specifying the exclusion of shoes and jackets).

Global Outcome Measures

Treatment outcome assessment in ED research has also included investigator-rated global outcome measures. The SIAB includes a global outcome assessment. In addition, the Morgan Russell scale (Morgan & Hayward, 1988) is a global rating scale that has been widely used to classify treatment outcome status in AN studies, but has frequently been modified in research.

Quality of Life/Impairment Measures

Increasing attention has been devoted to assessing quality of life in ED treatment measurement, and several questionnaires have been developed that specifically focus on health-related quality of life, including the impact of ED symptoms on physical and psychosocial functioning (see Engel, Adair, Las Hayas, & Abraham, 2008; Hay & Mond, 2005).

Children and Adolescents

Although measurement of EDs in children and adolescents is challenging due to problems in defining and assessing symptoms accurately, several instruments have been developed or adapted that can be used in treatment studies (see reviews by Lask & Bryant-Waugh, 2007; Le Grange, 2005; Stice & Peterson, 2007). Most notably, the EDE has been adapted for use with children and adolescents in research investigations, including treatment outcome studies (Bryant-Waugh, Cooper, Taylor, & Lask, 1996; Tanofsky-Kraff et al., 2003).

Technology-Based Assessment in Treatment Efficacy Studies

Advances in technology have improved the ease with which treatment outcome measures can be administered and scored. For example, self-report questionnaires can be entered by the research participant or patient directly in the computer for scoring and interpretation—a task that can be accomplished from distal sites using secure Web-based database systems. This process prevents calculation errors as well as minimizes errors in data entry. In addition, portable technology can be utilized to minimize retrospective recall bias. For example, EMA is a technique in which research participants or patients record their symptoms, attitudes, and emotions in "real time" using handheld computer devices—an approach that reduces measurement error from recall biases (Engel, Wonderlich, & Crosby, 2005; Stone & Shiffman, 1994).

Data Quality, Training, and Monitoring

All staff members in treatment research who have patient interaction should be trained in advanced clinical skills. Although these skills are obviously required to conduct assessment interviews and implement treatment interventions, they are also important for staff who conduct phone screenings, administer questionnaires, and collect measurement materials.

The importance of clinical skills in conducting treatment assessment to enhance data quality cannot be overemphasized, especially in the context of ED research (Grilo, 2005; Peterson, 2005). The ability to establish and maintain rapport, express empathy, use reflective listening, manage defensiveness and hostility, and probe for detailed responses is as essential in research as it is in clinical settings. In particular, asking questions in a manner that reflects an understanding of ED symptoms and avoiding critical remarks are essential. When completing assessment instruments, participants should be given a rationale for their importance as well as an accurate estimate of how much time they will need to complete questionnaires and interviews. Participants should also be offered breaks during this process to minimize fatigue and enhance concentration.

In both research and clinical settings establishing and monitoring assessment quality is essential. Initial training is required to ensure that staff members are clear about concepts and procedures for administering, scoring, and interpreting assessment instruments. Trainees often find it helpful to observe more experienced staff in these types of interactions, role-play challenging scenarios and discuss ways to manage them, and meet regularly to discuss clinical issues that arise in the context of treatment outcome research with supervisory staff. In addition, interrater reliability should be established at the beginning and throughout the course of the study for interview-based measures. Interviews should be audiotaped or videotaped and a subset chosen at random for test–retest reliability rating. In addition, tapes should be rated by an expert assessor who can provide feedback to interviewers throughout the investigation. Assessment staff should meet on a regular basis throughout the study to prevent "drift" and to ensure consistency among staff and over the course of the study.

Conclusions

Assessing ED and associated symptoms in treatment outcome follows a series of steps that includes formulating hypotheses, defining variables, selecting instruments, and monitoring data quality. Regardless of the setting or the type of measure, assessment based on good clinical skills is essential to enhance the assessment process, improve the reliability and validity of data, and minimize attrition. Assessment is an integral part of treatment research as well as clinical practice.

References

Anastasi A, & Urbina S. (1997). *Psychological testing* (7th ed.). New York: Prentice-Hall.

Anderson DA, Lundgren JD, Shapiro JR, & Paulosky CA. (2004). Assessment of eating disorders: Review and recommendations for clinical use. *Behavior Modification*, 28:763–782.

Anderson DA, & Paulosky CA. (2004). Psychological assessment of eating disorders and related features. In JK Thompson (Ed.), *Handbook of eating disorders and obesity* (pp. 112–129). New York: Wiley.

Baron RM, & Kenny DA. (1986). The moderator–mediator variable distinction in social psychology research: Conceptual, strategic and statistical considerations. *Journal of Personality and Social Psychology*, 51:1173–1182.

Berg K, Peterson CB, & Crow SJ. (2008). *Psychometric properties of the Eating Disorder Examination and the Eating Disorder Examination—Questionnaire.* Unpublished manuscript.

Bryant-Waugh RJ, Cooper PJ, Taylor CL, & Lask BD. (1996). The use of the Eating Disorder Examination with children: A pilot study. *International Journal of Eating Disorders*, 19:391–397.

Celio AA, Wilfley DE, Crow SJ, Mitchell JE, & Walsh BT. (2004). A comparison of the Binge Eating Scale, Questionnaire for Eating and Weight Patterns—Revised, and Eating Disorder Examination—Questionnaire with instructions with the Eating Disorder Examination in the assessment of binge eating disorder and its symptoms. *International Journal of Eating Disorders*, 36:434–444.

Couturier JL, & Lock J. (2006). Denial and minimization in adolescents with anorexia nervosa. *International Journal of Eating Disorders*, 39:212–216.

Elder KA, & Grilo CM. (2007). The Spanish language version of the Eating Disorder Examination—Questionnaire: Comparison with the Spanish language version of the Eating Disorder Examination and test–retest reliability. *Behaviour Research and Therapy*, 45:1369–1377.

Engel SG, Adair CE, Las Hayas C, & Abraham S. (2009). Health-related quality of life and eating disorders: A review and update. *International Journal of Eating Disorders*, 42:179–187.

Engel SG, Wonderlich SA, & Crosby RD. (2005). Ecological momentary assessment. In JE Mitchell & CB Peterson (Eds.), *Assessment of eating disorders* (pp. 203–220). New York: Guilford Press.

Fairburn CG. (2008). *Cognitive behavior therapy and eating disorders.* New York: Guilford Press.

Fairburn CG, & Cooper Z. (1993). The Eating Disorder Examination (12th ed.). In CG Fairburn & GT Wilson (Eds.), *Binge eating: Nature, assessment, and treatment* (pp. 317–360). New York: Guilford Press.

Fichter MM, Herpertz S, Quadflieg N, & Herpertz-Dahlmann B. (1998). Structured Interview for Anorexia and Bulimic Disorders for DSM-IV and ICD-10: Updated (3rd) revision. *International Journal of Eating Disorders*, 24:227–249.

Fichter MM, & Quadflieg N. (2001). The Structured Interview for Anorexic and Bulimic Disorders for DSM-IV and ICD-10 (SIAB-EX): Reliability and validity. *European Psychiatry*, 16:38–48.

First MB, Spitzer RL, Gibbon M, & Williams JBW. (1997). *User's guide for the Structured Clinical Interview for DSM-IV Personality Disorders (SCID-II).* Washington, DC: American Psychiatric Press.

First MB, Spitzer RL, Gibbon M, & Williams JBW. (2002). *Structured Clinical Interview for DSM-IV-TR Axis I Disorders—Patient Edition (SCID-I/P)*. New York: Biometrics Research, New York State Psychiatric Institute.

Garner DM. (2004). *Eating Disorder Inventory–3*. Lutz, FL: Psychological Assessment Resources.

Goldfein JA, Devlin MJ, & Kamenetz C. (2005). Eating Disorder Examination—Questionnaire with and without instruction to assess binge eating in patients with binge eating disorder. *International Journal of Eating Disorder*, 37:107–111.

Grilo CM. (2005). Structured instruments. In JE Mitchell & CB Peterson (Eds.), *Assessment of eating disorders* (pp. 79–97). New York: Guilford Press.

Grilo CM, Lozano C, & Elder KA. (2005). Inter-rater and test–retest reliability of the Spanish language version of the Eating Disorder Examination interview: Clinical and research implications. *Journal of Psychiatric Practice*, 11:231–240.

Grilo CM, Masheb RM, Lozano-Blanco C, & Barry DT. (2004). Reliability of the Eating Disorder Examination in patients with binge eating disorder. *International Journal of Eating Disorders*, 35:80–85.

Grilo CM, Masheb RM, & Wilson GT. (2001). A comparison of different methods for assessing the features of eating disorders in patients with binge eating disorder. *Journal of Consulting and Clinical Psychology*, 69:317–322.

Grilo CM, Masheb RM, & Wilson GT. (2006). Rapid response to treatment for binge eating disorder. *Journal of Consulting and Clinical Psychology*, 74:602–613.

Keel PK, Crow S, Davis TL, & Mitchell JE. (2002). Assessment of eating disorders: Comparison of interview and questionnaire data from a long-term follow-up study of bulimia nervosa. *Journal of Psychosomatic Research*, 53:1043–1047.

Kraemer HC, Wilson GT, Fairburn CG, & Agras WS. (2002). Mediators and moderators of treatment effects in randomized clinical trials. *Archives of General Psychiatry*, 59:877–883.

Lask B, & Bryant-Waugh R. (Eds.). (2007). *Eating disorders in children and adolescents*. London: Routledge.

Laurenceau J, Hayes AM, & Feldman GC. (2007). Some methodological and statistical issues in the study of change processes in psychotherapy. *Clinical Psychology Review*, 27:682–695.

Le Grange D. (2005). Family assessment. In JE Mitchell & CB Peterson (Eds.), *Assessment of eating disorders* (pp. 148–174). New York: Guilford Press.

Loeb KL, Pike KM, Walsh BT, & Wilson GT. (1994). Assessment of diagnostic features of bulimia nervosa: Interview versus self-report format. *International Journal of Eating Disorders*, 16:75–81.

Loeb KL, Wilson GT, Labouvie E, Pratt EM, Hayaki J, Walsh BT, et al. (2005). Therapeutic alliance in two interventions for bulimia nervosa: A study of process and outcome. *Journal of Consulting and Clinical Psychology*, 73:1097–1107.

Mitchell JE, Crow S, Peterson CB, Wonderlich S, & Crosby RD. (1998). Feeding laboratory studies in patients with eating disorders: A review. *International Journal of Eating Disorders*, 24:115–124.

Morgan HG, & Hayward AE. (1988). Clinical assessment of anorexia nervosa: The Morgan–Russell Outcome Assessment Schedule. *British Journal of Psychiatry*, 152:367–371.

Peterson CB. (2005). Conducting the diagnostic interview. In JE Mitchell & CB Peterson (Eds.), *Assessment of eating disorders* (pp. 32–58). New York: Guilford Press.

Peterson CB, & Miller KB. (2005). Assessment of eating disorders. In S Wonderlich, JE Mitchell, M de Zwaan, & H Steiger (Eds.), *Eating disorders review: Part I* (pp. 105–126). Oxford, UK: Radcliffe.

Pike KM, Wolk SL, Gluck M, & Walsh BT. (2000). Eating disorders measures. In *American Psychiatric Association handbook of psychiatric measures* (pp. 647–671). Washington, DC: American Psychiatric Association.

Reas DL, Grilo CM, & Masheb RM. (2006). Reliability of the Eating Disorder Examination—Questionnaire in patients with binge eating disorder. *Behaviour Research and Therapy*, 44:43–51.

Rock CL. (2005). Nutritional assessment. In JE Mitchell & CB Peterson (Eds.), *Assessment of eating disorders* (pp. 129–149). New York: Guilford Press.

Schacter DL. (1999). The seven sins of memory: Insights from psychology and cognitive neuroscience. *American Psychologist*, 54:182–203.

Stice E. (1998). Relations of restraint and negative affect to bulimic pathology: A longitudinal test of three competing models. *International Journal of Eating Disorders*, 23:243–260.

Stice E, Fisher M, & Lowe MR. (2004). Are dietary restraint scales valid measures of acute dietary restriction?: Unobtrusive observational data suggest not. *Psychological Assessment*, 16:51–59.

Stice E, & Peterson CB. (2007). Eating disorders. In EJ Mash & RA Barkley (Eds.), *Assessment of childhood disorders* (4th ed., pp. 751–780). New York: Guilford Press.

Stone AA, & Shiffman S. (1994). Ecological momentary assessment (EMA) in behavioral medicine. *Annals of Behavior Medicine*, 16:199–202.

Strauman TJ, & Merrill KA. (2004). The basic science/clinical science interface and treatment development. *Clinical Psychology: Science and Practice*, 11:263–266.

Stunkard AJ, & Messick S. (1985). The Three-Factor Eating Questionnaire to measure dietary restraint, disinhibition, and hunger. *Journal of Psychosomatic Research*, 9:71–83.

Sysko R, Walsh BT, & Fairburn CG. (2005). Eating Disorder Examination—Questionnaire as a measure of change in patients with bulimia nervosa. *International Journal of Eating Disorders*, 27:100–106.

Tanofsky-Kraff M, Morgan CM, Yanovski SZ, Marmarosh C, Wilfley DE, & Yanovski JA. (2003). Comparison of assessment of children's eating-disordered behaviors by interview and questionnaire. *International Journal of Eating Disorders*, 33:213–224.

Thompson JK. (2004). The (mis)measurement of body image: Ten strategies to improve assessment for applied and research purposes. *Body Image*, 1:7–14.

Thompson JK, Roehrig M, Cafri G, & Heinberg L. (2005). Assessment of body image disturbance. In JE Mitchell & CB Peterson (Eds.), *Assessment of eating disorders* (pp. 175–202). New York: Guilford Press.

van Strien T, Frijters JER, Bergers GPA, & Defares PB. (1986). The Dutch Eating Behavior Questionnaire (DEBQ) for assessment of restrained, emotional, and external eating behavior. *International Journal of Eating Disorders*, 5:295–315.

Vitousek KB, Daly J, & Heiser C. (1991). Reconstructing the internal world of the eating-disordered individual: Overcoming denial and distortion in self-report. *International Journal of Eating Disorders*, 10:647–666.

Vitousek KB, & Stumpf RE. (2005). Difficulties in the assessment of personality traits and disorders in eating-disordered individuals. *Eating Disorders*, 13:37–60.

Wilson GT, Fairburn CG, Agras WS, Walsh BT, & Kraemer HC. (2002). Cognitive-behavioral therapy for bulimia nervosa: Time course and mechanisms of change. *Journal of Consulting and Clinical Psychology*, 70:267–274.

Wilson GT, & Vitousek KM. (1999). Self-monitoring in the assessment of eating disorders. *Psychological Assessment*, 11:480–489.

Zanarini MC, Skodol AE, Bender D, Dolan RL, Sanislow C, Schaefer E, et al. (2000). The Collaborative Longitudinal Personality Disorders Study: Reliability of Axis I and II diagnoses. *Journal of Personality Disorders*, 14:291–299.

Zimmerman M, McGlinchey JB, Chelminski I, & Young D. (2008). Diagnostic co-morbidity in 2300 psychiatric outpatients presenting for treatment evaluated with a semi-structured diagnostic interview. *Psychological Medicine*, 38:199–210.

CHAPTER 33

What Treatment Research Is Needed for Anorexia Nervosa?

W. Stewart Agras and Athena Hagler Robinson

There has been remarkably little change in our ability to treat anorexia nervosa (AN) over the past 25 years, despite the research that has been accomplished. A recent review of randomized controlled trials for this time period found weak evidence for treatment efficacy in both psychotherapy and pharmacological studies (Bulik, Berkman, Brownley, Seway, & Lohr, 2007). One exception is a family therapy for adolescents, the "Maudsley approach" or "behavioral family therapy," which focuses on enabling parents to refeed their child and appears promising (Lock, Agras, Bryson, & Kraemer, 2005; Eisler, Lock, & Le Grange, Chapter 8, this volume). However, it is unclear whether this approach is superior to other types of family therapy or to individual therapy; hence it cannot be recommended as an evidence-based treatment at this point. To answer the question "What research is needed for the treatment of AN?", it is necessary to first understand the causes for the present state of affairs in AN treatment research.

General Problems in AN Treatment Research

Insufficient Sample Size

For the 11 controlled psychotherapy studies reviewed in the paper referenced above (Bulik et al., 2007), the median sample size per group was 15 with a range from 12 to 43. Calculations reveal that the minimum sample size needed to power reliable and valid statistical analyses would be closer to 40 participants per cell. Only one study approached this cell size (Lock et al., 2005). For the eight controlled medication trials reviewed, the median sample size was 20 with a range from 7 to 27. Hence, with one exception both medication and psychotherapy trials were underpowered, raising the possibility that effective treatments were overlooked.

Dropout Rates

Further compromising the small sample sizes are the often sizeable dropout rates reported from the same studies. The median dropout rate for the psychotherapy studies was 13% with a range from 0 to 38%, and for medication trials 18% with a range from 0 to 66%. Two of the largest trials were not included in the review study noted above. The first was a psychotherapy trial that enrolled 122 participants and had a dropout rate of 46% (Halmi et al., 2005), and the second was a medication trial that enrolled 93 participants and had a dropout rate of 57% (Walsh et al., 2006). As one of these studies noted and demonstrated (Halmi et al., 2005), such high dropout rates suggest that the characteristics of dropouts are not randomly distributed among treatment groups. Although dropouts in some studies are likely to be random—for example, caused by participants having difficulty in attending treatment—others may not be—for example, dropouts due to a particular characteristic of treatment, or an interaction between particular participant features and a particular therapy. In the case of random dropouts that are distributed equally among treatment groups, imputation methods such as carrying forward the last value appear reasonable. However, the higher the dropout rate, the greater the risk that imputation will distort the results, although mixed models analysis may mitigate this problem to some extent. With nonrandom dropout one must assume that participant characteristics are no longer randomly distributed among treatment groups, especially when there is differential dropout between treatments. Hence, an outcome analysis (that assumes a random distribution of variables among treatment groups) is not appropriate. In the Halmi and colleagues (2005) paper this was recognized, and the analysis sought instead to explore the reasons for low treatment acceptance.

Recruitment Difficulties

Compounding dropout rates is the low acceptance rate of individuals eligible to enter a trial. In one multisite study, those with some form of barrier to acceptance equaled or exceeded the number that finally entered to the trial (McDermott et al., 2004). In another study almost twice as many refused to participate as were randomized (Kaye et al., 2001). This relatively low acceptance rate of entry to studies, combined with the relative rarity of AN, makes recruitment of individuals with AN to clinical trials very difficult. In the multisite study noted above (McDermott et al., 2004), three sites specializing in the treatment of AN failed to recruit their target sample size. Each site demonstrated a large decline in the number of eligible patients over a 4-year period with corresponding declines in entered subjects. After 4 years very few participants were entered in the study, suggesting that the pool of available participants had been exhausted at each site and that it was not cost-effective to continue the trial after about 3 years of recruitment. These results were for a study of adult (more chronic) patients with AN. It seems that it is easier to recruit adolescent individuals with AN to studies, although the low sample sizes of many adolescent studies suggests otherwise. Nonetheless, the involvement of parents who are anxious about their child's illness is likely to help in recruiting and retaining adolescent participants.

Placebo Controls

Given the severity of the disorder, it is neither ethical nor feasible to offer potential participants with AN a placebo condition, even though the evidence for the effectiveness of any treatment is weak. This limitation complicates the design of treatment studies. For example, medication studies must be carried out in the context of ongoing treatment with medication/placebo added. In these research reports, the base treatment is often not described adequately, and is therefore not replicable, nor are such treatments standardized between subjects. Similarly, psychotherapy studies cannot use the equivalent of placebo controls. Hence psychotherapy studies must compare a new treatment to some form of active treatment (including treatment as usual). The result for both medication and psychotherapy trials is a need for larger studies in order to obtain adequate power. The need for larger samples, in turn, militates against recruitment of an adequate number of participants to these studies.

Summary

The problems associated with the successful accomplishment of well-designed treatment trials for AN are many, and hence few adequate trials have been reported in the literature. The majority suffers from inadequate sample sizes often compounded by high dropout rates. Recruitment is difficult because of the relative rarity of the disorder, the reluctance of individuals to enter controlled trials, and the ease with which pools of potential participants are exhausted.

Approaches to Future Research

The recruitment and retention problems discussed above essentially mean that single-site studies, particularly of adult patients with AN, will have inadequate power. Hence, multisite studies are needed. Because of the rarity of controlled treatment studies of AN, particularly in the United States (Agras et al., 2004), few sites have had experience in recruitment of either adult or adolescent participants to treatment trials. Although sites without such experience can develop reasonable recruitment plans, it is likely that in any multisite study some sites will fail to recruit an adequate number of participants despite such plans. This probability will threaten the viability of any proposed study. Hence, it will be necessary to identify sites that are able to recruit adequate samples of adult and/or adolescent participants, possibly by trial and error. The ultimate aim would be to identify a relatively large number of sites able to participate in treatment trials, thus forming a collaborative group. Without such a group of expert sites it would be difficult, if not impossible, to move the quest for evidence-based treatments for AN forward. Does this mean that single-site studies should not be done? Not necessarily. Single-site small-scale studies are still needed to identify promising treatments that can then be studied in a more definitive manner. For the purpose of clarity, treatment research in adults and adolescents is considered separately in the next two sections.

Future Research in Adults

Understanding Poor Compliance

From the brief review of the literature presented so far it is clear that poor compliance with treatment leading to nonacceptance of randomization, poor acceptance of treatment, and treatment and assessment dropout, needs to be better understood and methods for remediation tested. In a recent multisite study of 167 adolescents with AN 25%, 31%, and 51% of participants in the three treatment groups did not receive the treatment to which they were allocated, largely because of poor compliance (Gowers et al., 2007). Given the differential dropout from treatment groups, it is probable that such refusals did not occur randomly.

Poor compliance is the most difficult barrier to treatment research in adult (more chronic) patients with AN. Without a solution to this problem, it is wasteful to squander resources on treatment trials doomed to failure. The authors of one failed multisite treatment study suggested that no further treatment studies in adult patients with AN should be carried out until poor acceptance and poor compliance with treatment were understood and successful remediation methods had been found (Halmi et al., 2005).

Most clinicians have encountered the resistance to treatment, fear of weight gain, and inflexibility demonstrated by many patients with AN. The causes of such resistance and well-known phenomenon of ambivalence to getting well, however, are less evident and have not been studied extensively. One study, using a self-report questionnaire approach to examine this issue, found that patients reported that aspects of their AN provided safety and structure to their lives as well as stifling their emotions (Gowers et al., 2007). These factors appear to be important underpinnings of poor compliance with treatment and offer potential treatment targets. In addition, it is clear that cognitive function is affected in AN and that, in turn, disordered cognitive function may lead to poor treatment compliance. Studies suggest that rigidities in cognitive function, including deficient set shifting and an excessively detailed information processing style, may be long-lasting and independent of weight regain (Tchanturia, Davies, & Campbell, 2007; Tchanturia et al., 2004). These problems also offer targets for potential treatment. At this point, identification of the causes of poor compliance and development of specific therapies to overcome such causes would appear to be the most pressing and fruitful approach to research with adult patients. Such studies could be small in scale, conducted in single sites, and aimed at reducing poor compliance with treatment.

Rehabilitation Rather Than a Focus on Weight

One possible reason for poor compliance is that the focus on weight gain, a central aspect of most treatment approaches for AN, sets up a struggle with patients by increasing their intense fears of weight gain. An alternative tactic would be to recognize that many patients with AN who have failed multiple treatments have a chronic illness, and that an approach promoting and enabling them to live fuller lives in the context of a chronic illness may be more successful and acceptable. Such a treatment strategy would leave medical issues such as weight gain and nutritional status to patients' physicians, allowing patients with AN to concentrate on moving forward in life with the help of a rehabilitation specialist. This treatment would select rehabilitation goals based on patients' functional disabilities.

What about Psychotherapy?

Because the treatment trials to date are difficult to interpret due to small sample sizes, often compounded by high dropout rates, it is possible that some treatments that are well established for other eating disorders (EDs) may be effective in the treatment of AN. For example, McIntosh and colleagues (2005) report that supportive clinical management was more effective than interpersonal psychotherapy (IPT), with cognitive-behavioral therapy (CBT) in an intermediate position for global outcome. However, there were no differences between groups for weight gain. Moreover, 37% of participants dropped out of the study, leaving 12 participants in each of the CBT and IPT groups and 11 participants in supportive clinical management. These findings raise the question of whether treatments such as CBT, IPT, and clinical management should be investigated further. It would be possible if an adequate number of treatment sites able to recruit participants were identified, to conduct a multisite study testing the effectiveness of such treatments. Whether such a course would be wise, given the compliance barriers discussed earlier, is a matter for serious debate.

Pharmacological Studies

The outlook for a successful medication trial in adult patients with AN appears no better than that for psychotherapy trials. The majority of medication trials in the literature has been plagued by small sample sizes (Bulik et al., 2007), high rates of refusal to participate (Kaye et al., 2001), and high dropout rates (Walsh et al., 2006). At this point there is no evidence-based medication treatment for AN either for the weight restoration phase of the illness (Attia, Haiman, Walsh, & Flater, 1998; Bulik et al., 2007) or for maintenance following weight restoration (Bulik et al., 2007; Walsh et al., 2006). Moreover, the effectiveness of some medications may vary according to the nutritional status of the patient, further complicating the design of pharmacological studies.

As is the case for psychotherapy studies, compliance with treatment is a major problem, leading to difficulty in recruiting adequate sample sizes, over and above the relative rarity of the disorder, and high dropout rates. It is possible that the underlying causes for poor compliance to medication differ from those for psychotherapy; hence investigations into the causes of poor compliance for medications may be as useful to medication trials as to psychotherapy research. Small-scale trials of novel agents may be useful as a precursor to larger trials, particularly if they target some of the problems associated with poor compliance, such as cognitive difficulties that inhibit successful learning. Whether or not genetic studies will lead to a better understanding of the biological mechanisms underlying AN remains to be seen. Ideally, such studies might eventually point the way to the use of specific medications in research.

Endophenotypes

Both psychotherapy and psychopharmacological research may benefit from the identification of endophenotypes and, in turn, lead to a better understanding of the genetic factors underlying AN. Endophenotypes are heritable correlates of AN that are independent of the state of the illness, in that they are present whether or not the illness is active, and are likely to be found in relatives not affected by the disorder and in childhood before the disorder develops (Treasure, 2007). Endophenotypes can be identified using a variety of research methods, including treatment research. For example, one approach in treatment research, and one that should be routine in any large-scale treatment trial, is to identify moderators of outcome (Kraemer, Wilson, Fairburn, & Agras, 2002). When a moderator is identified and appears to be of theoretical interest when viewed in the larger context of the research literature, it may be useful to determine whether it may lead to identification of a gene. This raises the issue of whether blood for future genetic studies should be collected in any large-scale treatment outcome study.

Future Research in Children and Adolescents

Recruitment and Compliance

Both recruitment and compliance may be less of a problem in children and adolescents with AN, as noted. Dropout rates appear lower in adolescents, with a median rate of 10% compared with 20% in adult studies (Bulik et al., 2007), and one moderately large-scale trial in adolescents conducted at a single site has been published (Lock et al., 2005). Two other multisite studies are ongoing, one comparing individual psychotherapy with behavioral family therapy at two sites and the other comparing two different types of family therapy at six sites, both with adolescents with AN. Family involvement and the child's dependence on the family probably contribute to the greater ease of recruitment and to better retention rates. These impressions, however, are based on very few studies and may prove erroneous as further studies are completed.

Psychotherapy Research

The status of psychotherapy research in children and adolescents is also somewhat more promising than in the case of adults. As noted earlier several small-scale studies and one larger study suggest that a specific type of family therapy is effective both at the end of treatment and at follow-up (Eisler et al., 2000; Lock, Couturier, & Agras, 2006). However, only small-scale comparisons with individual therapy or another form of family therapy have been published to date. Hence, the studies investigating the specificity of this form of family therapy by comparing it with another type of family therapy and with individual therapy are critical in pointing the path forward for psychotherapy research in children and adolescents with AN. If there is a lack of specificity, then the common factors between the various types of therapy must be considered, and in both cases research aimed at improving the results of therapy would be important. Moderators of family therapy outcomes have been found (Lock et al., 2005) and require replication and extension. Such moderators may eventually be useful in developing treatment algorithms that point toward individualized treatments.

Pharmacological Research

There is presently a dearth of pharmacological studies in children and adolescents. For the most part, pharmacological treatment studies in children and adolescents tend to follow from positive findings in adults with the same or allied disorder, as has been the case, for example, in depression and anxiety disorders. At this point, given that there are no evidence-based studies for adults with AN, large-scale pharmacological research in children and adolescents with AN should be put on hold until promising and acceptable agents have been identified in replicated studies with adults.

Early Identification of the Disorder

At this point treatment research in AN can be usefully partitioned into children and adolescents (low chronicity) and adults (high chronicity). The ideal approach to management of AN would be to identify cases as early as possible and treat them effectively in order to reduce the number of chronic cases, which are expensive to manage and are associated with both psychological and physical disabilities and a high death rate. As one part of this aim, research should be directed at methods to shorten the time from onset of the disorder to treatment. Such research may involve parent and teacher education, as well as education of health professionals.

Medical Safety

The safety measures used in treatment studies of patients with AN are rarely mentioned, and adverse events are often omitted from such reports. This reality suggests that there is no accepted practice regarding the medical and psychiatric safety measures used for children, adolescents, or adults with AN who are participating in treatment trials. Yet both groups of patients are at risk to suffer adverse events in the course of treatment trials due to their low weight. The first safety measure would be to ensure that each participant has adequate expert medical care throughout a treatment trial. Given the number of individuals in the United States who do not have any or adequate health insurance, this requirement would raise the dilemma of either not entering participants without adequate health insurance to a treatment trial or providing such medical care within the trial. The first choice risks compromising recruitment, whereas the second choice would increase the costs associated with the trial. This issue is particularly salient for children and adolescents with AN who may be more likely than adults to demonstrate physiological instability, and proposed safety measures for this group have been well documented (American Academy of Pediatrics, 2003; Katzman, 2005). The issue is somewhat less salient for adults because of the longer duration of the illness and less likelihood of physiological instability. On the other hand, purging frequency is higher among adults, requiring careful electrolyte and cardiovascular monitoring.

Summary and Conclusions

Careful planning is needed to move the field of treatment research in AN forward in a more fruitful way than has occurred in the past quarter century. It is suggested that the identification of a group of sites that has demonstrated ability to recruit both adolescent and adult participants for clinical trials may be one method to achieve this result.

The critical stumbling block to further treatment research in AN is poor acceptance of, and poor compliance with, treatment, affecting recruitment and retention of participants to clinical trials. This problem may affect children and adolescents less than adult participants, given children's dependence on their families and the positive influence of families on recruitment and retention. Until the problems of poor acceptance and compliance in adults with AN are understood, and effective means to overcome them have been developed and tested, it is unlikely that either psychotherapy or pharmacological studies in adult individuals with AN will be any more successful than those already published. Hence, the first priority is to encourage further studies to pinpoint the reasons for noncompliance in adults with AN. Small-scale studies, particularly those investigating therapies to overcome specific behaviors or processes associated with poor acceptance and compliance, are needed with adults with AN as precursors to larger trials. Similarly, small-scale studies of novel pharmacological agents may be useful. The potential usefulness of a specific form of family therapy in children and adolescents may point the way forward for psychotherapy research in this area. However, pharmacological research with adolescents may have to await positive results from novel agents in adult populations. Understanding of endophenotypes and their genetic underpinnings may be facilitated by carefully conducted treatment research designed to allow examination of moderators. Such moderators, when set in the larger context of the research literature, may well be endophenotypes. A recommendation was made to consider blood collection in all large-scale treatment studies to facilitate the identification of genetic factors in AN.

Acknowledgment

This chapter was supported in part by Grant Nos. MH076290 and MH076287 from the National Institute of Mental Health.

References

Agras WS, Brandt HA, Bulik CM, Dolan-Sewell R, Fairburn CG, Halmi KA, et al. (2004). Report of the National Institutes of Health workshop on overcoming barriers to treatment research in anorexia nervosa. *International Journal of Eating Disorders*, 35:509–521.

American Academy of Pediatrics. (2003). Position statement: Identifying and treating eating disorders. *Pediatrics*, 111:204–211.

Attia E, Haiman C, Walsh T, & Flater SR. (1998). Does fluoxetine augment the inpatient treatment of anorexia nervosa? *American Journal of Psychiatry*, 155:548–551.

Bulik CM, Berkman ND, Brownley KA, Seway JA, & Lohr KN. (2007). Anorexia nervosa treatment: A systematic review of randomized controlled trials. *International Journal of Eating Disorders*, 40:310–320.

Eisler I, Dare C, Hodes M, Russell G, Dodge E, & Le Grange D. (2000). Family therapy for adolescent anorexia nervosa: The results of a controlled comparison of two family interventions. *Journal of Child Psychology and Psychiatry*, 41:727–736.

Gowers S, Clark A, Roberts C, Griffiths A, Edwards V, Bryan C, et al. (2007). Clinical effectiveness of treatments for anorexia nervosa in adolescents: Randomised controlled treatment trial. *British Journal of Psychiatry*, 191:427–435.

Halmi K, Agras WS, Crow S, Mitchell J, Wilson GT, Bryson SW, et al. (2005). Predictors of treatment acceptance and completion in anorexia nervosa: Implications for future research. *Archives of General Psychiatry*, 62:776–781.

Katzman DK, (2005). Medical complications in adolescents with anorexia nervosa: A review of the literature. *International Journal of Eating Disorders*, 37:952–959.

Kaye WH, Nagata T, Weltzin TE, Hsu LKG, Sokol MS, McConaha C, et al. (2001). Double-blind placebo-controlled administration of fluoxetine in restricting and restricting-purging-type anorexia. *Biological Psychiatry*, 49:644–652.

Kraemer HC, Wilson GT, Fairburn CG, & Agras WS. (2002). Mediators and moderators of treatment effects in randomized controlled trials. *Archives of General Psychiatry*, 59:877–883.

Lock J, Agras WS, Bryson S, & Kraemer HC. (2005). A comparison of short and long-term family therapy for adolescent anorexia nervosa. *Journal of the American Academy of Child and Adolescent Psychiatry*, 44:632–639.

Lock J, Couturier J, & Agras WS. (2006). Comparison of long-term outcomes in adolescents with anorexia nervosa treated with family therapy. *Journal of the American Academy of Child and Adolescent Psychiatry*, 4:666–672.

McDermott C, Agras WS, Crow SJ, Halmi K, Mitchell JE, & Bryson S. (2004). Participant recruitment for an anorexia nervosa treatment study. *International Journal of Eating Disorders*, 35:33–41.

McIntosh VV, Jordan J, Carter FA, Luty SE, McKenzie JM, Bulik CM, et al. (2005). Three psychotherapies for anorexia nervosa: A randomized, controlled trial. *American Journal of Psychiatry*, 162:741–747.

Tchanturia K, Davies H, & Campbell IC. (2007). Cognitive remediation therapy for patients with anorexia nervosa: Preliminary findings. *Annals of General Psychiatry*, 6:14–16.

Tchanturia K, Morris RG, Anderluh MB, Collier DA, Nikolaou V, & Treasure J. (2004). Set shifting in anorexia nervosa: An examination before and after weight gain, in full recovery and relationship to childhood and adult OCPD traits. *Journal of Psychiatric Research*, 38:545–542.

Treasure JL. (2007). Getting beneath the phenotype of anorexia nervosa: The search for viable endophenotypes and genotypes. *Canadian Journal of Psychiatry*, 52:212–219.

Walsh BT, Kaplan AS, Attia E, Olmsted M, Parides M, Carter JC, et al. (2006). Fluoxetine after weight restoration in anorexia nervosa: A randomized controlled trial. *Journal of the American Medical Association*, 295:2605–2612.

CHAPTER 34

What Treatment Research Is Needed for Bulimia Nervosa?

G. Terence Wilson

Bulimia nervosa (BN) can be treated effectively using both psychological and pharmacological interventions (Wilson & Fairburn, 2007). Currently available evidence clearly indicates that the most extensively researched and most effective treatment is cognitive-behavioral therapy (CBT) (Wilson & Shafran, 2005). As we look to the future three pressing and major challenges can be identified: First, treatment, as effective as it has been shown to be, is still not good enough. For example, the current treatment of choice, CBT, eliminates both binge eating and purging in approximately 30–50% of all cases. Of the remaining patients, many show varying degrees of improvement, whereas others drop out of treatment prematurely or do not improve. Second, effective treatment must be developed for hitherto understudied populations (e.g., adolescents and minority group members). Third, the evidence in North America and elsewhere shows that effective treatment such as CBT is relatively rarely provided to patients in service settings. There exists a compelling need to develop efficient means of training therapists to competently deliver evidence-based treatment in routine clinical practice.

Improving Therapeutic Efficacy

Nonspecific Predictors, Moderators, Mechanisms, and Treatment Integrity

Research priorities that will likely lead to still more effective treatments include studies that identify nonspecific predictors of outcome, moderators of treatment outcome, and mechanisms of change (Kraemer, Wilson, Fairburn, & Agras, 2002) and develop ways of assessing treatment integrity (Perepletchikova, Treat, & Kazdin, 2007).

Nonspecific Predictors of Outcome

Identifying reliable predictors of response to treatment will facilitate a targeted focus on treatment-resistant patients. Yet identifying robust predictors of treatment outcome for BN has proven elusive. Comorbid psychiatric and personality disorders are common in those with BN, but they do not necessarily predict a poorer outcome or improve treatment planning. It is widely believed in clinical circles that personality disorders, and borderline personality disorder in particular, are associated with a worse treatment outcome (e.g., American Psychiatric Association, 2006). The evidence from randomized controlled trials (RCTs), however, is inconsistent (National Institute for Health and Clinical Excellence [NICE], 2004). In a large treatment outcome study, Rowe and colleagues (2008) found that borderline personality disorder had no impact on response to CBT. Moreover, a major prospective repeated-measures study of women with BN or eating disorder not otherwise specified (EDNOS) showed that over a time span of 5 years, the natural course of both BN and EDNOS was not "influenced significantly by the presence, severity, or time-varying changes of co-occurring PD psychopathology" (Grilo et al., 2007, p. 738).

Two variables have emerged thus far as clinically useful predictors of BN outcomes. One is *negative affect*, derived from cluster-analytic studies of patients (Stice & Agras, 1999). The finding that patients can be divided into two subgroups as a function of a dimensional measure of depressed mood and low self-esteem has been replicated in clinical and community studies of BN (Grilo, Masheb, & Berman, 2001; Stice & Fairburn, 2003), and in studies of binge-eating disorder (BED) (Masheb & Grilo, 2008). The negative affect subtype has more eating disorder (ED) psychopathology, associated psychiatric problems, and social maladjustment, and appears to be a negative prognostic factor. Future studies will be able to target the presence of this construct of negative affect with explicitly focused interventions (see below).

A second predictor is not a pretreatment patient characteristic but *early response to treatment*. Two large multisite RCTs for BN found that early response to manual-based CBT (a significant reduction in purging by week 4) was a strong predictor of outcome at posttreatment (Agras, Crow, et al., 2000) and 1-year follow-up (Fairburn, Agras, Walsh, Wilson, & Stice, 2004). A similar finding has been found for BN treatment outcomes with antidepressant medication (Walsh, Sysko, & Parides, 2006). The full theoretical, methodological, and practical ramifications of this robust finding have yet to be systematically explored, although its significance has been built into Fairburn's (2008) enhanced cognitive-behavior therapy (CBT-E). The therapy requires therapists to "take stock" after the initial seven sessions of treatment: namely, evaluate progress and identify obstacles to improvement if insufficient improvement has been made.

Moderators of Treatment Outcome

Identifying moderators answers the "clinical matching" question: What treatments work best for whom? Evidence from RCTs on this clinically crucial question is sorely lacking. Part of the problem here, as with nonspecific predictors, is that large sample sizes are required. Encouraging research findings are beginning to emerge, however. For example, Fairburn and colleagues (2009) compared two forms of CBT-E in the treatment of patients with either BN or EDNOS. The "focused" form (CBT-EF) concentrated on specific ED psychopathology, whereas in the "broader" form (CBT-EB) particular treatment modules were used to address additional psychopathology, namely, mood intolerance (which is a feature of negative affect, as discussed above), perfectionism, low self-esteem, and interpersonal problems. Both treatments were significantly superior to a wait-list control group after 8 weeks. At posttreatment (20 weeks) and follow-up (60 weeks) the two treatments were comparably effective. Moderator analysis, however, suggested that they might have differential effects on subgroups of patients. As predicted, the more complex subgroup, with additional psychopathology, appeared to fare better with CBT-EB, whereas the less complex subgroup without this level of psychopathology appeared to respond more favorably to CBT-EF. The authors caution that the moderator analysis was exploratory, and that the individual statistical tests fell short of significance, despite the consistent pattern. The study calls for replication and extension in future RCTs with theory-driven hypotheses about likely moderators. Accomplishing such goals will require large, expensive, multisite studies—but there can be no short-cuts. Given the theoretical and practical implications, the necessary research must be completed.

The "dodo bird" verdict on psychological treatments is as dead as the bird itself. No longer can it be argued that all psychotherapies are equally effective or reducible to some "common factors" notion. The evidence for specificity in treatment outcome in BN and BED is beginning to mount and will be further advanced by the study of moderators (Wilson, Grilo, & Vitousek, 2007; Wilson, Wilfley, Agras, & Bryson, in press).

Mechanisms of Change

If research on moderators of outcome has lagged behind the development and evaluation of treatment packages (e.g., CBT), we know even less about the mechanisms of change underpinning evidence-based therapies. It is essential that we learn more about mechanisms of change because this knowledge will allow active therapeutic elements of current treatment packages to be identified and then refined, which in turn will promote more efficient and effective interventions. And such knowledge will advance our understanding of the nature of the EDs we treat (Kazdin & Weisz, 1998; Kraemer et al., 2002).

At present we have minimal research and only a few isolated findings regarding possible mechanism of change for BN. There is suggestive evidence that the early reduction of dysfunctional dietary restraint is a partial mediator of CBT and possibly interpersonal psychotherapy (IPT) (Wilson, Fairburn, Agras, Walsh, & Kraemer, 2002). Mediators identified in RCTs are fundamentally correlational in nature, being associated with a significant part of the effects of the treatment in question. To establish causality, the next step would be to manipulate the mediator in an experimental design (Kraemer et al., 2002).

Studying mediators of change in psychological therapies poses particular challenges. As Murphy, Cooper, Hollon, and Fairburn (2009) point out, most evidence-based psychological treatments comprise different components. Do we focus on a unified conceptualization of the different components or evaluate each individually? Another obstacle is that even structured manual-based treatments must be tailored to the individual patient. There is a balance between flexibility and focus such that different patients may be treated differently even within the same therapy framework. Murphy and colleagues (2009) have provided a blueprint for how to address these conceptual and practical problems in future research on mediators. The approach relies on hypothesizing putative mediators of four specific procedural elements that are designed to address psychopathological processes thought to maintain BN. In addition, they offer guidance on how to assess the required temporal precedence of the mediator over treatment outcome.

Treatment Integrity

Treatment integrity is the degree to which a particular intervention is delivered as intended. Two key components of treatment integrity are (1) adherence—the extent to which the therapist implements the prescribed procedures and avoids those that are not; and (2) competence—the skill with which the therapist delivers the treatment. Problems with treatment integrity pose threats both to internal validity and external validity of a treatment outcome study. Determining whether specific treatment procedures are causally related to treatment outcome depends in part on adequate treatment integrity. Assessing therapist competence is a major challenge in disseminating evidence-based treatments, as noted below.

In their searching analysis of treatment integrity, Perepletchikova and colleagues (2007) found that systematic evaluations of this critically important aspect of treatment studies have been "extremely rare" in the psychotherapy research literature in general. One factor associated with assessment of treatment integrity was the degree to which a therapy emphasized specific skill building. Evidence-based treatments such as CBT in part comprise skill building through explicit techniques, but this dimension alone hardly suffices to capture therapist expertise in selecting, timing, and implementing diverse treatment strategies within a positive and collaborative therapeutic relationship. RCTs of BN have typically used treatment manuals, prestudy training, and continuing supervision throughout the study to ensure integrity. However, even in these cases the assessment of competence has been limited to the mainly subjective judgment of an expert in the use of a particular treatment. How best to assess treatment integrity in a way that is effective but also realistic should be a focus of future research in this area.

Future Research Agendas

This chapter is focused on evidence-based treatments using the widely accepted scientific criteria articulated in the NICE (2004) guidelines. The often heard objection from practitioners is that because a treatment has not been studied in an RCT does not mean it is ineffective. Of course this is so, but to take nonempirically supported therapies seriously, they will have to be evaluated in methodologically rigorous studies. Future research on such therapies is essential, given that there is some evidence that treatments naturalistically delivered by practicing clinicians in representative treatment settings may not be as effective as claimed (Ben-Tovim et al., 2001).

Improving CBT for BN

Given that manual-based CBT is currently the most effective treatment for BN, it makes sense to try to make it better still. Three approaches have been discussed in the literature (Wilson et al., 2007) and are briefly noted here.

Combining CBT with Antidepressant Medication

Thus far concurrent combined treatment does not seem to be reliably more effective in addressing specific ED psychopathology than CBT alone, although combined treatment may successfully address comorbid psychopathology (e.g., depression) (Wilson & Fairburn, 2007).

Integrating CBT with Other Psychological Therapies

The long-held view that "psychotherapy integration" will produce more effective treatment is still widely endorsed. In the United States it often means blending CBT with some form of psychodynamic therapy. For example, the American Psychiatric Association (2006) guidelines stated that "using psychodynamic interventions in conjunction with CBT and other psychotherapies may yield better global outcomes (e.g., comorbidity and quality of life) versus binge eating and purging" (p. 19). Yet research showing that some form of integrated psychotherapy is effective with BN, let alone more effective than CBT, is lacking.

A major concern for trying to integrate different and potentially incompatible psychological therapies is that we know little about mechanisms of action and hence active therapeutic ingredients. Accordingly, what might be premature attempts at integration could simply combine redundant procedures, if not undermine CBT altogether by diluting the focus on essential mechanisms and targets of change. A working guideline might be that caution must be taken to ensure that so-called integrated treatments are conceptually and clinically consistent.

Enhancing Manual-Based CBT

Another option would be to improve the efficacy of existing manual-based CBT for BN. The original Fairburn, Marcus, and Wilson (1993) treatment protocol represented a limited range of available CBT principles and procedures. As previously advocated (Fairburn, Cooper, & Shafran, 2003; Wilson, 1999), it is an inviting prospect to incorporate into treatment for those with BN, CBT strategies that are not only conceptually consistent with the established protocol, but also have been demonstrated to be effective in the treatment of related clinical problems such as anxiety and mood disorders.

The current state-of-the-art CBT approach is Fairburn's (2008) CBT-E, a comprehensive, principle-driven treatment that draws upon a broader range of mechanisms believed to maintain BN as well as a wider array of behavioral and cognitive interventions. Based on the first controlled evaluation of the treatment, Fairburn and colleagues (2009) suggest that it might be more effective than the original manual-based treatment. Whether this is so remains to be determined in future studies. The general theme of CBT-E, which introduces greater flexibility and individualization of treatment via a menu of optional modules for enhancing the core focal treatment, with guidelines for when and how to adapt treatment, will prove clinically appealing and will likely drive much of the treatment research agenda. The details of some of the additional treatment modules might differ, but the overarching framework will be similar.

One of the advantages of CBT-E is the more intensive and systematic focus on dysfunctional body shape and weight concerns. One facet of this focus is the experience reported by so many patients with BN about "feeling fat." As Fairburn (2008) observes, there has been little research on this pervasive and distress-inducing phenomenon. In addition to the expanded therapeutic focus of CBT-E, other applications of current developments in CBT, including mindfulness and acceptance and commitment-based approaches, can be anticipated (Wilson, 2004).

The Generalizability of Evidence-Based Treatments

Increasingly, the evidence rebuts the criticism that evidence-based treatments, established via RCTs, are of little or limited relevance to "real-world" therapy and settings (e.g., Weisz, Weersing, & Henggeler, 2004; Westen, Novotny, & Thompson-Brenner, 2004). Dimensions along which generalizability must be directly assessed in studies of dissemination include heterogeneous patient groups, diverse clinical settings, and levels of therapist training and competence. The ED field lags behind progress made in other areas where innovative research strategies, including quasi-experimental and nonexperimental designs, have shown that the results of RCTs are generalizable to treatment in routine clinical settings (Wilson, 2007). The available evidence, albeit sparse, is promising. Tuschen-Caffier, Pook, and Frank (2001) obtained favorable results in treating an unselected sample of patients with BN in a clinical service setting. Similarly, Fairburn and colleagues (2009) imposed few inclusion criteria in their clinically relevant sample drawn from two catchment area clinics.

Whereas some critics have questioned the applicability of current empirically supported treatments for minority groups (Hall & Nagayama, 2001), emerging evidence shows that CBT appears comparably effective with minority group members in the treatment of depression (Miranda et al., 2005; Roselló, Bernal, & Rivera-Medina, 2008). Consistent with this broader pattern of results, a preliminary study investigating how ethnicity may affect treatment outcome in BN found that across all ethnic groups, CBT showed significantly greater abstinence rates compared with IPT (Chui, Safer, Bryson, Agras, & Wilson, 2007). These findings are consistent with the earlier Agras, Walsh, and colleagues (2000) report that CBT is the preferred form of treatment for patients with BN. Replication and extension with minority group populations is needed.

It is important to study BN in adolescence because developmental factors have been implicated in its onset. Lock (2005) and Wilson and Sysko (2006) have described adaptations of CBT that take into account the specific developmental features of adolescence. Preliminary findings suggest that the treatment will prove effective when it is investigated in future studies. For example, Schmidt and colleagues (2007) compared family therapy (based on the Maudsley model) with guided self-help based on cognitive-behavioral principles (CBTgsh) in the treatment of adolescents with BN or EDNOS. CBTgsh resulted in a more rapid response, greater acceptability, and lower cost than family therapy. Le Grange, Crosby, Rathouz, and Leventhal (2007) showed that the same Maudsley family therapy was more effective than supportive psychotherapy in an adolescent sample with BN.

Dissemination Research

The relative unavailability of adequately administered evidence-based treatment for EDs in general routine clinical practice has been well documented. The following are two of the barriers to dissemination that are high priority for future research.

Therapist Training in Evidence-Based Treatment

Adequate training in evidence-based treatments for BN and EDs more generally is simply not available to the many clinicians interested in acquiring the expertise. Developing more efficient and effective ways of training therapists to deliver these treatments in the form that they were shown to be effective (i.e., we must ensure integrity in dissemination) is imperative. There is reason to believe that therapists may choose components of evidence-based treatment protocols based on subjective preference or ease of administration, thereby possibly omitting or diluting what may be the most effective therapeutic elements (Von Ranson & Robinson, 2006).

Referring to psychological therapy as a whole, Holloway and Neufeldt (1995) observed that "just as supervision demands of trainees a systematic and deliberate delivery of treatment to the client, so it must be demanded of supervisors that they deliver the requisite skills to the trainee. To accomplish this goal, researchers must now devise clear methods of training, standardized manuals for its delivery, and empirical studies that will test its effectiveness as a contributing component in psychotherapy training" (p. 208). This call to action has gone unheeded despite its obvious importance. The literature on supervision and training is consistent in noting the absence of evidence for the effectiveness of different formats of supervision and clinical training. We need to determine the minimal or optimal level of therapist training, experience, and expertise needed for effective delivery of evidence-based treatments.

Simply providing therapists with a manual is insufficient, just as are 1- or 2-day workshops or training institutes. The scant research that exists shows that didactic introductory work needs to be followed up in supervised casework in which trainees receive feedback on their performance of specific skills (Miller, Yahne, Moyers, Martinez, & Pirritano, 2004; Sholomskas et al., 2005). Looking to the future, we can anticipate that the tools of instructional design and technology will be harnessed to translate current text-based, manualized therapies into various interactive and Web-based applications (Cucciare, Weingardt, & Villafranca, 2008; Weingardt, 2004).

Modifying (Simplifying) Treatments to Make Them More Disseminable

To make evidence-based treatments more readily adopted by a wide range of mental health professionals, they would ideally be made less complex so that training requirements were reduced. Knowing the basic principles and mechanisms of therapeutic change would make it easier to teach essential treatment strategies. Alternatively, CBTgsh—which combines a self-help manual with a limited number of brief therapy sessions—is a readily disseminable intervention that is effective for at least a subset of adult and adolescent patients with BN (Ljotsson et al., 2007; Schmidt et al., 2007). Where, how, and by whom CBTgsh should be delivered should be the focus of future research (Wilson et al., 2007). Perkins, Murphy, Schmidt, and Williams (2006) concluded that CBTgsh may be useful as a first intervention in a stepped-care framework and may be an alternative to conventional therapist-delivered psychological therapy. Studies of CBTgsh that include health economic analyses are strongly indicated.

References

Agras WS, Crow SJ, Halmi KA, Mitchell JE, Wilson GT, & Kraemer H. (2000). Outcome predictors for the cognitive-behavioral treatment of bulimia nervosa: Data from a multisite study. *American Journal of Psychiatry*, 157:1302–1308.

Agras WS, Walsh BT, Fairburn CG, Wilson GT, & Kraemer HC. (2000). A multicenter comparison of cognitive-behavioral therapy and interpersonal psychotherapy for bulimia nervosa. *Archives of General Psychiatry*, 57:459–466.

American Psychiatric Association. (2006). Practice guideline for treatment of patients with eating disorders (3rd ed.). *American Journal of Psychiatry*, 163:4–54.

Ben-Tovim DI, Walker K, Gilchrist P, Freeman R, Kalucy R, & Esterman A. (2001). Outcome in patients with eating disorders: A 5-year study. *Lancet*, 357:1254–1257.

Chui W, Safer D, Bryson SW, Agras WS, & Wilson GT. (2007). A comparison of ethnic groups in the treatment of bulimia nervosa. *Eating Behaviors*, 8:485–491.

Cucciare MA, Weingardt KR, & Villafranca S. (2008). Using blended learning to implement evidence-based psychotherapies. *Clinical Psychology: Science and Practice*, 15:299–307.

Fairburn CG. (Ed.). (2008). *Cognitive behavior therapy and eating disorders.* New York: Guilford Press.

Fairburn CG, Agras WS, Walsh BT, Wilson GT, & Stice E. (2004). Prediction of outcome in bulimia nervosa by early change in treatment. *American Journal of Psychiatry*, 161:2322–2324.

Fairburn CG, Cooper Z, Doll HA, O'Connor ME, Bohn K, Hawker DM, et al. (2009). Transdiagnostic cognitive-behavioral therapy for patients with eating disorders: A two-site trial with 60-week follow-up. *American Journal of Psychiatry*, 166:311–319.

Fairburn CG, Cooper Z, & Shafran R. (2003). Cognitive behaviour therapy for eating disorders: A "transdiagnostic" theory and treatment. *Behaviour Research and Therapy*, 41:509–529.

Fairburn CG, Marcus MD, & Wilson GT. (1993). Cognitive-behavioral therapy for binge eating and bulimia nervosa: A comprehensive treatment manual. In CG Fairburn & GT Wilson (Eds.), *Binge eating: Nature, assessment, and treatment* (pp. 361–404). New York: Guilford Press.

Grilo CM, Masheb RM, & Berman RM. (2001). Subtyping women with bulimia nervosa along dietary and negative affect dimensions. *Eating and Weight Disorders*, 6:53–58.

Grilo CM, Pagano ME, Skodol AE, Sanislow CA, McGlashan TH, Gunderson JG, et al. (2007). Natural course of bulimia nervosa and eating disorder not otherwise specified: 5-year prospective study of remissions, relapses, and the effects of personality disorder psychopathology. *Journal of Clinical Psychiatry*, 68:738–746.

Hall GC. (2001). Psychotherapy research with ethnic minorities: Empirical, ethical, and conceptual issues. *Journal of Consulting and Clinical Psychology*, 69:502–510.

Holloway EL, & Neufeldt SA. (1995). Supervision: Its contributions to treatment efficacy. *Journal of Consulting and Clinical Psychology*, 63:207–213.

Kazdin AE, & Weisz JR. (1998). Identifying and developing empirically supported child and adolescent treatments. *Journal of Consulting and Clinical Psychology*, 66:19–36.

Kraemer HC, Wilson GT, Fairburn CG, & Agras WS. (2002). Mediators and moderators of treatment effects in randomized clinical trials. *Archives of General Psychiatry*, 59:877–883.

Le Grange D, Crosby RD, Rathouz PJ, & Leventhal BL. (2007). A randomized controlled comparison of family-based treatment and supportive psychotherapy for adolescent bulimia nervosa. *Archives of General Psychiatry*, 64:1049–1056.

Ljotsson B, Lundin C, Mitsell K, Carlbring P, Ramklint M, & Ghaderi A. (2007). Remote treatment of bulimia nervosa and binge eating disorder: A randomized trial of Internet assisted cognitive behavioural therapy. *Behaviour Research and Therapy*, 45:649–661.

Lock J. (2005). Adjusting cognitive behavior therapy for adolescents with bulimia nervosa. *American Journal of Psychotherapy*, 59:267–281.

Masheb RM, & Grilo CM. (2008). Prognostic significance of two sub-categorization methods for the treatment of binge eating disorder: Negative affect and overvaluation predict, but do not moderate, specific outcomes. *Behaviour Research and Therapy*, 46:428–437.

Miller WR, Yahne CE, Moyers TB, Martinez J, & Pirritano M. (2004). A randomized trial of methods to help clinicians learn motivational interviewing. *Journal of Consulting and Clinical Psychology*, 72:1050–1062.

Miranda J, Bernal G, Kohn A, Hwang, W.-C., & La Fromboise T. (1995). Psychosocial interventions for minorities. In S Nolen-Hoeksema (Ed.), *Annual review of clinical psychology* (Vol. 1, pp. 113–142). Palo Alto, CA: Annual Reviews.

Murphy R, Cooper Z, Hollon SD, & Fairburn CG. (2009). How do psychological treatments work?: Investigating mediators of change. *Behaviour Research and Therapy*, 47:1–5.

National Institute for Health and Clinical Excellence. (2004). *Eating disorders: Core interventions in the treatment and management of anorexia nervosa, bulimia nervosa and related eating disorders* (Clinical Guideline No. 9). London: Author. Available online at *www.nice.org.uk*.

Perepletchikova F, Treat T, & Kazdin AE. (2007). Treatment integrity in psychotherapy research: Analysis of the studies and examination of the associated factors. *Journal of Consulting and Clinical Psychology*, 75:829–841.

Perkins SJ, Murphy R, Schmidt U, & Williams C. (2006). Self-help and guided self-help for eating disorders. *Cochrane Database of Systematic Reviews*, Issue 3 (Article No. CD004191), DOI: 10/1002/14651858.CD004191.pub2.

Roselló J, Bernal G, & Rivera-Medina C. (2008). Individual and group CBT and IPT for Puerto Rican adolescents with depressive symptoms. *Cultural Diversity and Ethnic Minority Psychology*, 14:234–245.

Rowe SL, Jordan J, McIntosh V, Carter FA, Bulik C, & Joyce PR. (2008). Impact of borderline personality disorder on bulimia nervosa. *Australian and New Zealand Journal of Psychiatry*, 42:1021–1029.

Schmidt U, & Grover M. (2007). Computer-based intervention for bulimia nervosa and binge eating. In JD Latner & GT Wilson (Eds.), *Self-help approaches for obesity and eating disorders: Research and practice* (pp. 166–175). New York: Guilford Press.

Schmidt U, Lee S, Beecham J, Perkins S, Treasure J, Yi I, et al. (2007). A randomized controlled trial of family therapy and cognitive-behavioral guided self-care for adolescents with bulimia nervosa or related disorders. *American Journal of Psychiatry*, 164:73–81.

Sholomskas DE, Syracuse-Siewert G, Rounsaville BJ, Ball SA, Nuro KF, & Carroll KM. (2005). We don't train in vain. *Journal of Consulting and Clinical Psychology*, 73:106–115.

Stice E, & Agras WS. (1999). Subtyping bulimics along dietary restraint and negative affect dimensions. *Journal of Consulting and Clinical Psychology*, 67:460–469.

Stice E, & Fairburn CG. (2003). Dietary and dietary-depressive subtypes of bulimia nervosa show differential symptom presentation, social impairment, comorbidity and course of illness. *Journal of Consulting and Clinical Psychology*, 71(6):1090–1094.

Tuschen-Caffier B, Pook M, & Frank M. (2001). Evaluation of manual-based cognitive-behavioral therapy for bulimia nervosa in a service setting. *Behaviour Research and Therapy*, 39:299–308.

Von Ranson K, & Robinson K. (2006). Who is providing what type of psychotherapy to eating disorder clients?: A survey. *International Journal of Eating Disorders*, 39:27–34.

Walsh BT, Sysko R, & Parides MK. (2006). Early response to desipramine among women with bulimia nervosa. *International Journal of Eating Disorders*, 39:72–75.

Weingardt KR. (2004). The role of instructional design and technology in the dissemination of empirically supported manual-based therapies. *Clinical Psychology: Science and Practice*, 11:313–333.

Weisz JR, Weersing VR, & Henggeler SW. (2005). Jousting with straw men: Comment on Westen, Novotny, and Thompson-Brenner (2004). *Psychological Bulletin*, 131:418–426.

Westen D, Novotny CM, & Thompson-Brenner H. (2004). The empirical status of empirically supported psychotherapies: Assumptions, findings, and reporting in controlled clinical trials. *Psychological Bulletin*, 130:631–663.

Wilson GT. (1999). Cognitive behavior therapy for eating disorders: Progress and problems. *Behaviour Research and Therapy*, 37:579–596.

Wilson GT. (2004). Acceptance and change in the treatment of eating disorders: The evolution of manual-based cognitive-behavioral therapy (CBT). In SC Hayes, VM Follette & M Linehan (Eds.), *Mindfulness and acceptance: Expanding the cognitive-behavioral tradition* (pp. 243–266). New York: Guilford Press.

Wilson GT. (2007). Manual-based treatment: Evolution and evaluation. In TA Treat, RR Bootzin, & TB Baker (Eds.), *Psychological clinical science: Papers in honor of Richard M McFall* (pp. 105–132). Mahwah, NJ: Erlbaum.

Wilson GT, & Fairburn CG. (2007). Eating disorders. In PE Nathan & JM Gorman (Eds.), *Treatments that work* (3rd ed., pp. 579–611). New York: Oxford University Press.

Wilson GT, Fairburn CG, Agras WS, Walsh BT, & Kraemer H. (2002). Cognitive behavior therapy for bulimia nervosa: Time course and mechanisms of change. *Journal of Consulting and Clinical Psychology*, 70:267–274.

Wilson GT, Grilo CM, & Vitousek K. (2007). Psychological treatment of eating disorders. *American Psychologist*, 62:199–216.

Wilson GT, & Shafran R. (2005). Eating disorders guideline from NICE. *Lancet*, 365:79–81.

Wilson GT, & Sysko R. (2006). Cognitive-behavioral therapy for adolescents with bulimia nervosa. *European Eating Disorders Review*, 14:8–16.

Wilson GT, Wilfley DE, Agras WS, & Bryson SW. (in press). Psychological treatments for binge eating disorder. *Archives of General Psychiatry*.

CHAPTER 35

What Treatment Research Is Needed for Eating Disorder Not Otherwise Specified and Binge-Eating Disorder?

Carlos M. Grilo

Eating disorders not otherwise specified (EDNOS) is a heterogeneous and poorly defined eating disorder (ED) diagnostic category. EDNOS is defined in the *Diagnostic and Statistical Manual of Mental Disorders* (4th ed.; DSM-IV; American Psychiatric Association, 1994) as clinically significant "disorders of eating that do not meet the criteria for any specific eating disorder" (p. 550). Thus, EDNOS includes an admixture of variations in bulimia nervosa (BN), anorexia nervosa (AN), and "mixed" EDs containing features of both BN and AN (Keel et al., 2004; Mitchell et al., 2007), as well as other eating problems. EDNOS also includes a specific ED—binge-eating disorder (BED)—for which provisional research diagnostic criteria were included in Appendix B of the DSM-IV. BED is defined primarily by recurrent binge eating without the regular use of inappropriate compensatory weight control methods that characterize BN. A recent critical review concluded that there is sufficient empirical evidence supporting the inclusion of BED as a distinct and formal ED diagnosis in the DSM-V (Striegel-Moore & Franko, 2008), whereas the remaining problems that comprise EDNOS remain poorly understood and thus represent a major priority for research.

Epidemiological studies have found that EDNOS (Favaro, Ferrara, & Santonastaso, 2003) and BED (Hudson, Hiripi, Pope, & Kessler, 2007) are both more prevalent than AN and BN combined. EDNOS is the most common ED diagnosis encountered in routine clinical practice (Zimmerman, Francione-Witt, Chelminski, Young, & Tortolani, 2008) and in specialized ED centers (Rockert, Kaplan, & Olmsted, 2007), including those for adolescents (Eddy, Doyle, Hoste, Herzog, & Le Grange, 2008). EDNOS and BED, like AN and BN, tend to be clinically severe (Schmidt et al., 2008) and are both associated with increased morbidity and high levels of health care utilization (Hudson et al., 2007; Striegel-Moore et al., 2008). EDNOS and BED are characterized by a variable course of illness, including symptom fluctuations, remissions, and relapses. Recent long-term longitudinal studies have documented that the courses of EDNOS (Ben-Tovim et al., 2001; Grilo, Pagano, et al., 2007) and BED (Fichter, Quadflieg, & Hedlund, 2008) are similar to that of BN.

Treatment Research on EDNOS and BED

Despite the prevalence and clinical severity of EDNOS and BED, controlled treatment research for these two ED variants has lagged behind research for the other EDs. To date, there is only one published randomized controlled trial (RCT) performed specifically with EDNOS (Fairburn et al., 2009), although other research has used subsyndromal variants of AN and BN. In contrast, treatment research with BED has progressed substantially since its early evolutions from the obesity and BN treatment literatures (Yanovski, 1993), although relatively few well-controlled studies have been performed, and many unanswered questions remain (Wilson, Grilo, & Vitousek, 2007). This chapter provides a brief overview of what is known about the treatment of EDNOS and BED as context for outlining the major challenges and future research in order to improve treatments.

Treatment of EDNOS

Little is known about the treatment of EDNOS. During a wait-list control condition EDNOS showed little change (Fairburn et al., 2009), and naturalistic outcome studies reveal both the seriousness of EDNOS and the limited effectiveness of existing "treatments as usual" (Ben-Tovim et al., 2001). Although recent controlled trials have specifically included patients with EDNOS as part of their overall study group (Le Grange, Crosby, & Lock, 2008; Mitchell et al., 2008; Schmidt et al., 2008; Walsh, Fairburn, Mickley, Sysko, & Parides, 2004), this involved "subthreshold" cases of BN, not the broader admixture of ED cases that comprise EDNOS. Since all of these studies, except for one (Schmidt et al., 2008), reported improvements for the overall ED study group only, it is unknown whether EDNOS and BN benefit differently from existing treatments.

Two recent RCTs with adolescents with EDs have produced relevant data regarding EDNOS (Le Grange et al., 2008; Schmidt et al., 2008) and serve as excellent models for how future treatment research (outlined later in this chapter) should integrate planned analyses to examine predictors and moderators of outcomes (see Kraemer, Wilson, Fairburn, & Agras, 2002). An RCT comparing family therapy (FT) and cognitive-behavioral therapy (CBT) for adolescents found that a significantly higher proportion of patients with EDNOS than with BN were abstinent from binge–purge behaviors at follow-up; ED diagnosis (EDNOS or BN), however, did not moderate treatment outcomes (Schmidt et al., 2008). An RCT comparing FT and individual supportive therapy for adolescents found that lower frequency of binge–purge episodes predicted higher likelihood of posttreatment partial remission, and that lower levels of ED psychopathology moderated treatment outcomes (i.e., patients with less severe ED were more likely to achieve partial remission if they received family-based treatment rather than individual supportive psychotherapy) (Le Grange et al., 2008). Lastly, one RCT with adults tested the efficacy of naltrexone versus placebo in combination with cognitive-behavioral coping skills therapy for alcohol-dependent women recruited and stratified by the presence or absence of coexisting ED psychopathology (O'Malley et al., 2007). In the subgroup of alcoholic women with broad ED psychopathology (reflecting EDNOS), a 70% reduction in binge eating and 35% reduction in associated ED psychopathology were achieved with treatment, although there were no significant differences between naltrexone versus placebo added to the coping skills treatment.

Collectively, these findings suggest that patients with EDNOS (O'Malley et al., 2007; Schmidt et al., 2008) or subthreshold BN (Le Grange et al., 2008) benefit from certain specific manualized treatments. Thus, existing evidence-based psychological treatments appear potentially adaptable to subgroups of patients with EDNOS. This possibility recently received strong support from the sole RCT performed to date specifically with EDNOS (Fairburn et al., 2009).

Fairburn and colleagues (2008) refined their evidence-based CBT (National Institute for Health and Clinical Excellence [NICE], 2004; Wilson et al., 2007) and developed a second-generation manual-based "enhanced CBT" (CBT-E) version developed for the full range of EDs. Fairburn and colleagues (2009), in a two-site RCT, tested the efficacy of two versions of CBT-E; CBT-Ef, a focused form designed to target ED psychopathology, versus CBT-Eb, a more complex broader form that can be tailored to individual patients' needs in order to target additional psychopathology (e.g., mood intolerance, perfectionism) thought to either maintain ED or complicate treatment. This RCT enrolled 154 patients with diverse EDs (except for extremely underweight cases) from two catchment area clinics and used few exclusion criteria, thus enhancing clinical relevance and generalizability. Both CBT-E versions were significantly superior to a delayed-treatment condition and produced substantial and "equivalent" improvements in ED psychopathology that were well maintained during a 60-week closed period of follow-up. Overall, at posttreatment roughly 51% of patients (61.4% of EDNOS and 45.7% of BN) had ED levels less than one standard deviation above community norms. Patients with EDNOS and BN did not differ significantly at pretreatment, posttreatment, or follow-up, nor did diagnosis moderate treatment outcomes. An exploratory analysis revealed trends suggesting that patients with higher levels of associated psychopathology appeared to benefit more from CBT-Eb, whereas patients without additional psychopathology benefited more from the "simpler" CBT-Ef approach (Fairburn et al., 2009). Thus, CBT-E appears to have efficacy not just for BN but for EDNOS (i.e., for the majority of patients with ED who present for treatment). These findings should be replicated and extended by other research groups. A major question for future research is whether the more complex CBT-Eb can be widely disseminated and mastered by clinicians and whether the added complexity reliably produces enhanced outcomes (see discussion below on "Is More Better?").

Treatment of BED

Pharmacotherapy Only

To date, most—but not all—RCTs testing pharmacotherapy for BED have reported statistically significant findings relative to placebos and have concluded that pharmacotherapy has efficacy for BED. However, a more circumspect view of the literature seems indicated to inform future treatment research priorities.

A recent meta-analysis of controlled trials (14 studies with 1,279 patients) evaluating pharmacotherapy-only for BED concluded that pharmacotherapy treatments have a clinically significant advantage over placebo for producing short-term remission from binge eating (Reas & Grilo, 2008). Overall, across different medication classes (mean attrition rate of 30%), 48.7% of patients receiving pharmacotherapy versus 28.5% of patients receiving placebo stopped binge-eating (based on last week endpoint data). The relative risk (RR) of 0.74 (95% confidence interval = 0.66–0.84) for this analysis, which can be interpreted as an effect size measure, indicates that pharmacotherapy reduces the risk of nonremission by 26%. Effect sizes for different classes of medication for achieving binge-eating abstinence varied somewhat. For selective serotonin reuptake inhibitor (SSRI) medications, the RR was 0.81, for sibutramine the RR was 0.80, and for antiepileptic medications the RR was 0.63. Overall, pharmacotherapy also showed evidence of a significant additional weight reduction of 3.4 kg compared to placebo (i.e., mean weight losses = 3.56 kg vs. 0.08 kg) as indicated by a significant effect size (weighted mean difference [WMD] = −3.42). This mean weight loss translates roughly to only 3.2% of original body weight for the average patient in these studies. The effect sizes varied considerably across the different medication classes, ranging from modest effects (WMD = −1.7) for SSRIs to larger effects for the antiepileptics (WMD = −4.6) and for sibutramine (WMD = −3.6) medications.

In terms of clinical implications, these recent meta-analytic findings may suggest changes to the specific recommendations offered previously in the NICE (2004) guidelines. Specifically, these findings highlight the potential efficacy of an antiobesity agent (sibutramine) and antiepiletic medications (particularly topiramate) but may suggest more limited utility of SSRIs, given their smaller effects on binge eating and essentially no effect on weight. More broadly in terms of clinical implications, these meta-analytic findings suggest caution in what can be told to patients. At this point, obese patients with BED can be told that certain medications enhance their chances of stopping binge-eating in the short term, and some weight loss may occur, but it is unlikely to be substantial, and that the longer-term effects of these medications are unknown.

In terms of research implications, the most pressing issue is the need for longer-term studies and especially for follow-up data. The longer-term effects of pharmacotherapy-only for BED are unknown. The sole placebo-controlled RCT of pharmacotherapy-only (with a medication subsequently withdrawn from the market) with a follow-up design reported rapid and high relapse rates after medication discontinuation (Stunkard, Berkowitz, Tanrikut, Reiss, & Young, 1996). In addition, one controlled but open-label trial reported that two SSRIs (fluoxetine and fluvoxamine) failed to significantly reduce binge eating or weight and were significantly inferior to CBT, CBT plus fluoxetine, and CBT plus fluvoxamine at posttreatment and 12-month follow-up (Ricca et al., 2001). Lastly, although the findings for the short-term efficacy of antiepileptics, notably topiramate for BED, are promising, a recent open-label extended treatment study reported nearly universal noncompliance due primarily to difficulties with side effects (McElroy et al., 2004). Such concerns regarding the durability of pharmacotherapy following discontinuation plus the modest support suggested by the meta-analysis (Reas & Grilo, 2008) highlight the need for continued research on pharmacotherapy approaches for BED. Such research studies should consider longer treatment trials (unlike the obesity literature, pharmacotherapy trials for BED have been of relatively short duration) and should include repeated follow-up assessments. Such studies are needed not just to determine overall durability of outcomes but to identify predictors of relapse (i.e., which patients are most at risk) and the time when the risk for relapse is heightened.

A final issue concerning future pharmacotherapy research concerns potential conflicts of interest. Twelve of the 14 published RCTs testing pharmacotherapy-only were funded by the drug manufacturer, and all but one (i.e., a trial with only 20 participants) reported that the tested medication demonstrated short-term efficacy. Industry sponsorship may be an important relevant context for interpreting the existing literature. Perlis and colleagues (2005) recently examined the extent and implications of industry sponsorship and financial conflict of interest in the reporting of RCTs in psychiatry. The authors identified 162 randomized double-blind placebo-controlled studies published in four leading psychiatry journals between 2001 and 2003. RCTs with reported conflict of interest were 4.9 times more likely to report positive results, an association that was significant only among the pharmaceutical industry funded studies (Perlis et al., 2005). Such findings are not specific or limited to psychiatry. Systematic reviews of the potential impact of financial conflicts on biomedical research have concluded that studies funded by the pharmaceutical industry are selectively published (Chan, Hrobjartsson, Haahr, Gotzsche, & Altman, 2004) and were significantly more likely to report positive outcomes than nonprofit organizations (Als-Nielsen, Chen, Glund, & Kjaergard, 2003; Bekelman, Li, & Gross, 2003). For example, Als-Nielsen and colleagues (2003) found that pharmacotherapy RCTs funded by for-profit organizations were 5.3 times more likely to recommend a medication, compared to RCTs funded by nonprofit organizations. Chan and colleagues (2004) previously urged that readers of original reports of RCTs, as well as of reviews, should be cautious in interpreting conclusions, given the potential for overestimation of efficacy. This state of affairs produces a quandary for clinicians and consumers of the literature and suggests the need for additional RCTs conducted without ties to industry. Of course, potential conflicts of interest also pertain to psychological treatments where such potential "allegiance" effects might occur. These issues highlight the need for replication and extension studies to be conducted by multiple research groups beyond just the developers of treatments (regardless of whether pharmacological or psychological methods are tested).

Psychological Treatment

NICE (2004) concluded that CBT-BED, a slightly adapted version of CBT-BN (Fairburn, Jones, Peveler, Hope, & O'Connor, 1993), is the treatment of choice. This clinical recommendation was assigned a grade of A, reflecting strong supporting empirical evidence for CBT-BED. Subsequent research has further supported this recommendation. Studies of CBT-BED consistently report remission rates (defined as 1-month abstinence from binge eating) of 50% or greater, along with broad improvements in associated psychological and psychosocial functioning, although weight loss tends to be minimal (Wilson et al., 2007). Different research groups have documented that the benefits of CBT-BED are well maintained through 12-month (Grilo, Masheb, Brownell, Wilson, 7 White, 2007; Munsch et al., 2007; Wilfley et al., 2002) and 24-month (Wilson, Wilfley, Agras, & Bryson, in press) follow-up. Recent RCTs have produced evidence for the specificity of CBT-BED, including superiority relative to fluoxetine (Grilo, Masheb, & Wilson, 2005; Ricca et al., 2001) and to behavioral weight loss in some studies (Wilson et al., in press).

Emerging research has supported the utility of self-help and guided-self-help CBT-based interventions, which is important in light of the limited availability of clinical specialists in the treatment of CBT. The NICE (2004) review and guidelines concluded that, with a methodological grade of B, patients with BED could be encouraged to attempt such an evidence-based CBT self-help program. Although the empirical support for CBT guided self-help methods from research conducted at specialty clinics is robust (Grilo & Masheb, 2005), research conducted in generalist settings is mixed (Ghaderi & Scott, 2003; Walsh et al., 2004). This difference highlights the need for broader "effectiveness" treatment research conducted in generalist clinical settings.

Two alternative specialized psychological treatments, interpersonal psychotherapy (IPT) and dialectical behavior therapy (DBT), have shown promise for the treatment of BED. The NICE (2004) review assigned a grade of B for the use of these two focal manualized treatments for BED. IPT has robust short-term and longer-term outcomes that are essentially identical to those for CBT (Wilfley et al., 2002) and may be especially relevant for BED patients with low self-esteem and high levels of ED psychopathology (Wilson et al., in press). Like CBT, these two psychological treatments fail to produce significant weight loss. Future research by other groups is needed to replicate and extend these promising findings and to determine whether these interventions can be widely disseminated and mastered by practicing clinicians.

Behavioral Weight Loss Therapy

Recent reviews (e.g., NICE, 2004) have suggested that behavioral weight loss (BWL) with moderate caloric restriction has utility for those with BED, particularly given the need to reduce excess weight, which other psychological treatments fail to achieve. However, research has not yet conclusively answered two pressing questions: (1) whether obese patients with BED benefit less from BWL treatments than obese patients who do not binge-eat; and (2) the relative efficacy of BWL compared to other psychological treatments.

Blaine and Rodman (2007) recently performed a meta-analysis of 36 studies of weight loss treatments that included analyses testing the potential moderating effects of binge eating on outcomes. Overall, across studies, binge-eating status moderated weight loss outcomes, but not psychological outcomes. Overall, average weight losses for obese binge eaters were negligible (1.3 kg) and substantially less than for obese non-binge-eaters (10.5 kg). These findings, however, must be viewed cautiously in light of methodological limitations (e.g., most notably, the weak assessment methods) that characterize most of that literature from which data were extracted to perform this meta-analysis.

A recent secondary analysis from the Look AHEAD (Action for Health in Diabetes) Trial aimed to test the potential moderating effects of binge eating on weight loss outcomes in overweight patients with Type II diabetes mellitus (Gorin et al., 2008). The authors characterized patients into four groups based on whether they reported any episodes of binge eating during the past 6 months on a self-report questionnaire. Most (85.4%) did not report binge eating at pretreatment or posttreatment, 7.5% reported binge eating at pretreatment but not posttreatment, 3.7% reported binge eating at both pretreatment and posttreatment, and 3.4% reported no binge eating at pretreatment but binge eating at posttreatment. The authors noted that patients who reported not binge-eating and patients who stopped binge-eating lost statistically significantly more weight (4.8 kg and 5.3 kg, respectively) than patients who continued to binge-eat (3.1 kg) or who started to binge-eat (3.0 kg). The authors concluded that overweight patients with Type II diabetes who stop binge-eating lose weight as successfully as non-binge-eaters. Unfortunately, this secondary reanalysis from this major NIH-funded study fails to shed any light on this important clinical question. Categorization of binge-eating status based on a self-reported endorsement of having "any" binge-eating episode during the past 6 months on a questionnaire (of uncertain diagnostic efficiency) essentially makes interpretation impossible.

Emerging evidence from recent carefully conducted and relatively large RCTs regarding the relative efficacy of BWL versus other psychological treatments is mixed. IPT (Wilson et al., in press) and CBT guided self-help were found to be significantly superior to BWL (Grilo & Masheb, 2005), although all of these RCTs reported minimal weight losses. Conversely, two RCTs reported that CBT produced significantly greater reductions in binge eating, whereas BWL produced significantly greater, albeit modest, weight loss at posttreatment, although both CBT and BWL had durable outcomes that differed little by 12-month follow-ups (Grilo, Masheb, et al., 2007; Munsch et al., 2007). Future research with BWL must focus on understanding reasons for the low levels of observed weight loss in many BWL trials with obese patients with BED. Future research comparing BWL and other psychological treatments could be enhanced by focused analyses of moderators and mediators of outcomes (see below).

Is More Better: Does Combining or Sequencing Treatments Enhance Outcomes?

A frequent "commonsense" clinical practice is to combine or sequence different approaches in the hopes of enhancing outcomes or helping refractory patients. Two seminal studies in this regard were conducted by Agras and colleagues, who tested sequenced manualized treatments with some degree of evidence base. Agras and colleagues (1994), in the first study of sequenced approaches, found that providing BWL following CBT produced little weight loss (mean 2.0 kg) or additional benefit of any kind. Agras and colleagues (1995) found that IPT delivered to patients with BED who failed to respond to CBT resulted in no further improvements. Various other combined approaches have been tested but overall have yielded disappointing findings. Indeed, NICE (2004) concluded that little is known about combination or sequenced approaches for BED, especially with regard to managing obesity, and provided a methodological grade of C. Some notable recent trials have found relatively little advantage to "adding more." Devlin and colleagues (2005) found that the addition of CBT—but not antidepressant medication—to BWL enhanced reduction in binge eating, but not weight. de Zwaan and colleagues (2005) reported that a comprehensive BWL combined with very low calorie diet (VLCD) resulted in 55% binge abstinence rates and an impressive average weight loss of 16.1%. Unfortunately, rapid and substantial regain of weight was common following treatment, with 29% of patients weighing more at 1-year follow-up than they did prior to the combined BWL-VLCD treatment. We reported that a sequential CBT plus BWL treatment was not superior to either CBT or BWL (Grilo, Masheb, et al., 2007).

Combining pharmacotherapy with psychological treatments has also resulted in disappointing findings. We reviewed eight studies ($N = 683$) that tested pharmacotherapy combined with psychological interventions using a variety of designs (Reas & Grilo, 2008). Combining medications with psychological or behavioral interventions failed to significantly enhance binge-eating outcomes in any study, nor did the addition of various antidepressant medications enhance weight loss. In contrast, recent double-blind RCTs found that adding topiramate (Claudino et al., 2007) or orlistat (Grilo, Masheb, & Salant, 2005) to CBT or adding orlistat to BWL (Golay et al., 2005) significantly, albeit clinically only modestly, enhanced weight loss. Thus, adding specific medications that are complementary to the CBT or BWL to specifically target weight loss may yield some additional benefits.

Targeted Research Needed to Improve Treatments

Although progress has been made and promising treatments for EDNOS and BED have been identified in recent years, many patients fail to improve sufficiently, and roughly half do not remit with the best available treatments. Moreover, little is known about (1) how to help nonresponders; (2) whether existing treatments are effective with certain groups underrepresented in RCTs (minority groups, younger patients, adolescents, patients with medical or psychiatric comorbidities frequently excluded from RCTs) (Guerdjikova & McElroy, 2009); (3) treatments naturalistically delivered in nonresearch clinical settings (Crow, Peterson, Levine, Thuras, & Mitchell, 2004); (4) effective training and dissemination of evidence-based treatments (Wilson et al., 2007); and (5) whether generalists can effectively deliver specialty-based treatments (Walsh et al., 2004).

One encouraging development is the recent refinement and extension of CBT, the best-established treatment for BN and BED, to also include the broader range of EDNOS. This refinement also integrates recent empirical advances in understanding psychological factors thought to play a role in the maintenance of EDs and to complicate treatment. Alternatively, this "enhanced" complex treatment requires replication and extension beyond the initial Fairburn and colleagues (2009) two-site RCT. Although CBT-E (Fairburn et al., 2009) represents a conceptually coherent theory- and evidence-based approach, enhanced based on empirical studies of putative maintaining factors, this complexity results in challenges that may make it more difficult for clinicians to master. It remains uncertain whether the added complexity results in substantially improved outcomes.

The broader literature on combined treatments for BED, reviewed above, suggests that the answer to the question "Is more better?" appears to be no! This answer may not be specific to BED. The alternative to trying to deliver more is to deliver less but more rigorously. One important demonstration of this point is found in the depression literature. In a large RCT, Dimidjian and colleagues (2006) found that among more severely depressed patients, behavioral activation (identified by component analysis of CBT for depression as an effective focused intervention) was comparable to antidepressant medication, and both were significantly superior to full CBT. A subsequent 24-month follow-up of treatment responders revealed that the acute treatments of behavioral activation and CBT differed little in their longer-term durability, and both were superior to antidepressant medication if discontinued and similar to continued medication (Dobson et al., 2008). These findings suggest that research on treatments for EDNOS and BED should begin to probe these treatments in order to determine the key ingredients.

More broadly, this point supports the astute warning by Hayes, Luoma, Bond, Masuda, and Lillis (2005) who recently stated:

> Focusing merely on validation of an ever-expanding list of multi-component manuals designed to treat a dizzying array of topographically defined syndromes and sub-syndromes creates a factorial research problem that is scientifically impossible to mount. Such a "brute force" empirical approach makes it increasingly difficult to teach what is known or to focus on what is essential. (p. 2)

Thus, more targeted treatment research is needed on our existing treatments.

Predictors, Moderators, Mediators, and Mechanisms of Change

Kraemer and colleagues (Kraemer et al., 2002) cogently argued that not only are RCTs the gold standard for evaluating the effectiveness of treatments, but they can also provide valuable information about predictors, moderators, and mediators of outcomes. Nonspecific "predictors" refer to pretreatment variables that predict treatment response across treatments (i.e., a main effect), and if identified, could provide clinicians with a signal about which patients might require a special or targeted focus. "Moderators" refer to pretreatment variables (uncorrelated with treatment) that interact with and influence the magnitude of treatment outcome (i.e., they differentially predict treatment outcomes) and provide information about what kinds of circumstances produce differing effects on treatments and for whom. If identified, moderators could inform rationale treatment prescription (i.e., "matching" treatments to patients) and might be relevant to mediators (and vice versa) to the extent that they suggest different processes might be involved for patients with or without those features. "Mediators" refer to intervening variables (during treatment) that statistically account, at least to some extent, for the relationship between treatment and outcome. Mediators are correlated with treatment, are changed during treatment, and the changes must precede the treatment effects on outcome. It is important to emphasize that mediators reflect statistical associations but do not establish causality. Thus, although mediators of change provide potential clues for how might treatments work, they do not necessarily reflect the actual casual *mechanisms* or processes through which the therapeutic changes actually occurred (Kazdin, 2007). "Mechanisms" refer to why treatments work and through what processes the therapeutic changes come about (Kazdin, 2007). Once mediators are found, experimental manipulations are needed in order to test potential causality and identify potential mechanisms.

To date, reliable predictors of BED/EDNOS outcome have yet to be conclusively identified, although recent studies have identified a few patient characteristics, including negative affect, ED psychopathology, self-esteem, and interpersonal problems (Hilbert et al., 2007; Masheb & Grilo, 2008). Although not a patient (or pretreatment) factor, rapid response to treatment has been identified as a reliable, clinically significant predictor of treatment outcome (Grilo & Masheb, 2007; Grilo, Masheb, & Wilson, 2006; Masheb & Grilo, 2007). Even less is known about moderators of outcome. Two RCTs (Hilbert et al., 2007; Masheb & Grilo, 2007) were unable to identify moderators of outcomes for BED, although a recent study (Wilfley et al., 2008) found that low-self esteem and higher ED psychopathology moderated treatment outcomes (IPT more effective for those patients). One promising cognitive variable for research to test as a predictor/moderator of treatment is overvaluation of shape/weight (Grilo et al., 2008), which characterizes roughly half of patients with BED and is strongly associated with increased ED psychopathology. For EDNOS, Fairburn and colleagues (2009) reported that higher levels of associated psychopathology moderated CBT-E outcomes (CBT-Eb more effective for those patients). Virtually nothing is known about mediators of treatment for BED or EDNOS. We reported that rapid response (early reductions in the frequency of binge eating during the first month of treatment) prospectively predicted significant subsequent weight loss during the remaining course of treatment (Grilo et al., 2006). This finding sheds further light on other reports that abstinence from binge eating is associated with significant, albeit modest, weight loss in those with BED (Devlin et al., 2005; Wilfley et al., 2002). This dearth of knowledge highlights the need for future research to make these types of analyses a priority. Another possibility for future research involves the "pooling" of data by different research groups who test the same manualized treatments using comparable assessment batteries. This strategy might be relevant to overcome the statistical power challenges inherent in these types of analyses.

Improved and Expanded Assessments

Assessment Instruments and Methods

Improving assessments, particularly for eating behaviors, represents a major research priority for the field (Grilo, Masheb, & Wilson, 2001). For example, dietary restraint (broadly speaking) occupies a central role in ED research yet remains a conceptual and measurement problem. The major dietary restraint scales used in treatment research appear to be unrelated to acute dietary restriction (Stice, Fisher, & Lowe, 2004) or to longer-term dietary restriction based on objective biological (doubly-labeled water estimates of energy intake) or observational behavioral data (Stice, Cooper, Schoeller, Tappe, & Lowe, 2007). The field has neglected to perform sufficient basic psychometric research on some of the major measures used in treatment research, such as the Eating Disorder Examination (EDE) interview and questionnaire (EDE-Q) versions (Grilo et al., 2001). For example, the factor structure of the EDE-Q has been tested in only two studies—both of which reported alternative structures (see Hrabosky et al., 2008), and there exist only three small published reports of the test–retest reliability of the EDE (see Grilo, Lozano, et al., 2005).

Although studies have reported various forms of disordered eating and overeating behaviors in BED (Masheb & Grilo, 2006a, 2006b) that differ from other eating-disordered and obese patient groups (Allison, Grilo, Masheb, & Stunkard, 2006), research has provided little guidance about how best to address these behaviors, and—not surprisingly—they receive little attention in existing CBT and BWL protocols. This lacuma suggests the need for more laboratory studies (Walsh & Boudreau, 2003) that may shed further light on basic processes such as hunger and satiety in BED (Samuels, Zimmerli, Devlin, Kissileff, & Walsh, 2009; Sysko, Devlin, Walsh, Zimmerli, & Kissileff, 2007). More broadly speaking, a greater emphasis is needed on *translational* research, in which basic science investigations on eating-related behaviors and cognitions may yield discoveries for novel interventions.

Assessment Protocols

Research on mediators (intervening variables that occur during treatment but before outcome) requires that repeated assessments be conducted during the course of treatment to ascertain changes in *both* the hypothesized mediator variables and the outcome variables. To date, most RCTs in BED—particularly the pharmacotherapy RCTs—have focused on pre- and postassessments but minimized assessments during the course of treatment (except for binge-eating and weight measures reflecting outcomes). Recent research has found that substantial and meaningful therapeutic changes can occur rapidly during the early stages of treatment for BED (Grilo & Masheb, 2007; Grilo et al., 2006; Masheb & Grilo, 2007). This finding highlights the need for treatment assessment protocols to repeatedly capture data during the first few weeks of treatment as well as during repeated time points throughout the course of treatment. Murphy, Cooper, Holon, and Fairburn (2009) recently outlined additional assessment strategies for studying mediators across different treatments as well as how to plan assessments for treatments comprising different components.

Biological and Neural Measurements

Treatment research with EDNOS and BED should begin to integrate biological measures for putative mechanisms involved in appetitive processes and energy balance and for broader health outcomes (e.g., glycemic control, metabolic syndrome). Another promising area of research includes recent studies of appetitive and motivational neurocircuitry in obesity (Abizaid, Gao, & Horvath, 2006; Wang et al., 2004). Studies have suggested brain function abnormalities underlying pathways implicated in reward processing in response to food intake in obese relative to lean persons (Stice, Spoor, Bohon, Veldhuizen, & Small, 2008). A recent study reported differential brain activation patterns in response to visual food stimuli across BED, BN, obese, and normal-weight groups (Schienle, Schafer, Hermann, & Vaitl, 2009). Abnormalities in the neural correlates of reward processing could be examined with respect to treatment outcome. An example of this potential avenue for research can be found in a recent Request for Applications issued by the National Institutes of Drug Abuse (Neurobiology of Behavioral Treatment: Recovery of Brain Structure and Function; DA-05-006; *grants.nih.gov/grants/guide/rfa-files/RFA-DA-05-006.html*), calling for interdisciplinary investigations into the neural mechanisms predicting and moderating effective treatments for drug abuse.

References

Abizaid A, Gao Q, & Horvath TL. (2006). Thought for food: Brain mechanisms and peripheral energy balance. *Neuron*, 51:691–702.

Agras WS, Telch CF, Arnow B, Eldredge K, Detzer MJ, Henderson J, et al. (1995). Does interpersonal therapy help patients with binge eating disorder who fail to respond to cognitive-behavioral therapy? *Journal of Consulting and Clinical Psychology*, 63:356–360.

Agras WS, Telch CF, Arnow B, Eldredge K, Wilfley DE, Raeburn SD, et al. (1994). Weight loss, cognitive-behavioral, and desipramine treatments in binge eating disorder: An additive design. *Behavior Therapy*, 25:225–238.

Allison KC, Grilo CM, Masheb RM, & Stunkard AJ. (2005). Binge eating disorder and night eating syndrome: a comparative study of disordered eating. *Journal of Consulting and Clinical Psychology*, 73:1107–1115.

Als-Nielsen B, Chen W, Gluud C, & Kjaergard LL. (2003). Association of funding and conclusions in randomized drug trials: A reflection of treatment effect or adverse events? *Journal of the American Medical Association*, 290:921–928.

American Psychiatric Association. (1994). *Diagnostic and statistical manual of mental disorders* (4th ed.). Washington, DC: Author.

Bekelman JE, Li Y, & Gross CP. (2003). Scope and impact of financial conflicts of interest in biomedical research: A systematic review. *Journal of the American Medical Association*, 289:454–465.

Ben-Tovim DI, Walker K, Gilchrist P, Freeman R, Kalucy R, & Esterman A. (2001). Outcome in patients with eating disorders: A 5-year study. *Lancet*, 357:1254–1257.

Blaine B, & Rodman J. (2007). Responses to weight loss treatment among obese individuals with and without BED: A matched-study meta-analysis. *Eating and Weight Disorders*, 12:54–60.

Chan AW, Hrobjartsson A, Haahr MT, Gotzsche PC, & Altman DG. (2004). Empirical evidence for selective reporting of outcomes in randomized trials: Comparison of protocols to published articles. *Journal of the American Medical Association*, 291:2457–2465.

Claudino AM, de Oliveira IR, Appolinario JC, Cordas TA, Duchesne M, Sichieri R, et al. (2007). Double-blind, randomized, placebo-controlled trial of topiramate plus cognitive-behavior therapy in binge eating disorder. *Journal of Clinical Psychiatry*, 68:1324–1332.

Crow SJ, Peterson CB, Levine AS, Thuras P, & Mitchell JE. (2004). A survey of binge eating and obesity treatment practices among primary care providers. *International Journal of Eating Disorders*, 35:348–353.

Devlin MJ, Goldfein JA, Petkova E, Jiang H, Raizman PS, Wolk S, et al. (2005). Cognitive behavioral therapy and fluoxetine as adjuncts to group behavioral therapy for binge eating disorder. *Obesity Research*, 13:1077–1088.

De Zwaan M, Mitchell JE, Crosby RD, Mussell MP, Raymond NC, Specker SM, et al. (2005). Short-term cognitive behavioral treatment does not improve outcome of a comprehensive very-low-calorie diet program in obese women with binge eating disorder. *Behavior Therapy*, 36:89–99.

Dimidjian S, Hollon SD, Dobson KS, Schmaling KB, Kohlenberg RJ, Addis ME, et al. (2006). Randomized trial of behavioral activation, cognitive therapy, and antidepressant medication in the acute treatment of adults with major depression. *Journal of Consulting and Clinical Psychiatry*, 74:658–670.

Dobson KS, Hollon SD, Dimidjian S, Schmaling KB, Kohlenberg RJ, Gallop RJ, et al. (2008). Randomized trial of behavioral activation, cognitive therapy, and antidepressant medication in the prevention of relapse and recurrence in major depression. *Journal of Consulting and Clinical Psychology*, 76:468–477.

Eddy KT, Doyle AC, Hoste RR, Herzog DB, & Le Grange D. (2008). Eating disorder not otherwise specified. *Journal of the American Academy of Child and Adolescent Psychiatry*, 47:156–164.

Fairburn CG, Cooper Z, Doll HA, O'Connor ME, Bohn K, Hawker DM, et al. (2009). Transdiagnostic cognitive-behavioral therapy for patients with eating disorders: A two-site trial with 60-week follow-up. *American Journal of Psychiatry*, 166:311–319.

Fairburn CG, Jones R, Peveler RC, Hope RA, & O'Connor M. (1993). Psychotherapy and bulimia nervosa: Longer-term effects of interpersonal psychotherapy, behavior therapy, and cognitive behavior therapy. *Archives of General Psychiatry*, 50:419–428.

Favaro A, Ferrara S, & Santonastaso P. (2003). The spectrum of eating disorders in young women: A prevalence study in a general population sample. *Psychosomatic Medicine*, 65:701–708.

Fichter MM, Quadflieg N, & Hedlund S. (2008). Long-term course of binge eating disorder and bulimia nervosa: Relevance for nosology and diagnostic criteria. *International Journal of Eating Disorders*, 41:577–586.

Ghaderi A, & Scott B. (2003). Pure and guided self-help for full and subthreshold bulimia nervosa and binge eating disorder. *British Journal of Clinical Psychology*, 42:257–269.

Golay A, Laurent-Jaccard A, Habicht F, Gachoud JP, Chabloz M, Kammer A, et al. (2005). Effect of orlistat in obese patients with binge eating disorder. *Obesity Research*, 13:1701–1708.

Gorin AA, Niemeier HM, Hogan P, Coday M, Davis C, DiLillo VG, et al., for the Look AHEAD Research Group. (2008). Binge eating and weight loss outcomes in overweight and obese individuals with type II diabetes. *Archives of General Psychiatry*, 65:1447–1455.

Grilo CM, Hrabosky JI, Allison KC, Stunkard AJ, & Masheb RM. (2008). Overvaluation of shape and weight in binge eating disorder and overweight controls: Refinement of a diagnostic construct. *Journal of Abnormal Psychology*, 117:414–419.

Grilo CM, Lozano C, & Elder KA. (2005). Inter-rater and test–retest reliability of the Spanish language version of the Eating Disorder Examination interview: Clinical and research implications. *Journal of Psychiatric Practice*, 11:231–240.

Grilo CM, & Masheb RM. (2005). A randomized controlled comparison of guided self-help cognitive behavioral therapy and behavioral weight loss for binge eating disorder. *Behaviour Research and Therapy*, 43:1509–1525.

Grilo CM, & Masheb RM. (2007). Rapid response predicts binge eating and weight loss in binge eating disorder: Findings from a controlled trial of orlistat with guided self-help cognitive behavioral therapy. *Behaviour Research and Therapy*, 45:2537–2550.

Grilo CM, Masheb RM, Brownell KD, Wilson GT, & White MA. (2007). *Randomized comparison of cognitive behavioral therapy and behavioral weight loss treatments for obese patients with binge eating disorder: 12-month outcomes*. Paper presented at the World Congress of Behavioural and Cognitive Therapy, Barcelona, Spain.

Grilo CM, Masheb RM, & Salant SL. (2005). Cognitive behavioral therapy guided self-help and orlistat for the treatment of binge eating disorder: A randomized, double-blind, placebo-controlled trial. *Biological Psychiatry*, 57:1193–1201.

Grilo CM, Masheb RM, & Wilson GT. (2001). Comparison of different methods for assessing the features of eating disorders in patients with binge eating disorder. *Journal of Consulting and Clinical Psychology*, 69:317–322.

Grilo CM, Masheb RM, & Wilson GT. (2005). Efficacy of cognitive behavioral therapy and fluoxetine for the treatment of binge eating disorder: A randomized double-blind placebo-controlled comparison. *Biological Psychiatry*, 57:301–309.

Grilo CM, Masheb RM, & Wilson GT. (2006). Rapid response to treatment for binge eating disorder. *Journal of Consulting and Clinical Psychology*, 74:602–613.

Grilo CM, Pagano ME, Skodol AE, Sanislow CA, McGlashan TH, Gunderson JG, et al. (2007). Natural course of bulimia nervosa and of eating disorder not otherwise specified: 5-year prospective study of remissions, relapses, and the effects of personality disorder psychopathology. *Journal of Clinical Psychiatry*, 68:738–746.

Guerdjikova AI, & McElroy SL. (2009). Binge eating disorder pharmacotherapy clinical trials: Who is left out? *European Eating Disorders Review*, 17:101–108.

Hayes SC, Luoma JB, Bond FW, Masuda A, & Lillis J. (2006). Acceptance and commitment therapy: Model, processes and outcomes. *Behaviour Research and Therapy*, 44:1–25.

Hilbert A, Saelens B, Stein R, Mockus D, Welch R, Matt G, et al. (2007). Pretreatment and process predictors of outcome in interpersonal and cognitive behavioral psychotherapy for binge eating disorder. *Journal of Consulting and Clinical Psychology*, 75:645–651.

Hrabosky JI, White MA, Masheb RM, Rothschild BS, Burke-Martindale CH, & Grilo CM. (2008). Psychometric evaluations of the Eating Disorder Examination—Questionnaire for bariatric surgery candidates. *Obesity*, 16:763–769.

Hudson JI, Hiripi E, Pope HG, Jr, & Kessler RC. (2007). The prevalence and correlates of eating disorders in the National Comorbidity Survey Replication. *Biological Psychiatry*, 61:348–358.

Kazdin AE. (2007). Mediators and mechanisms of change in psychotherapy research. *Annual Review of Clinical Psychology*, 3:1–27.

Keel PK, Fichter M, Quadflieg N, Bulik CM, Baxter MG, Thornton L, et al. (2004). Application of a latent class analysis to empirically define eating disorder phenotypes. *Archives of General Psychiatry*, 61:192–200.

Kraemer HC, Wilson GT, Fairburn CG, & Agras WS. (2002). Mediators and moderators of treatment effects in randomized clinical trials. *Archives of General Psychiatry*, 59:877–883.

Le Grange D, Crosby RD, & Lock J. (2008). Predictors and moderators of outcome in family-based treatment for adolescent bulimia nervosa. *Journal of the American Academy of Child and Adolescent Psychiatry*, 47:464–470.

Masheb RM, & Grilo CM. (2006a). Eating patterns and breakfast consumption in obese patients with binge eating disorder. *Behaviour Research and Therapy*, 44:1545–1553.

Masheb RM, & Grilo CM. (2006b). Emotional overeating and its associations with eating disorder psychopathology among overweight patients with binge eating disorder. *International Journal of Eating Disorders*, 39:141–146.

Masheb RM, & Grilo CM. (2007). Rapid response predicts treatment outcomes in binge eating disorder: Implications for stepped care. *Journal of Consulting and Clinical Psychology*, 75:639–644.

Masheb RM, & Grilo CM. (2008). Examination of predictors and moderators for self-help treatments of binge eating disorder. *Journal of Consulting and Clinical Psychology*, 76:900–904.

McElroy SL, Shapiro NA, Arnold LM, Keck PE, Rosenthal NR, Wu SC, et al. (2004). Topiramate in the long-term treatment of binge eating disorder associated with obesity. *Journal of Clinical Psychiatry*, 65:1463–1469.

Mitchell JE, Crosby RD, Wonderlich SA, Crow S, Lancaster K, Simonich H, et al. (2008). A randomized trial comparing the efficacy of cognitive-behavioral therapy for bulimia nervosa delivered via telemedicine versus face-to-face. *Behaviour Research and Therapy*, 46:581–592.

Mitchell JE, Crosby RD, Wonderlich SA, Hill L, Le Grange D, Powers P, et al. (2007). Latent profile analysis of a cohort of patients with eating disorders not otherwise specified. *International Journal of Eating Disorders*, 40S:S95–S98.

Munsch S, Biedert E, Meyer A, Michael T, Schlup B, Tuch A, et al. (2007). A randomized comparison of cognitive behavioral and behavioral weight loss treatment for overweight individuals with binge eating disorder. *International Journal of Eating Disorders*, 40:102–113.

Murphy R, Cooper Z, Hollon SD, & Fairburn CG (2009). How do psychological treatments work?: Investigating mediators of change. *Behaviour Research and Therapy*, 47:1–5.

National Institute for Health and Clinical Excellence (NICE). (2004). *Eating disorders: Core interventions in the treatment and management of anorexia nervosa, bulimia nervosa and related eating disorders* (Clinical Guideline No. 9). London: Author. Available online at *www.nice.org.uk*.

O'Malley SS, Sinha R, Grilo CM, Capone C, Farren CK, McKee SA, et al. (2007). Naltrexone and cognitive behavioral coping skills therapy for the treatment of alcohol drinking and eating disorder features in alcohol-dependent women: A randomized controlled trial. *Alcoholism: Clinical and Experimental Research*, 31:625–634.

Perlis RH, Perlis CS, Wu Y, Hwang C, Joseph M, & Nierenberg AA. (2005). Industry sponsorship and financial conflict of interest in the reporting of clinical trials in psychiatry. *American Journal of Psychiatry*, 162:1957–1960.

Reas DL, & Grilo CM. (2008). Review and meta-analysis of pharmacotherapy for binge eating disorder. *Obesity*, 16:2024–2038.

Ricca V, Mannucci E, Mezzani B, Moretti S, Di Bernardo M, Bertelli M, et al. (2001). Fluoxetine and fluvoxamine combined with individual cognitive-behavioral therapy in binge eating disorder: A one-year follow-up study. *Psychotherapy and Psychosomatics*, 70:298–306.

Rockert W, Kaplan AS, & Olmsted MP. (2007). Eating disorder not otherwise specified: The view from a tertiary care treatment center. *International Journal of Eating Disorders*, 40:S99–S103.

Samuels F, Zimmerli EJ, Devlin MJ, Kissileff HR, & Walsh BT. (2009). The development of hunger and fullness during a laboratory meal in patients with binge eating disorder. *International Journal of Eating Disorders*, 42:125–129.

Schienle A, Schafer A, Hermann A, & Vaitl D. (2009). Binge-eating disorder: Reward sensitivity and brain activation to images of food. *Biological Psychiatry*, 65:654–661.

Schmidt U, Lee S, Perkins S, Eisler I, Treasure J, Beecham J, et al. (2008). Do adolescents with eating disorder not otherwise specified or full-syndrome bulimia nervosa differ in clinical severity, comorbidity, risk factors, treatment outcome or cost? *International Journal of Eating Disorders*, 41:498–504.

Stice E, Cooper JA, Schoeller DA, Tappe K, & Lowe MR. (2007). Are dietary restraint scales valid measures of moderate- to long-term dietary restriction?: Objective biological and behavioural data suggest not. *Psychological Assessment*, 19:449–458.

Stice E, Fisher M, & Lowe MR. (2004). Are dietary restraint scales valid measures of acute dietary restriction?: Unobtrusive observational data suggest not. *Psychological Assessment*, 16:51–59.

Stice E, Spoor S, Bohon C, Veldhuizen MG, & Small DM. (2008). Relation of reward from food and anticipated food intake to obesity: A functional magnetic resonance imaging study. *Journal of Abnormal Psychology*, 117, 924–935.

Striegel-Moore RH, DeBar L, Wilson GT, Dickerson J, Rosselli F, Perrin N, et al. (2008). Health services use in eating disorders. *Psychological Medicine*, 38:1465–1474.

Striegel-Moore RH, & Frank DL. (2008). Should binge eating disorder be included in the DSM-V?: A critical review of the state of the evidence. *Annual Review of Clinical Psychology*, 4:305–324.

Stunkard AJ, Berkowitz R, Tanrikut C, Reiss E, & Young L. (1996). D-fenfluramine treatment of binge eating disorder. *American Journal of Psychiatry*, 153:1455–1459.

Sysko R, Devlin MJ, Walsh BT, Zimmerli E, & Kissileff HR. (2007). Satiety and test meal intake among women with binge eating disorder. *International Journal of Eating Disorders*, 40:554–561.

Walsh BT, & Boudreau G. (2003). Laboratory studies of binge eating disorder. *International Journal of Eating Disorders*, 34:S30–S38.

Walsh BT, Fairburn CG, Mickley D, Sysko R, & Parides MK. (2004). Treatment of bulimia nervosa in a primary care setting. *American Journal of Psychiatry*, 161:556–561.

Wang GJ, Volkow ND, Telang F, Jayne M, Ma J, Rao M, et al. (2004). Exposure to appetitive food stimuli markedly activates the human brain. *NeuroImage*, 21:1790–1797.

Wilfley DE, Welch RR, Stein RI, Spurell EB, Cohen LR, Saelens BE, et al. (2002). A randomized comparison of group cognitive-behavioral therapy and group interpersonal psychotherapy for the treatment of overweight individuals with binge-eating disorder. *Archives of General Psychiatry*, 59:713–721.

Wilson GT, Grilo CM, & Vitousek K. (2007). Psychological treatments for eating disorders. *American Psychologist*, 62:199–216.

Wilson GT, Wilfley DE, Agras WS, & Bryson SW. (in press). Psychological treatments of binge eating disorder. *Archives of General Psychiatry*.

Yanovski SZ. (1993). Binge eating disorder: Current knowledge and future directions. *Obesity Research*, 1:306–324.

Zimmerman M, Francione-Witt C, Chelminski I, Young D, & Tortolani C. (2008). Problems applying the DSM-IV eating disorders diagnostic criteria in a general psychiatric outpatient practice. *Journal of Clinical Psychiatry*, 69:381–384.

Author Index

Subject Index

Page numbers followed by *f* indicate figure, *t* indicate table

589